Biomedical Engineering

Biomedical Engineering

Edited by
Carlos Alexandre Barros de Mello

Biomedical Engineering

Edited by Carlos Alexandre Barros de Mello

CBS, Edition 2016

Published by InTech

Janeza Trdine 9, 51000 Rijeka, Croatia

Technical Editor Teodora Smiljanic

Cover Designer Dino Smrekar

Additional hard copies can be obtained from orders@intechopen.com

Biomedical Engineering, Edited by Carlos Alexandre Barros de Mello
p. cm.
ISBN 978-953-307-013-1

Preface

Biomedical Engineering can be seen as a mix of Medicine, Engineering and Science. In fact, this is a natural connection, as the most complicated engineering masterpiece is the human body. And it is exactly to help our "body machine" that Biomedical Engineering has its niche.

The link thus formed between Engineering and Medicine is so important that we cannot think of disassembling it anymore. From all Engineering subspecialties we see progress: from signal processing of heart and brain signals to mechanical human-like organs; from robust, precise and accurate devices for clinical analysis to devices for real-time applications in the surgical theater; and so on.

Nowadays, Biomedical Engineering has spread all over the world. There are many universities with strong undergraduate and post-graduate courses, well-established communities and societies and well-known conferences.

This book brings the state-of-the-art of some of the most important current research related to Biomedical Engineering. I am very honored to be editing such a valuable book, which has contributions of a selected group of researchers describing the best of their work. Through its 36 chapters, the reader will have access to works related to ECG, image processing, sensors, artificial intelligence, and several other exciting fields.

We hope you will enjoy the reading of this book and that it can be used as handbook to students and professionals seeking to gain a better understanding of where Biomedical Engineering stands today.

October, 2009

Editor

Carlos Alexandre Barros de Mello

Center of Informatics, Federal Univeristy of Pernambuco

Brazil

Contents

1

Microelectronic Biosensors: Materials and Devices

David P. Klemer, MD, PhD
University of Wisconsin-Milwaukee
Milwaukee, Wisconsin, U.S.A.

1. Introduction

The advent of novel materials for electronics, optoelectronics and nanoelectronics holds the promise for new microelectronic device designs and applications across all fields of science and technology. Furthermore, the increasing sophistication of fabrication processes and techniques used in the semiconductor industry has resulted in the ability to produce circuits of greater complexity at remarkably reduced costs, a trend which has been continuing over the past half-century. Application of progress made in the microelectronics industry to the biomedical and biotechnology fields is a research area rich in possibilities, given the rapid parallel growth in both microelectronics and biotechnology.

It is an unfortunate fact that new advances in biotechnology and biomedical engineering have historically tended to increase the costs of medicine and healthcare (Patel & Rushefsky, 2006). For example, a computed tomography (CT) scan is typically more expensive than traditional digital or "plain film" x-ray imaging, and a magnetic resonance (MR) scan is typically more expensive than a CT scan. Incorporation of the principles and techniques used in the microelectronics field has the potential for reversing this trend. Based on a batch-fabrication approach, mature processing techniques used in the semiconductor industry have the potential for dramatically reducing the cost of manufacture for diagnostic devices used for the detection, treatment and management of disease.

It is thus of critical importance to develop a knowledge base which spans the interdisciplinary boundary between microelectronics and biotechnology. In this chapter we will review the materials and devices which can serve to bridge the interdisciplinary boundary between microelectronics and biomedicine, and we will discuss some of the resulting novel biosensor designs which have been proposed for biomedical applications. The material will focus on so-called *in vitro* biosensors which are used to detect or sense the presence of specific biomolecule—such as proteins, peptides, nucleic acids (DNA or RNA), oligonucleotides, or peptide nucleic acids (PNAs)—in an analyte sample. We will not consider *in vivo* techniques which seek to diagnose disease within the body, typically using imaging modalities. Successful development of low-cost biosensors can facilitate screening programs for early diagnosis and treatment of disease, reducing the resulting morbidity and mortality and lowering the overall cost of healthcare.

2. Materials

This section provides a brief summary of various materials and material systems which have received significant attention for their potential for biological application, in specific, for sensing applications in molecular diagnostics. The list is by no means exhaustive, but is intended to focus on a relevant subset of materials of interest. Table 1 summarizes a number of advantages and disadvantages of the major material systems to be discussed in the sections below.

Material system	Advantages	Disadvantages
Silicon	Low cost Mature processing techniques	Limits in operating frequency range
Compound semiconductors	High carrier mobility, high frequency operation Suitability for optoelectronics Capability for bandgap engineering and epitaxially-grown layers	Cost
Organic semiconductors	Ease of application (inkjet, spin casting) Suitability for flexible substrates Suitability for optoelectronics	Low carrier mobility Not amenable to standard process flows
Nanomaterials	Novel physicochemical and electronic properties	Not amenable to standard process flows Unproven safety profile

Table 1. Advantages and disadvantages associated with various relevant material systems.

2.1 Silicon

As a member of column IV of the periodic table of the elements, silicon manifests a unique set of properties which has resulted in profound technological advances over the last half-century. Silicon exhibits a crystal structure in which each silicon atom bonds covalently with four neighboring atoms in a tetrahedral arrangement, forming a so-called diamond lattice (Sze & Ng, 2006). At a temperature of absolute zero, all outer shell electrons are confined to covalent bonds, leaving no free electrons for conduction. As temperatures rise above absolute zero, thermal energy can result in the liberation of electrons available for conduction. Thus, silicon behaves neither as a perfect insulator nor a perfect conductor, but instead a 'semiconductor' whose electrical properties can be readily altered through the addition of a very small number of impurity atoms ('doping'). Doping of selected regions of a silicon substrate allows for the spatial definition of electronically-active devices which can then be interconnected to perform complex circuit functions.

Crystalline silicon also possesses properties which allow for the coupling of mechanical and electrical effects, as effectively illustrated by the development of devices for MicroElectroMechanical Systems (MEMS). An early example is given by silicon pressure sensors, in which a thin diaphragm etched into silicon is used to transduce applied mechanical stresses into resistance (and voltage) variations (Kim & Wise, 1983). Likewise, the resonance frequency of appropriately-designed thin silicon cantilever structures is sensitive to small changes in mass loading; this effect has been used in the detection of biomolecular binding events, discussed later in this chapter.

2.2 Compound semiconductors

Elements from column III and column V of the periodic table can be combined in a 1:1 stoichiometric ratio and used to form crystalline materials. Substrates from these III-V materials also exhibit semiconducting properties in a manner similar to the column IV semiconductors such as silicon and germanium (Williams, 1990). Numerous semiconductor materials are based on III-V compounds, most notably gallium arsenide (GaAs) and, more recently, gallium nitride (GaN). Compound semiconductor materials tend to be more expensive than their silicon counterparts, primarily due to the difficulties associated with the growth of high-purity crystals for large-diameter (150mm and higher) wafer substrates. Notwithstanding, these materials have the advantage of higher electron mobility and suitability for use at high frequencies. These materials also exhibit higher resistivity than silicon, allowing for their use in applications which demand very low leakage currents and high sensitivities; for this reason, some III-V materials have been termed "semi-insulators." In addition, III-V materials have unique optoelectronic properties which render them useful for photonic (and biophotonic) applications, such as fluorescence detection. The fact that III-V materials can be grown, layer-by-layer, into complex epitaxial structures has allowed for the development of novel "bandgap-engineered" devices such as high-electron-mobility transistors (HEMTs), heterojunction bipolar transistors (HBTs) and complex optoelectronic devices such as quantum well lasers (Golio, 1991). Although these materials have traditionally been used less frequently in biosensing applications, their high-frequency and optoelectronic capabilities make them good candidates for future innovations in microwave and optoelectronic device applications in biosensing.

2.3 Organic semiconductors

Intense research activity in semiconducting materials has recently focused on so-called organic semiconductors, typically based on carbon-containing compounds and polymers. The electron distribution in organic molecules composed of π-conjugated systems (i.e., carbon-containing molecules composed of repeating double-bond/single-bond units) is delocalized, allowing for relative ease of electron (current) flow in these materials. In addition, proper selection of the conjugation length allows for interesting optoelectronic activity, hence these materials have found great use as organic light-emitting diodes (OLEDs) and as photovoltaic materials (Shinar, 2003; Brabec et al., 2008). Figure 1 illustrates a monomer of one such material used in organic semiconducting applications, 2-methoxy-5-(3',7'-dimethyloctyloxy)-1,4-phenylenevinylene, or MDMO-PPV (Sigma-Aldrich Corp, Milwaukee, WI, U.S.A.); the conjugated nature of the molecule is evident.

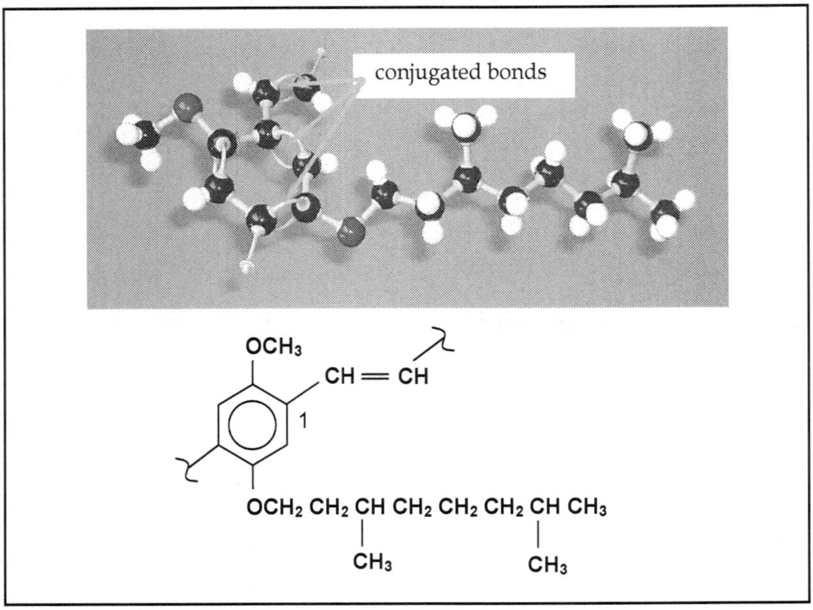

Fig. 1. The organic semiconducting monomer MDMO-PPV.

The design and fabrication of devices based on organic semiconductors varies significantly from traditional solid-state devices based on silicon or compound semiconductors, at once both an advantage and a disadvantage. Organic semiconducting materials may be deposited onto rigid or flexible substrates using low-cost inkjet printing or spin-casting techniques, but these materials are relatively less amenable to traditional photolithographic techniques for patterning and device definition. Although this may be advantageous for simple devices, it can complicate the processing for more complex devices or integrated circuits.

2.4 Nanomaterials

The term 'nanomaterials' has been applied to materials that incorporate structures having dimensions in the range 1-100 nm, and whose electrical and/or chemical properties are also influenced by their small dimensional scale. These materials have a wide variety of morphologies, including nanotubes, nanowires, nanoparticles (also termed quantum dots), and sheet-like two-dimensional structures (Vollath, 2008). The unique optical, electrical, mechanical and chemical properties of nanomaterials have attracted considerable interest—these properties are influenced by quantum mechanical effects, and may vary from those of the individual constituent atoms or molecules, as well as those of the corresponding bulk material. As the prototypical example, carbon nanotubes have been the subject of great research focus, given their great strength, high thermal and electrical conductivity, and chemical stability. The number of new nanomaterial systems is growing rapidly, from carbon-based structures (nanotubes and fullerines) to those based on compound semiconductors (CdSe, CdTe quantum dots and ZnO nanowires) and metallic nanoparticles such as colloidal gold.

Material systems based on combinations of nanomaterials (so-called hybrid nanomaterials) have also received a great deal of attention in the research community based on the proposed synergistic effects of nanomaterials of different compositions and morphologies in close proximity. Hybrid nanomaterial systems may exhibit great sensitivity to variations in the local electrochemical milieu, and this has led to the design of novel sensing devices for biological and chemical applications.

The quantum effects associated with the small dimensional scale of nanostructures result in unique physicochemical properties which may be used to advantage in biosensing systems. Quantum dot nanoparticles, for example, produce a fluorescence emission which can be tuned by adjusting the particle diameter during synthesis (Rogach, 2008). The Stokes shift—the difference between the fluorescence emission wavelength and the excitation wavelength—can be much larger than for the organic fluorophores which have traditionally been widely used in fluorescence labeling, imaging and biomolecular sensing.

2.5 Photonic and optoelectronic materials

In addition to their useful electronic properties, many of the semiconducting materials and nanomaterial structures mentioned in the previous sections also have interesting optoelectronic properties which can be exploited in biophotonic applications. Light-emitting semiconductor diodes and diode lasers based on III-V compound semiconductors are ubiquitous (Chuang, 1995), although research continues into optoelectronic devices based on other compound semiconducting materials (e.g., II-VI materials such as ZnSe) and silicon-based optoelectronic devices. Likewise, a large percentage of the commercial organic semiconductor market is devoted to organic light-emitting diodes (OLEDs). Finally, as mentioned in the previous section, quantum dot nanomaterials fabricated from cadmium- and indium-based compounds also have interesting optical fluorescence properties which have been proposed for biophotonic applications.

The use of optoelectronic materials in biomedicine represents a very large and significant research field. Research and development in biophotonics is such a large and important area that it would require a chapter specifically devoted to the topic. Accordingly, the discussion of biophotonic devices in the remainder of this chapter will be limited, with primary focus on devices which are microelectronic, rather than optoelectronic, in nature.

3. Biosensor technologies

In the most common biosensor implementation, a probe molecule is affixed to a sensing platform and used to recognize or detect a target molecule which is complementary to the probe—it is this feature of biosensors which provides high specificity and a low false-positive rate in qualitative sensing applications (Prasad, 2003). As an example, a protein antibody may serve as the probe, used to detect a specific protein antigen, or a single stranded oligonucleotide may be used as a biorecognition probe for the complementary segment of single-stranded DNA. There are numerous candidates for biorecognition probes, including antigen and antibody molecules, protein lectins (which bind to specific carbohydrate or glycoprotein molecules), protein receptor molecules (which bind to a specific ligand), and nucleic acid (oligonucleotide) probes.

Various physicochemical properties of sensing structures have been used to detect the presence of a target molecule in analyte solution. Binding of a target with an immobilized probe molecule may result in changes which can be detected using electromagnetic energy across the spectrum—from low frequencies used in impedimetric sensors to very high frequencies involved in the detection of radiolabeled target molecules. As another example, changes in optical properties at the sensor surface may be used in various detection schemes—for example, a fluorescence emission or a change in optical reflectance at a sensor surface may be used to indicate the presence of a target molecule (Liedberg et al., 1995).

Other parameters, such as the acoustic properties of surface-acoustic wave devices or the mass of a resonant structure may be altered by probe-target binding, and these parameters may also serve to transduce a binding event into a detectable signal. This signal can then be further processed to provide a qualitative or quantitative metric of the presence of the target biomolecule. In the following sections, specific biosensor implementations are discussed, based on the material systems discussed in Section 2.

3.1 Quartz crystal (piezoelectric) microbalances

The piezoelectric properties of various materials have been exploited in electronic circuits and systems for decades. Perhaps the largest and best-known application of piezoelectric devices is their use in precision timing and frequency reference applications, from wristwatches to computer clock-generation circuits. The resonant frequency of a crystal piezoelectric resonator will vary inversely with mass, a fact which is routinely used to advantage in crystal thickness monitors used to indicate thicknesses in vacuum thin-film deposition systems. Figure 2 illustrates a small circular quartz disc with metalized gold electrodes deposited on opposite faces. The piezoelectric properties of the quartz material confer a resonance behavior which can be modeled by the equivalent circuit shown; embedding this crystal in an oscillator circuit allows variations in mass to be transduced into a change in oscillator frequency.

When used to sense very small changes in mass based on variations in resonance frequency, quartz crystal resonators have been termed 'quartz crystal microbalances,' and these devices have been used in the detection of biological molecules to complete unicellular organisms (Zeng et al., 2006). In practice, the piezoelectric disc would be coated with a probe biomolecule which is immobilized onto the surface, and the disc (placed in a suitable electrical mount) would be located in an analyte flow cell. Applications of these devices as molecular biosensors range across all specialties of medicine, including infectious disease, oncology, rheumatology, neurology and others.

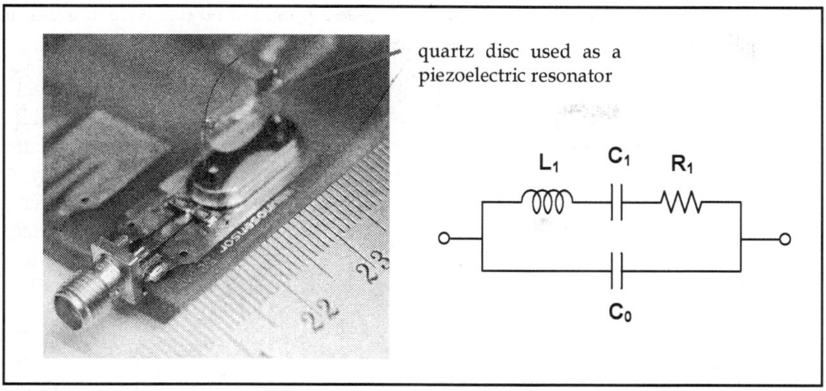

Fig. 2. A quartz disc with gold electrodes in a circuit mount. This device exhibits electrical resonance behaviour, modelled by the equivalent circuit shown. (Scale for size reference; small divisions represent 1mm.)

Applications of quartz crystal microbalances and related piezoelectric devices for biosensing are wide-ranging, and include the detection of *Mycobacterium tuberculosis* (He & Zhang, 2002), *Francisella tularensis* (Pohanka et al., 2007), *Escherichia coli* (Sung et al., 2006), as well as such tumor biomarkers as carcinoembryonic antigen (Shen et al., 2005) and alpha-fetoprotein (Ding et al., 2007).

3.2 Solid state biosensors

Most complex biomolecules (such as proteins and nucleic acids) have internal distributions of positive and negative charge; indeed, these charge distributions may determine the three-dimensional structure of the molecule. The distribution of this charge may influence current flow in solid state devices such as field-effect transistors, serving as a mechanism for direct transduction of binding events into an electrical signal. So-called ion-sensitive field effect transistors (ISFETs) have been designed and implemented based on this phenomenon. A typical ISFET device incorporates conductive (n-type) drain and source islands, and the flow of electrons between the drain and source is modulated by binding events between target and probe biomolecule. An external counterelectrode is used to establish a reference gating potential which biases the transistor device (Offenhäusser & Rinaldi, 2009).

Figure 3 illustrates the cross-sectional structure of an ISFET device; a protein antibody immobilized onto the surface region between the drain and source serves as the biorecognition molecule. An analyte solution which may contain target antigen is presented to the device via a microfluidic flow cell. Binding of the target antigen with immobilized antibody (shown for two of the molecules in Figure 3) modulates current flow from drain to source in a suitably-biased ISFET device.

ISFET sensors fabricated on silicon have been used to implement these types of biosensing devices, and arrays of ISFET sensors can be fabricated using standard silicon processing techniques. A major advantage of designing ISFET sensors in arrays is the ability to perform sensing of multiple different target biomolecules, using appropriately-immobilized probes. So-called multiplexed arrays are useful for rapid diagnosis involving multiple biomarkers, with applications in infectious disease diagnosis, genetic screening, and assays for drug development.

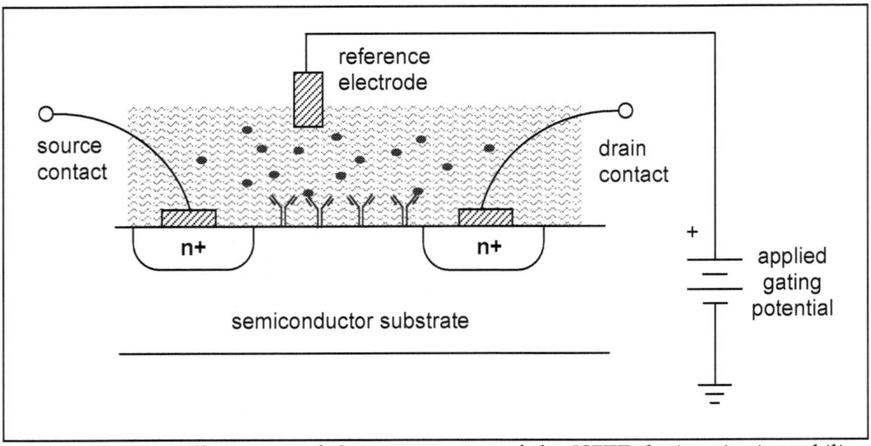

Fig. 3. A schematic illustration of the cross-section of the ISFET device. An immobilized biomolecule in the gate region between drain and source is used to recognize target molecules.

Arrays of solid-state field-effect devices have been fabricated using the same standard transistor fabrication techniques used to make complementary metal-oxide-semiconductor (CMOS) integrated circuits, and used for multiplexed DNA biosensing applications (Levine et al., 2009) as well as for biochemical detection (Chang et al., 2008).

Solid-state devices based on compound semiconductors are also receiving notable attention. ISFET devices have been made using a III-V (AlGaN/GaN) system and are being proposed for biosensing applications (Steinhoff et al., 2003). Solid-state diode and transistor structures have been fabricated on GaN and proposed for use as chemical and biological sensors (Pearton et al., 2004). Other investigations include the study of functionalization of GaAs surfaces with self-assembled monolayers of organic molecules (Voznyy & Dubowski, 2008).

3.3 MEMS devices

As discussed in Section 2.1, semiconductor devices having unique three-dimensional structures may be fabricated using standard processing techniques developed for the semiconductor and integrated circuit industry. MicroElectroMechanical Systems (MEMS) may be fabricated with structures having interesting electronic and mechanical properties; one such standard structure is a simple microcantilever which can be etched into silicon. Like piezoelectric sensors, such cantilevers have a resonance frequency which is mass-dependent; accordingly, they can also be used as sensitive detectors of biomolecular binding events. Figure 4 schematically illustrates a MEMS cantilever to which an antibody biorecognition element is attached. Binding of the corresponding antigen results in a mass change which can be detected as a change in frequency of a resonant circuit fabricated as part of the cantilever structure (Marie et al., 2002).

Other applications of MEMS devices as biosensors are based on other physicochemical properties of MEMS structures. These include thermally-sensitive MEMS devices for metabolic monitoring (Wang et al., 2008), MEMS devices for diagnosis of neoplastic disease (Ortiz et al., 2008), and a high-sensitivity acoustic-wave biosensor fabricated using MEMS technology (Valentine et al., 2007).

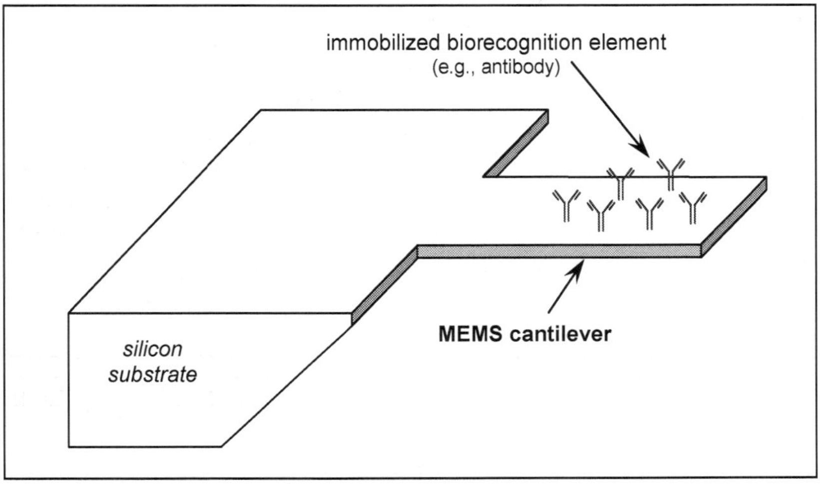

Fig. 4. A MEMS cantilever biosensor, based on mass changes which occur during binding.

3.4 Nanomaterial-based sensors

A wide variety of biosensing devices that are based on nanomaterials have been investigated, ranging from amperometric devices for quantification of glucose, to quantum dots as fluorescent probes. Colloidal gold nanoparticles have been used for several decades and can be readily conjugated to antibodies for use in immunolabeling and immunosensing; in addition, these nanoparticles also find application as a contrast agent for electron microscopy. Gold nanoparticles have also been used as probes for optoelectronic detection of nucleic acid sequences (Martins et al., 2007). Magnetic nanoparticles (based, for example, on iron) may also be used in immunolabeling applications as well as for cell separation under the influence of a magnetic field. Like gold nanoparticles, iron-based nanoparticles may also be used an a imaging contrast agent—specifically, for magnetic resonance imaging.

For biochemical sensing, zinc oxide nanostructures have been proposed for use as a cholesterol biosensor (Umar et al., 2009) and carbon nanotubes have been investigated as biosensors for glucose (Chen et al., 2008) and insulin quantification (Qu et al., 2006). In addition, hybrid nanomaterial systems consisting of two or more types of nanostructures are also receiving considerable attention for sensing (Figure 5).

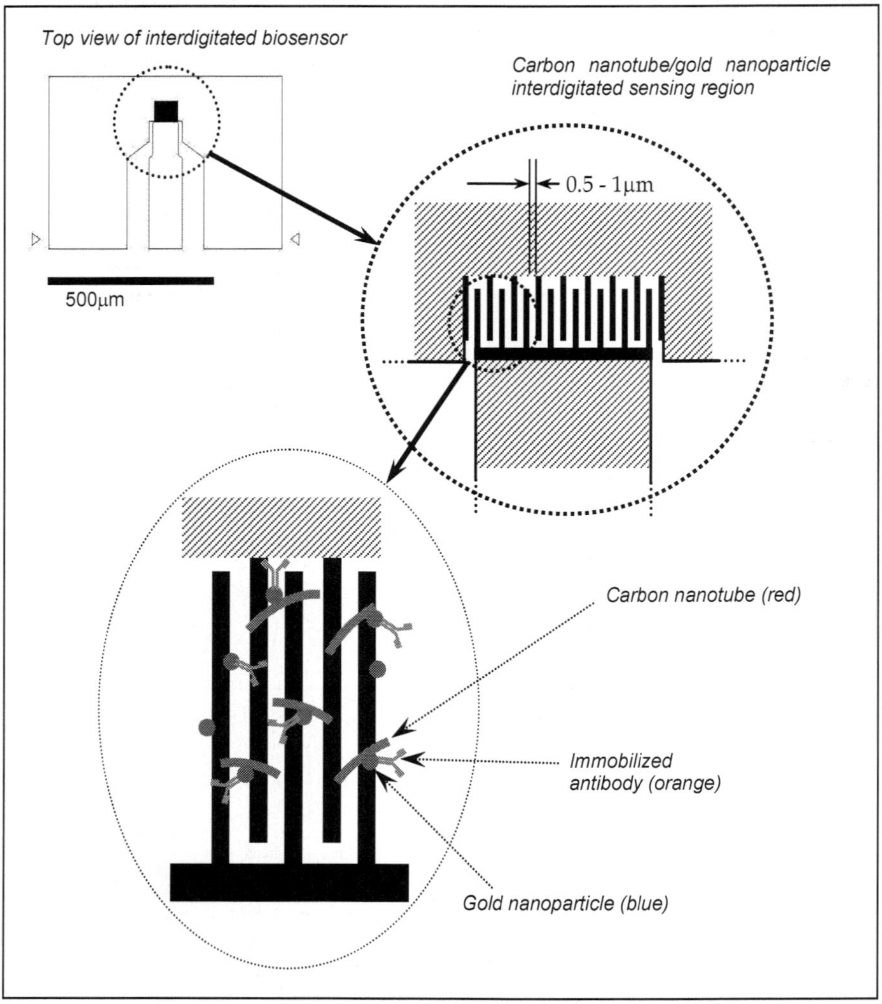

Fig. 5. A proposed carbon nanotube/gold-labeled antibody biosensor.

In this implementation, carbon nanotubes are coupled with gold nanoparticles attached to antibodies which serve as biorecognition molecules. The schematic illustration in Figure 5 (not drawn to scale) indicates this impedimetric biosensing approach, in which an interdigitated electrode is used to make electrical contact to the nanomaterial system consisting of carbon nanotubes with attached gold-conjugated antibody. Other hybrid systems employing carbon nanotubes and platimum nanowire structures, for example, have been investigated for glucose quantification (Qu et al., 2007) as well as for immunosensing.

In other "hybrid-material-system" approaches, nanomaterials have also been investigated for their ability to enhance sensitivity in a material system which includes an organic semiconductor component. In addition, systems which incorporate carbon nanostructures into MEMS systems ("C-MEMS devices") have also been proposed for arrays for detection of DNA (Wang & Madou, 2005).

3.5 Organic semiconductor-based sensors

Organic semiconductors find their greatest application in photonics, as a result of extensive development of organic light-emitting diodes (OLEDs) and photovoltaic devices. There has been relatively little investigation into the potential use of organic semiconductors as biosensing devices. This, despite the fact that it has been suggested (Cooreman et al., 2005) that the organic nature of conjugated polymer semiconductors may provide an ideal platform for the development of sensors suitable for biomolecular detection. Impedimetric biosensors based on organic semiconducting polymers have been investigated, including sensors which incorporate a hybrid organic semiconductor/gold nanoparticle sensing platform, shown in Figure 6 (Omari et al., 2007).

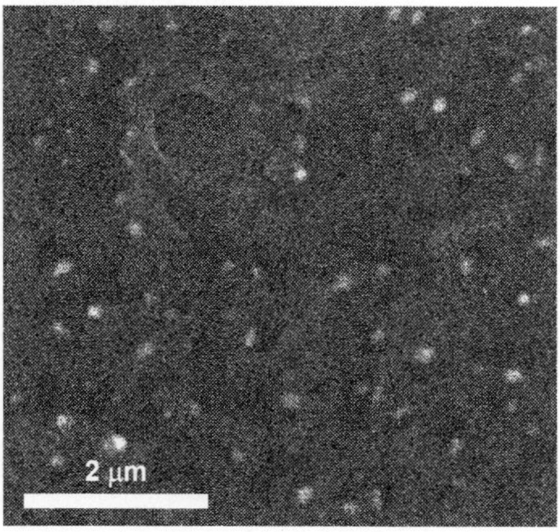

Fig. 6. Illustration of a hybrid material system consisting of gold nanoparticles applied to an organic semiconducting polymer layer, viewed by scanning electron microscopy.

This organic semiconductor/gold nanoparticle sensing platform has also been investigated as a platform for immunoassays (Li et al., 2008). The development of biosensors based on this material system is facilitated by the fact that the conjugation of gold nanoparticles to antibodies is a mature technology, with a large variety of gold-labeled antibodies commercially available.

4. Conclusion

Numerous material systems exist which can support the design and development of novel biosensing approaches for *in vitro* biomolecular diagnostic applications, ranging from traditional materials such as silicon and GaAs to novel materials such as conjugated organic polymer semiconductors. In addition, newly discovered nanomaterials offer the potential for increased sensitivity and lower cost, and the hope of reversing an unfortunate historic trend towards increased costs associated with new, more sophisticated advances in healthcare technology. Although microelectronic biosensors have great potential for facilitating the development of inexpensive devices for molecular diagnostics, this research requires a knowledge of materials science, electrical engineering, semiconductor device design and fabrication, chemistry and biochemistry, nanotechnology, biology and medicine. Developing an intellectual base which will aid this research requires an interdisciplinary teamwork approach. The fertile boundary at the intersection of these disparate fields of knowledge holds the potential for novel, interesting and useful developments in biomicroelectronics.

5. References

Brabec, C.; Scherf, U. & Dyakonov, V., eds. (2008). *Organic Photovoltaics: Materials, Device Physics, and Manufacturing Technologies,* Wiley-VCH, ISBN 978-3527316755, Weinheim, Germany

Chang, Y-W.; Tai, Y-T.; Huang, Y-T. & Yang, Y-S. (2008). A CMOS-based phototransistor for high-sensitivity biochemical detection using absorption photometry. *Proceedings of the 3rd International Conference on Sensing Technology, ICST 2008,* pp. 82-85, ISBN 9781424421770, Tainan, Taiwan, November-December 2008, IEEE, Piscataway, NJ

Chen, X.; Chen, J.; Deng, C.; Xiao, C.; Yang, Y.; Nie, Z. & Yao, S. (2008). Amperometric glucose biosensor based on boron-doped carbon nanotubes modified electrode. *Talanta,* Vol. 76, No. 4, (August 2008) pp. 763-767, ISSN 0039-9140

Chuang, S. L. (1995). *Physics of Optoelectronic Devices,* Wiley-Interscience, ISBN 978-0471109396, New York

Cooreman P.; Thoelen, R.; Manca, J.; vandeVen, M.; Vermeeren, V.; Michiels, L.; Ameloot, M. & Wagner, P. (2005). Impedimetric immunosensors based on the conjugated polymer PPV. *Biosensors & Bioelectronics,* Vol. 20, No. 10, (April 2005) pp. 2151-56, ISSN 0956-5663

Ding, Y.; Liu, J.; Wang, H.; Shen, G. & Yu R. (2007). A piezoelectric immunosensor for the detection of alpha-fetoprotein using an interface of gold/hydroxyapatite hybrid nanomaterial. *Biomaterials,* Vol. 28, No. 12, (April 2007) pp. 2147-54, ISSN 0142-9612

Golio, J. M. (1991). *Microwave MESFETs and HEMTs,* Artech House, ISBN 978-0890064269, Boston

He, F. & Zhang, L. (2002). Rapid diagnosis of M. tuberculosis using a piezoelectric immunosensor. *Analytical sciences,* Vol. 18, No. 4, (April 2002) pp. 397-401, ISSN 0910-6340

Kim, S-C. & Wise, K. D. (1983). Temperature sensitivity in silicon piezoresistive pressure transducers. *IEEE Transactions on Electron Devices,* Vol. ED-30, No. 7, (July 1983) pp. 802-810, ISSN 0018-9383

Levine, P. M.; Gong, P.; Levicky, R. & Shepard, K. L. (2009). Real-time, multiplexed electrochemical DNA detection using an active complementary metal-oxide-semiconductor biosensor array with integrated sensor electronics. *Biosensors & Bioelectronics,* Vol. 24, No. 7, (March 2009) pp. 1995-2001, ISSN 0956-5663

Li, F.; Klemer, D. P.; Kimani, J. K.; Mao, S.; Chen, J & Steeber, D. A. (2008). Fabrication and characterization of microwave immunosensors based on organic semiconductors with nanogold-labeled antibody. *Proceedings of the 30th Annual International Conference of the IEEE Engineering in Medicine and Biology Society,* pp. 2381-2384, ISBN 978-1424418152, Vancouver, Canada, August 2008, IEEE, Piscataway, NJ

Liedberg B.; Nylander, C. & Lundstrom, I. (1995). Biosensing with surface plasmon resonance - how it all started. *Biosensors & Bioelectronics,* Vol. 10, No. 8, i-ix, ISSN 0956-5663

Marie, R.; Jensenius, H.; Thaysen, J.; Christensen, C. B. & Boisen, A. (2002). Adsorption kinetics and mechanical properties of thiol-modified DNA-oligos on gold investigated by microcantilever sensors. *Ultramicroscopy,* Vol. 91, No. 1-4, (May 2002) pp. 29-36, ISSN 0304-3991

Martins, R.; Baptista, P.; Raniero, L.; Doria, G.; Silva, L.; Franco, R. & Fortunato, E. (2007). Amorphous/nanocrystalline silicon biosensor for the specific identification of unamplified nucleic acid sequences using gold nanoparticle probes. *Applied Physics Letters,* Vol. 90, No. 2, (2007) pp. 023903.1-3, ISSN 0003-6951

Offenhäusser, A. & Rinaldi, R. (2009). *Nanobioelectronics - for Electronics, Biology, and Medicine,* Springer, ISBN 978-0387094588, New York

Omari, E. A.; Klemer, D. P.; Steeber, D. A. & Gaertner, W. F. (2007). Polymer semiconductors as a biosensing platform: peroxidase activity of enzyme bound to organic semiconducting films. *Proceedings of the 29th Annual International Conference of the IEEE Engineering in Medicine and Biology Society,* pp. 107-110, ISBN 978-1424407880, Lyon, France, August 2007, IEEE, Piscataway, NJ

Ortiz, P; Keegan, N.; Spoors, J.; Hedley, J.; Harris, A.; Burdess, J.; Burnett, R.; Velten, T.; Biehl, M.; Knoll, T.; Haberer, W.; Solomon, M.; Campitelli, A. & McNeil, C. (2008). A hybrid microfluidic system for cancer diagnosis based on MEMS biosensors. *Proceedings of the 2008 Biomedical Circuits and Systems Conference,* pp. 337-340, ISBN 978-1424428793, Baltimore, MD, November 2008, IEEE, Piscataway, NJ

Patel, K. & Rushefsky, M. E. (2006). *Health Care Politics and Policy in America,* M. E. Sharpe, ISBN 978-0765614797, Armonk, New York

Pearton, S.J.; Kang, B.S.; Kim, S.; Ren, F.; Gila, B.P.; Abernathy, C.R.; Lin, J. & Chu, S.N.G. (2004). GaN-based diodes and transistors for chemical, gas, biological and pressure sensing. *Journal of Physics Condensed Matter,* Vol. 16, No. 29, (July 2004) pp. R961-R994, ISSN 0953-8984

Pohanka, M.; Pavlis, O. & Skládal, P. (2007). Diagnosis of tularemia using piezoelectric biosensor technology. *Talanta,* Vol. 71, No. 2, (February 2007) pp. 981-5, ISSN 0039-9140

Prasad, P. N. (2003). *Introduction to Biophotonics,* Wiley-Interscience, ISBN 978-0471287704, Hoboken, NJ

Qu, F.; Yang, M.; Lu, Y.; Shen, G. & Yu, R. (2006). Amperometric determination of bovine insulin based on synergic action of carbon nanotubes and cobalt hexacyanoferrate nanoparticles stabilized by EDTA. *Analytical and Bioanalytical Chemistry,* Vol. 386, No. 2, (September 2006) pp. 228-34, ISSN 1618-2642

Qu, F.; Yang, M.; Shen, G. & Yu, R. (2007). Electrochemical biosensing utilizing synergic action of carbon nanotubes and platinum nanowires prepared by template synthesis, *Biosensors & Bioelectronics,* Vol. 22, No. 8, (March 2007) pp. 1749-55, ISSN 0956-5663

Rogach, A., ed. (2008). *Semiconductor Nanocrystal Quantum Dots: Synthesis, Assembly, Spectroscopy and Applications,* Springer-Verlag, ISBN 978-3211752357, Vienna

Shen, G.Y.; Wang, H.; Deng, T.; Shen, G.L. & Yu, R.Q. (2005). A novel piezoelectric immunosensor for detection of carcinoembryonic antigen. *Talanta,* Vol. 67, No. 1, (July 2005) pp. 217-20, ISSN 0039-9140

Shinar, J., ed. (2003). *Organic Light-Emitting Devices: A Survey,* Springer-Verlag, ISBN 978-0387953434, New York

Steinhoff, G.; Purrucker, O.; Tanaka, M.; Stutzmann, M. & Eickhoff, M. (2003). $Al_xGa_{1-x}N$–a new material system for biosensors. *Advanced Functional Materials,* Vol. 13, No. 11, (November 2003) pp. 841-846, ISSN 1616-301X

Sung, J. H.; Ko, H. J. & Park, T. H. (2006). Piezoelectric biosensor using olfactory receptor protein expressed in Escherichia coli. *Biosensors & Bioelectronics,* Vol. 21, No. 10, (April 2006) pp. 1981-6, ISSN 0956-5663

Sze, S. M. & K. K. Ng (2006). *Physics of Semiconductor Devices, 3ed,* Wiley-Interscience, ISBN 978-0471143239, New York

Umar, A; Rahman, M. M.; Al-Hajry, A. & Hahn, Y.-B. (2009). Highly-sensitive cholesterol biosensor based on well-crystallized flower-shaped ZnO nanostructures. *Talanta,* Vol. 78, No. 1, (April 2009) pp. 284-9, ISSN 0039-9140

Valentine, J. E.; Przybycien, T. M. & Hauan, S. (2007). Design of acoustic wave biochemical sensors using micro-electro-mechanical systems. *Journal of Applied Physics,* Vol. 101, No. 6, (2007) Article 064508, ISSN 0021-8979

Vollath, D. (2008). *Nanomaterials: An Introduction to Synthesis, Properties and Applications,* Wiley-VCH, ISBN 978-3527315314, Weinheim, Germany

Voznyy, O. & Dubowski, J. J. (2008). Structure of thiol self-assembled monolayers commensurate with the GaAs (001) surface. *Langmuir,* Vol. 24, No. 23, (December 2008), pp. 13299-305, ISSN 0743-7463

Wang, C. & Madou, M. (2005). From MEMS to NEMS with carbon. *Biosensors & Bioelectronics,* Vol. 20, No. 10, (April 2005) pp. 2181-2187, ISSN 0956-5663

Wang, L.; Sipe, D. M.; Xu, Y. & Lin, Q. (2008). A MEMS thermal biosensor for metabolic monitoring applications. *Journal of Microelectromechanical Systems,* Vol. 17, No. 2, (April 2008) pp. 318-327, ISSN 1057-7157

Williams, R. E. (1990). *Modern GaAs Processing Methods,* Artech House, ISBN 978-0890063439, Boston

Zeng, H.; Wang, H.; Chen, F.; Xin, H.; Wang, G.; Xiao, L.; Song, K.; Wu, D.; He, Q. & Shen, G. (2006). Development of quartz-crystal-microbalance-based immunosensor array for clinical immunophenotyping of acute leukemias. *Analytical Biochemistry,* Vol. 351, No. 1, (April 2006) pp. 69-76, ISSN 0003-2697

2

Low-Power and Low-Voltage Analog-to-Digital Converters for wearable EEG systems

J. M. García González[1], E. López-Morillo[2], F. Muñoz[2], H. ElGmili[2] and R. G. Carvajal[2]

Micronas GmbH[1], Germany[1]

Electronic Engineering Department, Universidad de Sevilla, Spain[2]

1. Introduction

Electroencephalography (EEG) has traditionally placed a vital role in monitoring, diagnosis and treatment for certain clinical situations, such as epilepsy, syncope and sleep disorder; by measuring the patient's brainwaves (Casson et al., 2008). Recently, EEG has also merged as powerful tool for neuroscientist allowing the research of cognitive states and the enhancement task-related performance of an operative through computer mediated assistance (Erdogmus et al., 2005).

During monitoring electrodes are placed on scalp to detect the micro-Volt EEG signals that result outside the head due to the synchronised neurological action within the brain. In practice, long-term EEG monitoring is generally required either inpatient or ambulatory. The conventional EEG systems limit patient mobility due to bulk size because of the battery sized required for the long term operation of the constituent electronics. There is thus a strong need for development of lightweight, wearable and wireless EEG systems operation to enable long-term monitoring of patients in their everyday environment (Yates et al., 2007). In this way, wearable EEG is the evolution of ambulatory EEG units from the bulky, limited lifetime devices available today to small devices present only on the head that record the EEG for long time; however this method demands ultra-low power and low voltage circuit design because of the lifetime of the batteries.

One of the most power consuming building blocks of a wearable EEG front-end is the Analog to Digital Converter (ADC) required to process the signal in the digital domain. Therefore it is necessary an ultra-low power ADC (Yang & Sarpeshkar, 2006) for EEG applications.

This chapter presents the design of two extremely low power consumption ADCs that can be used for a wearable EEG system under a very low supply voltage environment. The architectures used for the converters are:

- A 10 bits second order Switched-Capacitor (SC) Sigma-Delta modulator.
- A 1.5-bit per stage 10-bit pipelined ADC.

To achieve both, the extremely low-power and the low voltage operation, a new design principle based on Quasi-Floating Gate (QFG) MOS transistors has been used. Moreover, the use of a class-AB operational amplifier (opamp) biased in weak inversion allows very low power consumption achieving the high open-loop gain requirements. The implementations in CMOS technology of data converters for EEG systems presented in this chapter confirm the usefulness of the proposed techniques for low-voltage and low-power applications.

2. EEG signal processing and front-end description

Typical EEG signals provided by the electrodes placed on the scalp are in the range 2-500 μV over a bandwidth of 0.5-30 Hz (Binnie et al., 1982). Present ambulatory systems typically have at least 16 channels and operate for around a day without recharging. Wireless systems offer around 8 EEG channels and last for 12 hours. Sampling frequencies higher than 200 Hz are typically specified, nevertheless the trend in EEG systems is for higher sampling frequencies and more recording channels, being not uncommon currently for inpatient monitors offer sampling frequencies of 1 kHz or more. Modern inpatient systems for epilepsy diagnosis may offer 256 channels (Casson et al., 2008). Furthermore, to avoid spatial aliasing towards 600 channels are needed.

Implementation of a low-power EEG system is not an easy task because of the nature of the signals. The reason is that the scalp electrodes drift with time superimposing a low frequency signal in the order of tens of milivolts (Cooper et al., 1974) to the desired EEG one. Two strategies can be followed to deal with this type of signals:

1. Digitalize the EEG signal and the drift signal together and remove the second one digitally. This signal processing requires a very accurate ADC with more than 20 bits of resolution, which would be very power consuming.
2. Filter the drift signal out in the front-end. This second strategy relaxes the ADC resolution at expense of tightening the requirements of the previous instrumentation amplifier because it is difficult to filter such a low-frequency signal out without affecting the desired one. ADCs being presented in this chapter are thought for this signal processing strategy. Because of the extremely low-power consumption of the ADC, there is more power budget available for the design of the filtering instrumentation amplifier (Yates et al., 2007).

Fig. 1. shows the basic block diagram of the low-power low-voltage front-end for wearable EEG systems. The front-end is made up of:

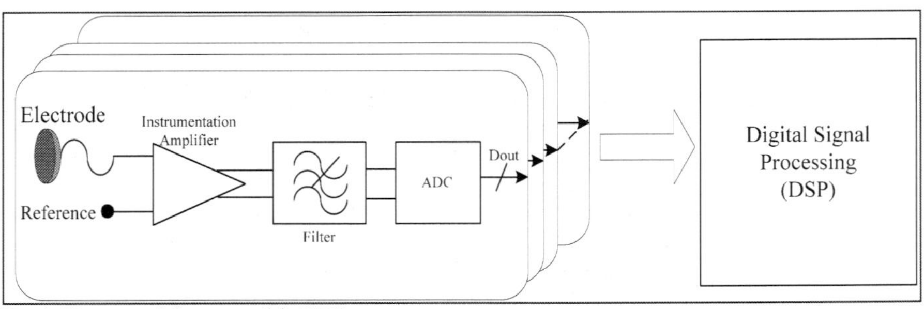

Fig. 1. Front-end for wearable EEG system.

1. An instrumentation amplifier. The instrumentation amplifier performs two tasks. It provides a gain of 175, which is required to accommodate the EEG signal to the

ADC input range. Simultaneously it provides high-pass filtering to remove undesired very low frequency signals hence reducing the effect of the electrode offset drift. Therefore it is possible the use of a moderate resolution ADC. In order to meet the noise specifications, chopper techniques are commonly used in the instrumentation amplifier (Menolfi & Huang, 1999). A chopper amplifier achieves exceptional noise performance and very low offset voltage by upconverting the signal before amplification through modulation with a square wave at chop frequency, f_{ch}. Ideally, the chop frequency is set to a frequency at which the flicker noise is negligible. After amplification at f_{ch} the signal is downconverted to baseband. However, the flicker noise and offset voltage are simultaneously upconverted to the chop frequency, where they can be filtered out (Yates & Rodriguez-Villegas, 2006).

2. An anti-aliasing filter.
3. A 10 bit ADC. The fact that the slowly-varying offset due to scalp electrodes' impedance drift is partially suppressed by the instrumentation amplifier allows relaxing the resolution requirements to only 10 bits.

If the volume of the overall device is assumed to be 1cm^3 and half of such volume is reserved for a battery of energy density of 200Wh/1 (Casson et al., 2008). For an operation of 30 days without recharging the average power consumption must be less than 140μW. Currently, 20-32 channels EGG systems are preferred. This implies that average power consumption per channel must be less than 5-3μW. The estimated power consumption of the digital signal processing is around 40μW. The power consumption of the entire system is:

$$P = N \cdot P_{ch} + P_{DSP} = N \cdot (P_a + P_f + P_{ADC}) + P_{DSP} \quad (1)$$

where N is the number of channels, P_{ch}, P_a, P_f, P_{ADC} and P_{DSP} are the power consumption of the channel, instrumentation amplifier, anti-aliasing filter, ADC and DSP respectively. A good design guideline is to reverse 50-66% of the complete analog power consumption (P_{ch}) for the ADC. Thus, a suitable ADC power consumption would be in the range of 3.3-2.5μW per channel for a 20 channels system, and 2-1.5μW for a 32 channel system.

The general specifications for ADCs used in the proposed EEG front-end are summarized in Table 1.

Maximum input frequency	25-100Hz
ADC sampling frequency	>1kHz
Resolution	>9 bits
Input Voltage Range	725mV differential
Supply Voltage	as low as possible (i.e. 1.2V)
Maximum power consumption	3.3-1.5μW

Table 1. General specifications for ADCs used in the EEG front-end.

In this chapter two different 10-bit ADC implementations are presented using a low supply voltage (1.2V).

1. The first ADC is implemented by using a pipelined architecture. Typically such ADC architecture is chosen for intermediate sampling frequencies, but this chapter shows how it is also possible and worthwhile to use a pipelined architecture to design a power efficient ADC for EEG applications.
2. The second ADC uses a switched-capacitor (SC) sigma-delta ($\Sigma\Delta$) architecture which is commonly used for biomedical applications (Goes et al., 2005), (Lee et al., 2005). The reduced number of operational amplifier of this architecture is an advantage for low-power specifications. However, the input signal bandwidth is limited due to the oversampling operation of $\Sigma\Delta$ ADCs.

Both ADCs have been designed using standard 0.5μm CMOS MOSIS technology. In this technology the MOS transistors have a relative high threshold voltage, V_{TP}=0.96V and V_{TN}=0.67V, which make increase the difficulty of achieve switch linearity and operational amplifiers open-loop gain requirements under a very low voltage supply with classical design techniques. Two strategies were adopted in order to solve these problems:

1. The use of CMOS switches based on quasi-floating gate transistors (QFG).
2. The use of sub-threshold biased class-AB operational amplifiers.

3. QFG transistors

A fundamental issue in SC circuits operating with a very low voltage supply is that not enough overdrive voltage can be provided to the gates of transistors acting as switches (Crols & Steyaert, 1994). In this way, the signal swing and linearity is limited. CMOS switches based on quasi-floating gate transistors are an alternative to the well known clock-boosting techniques and bootstrapped switches (Ramírez-Angulo et al., 2004).

A QFG transistor is a MOS transistor with its gate terminal weakly connected to a DC voltage through a very large resistor. This resistor is used to set the DC operating point of the gate terminal of the input MOS transistor. The resistor can be implemented by means of a MOS transistor in cut-off region.

Fig. 2. shows a QFG nMOS transistor with multiple inputs. A simple ac analysis reveals that the ac voltage at the quasi-floating gate is given by:

$$V_G = \frac{sR_{leak}}{1+sR_{leak}C_T} \cdot \left(\sum_{j=1}^{N} C_j V_j + C_{GS}V_S + C_{GD}V_D + C_{GB}V_B \right) \tag{2}$$

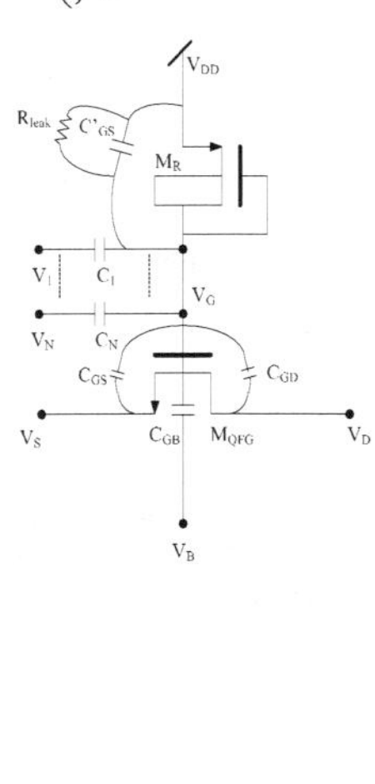

Fig. 2. QFG nMOS transistor.

where C_T is the total capacitance:

$$C_T = \sum_{j=1}^{N} C_j + C_{GS} + C_{GD} + C_{GB} + C'_{GD} \quad (3)$$

The factor $sR_{leak}/(1+sR_{leak}C_T)$ in (2), represents a high-pass filter. In this way, low-frequencies components of the input are filtered out with a cut-off frequency $1/(1+sR_{leak}C_T)$, which can be very low. Therefore, even for very low frequencies, (2) becomes a weighted averaging of the ac input voltages determined by capacitor ratios, plus some parasitic terms. The pull-up resistor R_{leak} sets the gate to a dc voltage equals to the positive rail, to which an ac voltage given by (2) is superimposed. Hence, the gate voltage can become higher than V_{DD}. An exact value of R_{leak} is not required, and its temperature and voltage dependence are not important, provided that R_{leak} value remains large enough not to influence the circuit operation at the lowest frequency required.

3.1 Rail to rail CMOS switch based on quasi-floating gate transistors

In low-voltage SC circuits there are some critical switches that need rail to rail signal swing operation. As the supply voltage is low, not enough overdrive is provided to the gates of transistors used as switches to be turned on over the whole signal range. A simple and very power efficient solution to this problem is the use of a QFG transistor as low-voltage rail-to-rail switch.

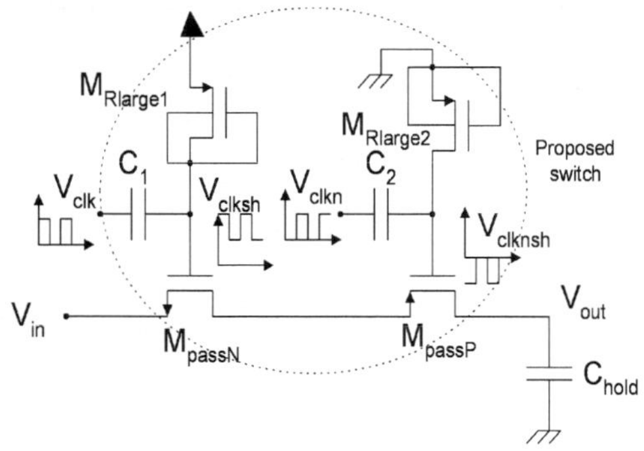

Fig. 3. A low voltage rail-to-rail T/H with a switch based on two complementary QFG transistors.

Fig. 3. shows how a T/H circuit is implemented using a low voltage analog switch based on two QFG transistors (Muñoz et al., 2003). The two complementary QFG transistors, M_{passN} and M_{passP}, are connected in series in order to get rail-to-rail operation.

The gate of M_{passN} is weakly tied to V_{DD} through a large nonlinear resistor implemented by transistor $M_{Rlarge1}$. The gate is also coupled to the clock signal through a small valued capacitor, C_1, so that the clock signal is transferred to the quasi-floating gate. The capacitor performs a level shift of approximately V_{DD}, which allows switching under very low-voltage restrictions. Note that the switch implemented by M_{passN} is not rail-to-rail because it is not possible to turn off the transistor for input signals near the negative rail. The rail-to-rail operation is achieved thanks to QFG transistor M_{passP} (driven by a complementary clock signal).

3.2 Low-voltage class-AB Operational Amplifier

At low supply voltages the signal dynamic range is reduced and makes not possible the use cascode transistors to get high-gain stages. In this context, two stage class-AB op-amps are the natural choice since they can have low power consumption, rail-to-rail output swing and high gain.

Fig. 4. shows the architecture of the operational amplifiers used in both implemented ADCs (Ramírez-Angulo et al., 2006).

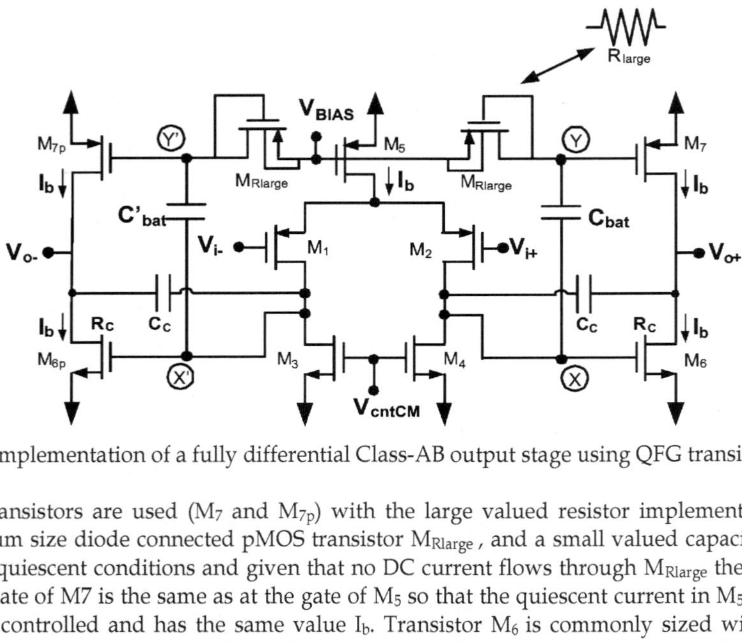

Fig. 4. Implementation of a fully differential Class-AB output stage using QFG transistors.

QFG transistors are used (M_7 and M_{7p}) with the large valued resistor implemented by a minimum size diode connected pMOS transistor M_{Rlarge}, and a small valued capacitor C_{bat}. Under quiescent conditions and given that no DC current flows through M_{Rlarge} the voltage at the gate of M7 is the same as at the gate of M_5 so that the quiescent current in M_5 and M_7 is well controlled and has the same value I_b. Transistor M_6 is commonly sized with W/L dimensions twice as large as those of M_3, M_4 so that the quiescent current in M_6 has also a value I_b. During dynamic operation, when the output of the op-amp is slewing, the voltage at node X is subject to a large change. Given that capacitor C_{bat} can not discharge/charge rapidly through M_{Rlarge} it acts as a floating battery and transfers the voltage variations at node X to node Y. This provides class AB (push pull) operation to the output stage. No additional circuitry to control the desired value of the quiescent output current is necessary due to the large resistor. The value of C_{bat} can be small as transistor M_{Rlarge} is intended to operate as a very large resistive element. The output stage has low supply requirements since it can operate with a supply voltage close to a transistor's threshold voltage:

$$V_{DD_{min}} = V_{GS6} + V_{SDsat2} + V_{SDsat5} \quad (4)$$

Amplifiers have been designed with transistors biased in weak inversion in order to minimize the power consumption and to achieve open-loop gain requirements. Bias current and transistor sizes are set to accomplish the settling requirements. An additional advantage of the used operational amplifier is that it presents enhanced phase margin and higher unity gain frequency as both transistors M6 and M7are active in the class-AB output stage.

4. Design of a low-power low-voltage 10-bit Pipelined ADC for wearable EEG systems

Multi-stage pipelined ADCs are one of the most popular architecture for high-speed applications. They consist of several cascaded stages, called multiplying digital-to-analog converter (MDAC), which contains a sample-and-hold (S/H), a low resolution ADC and a digital-to-analog converter (DAC). A digital delay line is required for output synchronisation to assure the correct operation.
The purpose of this section is to show how it is possible to use a classical power-consuming high-speed ADC architecture for low-power EEG applications by means of a deep understanding of pipelined ADC architecture and design techniques like quasi-static gate transistors. The target is to use this ADC for wearable EEG systems with more than 20 channels and performing simultaneously the analog-to-digital conversion of more than one channel.
Fig. 5 shows block diagram of the presented pipelined ADC. The whole system uses fully-differential architecture without a dedicated front-end S/H and consists of a cascade of 9 fully-differential MDACs stages with 1.5 bits of resolution at 4 kHz of sampling frequency. The last stage is just a 2-bit resolution flash ADC. Bit redundancy is used in order to correct offset errors in the digital domain. Each MDAC stage composes of a S/H, a low-resolution analog-to-digital sub-converter (sub-ADC), a digital-to-analog sub-converter (sub-DAC), and a gain block.

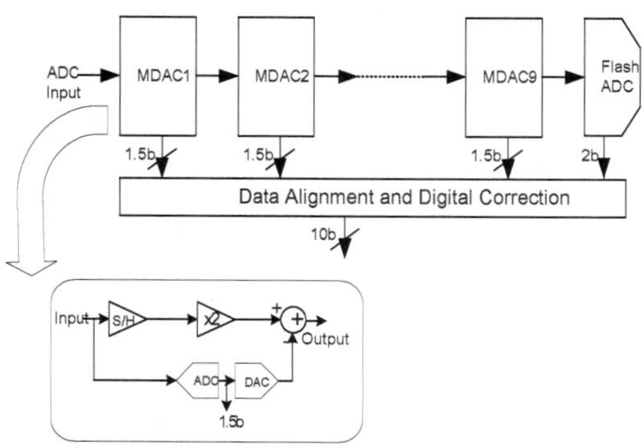

Fig. 5. 10-bit Pipelined ADC architecture.

Fig. 6. shows the architecture of the MDAC stage. In order to achieve low-power and low-voltage restrictions, the input common mode of the operational amplifier is different to the common mode of the input signal. The MDAC stage has two operation phases called *sampling phase* and *amplification phase*. During the *sampling phase* the input of the MDAC is sampled and stored in both capacitors C_f and C_S. The difference between the input and output common mode of the operational amplifier together with the offset and flicker noise, which were stored in C_m during the previous *amplification phase*, is corrected. During the amplification phase the sub-ADC provides the output bits and decides which signal must be supplied by the multiplexer.

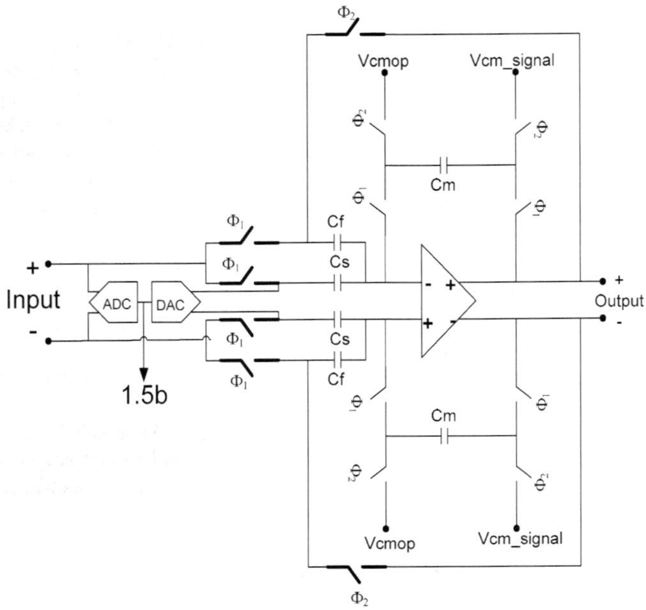

Fig. 6. MDAC architecture (critical switches are highlighted).

The critical switches (that are highlighted in Fig. 6) need rail-to-rail signal swing operation and they were implemented, as it was mentioned before, by means of QFG transistors of Fig. 3. The sampled input is amplified by the factor $1+(C_f/C_S)$, called gain of the MDAC, by connecting the top plate of the capacitor C with the output of the operational amplifier. In a traditional 1.5-bit MDAC stage both capacitor have the same value, so the MDAC has a gain of 2. The transfer function of a MDAC stage is given by:

$$\mathrm{Vout} = \left(1 + \frac{C_f}{C_S}\right) \cdot \mathrm{Vin} + \left(\frac{C_f}{C_S}\right) \cdot D \cdot \mathrm{Vref} \tag{5}$$

where Vref is the reference voltage of the pipelined ADC, Vin the input voltage of the MDAC stage, and:

$$D = \begin{cases} -1 & \text{if} \quad \mathrm{Vin} > \mathrm{Vref}/4 \\ 0 & \text{if} \quad -\mathrm{Verf}/4 \le \mathrm{Vin} \le \mathrm{Vref}/4 \\ 1 & \text{if} \quad \mathrm{Vin} < \mathrm{Vref}/4 \end{cases} \tag{6}$$

Only two comparators are required to implement the sub-ADC in a 1.5-bit MDAC stage. The output bits of the MDACs stages are aligned and digitally processed obtaining the final 10-bit output data. Bit redundancy is used in order to correct the comparator offsets of MDAC stages in the digital domain (Gorbatenko, 1966). Due to this redundancy, low resolution comparators can be used with offset up to $\pm Vref/2^{B+1}$, being B the bit resolution of the sub-ADC (Cho & Gray, 1994).

The correct operation of a pipelined ADC is fully dependent on which value the output voltage of each MDAC stage is settled at the end of the amplification phase which is processed by next pipeline stage. Errors in the MDAC output voltage limit the performance of the ADC. The maximum voltage error allowed at the output of an MDAC, without degradation in the ADC performance, specifies the MDAC building-blocks requirements. In this way, a deep understanding of the errors at the MDAC output voltage arises in knowledge regarding power saving in the right stage. In this section the error sources in pipelined ADC are described and such description is used to implement a behavioural simulator to obtain the requirements of the building-block of each MDAC stage of the ADC for a required resolution and sampling frequency.

The errors concerning to the value of the output voltage of a MDAC stage can be classified into three different groups:

- Static errors: these errors imply that the output voltage value of the MDAC differs, timely independent, from the ideal one. The dynamic of the MDAC stage is not considered.
- Dynamic errors: these are errors which imply that the output voltage of the MDAC does not achieve the static value in time. In this group, the dynamic of the MDAC is only considered as unique error source.
- Noise

4.1 Static errors in MDAC stages

The first important static error source in pipelined ADCs is the mismatch between the capacitors C_f, C_s of each stage. Considering a mismatch δC between both capacitors, C_f=C, C_s/C_f=1+δC; an error term (ε) appears at the residue voltage in (5):

$$Vout = \left(1 + \frac{C_s}{C_f}\right) \cdot Vin + \left(\frac{C_s}{C_f}\right) \cdot D \cdot Vref + \varepsilon \qquad (7)$$

where the error term ε is:

$$\varepsilon = \delta C \cdot (Vin + D \cdot Vref) \qquad (8)$$

Another source of error it the finite gain of the operational amplifier. Assuming an open-loop gain of A_0 for the operational amplifier of the MDAC stage the error term of (7) becomes:

$$\varepsilon = \varepsilon_{mismatch} - \frac{(2 + \delta C)}{A_0} \cdot \left(Vout_{ideal} + \varepsilon_{mismatch}\right) \qquad (9)$$

where $\varepsilon_{mismatch}$ is the error term written in (8) and $Vout_{ideal}$ is the output voltage of the MDAC stage at the end of the amplification phase when no error sources are considered. This equation shows that low open-loop gain of the operational amplifier increases the errors produced by the capacitor mismatch.

4.2 Dynamic errors in MDAC stages

Error sources related to the speed of the MDAC stage are considered in this section. The first dynamic error source which must be considered is the on-resistance of the switches, which are part of the switch capacitor network of the MDAC. During the sampling phase, the on-resistance of the input switches, together with the capacitors; introduces an error in the sampled input voltage (Carner & Un-Ku). The sampled input voltage at the end of the sampling phase is:

$$Vin_{sampled} = Vin \cdot (1 - \exp(-Ts / 2R_{ON}C)) \quad (10)$$

where R_{ON} and C are the switch on-resistance and capacitance where the analog input signal is sampled, and Ts the clock period. In order to achieve good enough settling, the time constant $R_{ON} \cdot C$ is designed to be several time smaller than the clock period. The drawback is that the equivalent noise bandwidth becomes larger than half of the sampling frequency and aliasing of the sampled noise spectra takes place. Thus, the value of the allowed switch on-resistance is defined in terms of the maximum error allowed in the sampled voltage:

$$\varepsilon_{sampled} = Vin - Vin_{sampled} < \frac{1}{2^{N_{stage}}} \Rightarrow R_{ON} < \frac{Ts}{2 \cdot C \cdot N_{stage} \cdot \ln(2)} \quad (11)$$

where N_{stage} is the required resolution of the stage where the switch is used.
Other dynamic error sources are related to the speed of the operational amplifier. In this way, the slew-rate (SR) of the operational amplifier limits the linear settling time, and a finite unity-gain frequency (GBW) makes the operational amplifier slower. The single-pole model of the MDAC stage shows that the output voltage at the end of the amplification phase is:

$$Vout = Vout_{static} \cdot (1 - \exp(-t_{set} \cdot 2\pi \cdot GBW \cdot \beta)) = Vout_{static}(1 + \varepsilon_{dynamic}) \quad (12)$$

where $Vout_{static}$ is the output voltage when only static error sources are considered (7), β is the feedback factor of the MDAC, and t_{set} is the linear settling time:

$$t_{set} = \frac{Ts}{2} - t_{SR} = \frac{Ts}{2} - \frac{(Vout_{static})}{SR} + \frac{1}{2\pi \cdot GBW \cdot \beta} \quad (13)$$

A two-pole system model for the complete MDAC describes a more accurately the settling behaviour. Considering that the system has a phase margin Φ_m, the damping factor is:

$$\zeta = \frac{1}{2 \cdot \sqrt{\cos(\Phi_m)}} \sqrt{1 - \cos^2(\Phi_m)} \quad (14)$$

and the natural frequency of the system is:

$$\omega_0 = \frac{2\pi \cdot GBW \cdot \beta}{\cos(\Phi_m)} \tag{15}$$

In this way, if $\zeta<1$, the MDAC output voltage at the end of the amplification phase is (Chuang, 1982):

$$\begin{aligned} Vout &\approx V_{SR} + (Vout_{static} - V_{SR}) \cdot \left(1 - \frac{1}{\sqrt{1-\zeta^2}} e^{-\omega_0 \cdot \zeta \cdot t_{set}} \sin\left(\sqrt{1-\zeta^2}\,\omega_0 \cdot t_{set} + \phi\right)\right) \\ &\approx Vout_{static} \cdot \left(1 - \frac{SR}{2\pi \cdot GBW \cdot Vout_{static}}\right) \end{aligned} \tag{16}$$

However, if $\zeta>1$, the MDAC output voltage at the end of the amplification phase is:

$$\begin{aligned} Vout &\approx Vout_{static}\left(1 - \frac{1}{2\sqrt{\zeta^2-1}} \cdot \left(\frac{e^{-\omega_0 \cdot \zeta \cdot t_{set} \cdot a}}{a} - \frac{e^{-\omega_0 \cdot \zeta \cdot t_{set} \cdot b}}{b}\right)\right) + \\ &+ V_{SR} \cdot \left(\frac{1}{2\sqrt{\zeta^2-1}} \cdot \left(\frac{e^{-\omega_0 \cdot \zeta \cdot t_{set} \cdot a}}{a} - \frac{e^{-\omega_0 \cdot \zeta \cdot t_{set} \cdot b}}{b}\right)\right) \\ a &= \zeta - \sqrt{\zeta^2 - 1} \\ b &= \zeta + \sqrt{\zeta^2 - 1} \end{aligned} \tag{17}$$

where V_{SR}, in (16) and (17), is the MDAC output voltage at the end of the slew-rate time:

$$V_{SR} = \frac{A_0 \cdot SR}{2\pi \cdot GBW}\left(1 - e^{-2\pi \cdot GBW \cdot t_{SR}/A_0}\right) \tag{18}$$

Other dynamic error sources are charge injection produced by the switches and clock feedthrough. Errors produced by charge injection can be minimized using dummy transistors in the switches. In addition, both errors are reduced using small transistor in the switches. The errors produced by charge injection and clock feedthrough can be modeled as a common mode offset in fully-differential switched capacitor circuits. This common mode offset is reduced by the Common Mode Rejection Ratio (CMRR) of the system.

Considering the whole error sources in an MDAC stage, the output voltage at the end of the amplification phase can be written as:

$$Vout = Vout_{ideal}(1 + \varepsilon_{static} + \varepsilon_{dynamic} + \varepsilon_{static} \cdot \varepsilon_{dynamic}) = Vout_{ideal}(1 + \varepsilon_{total}) \tag{19}$$

This total error worsens the signal-to-noise ratio (SNR) and will produce total harmonic distortion (THD) of the pipelined ADC. The total error of a MDAC stage can be referred to the input of the ADC. In this way, if the total error of each MDAC is referred to the ADC input, the effective number of bits (ENOB) of the pipelined ADC is:

$$ENOB = \left(20\log\left(\frac{V_{FS}}{2 \cdot \sum_{j=1}^{N} \prod_{i=1}^{j} \varepsilon_{total_j} / G_i} \right) - 1.76 \right) / 6.02 \tag{20}$$

where V_{FS} is the ADC full-scale, N the number of stages of the ADC, ε_{totalj} the total relative error of the stage "j" and G_i the ideal gain of the stage "i".

4.3 Noise in MDAC stages

The noise in each stage of the pipeline ADC is produced by the switches, the operational amplifier, and the reference voltage generator. As it has been described in the previous section, the unity gain frequency of the operational amplifier and the inverse of the *R C* time must be several times larger than the sampling frequency. The noise suffers from aliasing because the equivalent noise bandwidth, of the sampling network and the operational amplifier, is larger than the Nyquist frequency. However, a MDAC stage has a gain higher than unity which implies that noise contributions to the equivalent input noise are progressively reduced from the first stage to the last stage. In this way, the total input equivalent noise of the MDAC stages is:

$$\overline{Vin_n} = \sqrt{\sum_{i=1}^{N} \prod_{j=1}^{N} \frac{\overline{Von_i}^2}{Gj^2}} \tag{21}$$

$\overline{Von_i}$ being the total output noise of the MDAC stage-*i*. The total output noise of an MDAC stage is the sum of the output referred noise power in sampling and amplification phase. The total output noise of an MDAC is:

$$\overline{Von}^2 = \frac{G^2 kT}{C_{MDAC}} + 4ktR_{ON} BWn_{OPA} + Sn_{OPA} BWn_{OPA} + Snr BWn_{ref} \tag{22}$$

where k is the Boltzmann constant, *T* is the temperature, C is the sum of the capacitance connected to the analog input during the sampling phase, R_{ON} is the on-resistance of the switches connected to the output during the amplification phase, Sn_{OPA} is the output noise spectral density of the operational amplifier, Snr is the noise spectral density of the reference voltage generator, BWn is the equivalent noise bandwidth of the operational amplifier and BWn is the minimum between the equivalent noise bandwidth of the operational amplifier and the equivalent noise bandwidth of the amplifier which generates the reference voltages.

The complete equivalent input noise power of the whole pipeline ADC is the sum of the equivalent input noise power of the MDAC stages plus the equivalent input noise power of the S/H circuit. Another important noise source in pipeline ADC is the clock jitter. The clock jitter is originated by the phase noise of the clock generator. The noise power produced by the clock jitter when a sinusoidal signal with half full-scale amplitude is:

$$\overline{Vn_{jitter}^{2}} = \left(\pi \cdot V_{FS} \cdot f_{in} \cdot \sigma_{jitter}\right)^{2} / 2 \tag{23}$$

f_{in} being the input signal frequency, σ_{jitter} the sampling jitter standard deviation of the clock signal.

4.4 Behavioral simulation results

Statistical behavioral simulations were done using MATLAB by means of the equations presented in the previous section to get the minimum restriction of the building blocks and considering the low-power consumption requirement. These behavioral simulations provide the maximum capacitor mismatch (and thus the minimum capacitor values), the open-loop and unity-gain frequency for the operational amplifiers as well as noise restrictions for the reference voltages generator. These basic specifications are summarized in Table 2:

Stage	Capacitor Mismatch (5σ%)	Open Loop Gain(dB)	GBW (kHz)
1	0.5	76	24
2	0.7	73	22
3	1.4	70	21
4	2.25	68	20
5	3.9	64	19
6	6.5	60	18
7	12	58	16
8	21	55	15
9	25	48	10

Table 2. Statistical behavioral simulation results.

4.5. Implementation details

Due to low-voltage supply the use of cascade transistor is not possible to achieve high enough open-loop gain. In this way, only classical two stage architectures can be implemented. In order to increase the linearity of the output stage and the open-loop gain, class-AB output stages have been used. The architecture presented in section 4, Fig. 4., was used for each opamp of the pipelined ADC and following the requirements presented in Table 2. As it was also mentioned before, the transistors of the opamp are biased in weak inversion in order to achieve the open-loop gain requirements with the minimum power consumption.

The sub-ADC, required in each MDAC stage, was implemented by means of two SC comparators, Fig. 7. The SC comparator operates on two non-overlapping clock phases. Thus, during the sampling phase, the analog input voltage is sampled in the capacitors 3C and C, while the latch is reset. During the comparison phase, the comparator compares the sampled analog input with the previously sampled reference voltage. The latch provides the digital output whereas the switched capacitor network samples the reference voltage in the capacitor C for the following comparison.

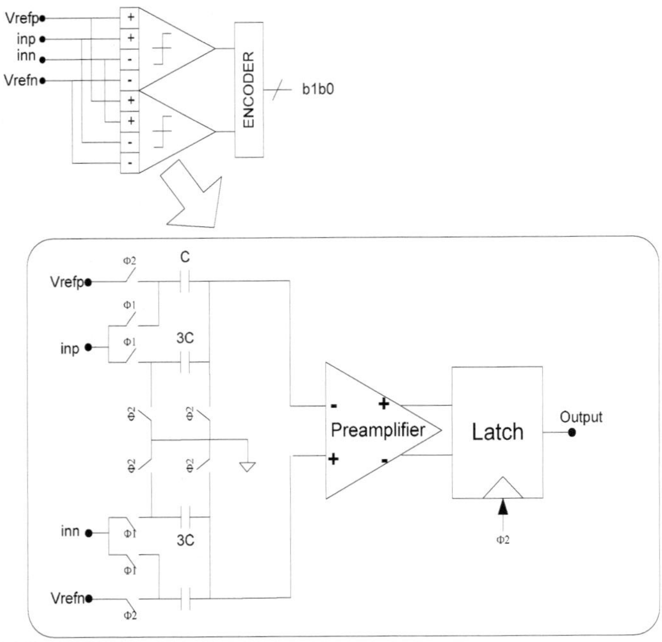

Fig. 7. Sub-ADC architecture.

The ADC was designed using an AMI (MOSIS) 0.5μm CMOS technology with PMOS and NMOS threshold voltages of about V_{TP}=-0.96V and V_{TN}=0.67V respectively. Table 3 summarizes the obtained post-layout simulation results of the complete pipelined ADC when a sinusoidal input signal of a -1dBFS and 93.75Hz is applied. The following figure of merit (FOM) was used:

$$FOM = \frac{P}{2^n f_n} \tag{24}$$

where n is the number of bits, P is the power consumption in Watts and f_n is the Nyquist frequency in Hz.

Sampling Rate	4kS/s
SNR (input 93.75Hz, 0.645Vpp)	61.5dB
THD (input 93.75Hz, 0.645Vpp)	-75.9dB
SINAD (input 93.75Hz, 0.645Vpp)	60.76dB
ENOB	9.8bits
Power Consumption	1.5μW
FOM	0.84pJ/state

Table 3. Simulation results.

Fig. 7. shows the spectrum of the reconstructed analog signal from the digital output bits of the pipelined ADC.
Simulation results are provided which shows 9.8 bits of resolution with 1.2 V supply voltage and only a power consumption of 1.5μW. The power efficiency is of 0.84pJ/state, being the most energy efficient converter of all the biomedical ADCs except (Yang et al., 2006).

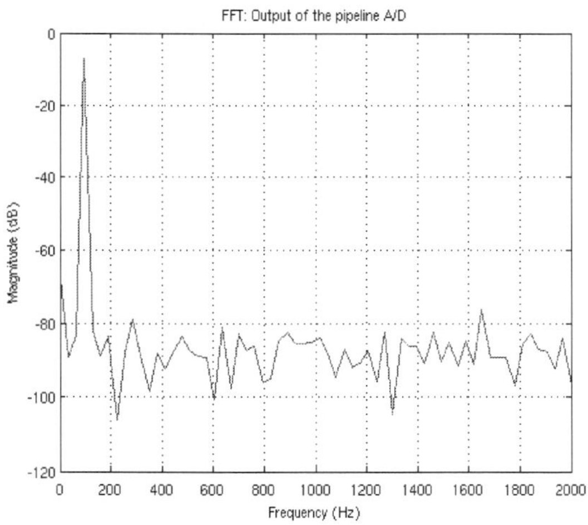

Fig. 8. Simulation results.

5. A 10-bit SC-ΣΔ modulator for EEG applications

Oversampling ΣΔ ADCs are based on the principle that the conversion error can be high-pass filtered and later remove by digital filters. The requirements on the analog parts are relaxed and high-resolutions can be achieved. The drawback is the relative small input signal bandwidth due to oversampling. A ΣΔ modulator consists of an analog filter, continuous or discrete time, and a coarse quantizer enclosed in a feedback loop. Together with the filter, the feedback loop acts to attenuate the quantization noise at low frequency while emphasizing the high frequency noise. Thus, the quantization noise is high-pass filtered while the input signal is only delayed. The high frequency noise can be removed by using digital low-pass filter (decimation), and a low-noise output signal is achieved.

A classical implementation of a single-bit second order SC-ΣΔ modulator is shown in Fig. 9. The most important building block in this architecture is the summing integrator.

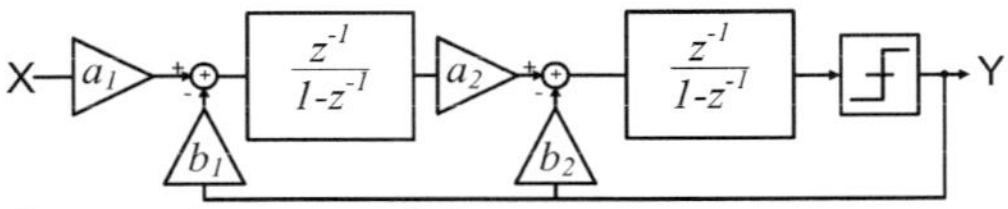

Fig. 9. Second-order discrete-time ΣΔ modulator.

The remaining building blocks in the analogy portion of the modulator are comparator and 1-bit DAC. The comparator circuit acts as a 1-bit ADC that maps its input into one of two digital output codes. The two digital output codes are then mapped back into analog levels by the DAC. If the two output codes of the comparator are defined as ±1/2, then the DAC, neglecting DAC, can be represented simply by gain block.
The ideal output of the second order ΣΔ modulator, when $b_2=2a_1a_2$ and $b_1=a_1$, which guarantee the loop stability; is described by:

$$Y(z) = z^{-2}X(z) + \left(1 - z^{-1}\right)^2 E(z) \tag{25}$$

where E(z) is the quantization noise in the quantizer and X(z) the input signal. Component mismatch, finite open-loop gain of the opamps, thermal noise and incomplete settling are the most important error sources in ΣΔ modulators which degrade the overall ADC performance. As it was previously mentioned, the most important building block of a ΣΔ modulator is the integrator. In this way, the error sources in such block must to be considered. The equation (20) corresponds to the following transfer function for an integrator:

$$H(z) = \frac{a_1 z^{-1}}{1 - z^{-1}} \tag{26}$$

where a_1 is the gain preceding the input to the integrator. Deviations in a_1 from its nominal value in the first integrator alter the noise shaping function of the modulator changing the ADC performance (Boser & Wooley, 1988). In SC ΣΔ modulators, these deviations are mainly a consequence of capacitor mismatch. Larger a_1 means higher gain in the forward path of the modulator and consequently greater attenuation of the quantization noise. However, if a1 is too large ($a_1>0.6$), the signal amplitudes at the integrator outputs increase rapidly and the system becomes unstable.
The ideal integrator DC gain is infinite. However, due to circuit constrains, the integrator DC gain is limited. This effect is called "integrator leak" and implies that only a fraction "P" of the previous output of the integrator is added to each new input sample. In this way, the DC gain of the integrator becomes:

$$H_0 = \frac{a_1}{1 - P} \tag{27}$$

and the new integrator transfer function:

$$H(z) = \frac{a_1 z^{-1}}{1 - Pz^{-1}} \tag{28}$$

The effect of the integrator leak is that limited gain at low frequencies reduces the attenuation of the quantization noise in the baseband increasing the in-band quantization noise.

In a general form, the in-band error power of a ΣΔ modulator can be expressed as (Medeiro et al., 1999):

$$P_{total} = P_Q + P_{noise} + P_{nl} + P_{set} \tag{29}$$

where P_Q is the quantization error, P_{noise} the noise circuit error, P_{nl} the non-linearity error and P_{set} the incomplete settling error. The design of the ADC can be made in such that quantization error is the dominant error source:

$$P_{noise} + P_{nl} + P_{set} << \frac{1}{12} \cdot \left[\frac{2 \cdot Vref}{2^B - 1}\right] \cdot \frac{\pi^{2L}}{(2 \cdot L + 1) \cdot M^{2L+1}} \tag{30}$$

where Vref is the reference voltage, L the modulator order and M the oversampling ratio. Every doubling of the sampling rate will provide L + 0.5 extra bits. The resolution can be increased by increasing the quantizator resolution and the modulator order. A problem with increasing the resolution of the quantizer is that the nonlinearities in the DACs will directly limit the ADC performance. Increasing the modulator order makes the stability of the loop more difficult, especially for order higher than 2.

Usually, the condition expressed in (25) implies a high amount of current consumption. Instead is more efficient to make the design such that $P_Q \cong P_{noise} + P_{nl} + P_{set}$.

In order to obtain an optimum design the following consideration were taken into account:

1. The value of the sampling capacitor at the modulator front-end is selected so that the error due to quantization noise and circuit noise is smaller than the maximum allowed in-band error. The amplifier noise, the switches noise and kT/C noise are the main contributor to the overall circuit noise (P_{noise}).
2. The error contribution due to incomplete settling is made a non-limiting factor by means of a high enough open-loop gain and GBW of the opamps. Anyway, the settling must not be limited by the slew-rate of the opamps. In addition, too high GBW will end ups with unnecessary extra power consumption. The GBW of the operational amplifiers must often be at least an order of magnitude greater than the sampling frequency. However, simulations show that the GBW of the operational amplifiers can be lower (Giustolisi. & Palumbo,2003). A good compromise for the GBW of the operational amplifiers is (Boser & Wooley, 1988):

$$GBW \geq \frac{1 + a_1}{\pi} \cdot f_s \tag{31}$$

3. Critical design parameter of the quantizer implemented by means of comparators must be considered. The speed of the comparator must be high enough for the desired sampling rate, and input offset, input referred noise and hysteresis must be low enough to not degrade the ADC performance.

5.1 ADC architecture and building blocks.

The second ADC implementation that is described in this chapter for EEG purposes is a 10-bit SC-ΣΔ modulator operating with a sampling frequency of 3.2 kHz and a full-scale range of 0.725 V (Lopez-Morillo et al., 2008). A simple and power efficient architecture for high resolution ADCs in the range of biomedical signals is the classical second-order ΣΔ modulator (Fig. 9). The main advantages of this architecture are simplicity, low sensitivity to component mismatch and stability.
System simulations have been performed using MATLAB/SIMULINK based on the models developed on (Boser & Wooley, 1988) and (Rabii & Wooly, 1999). As a result of these simulations (including the main non-idealities such as finite DC gain, bandwidth, and slew-rate of the amplifiers) a set of specifications for the most important building blocks have been obtained. These specifications are summarized in Table 2.

General Specifications	Oversampling ratio	64
	Sampling frequency	3.2kHz
Integrators' coefficients	a_1,b_1	0.25
	a_2	0.5
	b_2	0.25
First integrator's opamp	Output-Swing	2Vpp
	Slew-rate (SR)	15V/ms
	Unity-gain frequency	8kHz
	DC gain	30dB
Clock	Jitter	$0.1ms_{rms}$
Capacitor values	C_{s1}	125fF
	C_{cds}	500fF
	C_{i1}	500fF
	C_{s2}	50fF
	C_{i2}	200fF

Table 4. Specifications for building blocks.

Behavioral simulations show a Dynamic Range (DR) of 72dB with an oversampling ratio of 64, which is enough to achieve the 10 bit resolution. In order to get an unconditionally stable modulator and to maximize the integrators output swing, the coefficients have been chosen as $a_1=b_1=b_2=0.25$ and $a_2=0.5$ (Rabii & Wooly, 1999).

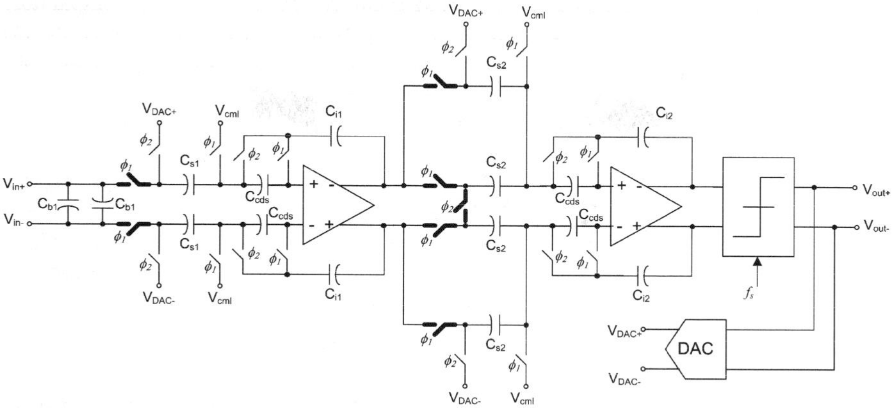

Fig. 10. Implementation of the second-order ΣΔ modulator (critical switches are highlighted).

Fig. 10 shows the SC implementation of the modulator of Fig. 9. The architecture is composed of two correlated double sampling (CDS) integrators, a comparator, and a 1-bit digital-to-analog converter. This implementation has been chosen attending to different implementation issues:

1. Flicker noise: as the desired signal bandwidth of the converter is low, the noise floor is dominated by flicker noise. Correlated Double Sampling has been used in order to shape the flicker noise outside of the signal band (Williams & Wooley, 1994). The basic operation of the CDS integrator is as follows. The amplifier flicker noise and offset is sampled across C_{CDS} during the first clock phase (ϕ_1). During the second clock phase (ϕ_2) the flicker noise and an offset are cancelled by the voltage stored in C_{CDS}.

2. Low-voltage operation: the use of a very low supply voltage introduces several issues that complicate the design of the Sigma-Delta modulator. The first problem to solve is the design of an operational amplifier with a large output swing that achieves sufficient gain and bandwidth. The other critical problem is the need of a rail-to-rail switch. These problems are solved using QFG techniques described in previous section 3 and 4.

3. Low-power operation: the main contributors to power consumption of a ΣΔ modulator are the operational amplifiers. Low-power operation is achieved by means of using the two-stage class-AB opamp based on QFG transistor and biased in weak inversion shown in section 4. Other measure to save power consumption is to minimize capacitor sizes which are limited either kT/C noise or capacitor mismatch specifications.

The 1-bit quantizer has been implemented using the architecture illustrated in Fig. 11. The dynamic latch operates as follows. When the clock ϕ_2 is low, the latch is reset, and its outputs are both pulled high. When ϕ_2 is high the latch enters in the regeneration phase because M3 and M4 form a positive feedback loop. The power consumption of the comparator is of only 32.5nW during normal operation. Capacitors C_{comp} perform a DC level shifting so that the input common mode voltage of the comparator is of V_{cmCOMP}=900mV. Moreover, by means of C_{comp}, the input signal is sampled at the end of clock phase ϕ_1.

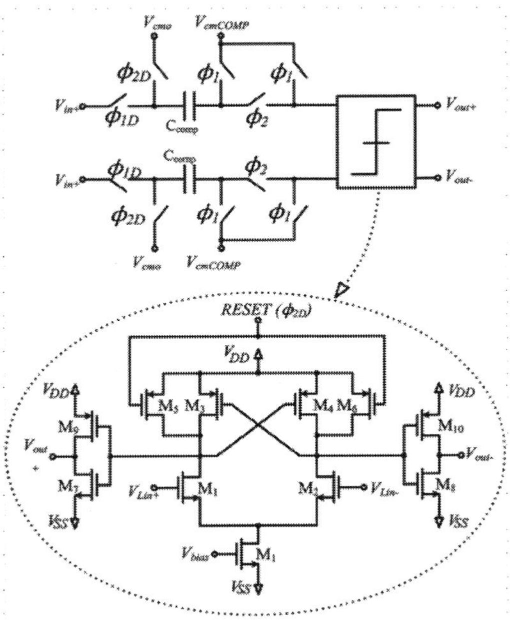

Fig. 11. 1-bit quantizer.

Switches connected to Vi_{n+} and Vi_{n-} are controlled by a delayed clock phase (ϕ_{1D}) in order to remove the input-dependent offset voltage due to the clock feedthrough.

The 1-bit digital-to-analog converter (DAC) has been implemented by switches controlled by the comparator outputs (Fig. 12). In order to maximize the dynamic range, the feedback reference voltages are equals to ±VFS/2, where V_{FS} is the Full-Scale Input Voltage of the ADC.

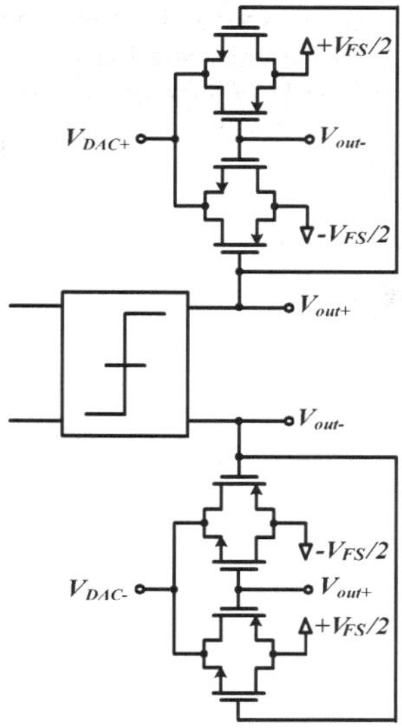

Fig. 12. 1-bit DAC.

5.2 Experimental results.

The Sigma-Delta modulator has been also implemented using an AMI (MOSIS) 0.5μm CMOS technology. The active area of the modulator is of 0.6 mm². A chip microphotograph is shown in Fig. 13. A sinusoidal input of 5Hz and 362 mV amplitude has been used to characterize the dynamic performance. Fig. 14 shows the output spectrum of the modulator, where a SNDR of 62.6 dB is demonstrated. Under these conditions, the power consumption is only of 140nW (90nW of static power consumption).

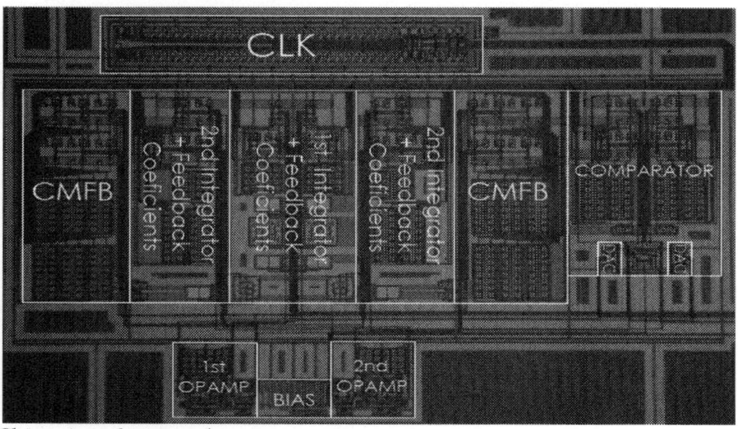

Fig. 13. Chip microphotograph.

Fig. 15(a) shows the SNDR and SNR versus the input amplitude normalized by the full scale input voltage (1.2V amplitude). It can be seen that the dynamic range is 67.4dB, which corresponds to 10.75 effective bits. Furthermore, in Fig. 15(b) the SNDR is shown, using input amplitude of 362mV, versus the frequency of the input signal. We can see that the modulator maintains its performance from DC to 25Hz.

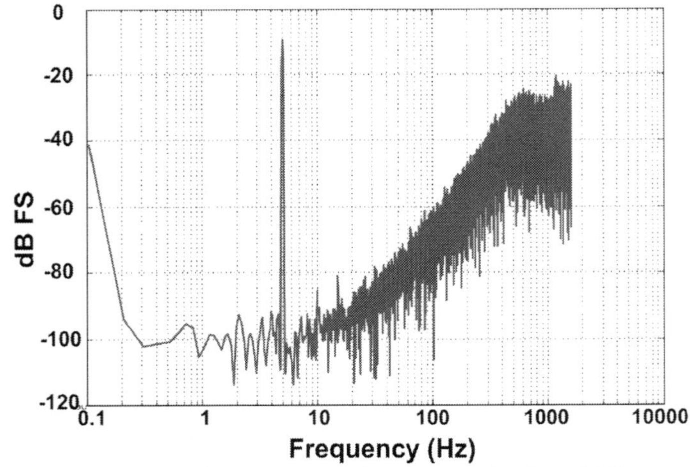

Fig. 14. Output spectrum with an input signal of 362mV amplitude and 5Hz.

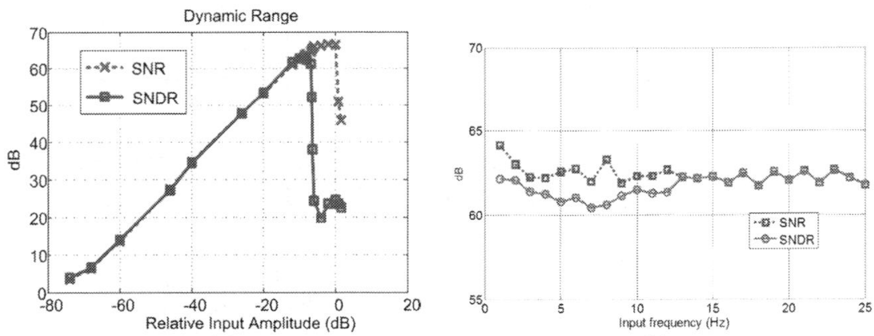

(a) (b)

Fig. 15. (a) SNDR and SNR versus the normalized input amplitude. (b) SNDR and SNR vs. input frequency (input signal of 362mV amplitude).

Table 5. summarizes the overall experimental results; (19) was used to calculate the ADC figure of merit.

Technology	MOSIS 0.5µm CMOS
Supply Voltage	1.2V
Full scale input signal	0.362V amplitude
Sampling rate	3.2kHz
Power consumption	140nW
Signal bandwidth	25Hz
ENOB	10.75 bits
Peak SNDR (362mV amplitude and 5Hz)	62.6dB
Peak SNR (950mV amplitude and 5Hz)	66.5dB
DR	67.4dB
Active area	$0.6mm^2$
FOM	1.6pJ/state

Table 5. ADC experimental results.

The reported low-power consumption and measured ENOB makes this ADC suitable for wearable EEG systems. In addition, the low area required makes possible to use this ADC in general purpose biomedical systems were more than one ADC in required.

6. Conclusions

Two 10-bit, low-voltage, low-power ADCs has been designed for wearable EEG systems. Innovative design techniques, circuit architectures based on QFG transistors, are described which allow circuit implementation at very low-voltage supply and low-power conditions. The first one uses pipeline architecture allowing higher input signal bandwidth showing 9.8 bits of resolution during by means of post-layout simulations. The second one uses a second-order SC-ΣΔ architecture with CDS, obtaining in measurements more than 10 bits of resolution.

In addition a deep understanding of the error mechanisms of both ADC architectures have been used to build up a behavioural simulator in order to obtain the design requirements of the ADCs building blocks.

In order to minimize the power consumption a novel weak-inversion biased class-AB operational amplifier based on QFG transistors has been used in both designs in order to achieve high-enough open-loop gain and output-swing under low-voltage conditions. Furthermore, QFG transistors have been used to solve the problem of the high-swing switches.

The presented ADCs have been implemented using MOSIS 0.5µm CMOS technology with high transistor threshold voltages (0.96V for p-MOS transistor). Simulations and experimental results show high enough performance for EEG signal processing with low-voltage supply and low-power consumption.

Table 6. shows a comparative study some of the most recently and relevant published state-of-the-art energy-efficient ADCs for biomedical applications.

Ref	ENOB (bits)	BW (kHz)	Power (μW)	V_{DD} (V)	Tech. CMOS	FOM (pJ/state)
(Yang & Sarpeshkar, 2006)	7.4	23	0.96	1.2	0.18μm	0.12
(Agah et al., 2007)	14	500	38000	1.8	0.18μm	2.3
(Yang & Sarpeshkar, 2005)	10	16	75	3	0.35μm	2.3
This work (Pipelined ADC)	9.8	2	1.5	1.2	0.5μm	0.84
This work (ΣΔ ADC)	10.75	0.025	0.14	1.2	0.5μm	1.6

Table 6. Comparative study of Biomedical ADCs.

We can be observed that the ΣΔ ADC converter described in this chapter is the less power consuming ADC reported so far. In addition, to the best authors' knowledge the energy efficient of both described ADCs are the best of all biomedical ADCs except (Yang & Sarpeshkar, 2006). However, their higher ENOB makes them more useful for modern and high-quality wearable EEG systems.

Finally, we can bring out that this work demonstrate the usefulness of using extensively the QFG technique for the design of very low-power and very low-voltage analog systems.

7. References

Casson, A. J.; Smith, S.; Duncan, J. S.& Rodriguez-Villegas, E. (2008). Wearable EEG: what is it needed and what does entail?, 30th *Annual International IEEE EMBS Conference*, pp. 5867-5870, Vancouver, British Columbia, Canada, August 20-24, 2008, ISSN 1557-170X

Erdogmus, D.; Adami, A.; Pavel, M.; Tian Lan; Mathan, S.; Whitlow, S. & Dorneich, M. (2005). Cognitive State Estimation Based on EEG for Augmented Cognition, *2nd International IEEE EMBS Conference on Neural Engineering*, pp. 566-569, ISBN 0-7803-8710-4, March 16-19, 2005

Yates, D.; López-Morillo, E.; Carvajal, R. G.; Ramirez-Angulo, J. & Rodriguez-Villegas, E. (2007). A Low-Voltage Low-Power Front-End for Wearable EEG Systems, *Proceedings of the 29th Annual International Conference of the IEEE EMBS*, pp. 5282-5285, ISBN 978-1-4244-0787-3, Cité Internationale, Lyon, France, August 23-26, 2007

Yang, H. Y. & Sarpeshkar, R. (2006). A Bio-Inspired Ultra-Energy-Efficient Analog-to-Digital Converter for Biomedical Applications. *IEEE Transactions on Circuits and Systems-I: Regular Papers*, Vol. 53, No. 11, pp. 2349-2356, November 2006 ISSN 1057-7122

Binnie, C. D.; Rowan, A. J. & Gutter, T. (1982). A manual of electroencephalographic technology. Cambridge University Press, ISBN 0521238471, Cambridge

Cooper, R.; Osselton, J. W.; & Shaw, J. C. (1974). EEG Technology, Second Edition, Butterworth & Co., ISBN 0407160027, London

Menolfi, C. & Huang, Q. (1999). A fully integrated untrimmed CMOS instrumentation amplifier with submicrovolt offset. *IEEE Journal of Solid-State Circuits*, Vol. 34, No. 3, pp. 415-420, March 1999, ISSN 0018-9200

Yates, D. & Rodriguez-Villegas, E. (2006). An Ultra Low Power Noise Chopper Amplifier for Wireless EEG, *49th IEEE International Midwest Symposium on Circuit and Systems, MWSCAS'06*, Vol. 2, pp. 449-452, August 6-9, 2006, ISSN 1548-3746

Goes, J.; Paulino, N.; Monteiro, R.; Vaz, B. & Garcao, A. S. (2005). Low-Power Low-Voltage CMOS A/D Sigma-Delta Modulator for Bio-Potential Signal Driven by a Single-Phase Scheme. *IEEE Transactions On Circuits and Systems –I: Regular Paper*, Vol. 52, No. 12, pp. 2595-2604, December 2005, ISSN 1057-7122

Lee, H.-Y.; Hsu, C.-M. & Huang, S.-C. (2005). Designing Low Power of Sigma-Delta Modulator for Biomedical Applications. *Biomedical Engineering applications, Basis & Communications*, No. 17, pp. 181-185, August 2005 ISSN 1016-2372

Crols, J. & Steyaert, M. (1994). Switch-Opamp: An approach to realize full CMOS switched-capacitor circuits at very low voltage supply voltages. *IEEE Journal of Solid-State Circuits*, Vol. 29, pp. 936-942, August 1994, ISSN 0018-9200

Ramírez-Angulo, J.; López-Martín, A. J.; González-Carvajal, R.; Muñoz-Chavero, F. (2004). Very Low-Voltage Analog Signal Processing Based on Quasi-Floating Gate Transistors. *IEEE Journal of Solid-State Circuits*, Vol. 39, Vol. 3, pp. 434-442, March 2004, ISSN 0018-9200

Muñoz, F.; Ramírez-Angulo, J.; Lopez-Martin, A.; Carvajal, R. G.; Torralbal, A., Palomo, B. & Kachare, M. (2003). Analogue switch for very-low volyage applications. *Electronic Letters*, Vol. 39, No. 9, pp. 701-702, May 1st 2003, ISSN 0013-5194

Ramírez-Angulo, J.; Carvajal, R. G.; Galan, J. A. & Lopez-Martin, A. (2006). A free but efficient low-voltage class-AB two-stage operational amplifier. *IEEE Transactions on Circuits and Systems-II: Express Briefs*, Vol. 53, Issue 7, pp. 568-571, July 2006, ISSN 1549-7747

Cho, T. B. & Gray, P. R. (1994). A 10-bit, 20-MS/s, 35-mW pipelined A/D converter, *Proceedings of the IEEE 1994 Custom Integrated Circuits Conference*, ISBN 0-7803-1886-2, pp. 409-502, 1-4 May 1994, San Diego, USA

Carnes, J. & Un-Ku, M. (2006). The effect of switch resistance on pipelined ADC MDAC settling time, *Proceedings of the 2006 IEEE International Symposium on Circuit and Systems, ISCAS 2006*, ISBN 0-7803-9389-9, pp. 5251-5254, 21-24 May 2006

Chuang, C. T. (1982). Analysis of the Settling Behaviour of an Operational Amplifier. *IEEE Journal of Solid-State Circuits*, Vol. SC-17; No. 1, pp. 74-80, February 1982

Medeiro, F.; Pérez-Verdú, B. & Rodríguez-Vázquez, A. (1999). Top-Down Design of High-Performance Sigma-Delta Modulators. Kluwer Academic Publishers, ISBN 978-0792383529, Norwood, MA.

Giustolisi,G. & Palumbo,G. (2003). A novel 1-V class-AB transconductor for improving speed performance in SC applications, *Proceedings of the 2003 International Circuits and Systems, ISCAS'03*, Vol. 1, ISBN 0-7803-7761-3 ,pp. 153-156, 25-28 May 2003

Boser, B. E. & Wooley, B. A. (1988). The design of sigma-delta modulation analog-to-digital converters. *IEEE Journal of Solid-State Circuits*, Vol. 23, No. 6, pp. 1298-1308, Dec. 1988, ISSN 0018-9200

Lopez-Morillo, E.; Carvajal, R. G.; Munoz, F.; ElGmili, H.; Lopez-Martin, A.; Ramirez-Angulo, J. & Rodriguez-Villegas, E. (2008). A 1.2-V 140-nW 10-bit Sigma-Delta Modulator for Electroencephalogram Applications. *IEEE Transactions on Biomedical Circuits and Systems*, Vol. 2, Issue 3, ISSN 1932-4545, pp. 223-230, September 2008

Rabii, S. & Wooly, B. A. (1999). The Design of Low-Voltage, Low-Power Sigma-Delta Modulator. Kluwer Academic Publisher, ISBN 0-7923-8361-3, Norwell, MA, USA

Williams, L. A. & Wooley, B. A. (1994). A Third-Order Sigma-Delta Modulator with Extended Dynamic Range. *IEEE Journal of Solid-State Circuits*, Vol. 29, No. 3, pp. 193-202, March 1994, ISSN 0018-9200

Gorbatenko, G. G. (1966). High-performance parallel-serial analog to digital converter with error correction. IEEE National Convention Record, New York, pp. 39-43, March 1966.

Agah, A.; Vleugels, K.; Griffin, P. B.; Ronaghi, M.; Plummer, J. D. & Wooley , B. A. (2007). A High-Resolution Low-Power Oversampling ADC with Extended-Range for Bio-Sensor Arrays, *IEEE Symposium on VLSI Circuits*, ISBN 978-4-900784-05-5, pp. 2628-2636, Dec. 2007

Yang, H. Y. & Sarpeshkar (2005). A time-based energy-efficient analog-to-digital converter. *IEEE Journal of Solid-State Circuits*, Vol. 40, Issue 8, pp. 1590-1601, Aug. 2005, ISSN 0018-9200

3

On-chip cell positioning and sorting using contactless methods: a comparison between different force-fields

Frénéa Marie[1] and Haddour Naoufel[2]
Laboratoire Ampère (UMR CNRS 5005), [1]Université de Lyon, [2]Ecole Centrale de Lyon France

1. Introduction

Controlling the motion of biological cells is one of the most important challenges of biomedical research. Cell positioning and separation are fundamental functions that have been widely studied in the past decades with the increased interest for stakes of micro total analysis system (μTAS) development. Major breakthroughs were achieved in this research area, thanks to the continuous improvement of micro fabrication techniques, now offering the possibility to design tools with feature sizes adapted to cell dimensions and to perform integration of cell handling devices. Moreover, micro fluidics has shown considerable promise as a tool for studying biological molecules and cells.
Our aim is to present recent developments in cell handling strategies, by focusing on dielectrophoretic, magnetic, optic and acoustic techniques, which, despite their specificities, present many similarities. To facilitate comparison, our study is deliberately restricted to contactless manipulation strategies. Contact-free manipulation techniques are intrinsically sterile and can provide fine control of exerted force. In the next section, we will present the forces and concepts used with the view of extracting common scientific bases. Then, we will illustrate their respective potential by presenting applications chosen to emphasize advantages and drawbacks of each technique. The characteristics and performances of the four methods will be summarized in the last part.

2. Contactless microparticle manipulation: forces and concepts

2.1 Dielectrophoresis

Dielectrophoresis (DEP) is defined as the motion of polarized particles subjected to non-uniform electric fields. Dielectrophoretic effects may arise from spatial non-uniformities of both magnitude and phase of AC electric fields, respectively interacting with the in-phase and out-of-phase components of the induced dipole moment (Wang *et al.* 1994; Wang *et al.* 1995).
cDEP: As first described by Pohl, conventional dielectrophoresis (cDEP) is the motion of polarized particle arising from the interaction of the electric field with the net induced

charges at the particle/medium interface(Pohl 1958). It implies a non-uniform spatial distribution of the field magnitude. The time-averaged DEP force experienced by a cell placed in an AC electric field $\overline{E}(\omega)$ can be written as:

$$< \mathbf{F}(t) >= 2\pi\varepsilon_m r^3 \,\mathrm{Re}\left[f_{CM}(\omega)\right] \nabla E_{RMS}^2 \qquad (1)$$

where r represents the cell radius, E_{RMS} and ω are the electric field RMS intensity and angular frequency, while f_{CM} is the Clausius-Mossotti factor, determined by the frequency-dependant polarisabilities of the particle and its surrounding medium:

$$f_{CM}(\omega) = \frac{\varepsilon_p^*(\omega) - \varepsilon_m^*(\omega)}{\varepsilon_p^*(\omega) + 2\,\varepsilon_m^*(\omega)} \qquad (2)$$

ε_p^* and ε_m^* are the complex permittivities of the particle and its immersion medium defined as $\varepsilon^* = \varepsilon - j\sigma/\omega$, ε and σ respectively denoting dielectric constant and conductivity.
Due to the field inhomogeneity, the forces acting on the opposite and equal charges of the induced dipole are unbalanced, which gives rise to a net force. Consequently, particles whose polarizability is greater than that of their surrounding medium ($\mathrm{Re}(f_{CM})>0$) are directed toward high field regions, (pDEP, Fig.1a), whereas particles whose polarizability is less than that of the medium ($\mathrm{Re}(f_{CM})<0$) move to the region of lowest field intensity (nDEP, Fig.1b).

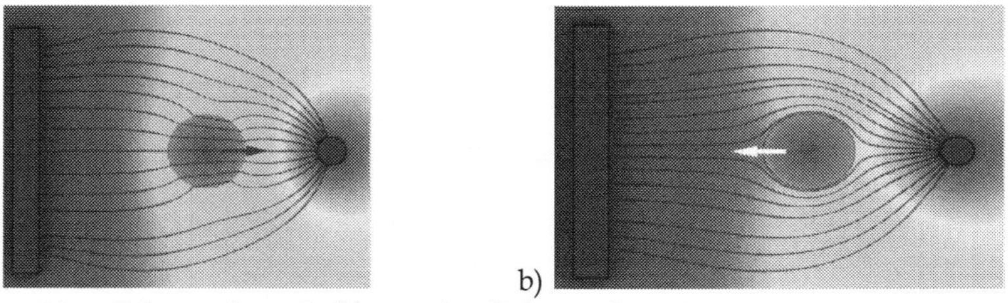

a) b)

Fig 1. a) positive dielectrophoresis, b) negative dielectrophoresis

twDEP: The twDEP force acts on a particle subjected to a travelling electric field. It is related to the phase non-uniformity of the electric field and arises from the interaction of the travelling field with the phase lagging component of the induced dipole moment. Such a field can be produced by planar electrodes arranged in rows and driven by a polyphase ac voltage. The resulting translational force propels the particle along the electrodes, with or against the field direction, depending on whether $\mathrm{Im}(f_{CM})$ is negative or positive, respectively (Jones 2003). In pratice, cDEP and twDEP effects can be observed simultaneously: while the particle translates, it is either pushed above the electrodes (nDEP) or attracted onto them (pDEP), depending on the sign of $\mathrm{Re}(f_{CM})$(Jones 2003).

2.2 Magnetophoresis

Magnetophoresis is the magnetic analogue of dielectropheresis and is defined as the translation of para or diamagnetic particles inside a non-uniform magnetic field. A non-spherical particle placed in a homogeneous magnetic field would experience a torque, so as to align with the field, but no translation should be observed. The difference between both methods lies in the fact that dielectrophoresis uses electric properties of matter while magnetophoresis exploits its magnetic properties. The magnetic force exerted on a particle depends on the volume of the particle (V), the difference in magnetic susceptibilities ($\Delta\chi$) between the particle (χ_p) and surrounding buffer medium (χ_m), as well as the strength and gradient of the applied magnetic field as shown below in equation (3):

$$F_{mag} = \frac{2\pi r^3(\chi_p - \chi_m)}{3\mu_0}\nabla|B|^2 \tag{3}$$

where r is the particle radius, μ_0 is the vacuum permeability and B is the magnetic flux density.
Therefore, the net magnetic force exerted on the particle increases with its volume and with the amplitude and the gradient of the field. The net magnetic force increases also with the difference in magnetic susceptibilities $\Delta\chi$ and the sign of the force depends on the sign of $\Delta\chi$. If $\Delta\chi$ is negative, the net magnetic force is negative and the particle is repelled from the maximum region to the minimum region of the magnetic field. Besides, if $\Delta\chi$ is positive, the net force is positive and the particle is attracted to the maximum field region.

2.3 Optical force

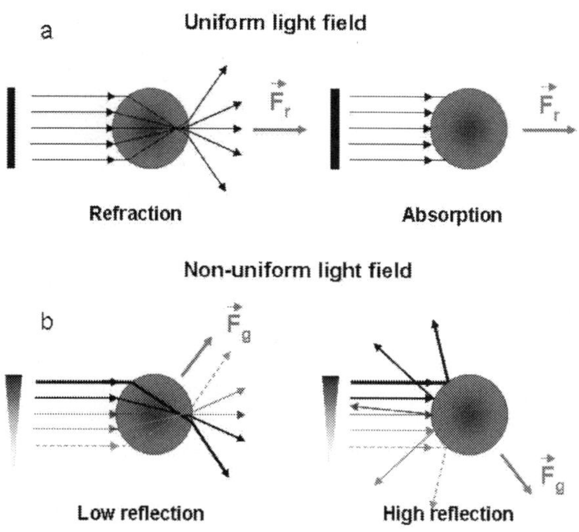

Fig. 2. a. Illustration of scattering force. b. gradient force.

Optical forces can also be used to trap and manipulate particles and biological cells. The light consists of photons having an energy $E= h\nu$ and a momentum $p= h\nu/c$, h denoting the Planck constant (6,626 x 10^{-34}J.s) and ν the frequency. Thus, when a photon is reflected by an object, it undergoes a variation of momentum that engenders a force on the reflecting

surface $F=dp/dt = nI/c$. n is the refractive index of the medium in which the photon propagates, I is the light beam intensity and c is the speed of light. In case where the lightened surface is a dielectric particle, the forces applied on the sphere can be divided into two components. The first is the scattering force (F_r) orientated in direction of light propagation and related to the absorption and the reflection of a uniform light field by the particle (Figure 2.a). The second is the gradient light force (F_g), which is related to interaction of the particle with a non-uniform light field. Photons distributed non-symmetrically around the centre of the particle result in a gradient force in the direction of the gradient field oblique with respect to the direction of light propagation (Figure 2.b). In the case of a little reflecting particle the gradient force tends to push the object towards the maximum of luminous intensity. However, if the particle is very reflecting, it can be expelled towards the minimal intensity areas.
Under the action of both scattering and gradient forces, a dielectric particle exposed to a focusing laser beam is attracted towards the axe of the beam and propelled in the direction of light propagation. For stable trapping in all three dimensions, the gradient component of the force pulling the particle towards the focal region must exceed the scattering component of the force pushing it away from that region. This condition necessitates a very high field gradient, produced by tightly focusing laser beam using an objective of high numerical aperture NA. Therefore, the force produced by the field gradient can overcome the forces due to gravity, Brownian motion and back-scattered light, resulting in a three-dimensional optical trap. The resulting optical tweezers allow to trap particles and to place them freely on a xy plane. Furthermore, when a highly condensed laser beam is used, the position of the particle can also be controlled in the z direction. Particles trapped by an optical tweezer can be divided into three regimes determined by the ratio of the incident light's wavelength λ to the diameter D of the irradiated particle. If the particle size is larger than the wavelength of the trapping laser, i.e., the radius $D>>\lambda$, the particle is in the Mie regime and optical forces can be computed from simple ray optics. If the trapped sphere is much smaller than the wavelength of the trapping laser, i.e., $D<<\lambda$, the conditions for Raleigh scattering are satisfied and optical forces can be calculated by treating the particle as a point dipole. In this approximation, the scattering and gradient force components are readily separated. When the particle sizes are comparable with the wavelength of the trapping laser, i.e $D\approx \lambda$, neither the ray optic nor the dipole approach is valid. Unfortunately, among objects that lie in this size range (0.1-10μm) are bacteria, yeast, organelles of larger cells and dielectric microspheres used alone or as handles to manipulate other biological objects. The calculation of optical forces requires the solution of Maxwell's equations with the appropriate boundary condition to supply an accurate description. Recently Nieminen et al. developed a computational toolbox implemented in Matlab ®, for the computational modelling of optical tweezers (Nieminen *et al.* 2007). The toolbox is designed for the calculation of optical forces and torques, and can be used for both spherical and nonspherical particles, in both Gaussian and other beams. However, in many research works, both the axial and the lateral trapping efficiencies for various configurations of optical tweezers are defined in terms of the constant Q of proportionality in an equation relating the incident laser power P at the focus to the resulting trapping force F (Svoboda *et al.* 1994).

$$F_{Trap} = \frac{Qn_m P}{c} \quad (4)$$

In equation 4, n_m is the refractive index of the suspending medium, c is the speed of light in vacuum and the quantity $n_m.P/c$ is simply the total linear momentum flux of the light beam. Q represents the fraction of power utilized to exert the force. Hence possible values of Q range between 0 and 1. For plane waves incident on a perfectly absorbing particle, Q = 1. Q value depends on the NA, laser wavelength, light polarization state, laser mode structure, relative index of refraction, and geometry of the particle.

2.4 Acoustic force

When exposed to an ultrasonic field, particles immersed in a liquid experience pressure fluctuations, arising from the displacement of the molecules of the medium. Acoustic forces exerted on the particle originate from acoustic pressure gradients.

The force experienced by particles in an acoustic standing wave is the result of two forces, namely the primary radiation force (PRF), originating from the standing wave, and the Bjerknes force (or secondary radiation force) due to the scattering of the incident sound waves by the particles. In most applications, the main force used is the acoustic PRF, since it is generally orders of magnitude stronger than the secondary forces, rapidly decreasing with interparticle distance. The axial component of the PRF, denoted by F_r (equ. 5), acts in the direction of the sound wave propagation and drives the particle toward the pressure nodes or antinodes, depending on the acoustic contrast factor ϕ (equ. 6).

$$F_r = -\left(\frac{\pi p_0^2 V_p \beta_m}{2\lambda}\right)\phi(\beta,\rho)\sin(2kx) \quad (5)$$

where $\phi(\beta,\rho)$ denotes for the acoustic contrast factor defined by :

$$\phi(\beta,\rho) = \frac{5\rho_p - 2\rho_m}{2\rho_p + 2\rho_m} - \frac{\beta_p}{\beta_m} \quad (6)$$

In the above equations, the parameters ρ_p and ρ_m respectively refer to the particle and medium densities, while β_p andβ_m represent their corresponding compressibilities. The axial PRF (equ. 5) is proportional to the acoustic pressure amplitude p_0 and to the particle volume V_p. λ represents the ultrasonic wavelength, k is the wave number defined by $2\pi/\lambda$ and x is the distance from a pressure node. The compressibility β is defined as: $\beta=1/(\rho c^2)$, where c denotes the sound velocity in the corresponding material.

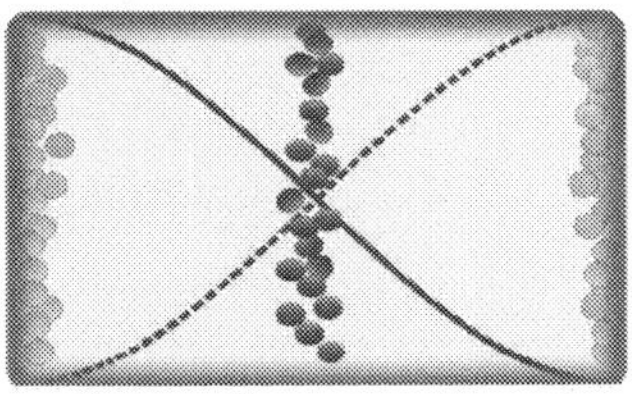

Fig. 3. Generation of an ultrasonic standing wave in a channel which length equals $\lambda/2$. Particles having a positive acoustic contrast factor ($\phi>0$) are directed to the chamber midplane toward the pressure node, whereas particles having $\phi<0$ collect at the chamber walls (pressure anti-nodes).

The technique of acoustic manipulation has been first used in macro-scaled systems, with chamber sizes comprised between a few mm and a few cm. It had already been applied to separate, filter or agglomerate bio particles from suspensions (Coakley 1997), before gaining increased attention over the last decade, with the recent development of chip integrated strategies (Laurell *et al.* 2007).

2.5 Shared principles

The four types of forces presented above obviously present common characteristics. To start with, they all rely on the existence of a field gradient. As can be deduced from the forces expression, when the field gradient is null (i.e. in uniform fields), the force cancels. In any case, when a particle is placed in a non-uniform field, it experiences a force F that drives it towards the regions where its potential energy U is minimized, according to the following relation: $\langle F \rangle = -\nabla \langle U \rangle$.

Moreover, particle manipulation can be performed as long as the contrast factor is not null, which indicates that the exploited properties of the particle must differ from the surrounding medium. In the case of DEP, the relevant properties are their frequency-dependant dielectric characteristics. When magnetophoresis is employed, the force factor reflects the cell/medium magnetic susceptibility contrast. Acoustophoretic motion is governed by mechanical characteristics of cells and their immersion medium, namely their respective densities and compressibilities. As regards optical cell handling, trapping or pushing effects may be observed, depending on the contrast between cell refractive index, dispersive properties and that of its surroundings. Concerning DEP and optical forces, it may also be pointed out that the DEP contrast factor f_{CM} is frequency-dependent and that the refractive indices and dispersions are wavelength-dependent.

3. Contactless micro particle manipulation: forces and concepts

3.1 A determinant parameter: the contrast factor

The force factor impacts not only the sign of the applied force, but also its magnitude. Accordingly, gaining knowledge about this factor and, when possible, being able to tune it, may be of great interest to control cell motion. To modulate the contrast factor, two strategies can be identified. The first one consists in influencing cell properties, by attaching functionalized beads to their surface, for instance. The second one consists in using the native properties of cells and adapting their immersion buffer composition. Of course, a combination of both these techniques can also be considered.

a. Cell properties

The dielectric properties of mammalian cells are usually described by the single-shell model, in which the cell interior is represented by an inner sphere of radius R surrounded by a thin envelope of thickness d, corresponding to the cell membrane.

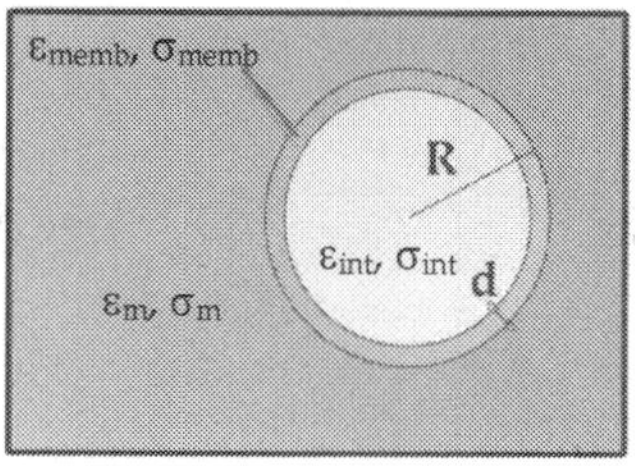

Fig. 4. Single-shell model of a spherical cell. Membrane capacitance, which is defined as ε_{memb}/d, ranges from 1.2 to 4 μF/cm² for most mammalian cells, whereas σ_{memb} is usually negligible (Gascoyne *et al.* 2004). Membrane thickness is generally comprised between 2 and 8 nm. As regards the cell interior, $0.1<\sigma_{int}<1.3$ S.m^{-1} and $50\varepsilon_0<\varepsilon_{int}<150\varepsilon_0$, where $\varepsilon_0 = 8.85 \times 10^{12}$ (Gascoyne *et al.* 1995).

Indeed, the complex permittivity of the cell (which appears in the DEP force factor expression, eqn. 2), reflects several aspects of its structure and composition, as demonstrated by Irimajiri (Irimajiri *et al.* 1979):

$$\varepsilon_p^* = \varepsilon_{memb}^* \left[\frac{\left(\frac{R}{R-d}\right)^3 + 2\left(\frac{\varepsilon_{int}^* - \varepsilon_{memb}^*}{\varepsilon_{int}^* + 2\varepsilon_{memb}^*}\right)}{\left(\frac{R}{R-d}\right)^3 - \left(\frac{\varepsilon_{int}^* - \varepsilon_{memb}^*}{\varepsilon_{int}^* + 2\varepsilon_{memb}^*}\right)} \right] \tag{7}$$

In equation 7, the subscripts *memb* and *int* refer to cell membrane and internal compartment, respectively. As can be understood from this equation, DEP offers a wide range of particle discrimination parameters, including compartment sizes, conductivities and dielectric constants. In the frequency range 5kHz-200 MHz, cell dielectric properties are mainly related to Maxwell-Wagner polarization resulting from the build up of ions at membrane interfaces under the influence of the electric field (Gascoyne *et al.* 2004). The time required for the polarization to take place depends on the field frequency, which confers to DEP one of its greatest advantages. Indeed, as the complex permittivity is related to the field frequency, this parameter can be varied to control the direction and magnitude of the DEP force. The evolution of cell dielectrophoretic behavior with respect to frequency may be perceived as the cell fingerprint. Different cell types can therefore be compared on the basis of their DEP spectra. Moreover, alterations in cell membrane integrity or various physiological changes induced in cells following specific treatment may be detected from modified DEP responses (Huang *et al.* 1999; Ratanachoo *et al.* 2002; Sudsiri *et al.* 2007). For example, DEP was used to discriminate between healthy and cancerous cells (Gascoyne *et al.* 1994) and to detect membrane changes of erythrocytes following malaria infection (Gascoyne *et al.* 1997; Gascoyne *et al.* 2002; Gascoyne *et al.* 2004). Cells exhibiting similar dielectrophoretic phenotypes may also be separated by DEP using marker-specific sorting. Hu used this technique in combination with nDEP deflection to illustrate affinity-based enrichment of rare bacteria labelled with polymeric beads from an excess of non target bacteria that did not express this marker (Hu *et al.* 2005).

The behaviour of a biological cell in presence of a magnetic field depends on its magnetic susceptibility. The magnetic susceptibility χ is the degree of magnetization of a material in response to an applied field. Magnetic susceptibility is negative for diamagnetic material (χ<0) and positive for paramagnetic objects (χ>0). Materials in which $|\chi| < 0.01$ are often considered non-magnetic, because their response to an applied magnetic field is negligible. Most cell types are non-magnetic with magnetic susceptibilities very close to that of their usual surrounding medium. Indeed, the susceptibility of vast majority of biological cells is in a narrow range of about ± 20% from that of water, $\chi_{H2O} = -9.05 \times 10^{-6}$ in SI units (Schenck 2000). Therefore, the difference of magnetic susceptibilities between cells and medium ($\Delta\chi$) is very small and the magnetic force exerted on the cells is too weak. To our knowledge, there exists a unique type of paramagnetic cells, which are the magnetotactic bacteria, as they enclose magnetite particles. Cell attraction to a magnetic field does not occur solely in paramagnetic cells. For instance, red blood cells have been separated from whole blood by magnetic attraction based on their native susceptibility (Han *et al.* 2004; Inglis *et al.* 2006). The deoxygenated red blood cells (erythrocytes), which contain high concentrations of paramagnetic haemoglobin, are diamagnetic cells but have a magnetic susceptibility (χ_{RBC} = -6.52×10^{-6} in SI units) higher than that of the water and the positive value of $\Delta\chi$ ($\Delta\chi = 2.52 \times 10^{-6}$) allows attraction of cells to regions of strong magnetic field. Magnetic labelling of non-magnetic cells can also be performed with commercially available magnetic markers such as superparamagnetic particles, magnetoliposomes or molecular magnetic labels. Detailed overview of magnetic labelling of cells with magnetic markers was documented by Safarik and Pamme. Magnetic labelling of cells allows increasing of their susceptibilities and permits their translation under non-uniform magnetic fields. This strategy has been widely used for separation and purification of cells by a selective magnetic labelling of the cell subpopulation target (Safarik *et al.* 1999; Pamme 2006).

In the case of optical force, the trapping force depends essentially on the Q-value. As previously mentioned, Q is determined experimentally and depends on both refraction index and geometry of the cell (Svoboda *et al.* 1994). These two physical properties respectively linked to the nature of the intracellular content and to the morphometry of the cell both contribute to the optical force. The strength of the gradient force increases with the refractive index of cells. However, the refractive index of most biological cells is in a narrow range of 1.3-1.4 (Balaev *et al.* 2001; Rappaz *et al.* 2005; Jin *et al.* 2006). Refractive indices of different cell types are reported in table 1. On the contrary, there is a large difference in the size and the shape of cells according to their nature, which can be exploited to distinguish between them (Paterson 2005).

Cell type	**Refractiveindex**
Escherichia coli bacteria	1.387 (Balaev *et al.* 2001)
Haemoglobin cytoplasm	1.387(Jin *et al.* 2006)
Blood plasma	1.351 (Jin *et al.* 2006)
Mammalian cells	1.38-1.41 (Rappaz *et al.* 2005)
Fibroblasts	1.358-1.374 (Rappaz *et al.* 2005)

Table 1. Refractive indices of different cell types

Refractive index of cells can be sensitively changed by labelling them with nano or microparticles having a very different refractive index such as polystyrene and silica

particles. For instance, Saxena et al. succeeded to enhance optical manipulation of biological cells by labelling them with polystyrene microparticles (Saxena 2003). This technique can be exploited to separate a specific subpopulation of cells. The cells with microspheres attached reacted to the optical landscape more strongly than cells without any attached beads due to the higher refractive index mismatch and resulting optical forces (Dholakia *et al.* 2007).
Acoustic properties of different cell types are reported in table 2. Most cell types present a higher density and lower compressibility than their usual suspension medium (Tsutsui *et al.* 2009), which gives a positive value of the acoustic contrast factor ϕ. As a result, the axial PRF drives them towards the standing wave pressure nodes. On the contrary, lipid vesicles and gaz bubbles are generally driven towards the pressure anti-node (ϕ<0) (Evander *et al.* 2007; Laurell *et al.* 2007).

Cell type	Mass density	Compressibility
Escherichia coli bacteria	1.160 g / cm^3(Godin *et al.* 2007)	-
Human red blood cells	1.139 g / cm^3 (Godin *et al.* 2007)	3.38x10^{-10} Pa^{-1} (Toubal *et al.* 1999)
HeLa cells	1.055 g / cm^3 (Park *et al.* 2008)	-
Water	0.997 g / cm^3	4.48x10^{-10} Pa^{-1}

Table 2. Mechanical properties of different biological particles and of water.

By gaining knowledge about cell properties, one can be able to predict the cell behavior when exposed to the force field under any given operating conditions (frequency, medium properties, etc.). Optimal separation conditions can therefore be estimated, for instance. Common strategies have been developed for the determination of the magnetic and dielectric properties of single cells. They rely on the fact that the force used to actuate cells may also be employed to probe their properties. These techniques imply the measurement of the solution properties (magnetic susceptibility or permittivity and conductivity and, in some cases, viscosity η). The technique of cell and particle tracking velocimetry for cell magnetization measurement was described by Moore (Moore *et al.* 2000; Moore *et al.* 2004) and Häfeli (Häfeli *et al.* 2002). A magnet assembly produces an unidimensional and constant energy density gradient over a region. The magnetic force exerted on a spherical particle therefore becomes:

$$F_m = V\Delta\chi \frac{d}{dx}\left(\frac{B^2}{2\mu_0}\right) \tag{8}$$

The opposing drag force exerted on the migrating particle is $F_d = 6\pi r\eta v$. Then, the measured cell speed v may be related to $\Delta\chi$ by the equation:

$$v = \frac{2r^2\Delta\chi}{9\eta}\frac{d}{dx}\left(\frac{B^2}{2\mu_0}\right) \tag{9}$$

Magnetophoretic mobility measurements were successfully performed on polystyrene (diamagnetic) beads placed in a solution containing paramagnetic ions. Wanichapichart has used a comparable method to determine cell dielectric properties by measuring the speed of cell translation in between a pair of cylindrical electrodes producing a well-characterized electric field (Wanichapichart *et al.* 2002). When the DEP and drag forces balance, the cell speed v is given by:

$$v = \frac{\varepsilon_m r^2 \operatorname{Re}(f_{CM})}{3\eta} \nabla E^2 \tag{10}$$

For each frequency point, v is plotted against ∇E^2 to obtain $\operatorname{Re}(f_{CM})$. It is therefore possible to deduce the dielectric properties of cell membrane and cytoplasm, by iterative method using the single-shell model presented in the previous section. Despite their similarities, there is a major difference between the techniques employed for magnetic and dielectric characterization of cells presented above, which lies in the fact that the first approach is static, while the second one implies frequency variation.

The technique of electrorotation (ROT) (De Gasperis *et al.* 1998) has also been intensively used to study the dielectric properties of various cells (Gascoyne *et al.* 1995; Huang *et al.* 1995). When a polarisable particle is placed in a rotating AC electric field, a dipole is induced. If the field frequency is sufficiently large, the dipole lags behind the applied field, which gives rise to a torque causing cell rotation. If this phase lag is more than 180°, cell rotates against the field direction. Otherwise the direction of rotation is with the field. ROT is therefore an analogue of twDEP, with electrodes arranged in a circle, rather than in line. At the equilibrium between induced torque and viscous drag, the rotation rate of the particle is:

$$R(\omega) = -\frac{\varepsilon_m \operatorname{Im}(f_{CM}) E^2}{2\eta} \tag{11}$$

Curve fitting procedures may be used to obtain the dielectric parameters of the cell, by minimizing the deviation between the experimental ROT spectrum (plot of the rotation rate with respect to the field frequency) and the theoretical spectrum predicted by the single-shell model. Electrorotation data are useful criterions to assess the feasibility of dielectrophoretic cell sorting (Yang *et al.* 1999).

Regarding optical force, as previously mentioned, Q parameter is the main determinant of trapping force. Q parameter can be experimentally determined using a calibration approach (Saxena 2003). This measure consists in placing the trapped particle in a laminar flow and increasing the hydrodynamic force until the particle escapes from the optical trap at some critical flow velocity. At this critical point, the trapping force (equ. 4) is equal to the drag force $F_d = 6\pi r \eta v$. It is therefore possible to calculate Q from measurement of this critical velocity.

b. Medium composition

The suspension medium composition is of great importance when using any of the contactless manipulation methods described above. Besides the need for operating under physiological conditions, the influence of medium properties on the force factor is also a concern.

Regarding DEP, while the expression of cell permittivity is rather intricate, the external electrolyte permittivity ε_m^* is wholly characterized by the bulk dielectric constant and conductivity. Apart from the electric field frequency, one of the variables that can be easily

adjusted to influence cell dielectric behavior is the medium conductivity. Changing this parameter enables to shift the DEP crossover frequency, which corresponds to the transition frequency between nDEP and pDEP regimes. Prior to DEP manipulation, cells are often resuspended in low conductivity buffers, in order to prevent Joule heating and undesirable electrothermal effects, and also because only nDEP can be observed in high-conductive media. pDEP-based assays require low-conductivity media, with σ_m usually ranging from 10 to 200 mS m^{-1} (Jaeger *et al.* 2008). In such cases, the medium osmolarity must be adapted by replacing the salts usually found in cell culture media by osmotically equivalent amounts of sugars. Buffers as conductive as culture media (0.2 to 2 S/m) has yet been employed for trapping (Park *et al.* 2009) or handling (Seger *et al.* 2004) of biological species using nDEP.
In magnetophoresis, the composition of the surrounding medium is also very important. Indeed, the amplitude and the sign of the magnetic force exerted on the cell depend on the difference of magnetic susceptibilities between cells and medium ($\Delta\chi$). As we described previously (section 3.2.a) the magnetic susceptibilities of the usual surrounding medium are very close to that of the most biological cell and $\Delta\chi$ is very small. However, it is possible to increase $\Delta\chi$ by increasing magnetic susceptibility of the medium. Indeed, the addition of paramagnetic molecules (such as Mn2+ or Gd3+ ions) to the medium increases its susceptibility (Kimura *et al.* 2004; Winkleman *et al.* 2004; Kimura *et al.* 2005). As a result, the obtained $\Delta\chi$ is negative with a large value and the non-magnetic cells experience a negative force that repels them form the magnetic field to the region of minimum field. This technique eliminates the need for cell labelling with magnetic markers for magnetic cell manipulation.

In the case of optical force, since biological cells are usually suspended in aqueous media that have almost the same refractive index, the dependence of optical trapping force on refractive index of the surrounding medium can rarely be exploited to achieve higher trapping forces (Sato *et al.* 1991).

As previously mentioned, in an aqueous medium, most solid particles have a positive acoustic contrast factor ϕ. Yet, Gupta et al. demonstrated that two particles with different compressibility or density could be separated by adjusting the medium properties in such a way that the sign of ϕ became different for the two particles (Gupta *et al.* 1995). A similar approach was used by Petersson to enable the fractionation of red cells, platelets, and leukocytes using a differential separation method based on the PRF force magnitude (see section 4.2). Cesium chloride was added into the suspending medium to modify its density and therefore reinforce the contrast between the cell ϕ factors (Petersson *et al.* 2007).

3.2 Field generation

High electric field gradients required for efficient cDEP cell handling can be obtained by using metal microelectrodes of appropriate design, fabricated via standard photolithography processing. Interelectrode gap reduction enables strong electric field generation without the need for applying high voltages. Various electrode designs are described in the literature, including large arrays of interdigitated rectangular electrodes (Inoue *et al.* 1988; Price *et al.* 1988; Burt *et al.* 1990; Pethig *et al.* 1992) and quadrupole electrode microstructures. Both bipolar and quadrupolar electrode configurations were investigated. On the one hand, the choice of bipolar structures simplifies the fabrication of large electrode arrays. On the other hand, quadrupole electrode structures provide increased focusing of cells under nDEP (Huang *et al.* 1991; Frénéa *et al.* 2003). 3-D field cages enabling accurate single cell trapping were also obtained using octupole arrangement of electrodes (Müller *et al.* 1999).

An alternative to electrode-based DEP is the technique of insulator-based DEP (iDEP), first employed by Masuda in the design of a cell fusion device (Masuda *et al.* 1989). It consists in using insulating features to create constrictions in the electric field produced by remote electrodes. It offers the advantage to solve problems inherent in the use of microelectrode, such as electrode deterioration due to electrolysis in the lower frequency range. The accessible frequency range can therefore be widened. This technique also owes its success to the advantages provided by the use of insulating materials, such as plastics, allowing low-cost and rapid fabrication technology (Lapizco-Encinas *et al.* 2004). A drawback is that a high-voltage power supply is needed to power the distant electrodes.

High magnetic field gradients can be obtained by designing micro magnet and micro electromagnet patterns on silicon or glass substrates. Generally, micro magnets are fabricated with ferromagnetic materials such as samarium cobalt (SmCo) or neodymium iron boron (NdFeB) via standard photolithography processing (Pamme 2006). Integrated micro-electromagnets can be manufactured by depositing micro-coil of conducting material such as cooper, gold or aluminium. Lee *et al.* have built several arrays of micro-electromagnetic coils for cell manipulation. Thanks to controlling independently each micro-electromagnetic coil with integrated circuit, they succeeded to turn on and off individually each coil, allowing the displacement of cells to a targeted location (Lee *et al.* 2004). Ramadan et al. described various designs of micro-coils to obtain high magnetic field gradients (Ramadan *et al.* 2009). This kind of systems requires utilization of a cooling system to keep the temperature of the surrounding medium at a survivable level for the cells. This makes the device less suitable for experiments that last for hours than other devices that do not generate heat during operation. Another approach to avoid heating problems associated to micro-electromagnetic coils and obtain precise control and strong gradients consists on using micro-patterns with magnetically susceptible features such as nickel, permalloy or soft iron. Then, micro-patterns can be magnetized with an external permanent magnet or electromagnet (Deng *et al.* 2002; Do *et al.* 2004; Ino *et al.* 2008). Such design present similarities with iDEP structures mentioned above.

To obtain a high optical gradient field, the conventional optical tweezers use a standard Gaussian laser beam. The most commonly used sources in optical tweezing are red and near infrared (IR) lasers due to their excellent beam quality and technological maturity. These lasers are ideally suited to biological applications as a consequence of their low absorption in water and biological tissue. This highly beneficial property allows biological material to be manipulated whilst minimizing the potential for damage (Ashkin *et al.* 1987). The classical Gaussian beam can be used to trap a single particle at one time. In order to perform multiple manipulations of different cells, the traditional gaussian beams were replaced by Non-Gaussian laser beams. Among these Non-Gaussian modes, we can mention a Bessel beam which consists of a bright centre spot surrounded by series of concentric rings of decreasing intensity. Through the use of such a beam as optical tweezer, it is possible to trap and manipulate, within perpendicular two-dimensional planes, many different particles distributed over a distance of approximately 3 mm simultaneously (Paterson 2005). A Laguerre–Gaussian mode has also been used to obtain a rotating asymmetric intensity profile. It is characterized by an intensity maxima spiral around a dark centre core, that is, a zero on-axis intensity. The presence of this dark centre core of weak intensity allows the trapping of reflecting particles, absorbent particles or particles with a low dielectric constant that could be expelled or degraded by standard Gaussian laser beam (O'Neil *et al.* 2001). Other optical tweezers systems were created to enable the manipulation of several cells simultaneously. Among them, we can mention the Acousto-optic deflectors (AODs) that is a powerful tool enabling creation and control of several (up to 100) independent optical tweezers only by deflecting one incoming laser beam. The AODs appear to be excellent for two-dimensional optical landscapes (Vossen *et al.* 2004). However, this technique is not convenient for the trapping of very small particles having a too fast Brownian movement. An alternative consists in using networks of laser diodes (Applegate *et al.* 2004) or *vertical cavity surface emitting laser* (VCSEL) to trap and manipulate microparticles (Ogura *et al.* 2002) or biological cells (Flynn *et al.* 2002). However, they have a relatively low power input. The limitation is that only cells smaller than 10 μm in size can be moved using the current VCSEL-driven optical tweezers. Other techniques use interference patterns with several laser beams to create several traps. MacDonald and al were able to build networks of three-dimensional traps by using interference patterns created with two Laguerre-Gauss beams called "doughnut" (MacDonald and coworkers, 2002). These interference patterns generate four individual tweezers that can be at the same time translated in three dimensions in the space. To achieve true three-dimensional multiple optical traps, one must choose holographic optical tweezers (HOT). HOTs offer complete flexibility in manipulating multiple particles independently (Curtis *et al.* 2002). A last way used for trapping and optical manipulation of cells consists in using evanescent fields. The first experiment in this domain was realized by Kawata and Sugiura (Kawata *et al.* 1992). The manipulation of particles by evanescent fields opens interesting perspectives for the design of innovative and compact systems for the manipulation, the detection and the sorting of particles or biological objects. It is also a step towards systems of optical positioning with very strong precision. Indeed, the volumes of traps defined by propagated fields are intrinsically limited by the diffraction phenomenon in free space, which is not the case for evanescent waves.

As regards micro scale acoustic manipulation, cells are subjected to an ultrasonic standing wave (USW) field generated by one or more on-chip integrated transducers. The USW is commonly generated throughout the fluid comprised between two parallel vertical walls of a rectangular resonator chamber etched in silicon (Nilsson *et al.* 2004) or glass (Laurell *et al.* 2007; Evander *et al.* 2008). The ultrasonic transducer can be placed underneath the channel, in which case the USW field induced in the fluid is orthogonal to the direction of transmission. This will result in particles collecting in planes perpendicular to the actuator and parallel to the chamber walls. Another design option consists in placing the actuator at one of the resonator walls (Hill *et al.* 2002; Lilliehorn *et al.* 2005). In this case, the induced USW is parallel to the direction of transmission and cells collect in planes parallel to both the transducer and the chamber walls. Higher force magnitudes scan be obtained by scaling down the channel dimensions. Indeed, the axial PRF is proportional to the frequency, which increases as the channel size decreases. The typical operating frequency ranges from 100 kHz to 10 MHz, with corresponding channel dimensions comprised between a millimeter to a few tens of micrometers (Laurell *et al.* 2007). The pressure amplitude may also be increased to obtain more important forces by adjusting the actuation voltage. The maximum applicable voltage is limited by the heating of the device, which is a particular concern in cell handling applications (Evander *et al.* 2007).

4. Applications

4.1 Cell positioning

Cell immobilization methods relying on contactless manipulation tools were recently reviewed by Johann (Johann 2006). As there is a wide range of applications requiring precise cell positioning, we have chosen to illustrate the possibilities offered by the different methods by focusing on the particularly challenging operation of cell arraying. Current diagnostic techniques or pharmacological screening require parallel analysis of millions of cells. Improving the technology for gathering cells into clumps make it possible to treat and control them differently while keeping them under observation. Precise positioning of individual cells is also required in many situations.

One of the advantages of DEP and laser tweezers is their high spatial accuracy suitable for 3-D manipulation of individual cells. Recent technological advances have enabled the fabrication of micro scale magnetic structures with well-defined features, which improved the spatial accuracy of magnetic manipulation tools. Acoustic manipulation is well suited for simultaneous handling of large groups of cells and less adapted to localized 3-D positioning of single cells, due to diffraction and absorption limitations for focused high-frequency ultrasonic field (Wiklund *et al.* 2006).

Figure 5 shows that both dielectrophoretic and diamagnetic trapping can be used to perform arraying of single cells or small groups of unlabelled cells. In the first case (fig. 5a), positioning accuracy is ensured by the use of quadrupole electrode sets symmetrically driven. Under nDEP, cells were repelled toward the center of the interelectrode gaps (Frénéa *et al.* 2003). In the second case (fig. 5b.), diamagnetic yeast cells were placed in a medium enriched in paramagnetic ions. They were confined at regularly spaced magnetic traps produced by permanent micro magnets under the effect of negative magnetophoresis, without any contact with the surface. Cell levitation height was estimated to 8 μm by simulation (Frenea-Robin *et al.* 2008).

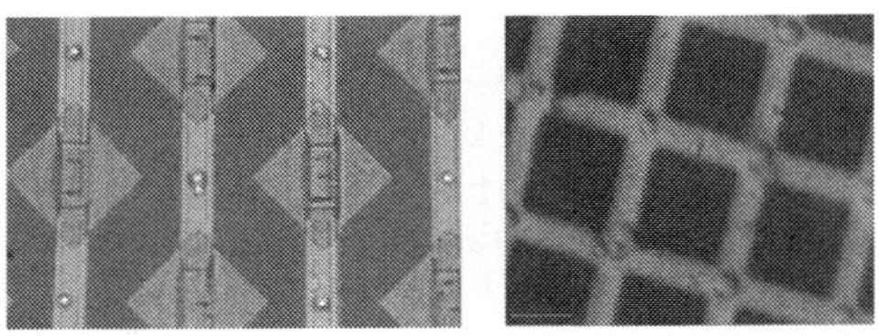

Fig. 5. a. Jurkat cells trapped at electric field minima by nDEP. b. 3-D trapping of yeast cells above an array of CoPt permanent micromagnets.

Compared with DEP, the use of permanent micro magnets offers the advantage to prevent Joule heating, but also poses the problem of later cell displacement, due to the static nature of the field. Diamagnetic levitation of micro droplets in air could also be performed with such micro magnet arrays, while nDEP required for dielectric levitation is non efficient in air. Tanase also described utilization of a 2-dimensional array of magnetized permalloy micro-ellipses for drawing magnetically labelled cells toward the tip of micro-ellipses and forming rows of cells (Tanase *et al.* 2005).

Lilliehorn et al. proposed to perform dynamic arraying of cells in a micro fluidic channel using an array of integrated ultrasonic micro transducers (Lilliehorn *et al.* 2005). This concept was validated on a one-dimensional array. The lateral extension of each trapping site was determined by the corresponding micro transducer dimensions (0.8 mm× 0.8 mm). Haake and coworkers have proposed a method for the controlled positioning of cells in one or two dimensions (i.e. in lines or points) based on the use of ultrasonic forces in a millimeter-scale device (Haake *et al.* 2004; Haake *et al.* 2005). To apply these forces, a sound field was generated into a layer of fluid comprised between a vibrating glass plate situated on top of the device and a reflecting surface at the bottom. Activating a piezo-transducer attached at one plate edge resulted in the formation of a one-dimensional standing wave in the plate. Therefore, an acoustic wave propagated between the plate and the reflecting surface. This induced in turn a 2-D standing-wave sound field in the intermediate liquid layer, resulting in cells forming bands parallel to the activated transducer. When two orthogonal transducers were activated, a 3-D sound field was induced in the fluid layer. As a result, cells were collected on a grid of oval points orientated in zigzag patterns dictated by the contours of minimum force potential. In order to improve cell confinement, Neild used another approach to generate the required field. Two orthogonally aligned strip electrodes were defined in the metallic coating of a piezoelectric actuator, which was located beneath the fluid cavity etched in a silicon wafer. These electrodes could be addressed individually to create two orthogonal ultrasonic fields. A grid of well-confined circular cell clumps could be obtained when two signals with slightly different frequencies were applied to the electrodes (Neild *et al.* 2006).

Optical trapping can also be used to assemble and organize cells in order to form a group of cells into a new structure with predefined configurations. Assembling and organizing cells require the utilization of computer-controlled SLMs (Spatial Light Modulators) built on holographic optical tweezers. This technique allows the manipulation of cells both laterally and axially over several tens of micrometres so that cells can be rearranged into 2D and 3D configurations. Therefore, Flynn and co-workers demonstrated 2D trapping of 2x2 arrays of Yeast cells and human red blood cells using a single VCSEL beam optical tweezers. They also indicated that maximum force in the VCSEL optical trap varies depending on the size and relative index of refraction of the trapped cells, as well as the scales of optical power (Flynn *et al.* 2002). Jordan *et al.* succeeded to fixe *E. coli* cells in liquid gelatine at predefined positions in a 3D structure (Jordan 2005). They anticipate that the ability to form such viable three dimensional structures will open a wide range of future applications, including the arrangement of various cell types in complex architectures, as motifs for promoting tissue differentiation and growth within the field of cell engineering. Akselrod *et al.* demonstrated the assembly of 3D heterotypic microarrays consisting of a Swiss 3T3 mouse fibroblast surrounded by a ring of Pseudomonas aeruginosa bacteria by using arrays of time-multiplexed holographic optical tweezers (Akselrod *et al.* 2006).

4.2 Cell sorting

a. Binary separation

A binary separation of a mixed cell population can be achieved if the medium properties are balanced in such a way that the contrast factors of the two cell types are of opposite signs. Indeed, the two fractions can be spatially separated, one being driven in the direction of the field gradient, and the other at the opposite. As an example, viable and non-viable cells were selectively isolated using positive and negative dielectrophoretic forces which respectively trapped them at the electrode edges or repelled them form the electrodes

(Markx *et al.* 1994). To perform such separation, the field frequency must fall between the DEP crossover frequencies of the two cell types. Physical separation of the two sub-populations is achieved by superimposing a liquid flow above the electrode array. Cells trapped at field minima (nDEP) can be eluted towards a device outlet, while those experiencing pDEP, held by a stronger force, remain attracted to the electrodes until the field is switched-off (Wang *et al.* 1993). For increased efficiency, flow separation can also be operated as a continuous process. In this case, the suspension is continuously flowing above the electrodes, and the cells are either trapped on the array by pDEP or collected at the outlet. The processing speed is limited by the ability of the electrodes to remove a passing particle from the fluid stream and retain it against the action of viscous drag (Hughes 2002). More than two particle sub-populations can be differentiated by performing several steps of frequency tuning and repeating the separation process.

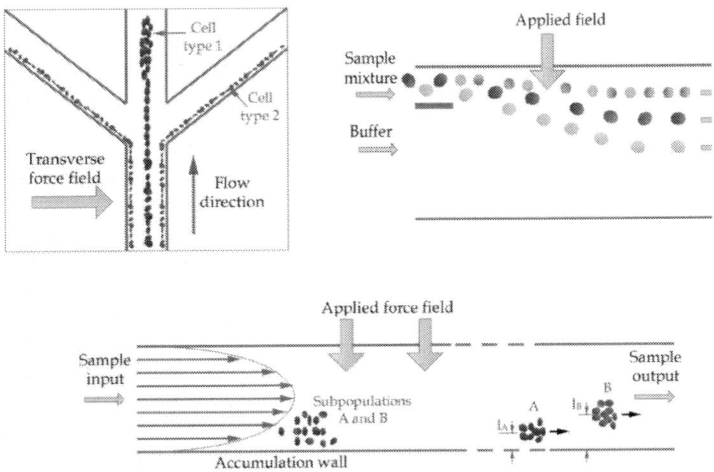

Fig. 6. a. and b. Continuous flow sorting based on the force sign (a) and/or magnitude (b), top view. c. Schematic representation of FFF (cross view). Sample B moves faster through the channel than A since $l_B > l_A$. Separation is performed in the flow direction.

Doh presented a continuous cell separation chip using three planar electrodes in a separation channel, where the pDEP cells moved away from the central streamline while the nDEP cells remained in the central streamline. The laminar nature of the flow enabled the collection of cell fractions through different outlets (Doh *et al.* 2005).
Using a comparable design (fig. 6a), Laurell and coworkers demonstrated acoustic binary separation of red blood cells ($\phi>0$) and lipid microemboli ($\phi<0$)(Nilsson *et al.* 2004; Petersson *et al.* 2005; Laurell *et al.* 2007). The RBCs accumulated into the channel midplane corresponding to the USW pressure node, while the lipid particles where driven towards the anti-nodal planes at the sidewalls.

Binary separation based on optical forces can be achieved via either the intrinsic properties of the cells, such as size, shape and refractive index with and without fluid flow. For instance, the Bessel beam has been used for flow-free optical separation of lymphocytes from erythrocytes using the difference in their shape (Paterson 2005). Therefore, the biconcave-shaped erythrocytes locked into outer rings of the Bessel beam, while spherically shaped lymphocytes rapidly moved directly to the beam centre and they were collected from the centre core.

Despite their simplicity and high efficiency, binary separation techniques are not applicable in all cases. The forces experienced by the two cell types must be of different signs and have a significant magnitude. This is not achievable if the cell properties are not sufficiently different, as it becomes difficult to adjust the medium properties in between.

b. Separation of polydisperse mixtures

When more than two cell types must be separated, it is possible to differentiate them based on the force magnitude. Such strategy has been employed in cell deflectors and Field Flow Fractionation (FFF) devices. The force magnitude depends on the particle size and on the contrast factor amplitude.

- **Cell deflectors**

The inherent laminar nature of micro scale fluid dynamics has enabled the design of new continuous-flow cell separators. A classical continuous flow sorter design is represented on figure 6.b. The particles in the mixture respond differently to the applied force field and are thus deflected from the direction of flow, which enable to collect them at different outlets.

Petersson et al. validated the concept of free flow acoustophoresis (FFA), where particle separation is achieved by acoustic standing wave force-induced lateral displacement in the laminar flow of a micro channel. A $\lambda/2$ USW generated between the side walls of the channel using a piezoceramic actuator gave rise to an acoustic force field perpendicular to the flow direction. At controlled flow rate, the particles that were most affected by the axial PRF reached the midplane of the channel while the others were dispersed between the sidewalls and the center. As the axial PRF is proportional to the particle volume, polystyrene particles sharing the same mechanical properties could be separated according to their size, which ranged from 2 to 10 μm (Petersson *et al.* 2007).

Cell separation using nDEP deflexion has also been reported recently by Hu. Cells introduced in a micro fluidic channel were deflected by the electric field into the collection stream if they were tagged with a dielectrophoretically responsive label or directed to the waste outlet otherwise (Hu *et al.* 2005).

Magnetic separation of cells can be achieved by labelling a specific cell subpopulation with magnetic particles through antigen–antibody interactions. Therefore, magnetically tagged cells can be separated from non-magnetic ones in continuous flow by applying magnetic forces perpendicularly to the flow direction in order to deflect cells into different trajectories. These systems require the creation of strong magnetic fields inside the micro fluidic channel. Inglis et al. described separation of magnetically labelled WBCs from blood cells by using nickel stripes integrated on a micro channel as magnetic deflector (Inglis *et al.* 2004). Xia et al succeeded to extract magnetically labelled E. coli from RBCs thanks to a strong magnetic field gradient generated by micro comb structures of NiFe integrated in a micro channel (Xia *et al.* 2006). Berger used ferromagnetic wires oriented at an angle of 45° to the flow of cells to develop a new magnetic sorting device. The sum of the hydrodynamic force and the magnetic field gradient created by wires constrains labelled cells to move along the magnetic wires where unlabelled cells flow into the central direction (Berger *et al.*

2001). Pamme et al. described separation of magnetic particles from non-magnetic ones in a flat separation chamber composed by a number of inlet and outlet, just by applying a magnetic field gradient perpendicularly to the direction of the flow. The magnetic deflection of cells depends on their magnetic susceptibilities and their size (Pamme 2006).
Optical deflectors have been also used for cell sorting and are based on targeting the specific subpopulation of cells with fluorescent markers (Dholakia *et al.* 2007). The mechanism for cell sorting is very similar to that of macroscopic FACS machines (Givan 2001). In micro fluidic regime, cells are chosen via an external decision through the fluorescence signal from the detection region. Optical force is used as an optical switch for cell deflection. Buican *et al.* were the first to use a deflection beam for cell sorting by deflecting out cells of interest into a reservoir of choice (Buican *et al.* 1987). Later, T and Y-types of micro channel junctions were designed and coupled with optical tweezers for trapping and delivering several target cells to a collection reservoir simultaneously (Ozkan *et al.* 2003; Enger *et al.* 2004). Optical separation can also be carried out by attaching silica microspheres to a specific subpopulation of cells via antibody–antigen binding. The cells with microspheres attached reacted to the optical landscape more strongly than cells without any attached beads due to the higher refractive index mismatch and accompanying optical forces(Dholakia *et al.* 2007). Within fluid flow, cells are sorted thanks to a size- and shape-dependent gradient force in competition with a size- and shape-dependent viscous drag force. Flowing particles through an optical potential energy landscape, such as two-dimensional (2D) or 3D interference pattern or holographically produced array, will facilitate the separation of cells according to their physical characteristics. MacDonald and coworkers demonstrated the separation of erythrocytes from lymphocytes based on shape difference by using an angled optical lattice (MacDonald *et al.* 2004).

- **Chromatographic separation**

Dielectrophoresis has also been widely applied as a force field in field-flow fractionation (FFF), a technique falling into the category of chromatographic separation methods. In FFF techniques, the field is applied at right angle to flow (fig. 6c) and serves to drive different types of particles into different stream laminae of the carrier fluid. As a result, different particles will travel at different velocities according to their distance from the bottom surface. Those particles, which are introduced to the channel inlet at the same point and time, will emerge from the outlet at different times according to their reaction to the applied field. In DEP-FFF, an electrode array is patterned onto the bottom surface and repels cells by nDEP towards a stable position. The resulting force on the particle results from both the nDEP effects and the buoyancy force. The levitation heights reached by different cell types (and therefore their velocity) will depend on both their dielectric properties (*via* $\mathrm{Re}(f_{CM})$) and densities. DEP-FFF has enabled the fractionation of various cell types and was even utilized to detect the effect of the differential expression of a single gene in genetically identical cells (Gascoyne *et al.* 2004).
twDEP can also be used to establish the chromatograph of a cell mixture, by introducing the sample at one end of the electrode array and then forcing cells to move along the tracks. The cell velocity is related to the dielectric properties of the particles, *via* $\mathrm{Im}\,(f_{CM})$. Hence some cell subpopulations will move more rapidly than others and will therefore be collected before at the opposite end. This technique is particularly interesting when cells present only slight differences. In such cases, long electrode arrays can be used to enable a clear separation of cell groups (Green *et al.* 1997).

Chromatographic separation requires precise sample injection prior to processing, which constitutes one of its main drawbacks compared to continuous flow devices (Pamme 2007). In tw-DEP devices, to ensure that particles start from one end of the electrode array simultaneously, sample precollection can be performed using cDEP electrodes that trap the particles by pDEP at the beginning of the tracks (Cui *et al.* 2001).

In the case of magnetic FFF, a magnetic field gradient is used as an external force passing at right angles to the channel, perpendicularly to the flow. The interaction of hydrodynamic and magnetic forces is used to separate the particles as they are carried along a separation channel according to their magnetic susceptibility and size. The controllability of both the field or gradient in field strength and the carrier flow rate contribute to the versatility of FFF. Other works described utilization of a ferromagnetic wire at the axis of channel placed perpendicular to a magnetic field that magnetized the wire allowing thus separation of particles (Carpinoa *et al.* 2005). Mitsuhashi *et al.* embedded ferromagnetic wires in both channel walls in the direction of fluid flow. The wires in each wall lay opposite spaces between wires in the other. An external field of 3T was applied. They were able to show slight retention of some transition metal salts, although band spreading was extremely high (Mitsuhashi *et al.* 2002). Recently, Carpino *et al.* reported utilization of a quadrupole magnet to obtain a field strength and field gradient relatively constant throughout an helical channel. They succeeded to retain many of the magnetic nanoparticles of interest and refer to the technique as Quadrupole magnetic field-flow fractionation (MgFFF) (Carpinoa *et al.* 2005).

Cell sorting can also be achieved using a balance between the viscous drag experienced by cells in fluid flow and the scattering force of a counter-propagating laser beam, termed 'optical chromatography' by Imasaka (Imasaka et al. 1995). When cells flow along the channel, the scattering force pushes them into the focal region of the laser beam. The net force between the scattering and drag forces results in different equilibrium positions for different cells. This method can be used to separate a range of cells including blood cells (Kaneta *et al.* 1997), bacterial spores and cells (Hart *et al.* 2007).

5. Comparison criteria

All the contactless forces described above depend on a force factor that changes according to the volume of manipulated cells. The capability of DEP to handle dielectric particles in a large range of size permits to obtain the larger force range in comparison with other contactless forces. Optical force exhibits the smaller force range due to tight focusing of the laser beam limiting the area over which the optical traps can be created and restricting the cell sizes that can be trapped. Numerous studies tend to show that acoustic manipulation can be considered to be non-lethal to cells (Hultström *et al.* 2007; Petersson *et al.* 2007). However, the majority of actuators employed for generating contactless forces (conductors, laser beams, electromagnets and piezoelectric transducers) may cause thermal damage, which restricts possibilities for long time cell exposition. Otherwise, dielectrophoresis may cause membrane breakdown, as a strong AC field is applied and a transmembrane potential induced (Lurquin 1997).The technique of iDEP presented in section 3.2 offers the possibility to avoid electrode fouling, which may also cause harm to cells.

No heat damages are induced by permanent micro magnets, which do not interfere with the ion concentration in aqueous solutions in contrary to dielectrophoresis. Moreover, highly selective separation of cells can be obtained using magnetic forces thanks to the large differences between magnetic susceptibilities of the magnetic labelled cells and non-magnetic ones. However, magnetophoresis has been limited until recently to cells that either have an intrinsic magnetic response or are tagged with magnetic beads but tagging protocols may not exist for all the cells of interest. DEP, acoustic and optic manipulations are generally based on tag-free protocols that do not require attaching cells to magnetic beads or other particles which are more attractive to biologists. Regarding elaboration of contactless manipulation systems, the integration of microelectrodes on microsystems remains easier than that of micro magnets. Optical tweezers are incorporated easily into a conventional microscope arrangement, the same objective lens being used for both focusing the laser beam and viewing the trapped object. Optical systems are suitable for single cell manipulation with high 3D precision but are not convenient for parallel manipulation owing to limited area over which the optical traps can be created. In the case of acoustic manipulation, the periodicity of the standing-wave can be exploited to handle many particles simultaneously. In many applications based on this technique, a single actuator is required to handle many cells simultaneously and generate a USW field throughout the whole channel. This may constitute an advantage over DEP, which uses a force field with short-range effects (Neild *et al.* 2007). But as a counterpart, until now, DEP has proven to offer more precision and versatility. Frequency-dependency of cell dielectric properties lends to DEP a dimension of discrimination that also constitutes an advantage of this widely used technique.

Method	DEP	Magnetic	Optic	Acoustic
Factor	f_{CM}	$\Delta\chi$	Q	$\phi(\beta,\rho)$
Force range (pN)	20-100000	10-10000	0.1-100	0.1-1000
Separation criteria	Complex permittivity	Magnetic susceptibility	Refractive index	Density and compressibility
Advantages	Frequency-dependency	Highly selective separation	Single cell 3D manipulation with high precision	Long-range effects
Disadvantages	Joule heating and modification of transmembrane potential	Magnetic labelling	Photodamage and thermal damage Not possible in optically opaque systems	Temperature increase

Table 3. Comparison of DEP, magnetic, optic and acoustic manipulation methods.

As each of the techniques presented above presents its own advantages and drawbacks, a potential for future research seem to be the development of new hybrid systems. For instance, Wiklund et al. combined DEP, acoustic and viscous drag forces to perform both high-precision handling of individual cells and high-throughput handling of groups of cells (Wiklund *et al.* 2006). As the use of ultrasound seem to be more appropriate than electric field for long-term exposition, DEP can be used for short-term accurate positioning, prior to long-term retention by acoustic forces.

By coupling optical force and dielectrophoresis, Chiou et al. presented for the first time a novel *optoelectronic tweezers (OET)* capable of trapping and transporting multiple biological cells (Chiou *et al.* 2004). This technique is based on focusing optical beam on a photoconductive surface to create a highly non-uniform electric field allowing optical addressing of dielectrophoresis forces with a spatial resolution of ~ 1μm. The optical intensity required is three orders of magnitudes lower than that of conventional optical tweezers. The OET does not require tight optical focusing and the trapping area can be tailored to match the cell size. It also offers the advantage of producing larger forces (several hundred picoNewtons) for cell manipulation (Choi *et al.* 2002; Hwang *et al.* 2008).

6. Conclusion

Various strategies of cell manipulation based on contactless forces were presented. Many contactless cell manipulations with batch and fluidic systems were described. Current research is concerned with the development of high performance micro fluidic systems in order to improve efficiency and throughput of cell manipulation with the aim to develop new solutions for clinical applications. Thanks to their similarities and differences, the contactless forces described in this chapter can be considered as elements of a toolbox that can be used according to the targeted cell species. The advantages and drawbacks of each contactless force can be evaluated as function of properties of manipulated cells as wells as working conditions. The combination of two or more manipulation tools will constitute a challenge for future research.

7. References

Akselrod, G. M., W. Timp, et al. (2006). "Laser-guided assembly of heterotypic three-dimensional living cell microarrays " Biophys J 91: 3465-3473.

Applegate, R., J. Squier, et al. (2004). "Optical trapping, manipulation, and sorting of cells ans colloids in microfluidic systems with diode laser bars." Optics express 12(19): 4390-4398.

Ashkin, A., J. M. Dziedzic, et al. (1987). "Optical trapping and manipulation of single cells using infrared beams." Nature (London) 330: 769-771.

Balaev, A. E., K. N. Dvoretski, et al. (2001). "Refractive index of escherichia coli cells " Saratov Fall Meeting: Optical Technologies in Biophysics and Medicine III 4707: 253-260.

Berger, M., J. Castelino, et al. (2001). "Design of a microfabricated magnetic cell separator." Electrophoresis 22: 3883-3892.

Buican, T. N., M. J. Smyth, et al. (1987). "Automated single-cell manipulation and sorting by light trapping." Appl. Opt. 26: 5311-5316.

Burt, J. P. H., R. Pethig, et al. (1990). "Dielectrophoretic characterisation of Friend murine erythroleukaemic cells as a measure of induced differentiation." Biochimica et Biophysica Acta, 1034: 93-101.

Carpinoa, F., L. R. Moorea, et al. (2005). "Analysis of magnetic nanoparticles using quadrupole magnetic field-flow fractionation." Journal of Magnetism and Magnetic Materials 293: 546-552.

Chiou, P. Y., W. Wong, et al. (2004). Cell adressing and trapping using novel optoelectronic tweezers. 17th IEEE International Conference on MEMS.

Choi, J.-W., J. Do, et al. (2002). Hybrid type on-chip magnetic particle separators for accurate positioning magnetic beads. Micro Total Analysis Systems, Nara, Japan.

Coakley, W. T. (1997). "Ultrasonic separations in analytical biotechnology." Trends in Biotechnology 15: 506-511.

Cui, L., D. Holmes, et al. (2001). "The dielectrophoretic levitation and separation of latex beads in microchips." Electrophoresis 22: 3893-3901.

Curtis, J. E., B. A. Koss, et al. (2002). "Dynamic holographic optical tweezers." Opt. Commun. 207: 169-175.

De Gasperis, G., X.-B. Wang, et al. (1998). "Automated electrorotation: dielectric characterization of living cells by real-time motion estimation." Meas.Sci.Technol. 9: 518-529.

Deng, T., M. Prentiss, et al. (2002). "Fabrication of magnetic microfiltration systems using soft lithography." Applied physics letters 80(3): 461-463.

Dholakia, K., W. M. Lee, et al. (2007). "Optical separation of cells on potential energy landscapes: enhancement with dielectric tagging." IEEE Journal of Selected Topics in Quantum Electronics 13(6): 1646-1654.

Do, J., J. Choi, et al. (2004). "Low-cost magnetic interdigitated array on a plastic wafer." Lab on a Chip 40: 3009-3011.

Doh, I. and Y.-H. Cho (2005). "A continuous cell separation chip using hydrodynamic dielectrophoresis (DEP) process." Sensors and Actuators A 121: 59-65.

Enger, J., M. Goksor, et al. (2004). "Optical tweezers applied to a microfluidic system." Lab Chip 4: 196-200.

Evander, M., L. Johansson, et al. (2007). "Noninvasive acoustic cell trapping in a microfluidic perfusion system for online bioassays." Anal Chem 79: 2984-2991.

Evander, M., A. Lenshof, et al. (2008). "Acoustophoresis in wet-etched glass chips." Anal Chem 80: 5178-5185.

Flynn, R. A., A. L. Birkbeck, et al. (2002). "Parallel transport of biological cells using individually addressable VCSEL arrays as optical tweezers. ." *Sensors and Actuators B* 87: 239-243.

Frénéa, M., S. P. Faure, et al. (2003). "Positioning living cells on a high-density electrode array by negative dielectrophoresis." Materials Science and Engineering: C 23: 597-603.

Frenea-Robin, M., H. Chetouani, et al. (2008). Contactless diamagnetic trapping of living cells onto a micromagnet array. IEEE Eng Med Biol Soc., Vancouver.

Gascoyne, P., C. Mahidol, et al. (2002). "Microsample preparation by dielectrophoresis: isolation of malaria." Lab Chip 2: 70-75.

Gascoyne, P., R. Pethig, et al. (1997). "Dielectrophoretic detection of changes in erythrocyte membranes following malarial infection." Biochem Biophys Acta 323: 240-252.

Gascoyne, P., J. Satayavivad, et al. (2004). "Microfluidic approaches to malaria detection." Acta Tropica 89: 357-369.

Gascoyne, P. R. C., F. F. Becker, et al. (1995). "Numerical analysis of the influence of experimental conditions on the accuracy of dielectric parameters derived from electrorotation measurements." Bioelectrochemistry and bioenergetics 36: 115-125.

Gascoyne, P. R. C., J. Noshari, et al. (1994). "Use of dielectrophoretic collection spectra for characterizing differences between normal and cancerous cells." IEEE transactions on industry applications 30: 829-834.

Gascoyne, P. R. C. and J. V. Vykoukal (2004). "Dielectroporesis-based sample handling in general-purpose programmable diagnostic instruments." Proceedings of the IEEE 92(1): 22-40.

Givan, A. L. (2001). Flow cytometry: first principles, Wiley-Liss, USA.

Godin, M., A. K. Bryan, et al. (2007). "Measuring the mass, density and size of particles and cells using a suspended microchannel resonator." Applied physics letters 91.

Green, N. G., M. P. Hughes, et al. (1997). "Large area multilayered electrode arrays for dielectrophoretic fractionation." Microelectronic Engineering 35: 421-424.

Gupta, S. and D. L. Feke (1995). "Fractionation of mixed particulate solids according to compressibility using ultrasonic standing wave fields." Chemical Engineering Science 50(20): 3275-3284.

Haake, A. and J. Dual (2004). "Positioning of small particles by an ultrasound field excited by surface waves." Ultrasonics 42: 75-80.

Haake, A., A. Neild, et al. (2005). "Positioning, displacement and localization of cells using ultrasonic forces." Biotechnology and Bioengineering 92(1): 8-14.

Häfeli, U. O., R. Ciocan, et al. (2002). "Characterization of magnetic particles and microspheres and their magnetophoretic mobility using a digital microscopy method." European Cells and Materials 3: 24-27.

Han, K. H. and B. Frazier (2004). "Continuous magnetophoretic separation of blood cells in microdevice format." Journal of Applied Physics 96(10): 5797-5802.

Hart, S. J., A. Terray, et al. (2007). "Sample concentration using optical chromatography." Opt. Express 15: 2724-2731.

Hill, M., Y. Shen, et al. (2002). "Modelling of layered resonators for ultrasonic separation." Ultrasonics 40: 385-392.

Hu, X., P. H. Bessette, et al. (2005). "Marker-specific sorting of rare cells using dielectrophoresis." PNAS 102(44): 15757-15761.

Huang, Y. and R. Pethig (1991). "Electrode design for negative dielectrophoresis." Meas.Sci.Technol.2: 1142-1146.

Huang, Y., X.-B. Wang, et al. (1999). "Membrane dielectric responses of human T-lymphocytes following mitogenic stimulation." Biochem Biophys Acta 1417: 51-62.

Huang, Y., X.-B. Wang, et al. (1995). "Electrorotational studies of the cytoplasmic dielectric properties of Friend murine erthroleukaemia cells." Phys. Med. Biol. 40: 1789-1806.

Hughes, M. P. (2002). "Strategies for dielectrophoretic separation in laboratory-on-a-chip systems." Electrophoresis 23: 2569-2582.

Hultström, J., O. Manneberg, et al. (2007). "Proliferation and viability of adherent cells manipulated by standing-wave ultrsaound in a microfluidic chip." Ultrasound in Medicine & Biology 33(1): 145-151.

Hwang, H., Y.-J. Choi, et al. (2008). "Interactive manipulation of blood cells using a lens-integrated liquid crystal display based optoelectronic tweezers system." Electrophoresis 29(6): 1203-1212.

Imasaka, T., Y. Kawabata, et al. (1995). "Optical chromatography." Anal Chem 67: 1763-1765.

Inglis, D. W., R. Riehn, et al. (2004). "Continuous microfluidic immunomagnetic cell separation." Appl. Phys. Lett. 85: 5093-5095.

Inglis, D. W., R. Riehn, et al. (2006). "Microfluidic high gradient magnetic cell separation." Journal of Applied Physics 99(8): 08K101.1-08K101.3.

Ino, K., M. Okochi, et al. (2008). "Cell culture arrays using magnetic force-based cell patterning for dynamic single cell analysis." Lab on a Chip 8: 134-142.

Inoue, T., R. Pethig, et al. (1988). "Dielectrophoretic behaviour of *micrococcuslysodeikticus* and its protoplast." Journal of electrostatics 21: 215-223.

Irimajiri, A., T. Hanai, et al. (1979). "A dielectric theory of multi-stratified shell model with its application to a lymphoma cell." J Theor Biol 78(2): 251-269.

Jaeger, M. S., K. Uhlig, et al. (2008). "Contact-free single-cell cultivation by negative dielectrophoresis." J.Phys.D, Apply.Phy 41.

Jin, Y. L., J. Y. Chen, et al. (2006). "Refractive index measurement for biomaterial samples by total internal reflection." Phys. Med. Biol. 51: 371-379.

Johann, R. M. (2006). "Cell trapping in microfluidic chips." Anal. Bioanal. Chem 385: 408-412.

Jones, T. B. (2003). "Basic theory of dielectrophoresis and electrorotation." IEEE Eng. Med. Biol. Magazine 33-42.

Jordan, P. (2005). "Creating permanent 3D arrangements if isolated cells using holographic optical tweezers " Lab Chip 5: 1224-1228.

Kaneta, T., Y. Ishidzu, et al. (1997). "Theory of optical chromatography." Anal Chem 69: 2701-2710.

Kawata, S. and T. Sugiura (1992). "Movement of micrometer-sized particles in the evanescent field of a laser beal." Optics Letters 17(11): 772-774.

Kimura, T., Y. Sato, et al. (2005). "Micropatterning of Cells Using Modulated Magnetic Fields." Langmuir 21: 830-830.

Kimura, T., M. Yamato, et al. (2004). "Particle Trapping and Undulation of a Liquid Surface Using a Microscopically Modulated Magnetic Field." 20: 572-574.

Lapizco-Encinas, B., B. A. Simmons, et al. (2004). "Insulator-based dielectrophoresis for the selective concentration and separation of live bacteria in water." Electrophoresis 25: 1695-1704.

Laurell, T., F. Petersson, et al. (2007). "Chip integrated strategies for acoustic separation and manipulation of cells and particles." Chem. Soc. Rev. 36: 492-506.

Lee, H., A. M. Purdon, et al. (2004). "Micromanipulation of biological systems with microelectromagnets." IEEE Transactions on magnetics 40(4): 2991-2993.

Lilliehorn, T., M. Nilsson, et al. (2005). "Dynamic arraying of microbeads for bioassays in microfluidic channels." Sensors and Actuators B 106: 851-858.

Lurquin, P. F. (1997). "Gene transfer by electroporation." Molecular Biotechnology 7: 5-35.

MacDonald, M. P., S. Neale, et al. (2004). "Cell cytometry with a light touch: sorting microsocpic matter with an optical lattice." Journal of Biological Regulators and Homeostatic Agents: 200-205.

MacDonald, M. P., L. Paterson, et al. (2002). "Creation and manipulation of three-dimensional optically trapped structures." Science 296(5570): 1101-1103.

Markx, G. H., M. S. Talary, et al. (1994). "Separation of viable and non-viable yeast using dielectrophoresis." J. Biotechnol. 32(1): 29-37.

Masuda, S., M. Washizu, et al. (1989). "Novel method of cell fusion in field constriction area in fluid integrated circuit." IEEE Trans. Industry Applicat. 25(4): 732-737.

Mitsuhashi, K., R. Yoshizaki, et al. (2002). "Retention of ions in a magnetic chromatograph using high-intensity and high gradient magnetic fields." Sep. Sci. Technol. 37: 3635-3645.

Moore, L. R., S. Milliron, et al. (2004). "Control of magnetophoretic mobility by susceptibility-modified solutions as evaluated by cell tracking velocimetry and continuous magnetic sorting." Anal. Chem. 76: 3899-3907.

Moore, L. R., M. Zborowski, et al. (2000). "The use of magnetite-doped polymeric microspheres in calibrating cell tracking velocimetry." J. Biochem. Biophys. Methods 44: 115-130.

Müller, T., G. Gradl, et al. (1999). "A 3-D microelectrode system for handling and caging single cells and particles." Biosensors and bioelectronics 14: 247-256.

Neild, A., S. Oberti, et al. (2007). "Design, modeling and characterization of microfluidic devices for ultrasonic manipulation." Sensors and Actuators B 121: 452-461.

Neild, A., S. Oberti, et al. (2006). "Simultaneous positioning of cells into two-dimensional arrays using ultrasound." Biotechnology and Bioengineering 97(5): 1335-1339.

Nieminen, T., V. Loke, et al. (2007). "Optical tweezers computational toolbox." J.Opt.A: Pure Appl. Opt. 9: S196-S203.

Nilsson, A., F. Petersson, et al. (2004). "Acoustic control of suspended particles in micro fluidic chips." Lab Chip 4: 131-135.

O'Neil, A. T. and M. J. Padgett (2001). "Axial and lateral trapping efficiency of laguerre-gaussian modes in inverted optical twezeers." *Optics Communications* 193: 45-50.

Ogura, Y., S. Nobuhiro, et al. (2002). "Optical levitation and translation of a microscopic particle by use of multiple beams generated by vertical-cavity-surface-emitting laser arrays sources." *Applied Optics* 41: 5645-5653.

Ozkan, M., M. Wang, et al. (2003). "Optical manipulation of objects and biological cells in microfluidic devices." Biomed. Microdevices 5: 61-67.

Pamme, N. (2006). "Magnetism and microfluidics." Lab on a Chip 6: 24-38.

Pamme, N. (2007). "Continuous flow separations in microfluidic devices." Lab on a Chip 7: 1644-1659.

Park, K., J. Jang, et al. (2008). "'Living cantilever arrays' for characterization of mass of single live cells in fluids." Lab Chip 8: 1034-1041.

Park, S., M. Koklu, et al. (2009). "Particle trapping in high-conductivity media with electrothermally enhanced negative dielectrophoresis." Anal Chem 81(6): 2303-2310.

Paterson, L. (2005). "Light-induced cell separation in a tailored optical landscape " Appl. Phys. Lett. 87.

Petersson, F., L. Aberg, et al. (2007). "Free flow acoustophoresis : microfluidic-based mode of particle and cell separation." Anal. Chem. 79: 5117-5123.

Petersson, F., A. Nilsson, et al. (2005). "Continuous separation of lipid particles from erythrocytes by means of laminar flow and acoustic standing wave forces." Lab on a Chip 5: 20-22.

Pethig, R., Y. Huang, et al. (1992). "Positive and negative dieletrophoretic collection of colloidal particles using interdigitated castellated microelectrodes." J.Phys.D, Apply.Phy 24: 881-888.

Pohl, H. A. (1958). "Some effects of non uniform fields on dielectrics." J. Apply. Phys. 29: 1182-1188.

Price, J. A. R., J. P. H. Burt, et al. (1988). "Applications of a new optical technique for measuring the dielectrophoretic behaviour of micro-organisms." Biochimica et Biophysica Acta, 964: 221-230.

Ramadan, Q., D. P. Poenar, et al. (2009). "Customized trapping of magnetic particles." Microfluid Nanofluid 6: 53-62.

Rappaz, B., P. Marquet, et al. (2005). "Measurement of the integral refractive index and dynamic cell morphometry of living cells with digital holographic microscopy." Optics Express 13: 9361-9373.

Ratanachoo, K., P. R. C. Gascoyne, et al. (2002). "Detection of cellular responses to toxicants by dielectrophoresis." Biochem Biophys Acta 1564: 449-458.

Safarik, I. and M. Safarikova (1999). "Use of magnetic techniques for isolation of cells." Journal of Chromatography B 722: 33-53.

Sato, S., M. Ishigure, et al. (1991). "Optical trapping and rotational manipulation of microscopic particles and biological cells using higher-order mode Nd:YAG laser beams." Electron. Lett 27: 1831-1832.

Saxena, V. (2003). "Polystyrene Microparticles as Handles for Optical Manipulation of CATH.a Cells" SURJ 2: 39-42.

Schenck, J. F. (2000). "Safety of strong, static magnetic fields." Journal of magnetic resonance imaging 12: 2-19.

Seger, U., S. Gawad, et al. (2004). "Cell immersion and cell dipping in microfluidic devices." Lab Chip 4: 148-151.

Sudsiri, J., D. Wachner, et al. (2007). "On the temperature dependance of the dielectric membrane properties of human red blood cells." Bioelectrochemistry 70: 134-140.

Svoboda, K. and S. M. Block (1994). "Biological applications of optical forces." Annu.Rev.Biophys.Biomol.Struct. 23: 247-285.

Tanase, M., E. J. Felton, et al. (2005). "Assembly of multicellular constructs and microarrays of cells using magnetic nanowires." Lab on a Chip 5: 598-605.

Toubal, M., M. Asmani, et al. (1999). "Acoustic measurement of compressibility and thermal expansion coefficient of erythrocytes." Phys. Med. Biol. 44: 1277-1287.

Tsutsui, H. and C.-M. Ho (2009). "Cell separation by non-inertial force fields in microfluidic systems." Mechanics Research Communications 36: 92-103.

Vossen, D. L. J., A. Van der Horst, et al. (2004). "Optical tweezers and confocal microscopy for simultaneous three-dimensional manipulation and imaging in concentrated colloidal dispersions." Rev. Sci. Instrum. 75: 2960-2970.

Wang, X.-B., M. P. Hughes, et al. (1995). "Non-uniform spatial distributions of both magnitude and phase of AC electric fields determine dielectrophoretic forces." Biochem Biophys Acta 1243: 185-194.

Wang, X.-B., H. Y, et al. (1994). "A unified theory of dielectrophoresis and travelling wave dielectrophoresis." J.Phys.D, Apply.Phy 27: 1571-1574.

Wang, X. B., Y. Huang, et al. (1993). "Selective dielectrophoretic confinement of bioparticles in potential energy wells." J.Phys.D, Apply.Phy 26: 1278-1285.

Wanichapichart, P., S. Bunthawin, et al. (2002). "Determination of cell dielectric properties using dielectrophoretic technique." ScienceAsia 28: 113-119.

Wiklund, M., C. Günther, et al. (2006). "Ultrasonic standing wave manipulation technology integrated into a dielectrophoretic chip." Lab on a Chip 6: 1537-1544.

Winkleman, A., K. L. Gudiksen, et al. (2004). "A magnetic trap for living cells suspended in a paramagnetic buffer." Applied physics letters 85(12): 2411-2413.

Xia, N., T. P. Hunt, et al. (2006). "Combined microfluidic-micromagnetic separation of living cells in continuous flow." Biomedical Microdevices 8: 299-308.

Yang, J., Y. Huang, et al. (1999). "Dielectric properties of human leukocyte subpopulations determined by electrorotation as a cell separation criterion." Biophysical Journal 76(6): 3307-3314.

Exploring Insight of User Needs: The First Stage of Biomedical Engineering Design

Jiehui Jiang, Adinda Freudenthal and Prabhu Kandachar
Delft University of Technology
Faculty of Industrial Design Engineering
The Netherlands

1. Introduction

1.1 What is design?

Compared with some fundamental sciences such as physics or mathematics, the history of industrial product design is much shorter and original from other subjects. To quote Herbert Simon (Simon, 1969) from his work on science of artificial: "Everyone designs who devises courses of action aimed at changing existing situations into preferred ones." Design is not fundamental research, which may be defined as a careful investigation or study. The design process needs research to accomplish the design task, but it typically involves the integration of fundamental knowledge, rather than the generation of fundamental knowledge.

On the other hand, design is not only craftsmanship (Paul and Richard, 2008). Creativity is an important skill in the design process. It is a brain activity as well as hand activity. Design work could be the manufacture of a physical device, and also could be a plan or a study to determine the process. It can range from the physical device level to the complete situation of product or manufacture related activities.

As a result, with the increased attention on interaction between product, user and environment (Hekkert and van Dijk, 2001; Tassul 2006; Hoog etc, 2008), the "product design" has widened from initial "arts, crafts and architecture" to the development of a complex system including aesthetics, ergonomics, economics, manufacture and so on (Roozenburg and Eekels , 1995; Muller, 2001; Roozenburg 2008). For most professional designers, their design activities are focusing on not only strict product development (Embodiment design, manufacture process (Pahl and Betiz, 1980)), but also product related behaviours such as user needs user experience or business model.

1.2 What is biomedical engineering design?

Biomedical engineering design means the design of biomedical devices and systems. As one part of healthcare design, biomedical devices and systems are much more complicated than common consumer products. They are characterized by such factors as reliability (hardware and software), mobility and affordability. Right now three kinds of biomedical engineering design can be recognized.

Healthcare devices, examples are:
- Stethoscope
- Blood pressure measurement device
- Blood sugar measurement device
- Defibrillator device
- Portable ultrasound device
- Surgery instruments
- Inject instruments
- Dental instruments

Healthcare service, examples are:
- Development of Computer Aided Design for screening diagnosis
- Development of Electrical Healthcare Records system
- Development of user friendly interfaces for special doctors
- Development of Hospital Information System
- Development of Picture and Communication System
- Development of disease database

Healthcare environment, examples are:
- Optimization of architecture of operation room
- Optimization of water purified system
- Development of indoor pollution filter system
- Optimization of drug delivery system

In certain cases, two issues or all three issues will be involved.

1.3 Role of user needs research in biomedical engineering design

User needs are usually considered as one part of in biomedical engineering design projects. (Paul and Richard, 2008) Each biomedical engineer has his/her personal experience to work with users. These users may include patient, doctor and industrial companies etc. It is an efficient way to prepare a biomedical design project from user needs research (Wiklund, 1995).

Recently, there are mainly two kinds industrial innovation models for healthcare: technical-original innovation and market (user) - original innovation (Robert and Tomas, 1998). Technical-original innovations are able to achieve success in medical devices, telemedicine and record management, based on Information and Communication Technology. Nevertheless, market (user) - original innovations are more general because they don't need to wait for the enabling technology development. (Enabling technology means core technologies for industrial innovations, like X-ray technologies for computerized tomography device design. One example is that the idea of Compact Disc initiated in 1980 by Philips and Sony research group, but the product did not appear until 1982, because laser technology was not available in 1980 (http://news.bbc.co.uk/2/hi/technology/6950845.stm).

As opposed to technical-original innovations, the key feature of market (user) - original innovations is that it is user-central. (Ronald and Everett, 1980)User needs are considered to be the start point of the innovation process and user's decision to purchase as the end of the process. The role of user needs research has been emphasized in this model and the interaction between users and engineers (or designers) is crucial. Of course, market (user) - original innovation is not the only one approach for designing a biomedical device and system.

1.4 Why do we write this article?

As biomedical engineer, the first author of this paper has been involved in several biomedical engineering design projects. The subject of "user needs research" was addressed in one of the cases: "Strategy design research for Rural China". After cooperative activities with students from industrial design engineering and market research, he personally found that "user needs research" was an interesting issue in biomedical engineering design. And he started to collect more knowledge about user research and analyzed past projects in the stand of industrial design engineering.

He found that the significance of user needs research has been ignored in several cases when he informally analyzed the cases from industrial biomedical engineers, academic biomedical staffs and students. Once he talked with biomedical engineers, he would like to ask the question "why will you design this device or system with this technology?" In most cases he got answers such as "increase the accuracy of the device (Reliability)", "cut down the device cost (Affordability)" or "suit for local situation (Usability)" will appear. But once he asked further "How did you prove your design is effective?", the feedback is uncompleted most of time.

As a result, the aim of this paper is to introduce a systemic process on user needs research, which can provide the higher goal with spirit of a professional industrial design.

Besides introduction and methodology at the beginning, this article includes three parts. In section 2 , firstly a case of user needs research of biomedical engineering design, named "Strategy design research for Rural China" will be described detailed; and then some tools and methods will be inducted from the case as one possible approach to conduct user centrered research; finally some discussions will follow about user needs research of biomedical engineering design.

This paper is an extended version based on the conference paper "New market, new challenge, new opportunity (2) -User context research" for 30th IEEE EMBS Conference in Canada, 2008 (http://ieeexplore.ieee.org/stamp/stamp.jsp?tp=&arnumber=4649474&isnumber=4649055) and the audios of this paper might be biomedical engineers, or related researchers and designer as well. (Jiehui and Kandachar, 2008)

1.5 Research objective and question

Open innovation includes several different type of innovation and user central innovation is one of them., Here it means involves users in the design process.(Henry etc, 2006) In this methodology, user needs are looked as the start points. The objective of user needs research is to explore insights of user needs, or with the word "Needs identification". Needs identification is the first stage to develop design opportunities and then result in function establishing and design hypothesis. In practice, user context research is frequently-used at the beginning, as presented in Figure 1.

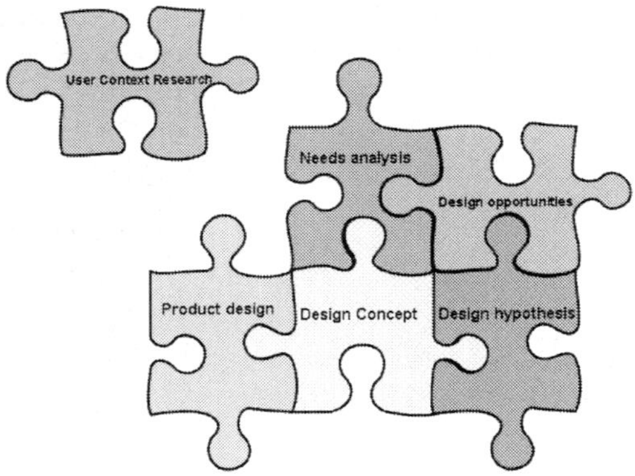

Fig. 1. Needs identification related design activities (first raw focus). User context research is often used in the beginning, and after needs analysis, design opportunities are the results of needs identification. Second raw is about concrete product development, and it provides feedback for the first raw, however, it won't be discussed here.

The aim of needs identification is to identify, define and clarify design objectives and subobjectives, and the relationships between them. In this paper, user context research needs analysis and design opportunities with published case will be discussed and the research question is "How the insights of the user needs were explored for biomedical engineering design?"

2. Methodology: Case study "searching for healthcare design opportunity for rural Shanghai"

This section will introduce a user central design case, which was meant as a first stage in product development: a preparation before the engineering phase of strict product development, Published earlier in EMBC. The major contests of the case come from the published conference paper (Jiehui and Kandachar, 2008).

2.1 Project motivation and research team

China has the largest population in the world (1.3 Billion) and 0.9 Billion is rural population (NBSC, 2007).They are composed of 0.75 Billion rural people who live in rural and 0.15 Billion who live in urban as migrant workers (John and Xinmin, 2006). Although their average income has increased every year to about 4000RMB/year (US$1.4/day) at the end of 2006 (NBSC, 2007), the income gap between rural and urban is becoming large year by year.

According to the World Bank, there are 4 billion people living on an income less than US$3 per day and 1 billion living less than even US$1 per day. This part of the population is often called "Base-of-the-Pyramid" (BoP), referred by Prahalad and Hart (Prahalad and Hart, 2007). And so more than 95% china rural belongs to BoP under this standard (NBSC, 2007).

Recently, some Multi National Companies (MNC) such as Hewlett-Packard (HP), Intel, Philips and Microsoft have been aware of the design opportunities of this market, as well as some design institutes such as Delft University of Technology (DUT) (Kandachar and Halm,

2008), Illinois Institute of Technology (IIT), Berkley and Standford which are partnering with MNCs for BoP design (Wilson and Wilson, 2006; Jamie and Niels, 2007).
As a result, this project is the strategy part of the research program "Provide healthcare solution for rural China" and the outputs are intended for industrial partners for future healthcare product design such as new business opportunities to sell simplified devices for rural hospitals.
The research team includes students form three academic stakeholders: Delft University of Technology, Erasmus University (Netherlands) and Shanghai University (China), which is sponsored by Philips Medical Systems and Applied Technologies. Related field work for user context researches are carried out through field study in rural Shanghai, by a student team of Tudelft and Shanghai University.(Jiang and Jennifer, 2007)

2.2 Research Process

For the case, a research process named "From Unstructured to Structured" has been designed by teammates Jan Pieter Adriaanse and Jaap Daalhuizen. (Figure 2)

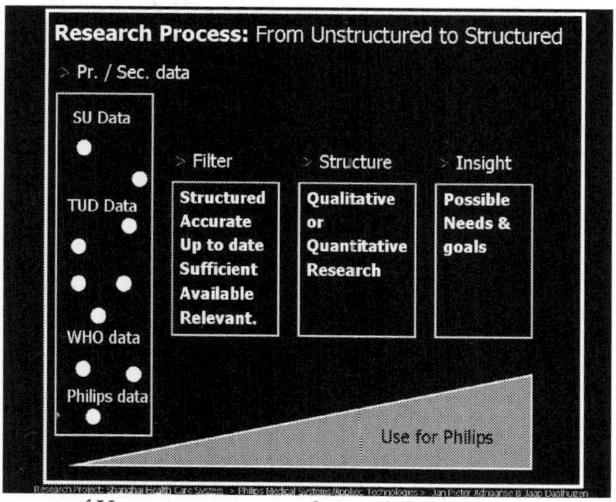

Fig. 2. Research Process of User context research in rural Shanghai

In this research process, Primary/Second hand data will be collected firstly through related research partners: Shanghai University, Tudelft and Philips and referred official data: statistic from World Health Organization.(WHO) (Carrin G, etc, 1999) These data are structured accurate up to date, which compose of background knowledge and well established tools of for researchers. Qualitative and Quantitative research will be done to analyze and structure research data and insight on possible needs and goals will be found through this research.

2.3 Research Details

2.3.1 Pre-work and information source identification

In this project, pre-work of user context research was done through Internet and literature reviews rather than practice as a user with a real product. The life style of local people has been studied by designer teams and information comes from three stakeholders: Academics, Non Government Organization and industrial companies. The tool "*brainstorm*" (workshop with stakeholders, see 3.4) was used at the beginning.

2.3.2 Qualitative research

After the first step, to gain initial insights on healthcare needs, a qualitative exploratory research in Shanghai was carried out in Chongmin island, rural Shanghai. The main approach was based upon the observation of the customs, habits and differences between people in everyday situations and four steps are used:

- Seeing through the eyes (*Initial Idea*)
- Unstructured observations *(Problem definition)*
- Diaries (*Data collection*)
- Semi structured interviews (*Interpretation and communication)*

To approach real life of target group, five rules are used for interviews:

- Develop empathy with the respondent
- Make sure the respondent is relaxed and comfortable
- Be personable to encourage and motivate respondents
- Note issues that interest the respondent and develop questions around these issues
- Not be happy to accept brief 'yes' or 'no' answers.

Target rural people are divided into five types in this research: elderly, farmer, worker, housing women and child. And the output of this step is 5 *personas (*introduced in 3.4*).*
Personas are archetypal users with specific goals and needs on real market and design research. They each represent a characteristic group of users, like 'workers' or 'farmers' (Thomas and James, 1995).

Following factors are included in our personas:

- A name
- A photograph
- Demographic characteristics
- Techno graphic characteristics
- Behavioural characteristics
- Barriers and/or challenges
- Specific goals and needs

Figure 3 shows a completed persona of elderly in Chongmin, which is composed of four parts: Introduction, Living conditions, Awareness and Needs. Pictures are added to help understand contents for readers and a special section: "I am quite satisfied with my life; it has always been like this. I hope my grandchildren have a better life." And this thought will be considered in an interaction healthcare design for rural China as culture factors. The needs of personas are looked as main outputs for future research and they are recorded as images.

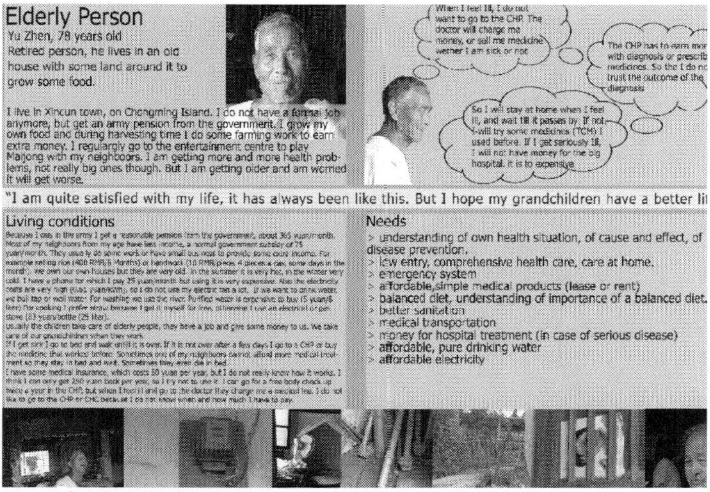

Fig. 3. Persona of elderly, Edited by Jan, Jaap and Jiang

2.3.3 Quantitative research

Quantitative research is used as the third step of this project. Here, the aim of quantitative research in this part is to prove hypothesis. Some hypotheses have been found through persona such as "care at home" for elderly; this hypothesis will be detected by other target elderly group. And then the factor or phenomena can be the evidence for researchers. *Questionnaires* (introduced in 3.4) are designed as quantitative research tools here.

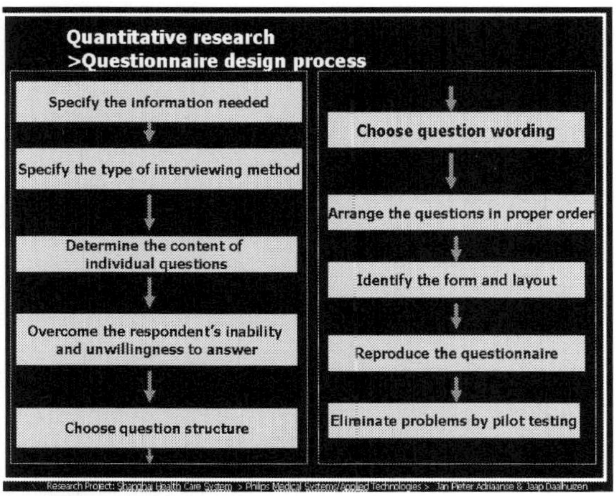

Fig. 4. Questionnaire design process

2.3.3.1 Questionnaire design

Three special objectives are confirmed before the design:

- It must translate the information needed into a set of specific questions that the respondent can and will answer;
- Must uplift, motivate and encourage the respondent to become involved in the interview;
- It must minimise response error.

Figure 4 shows the design process of questionnaires in this research. The contents of questions are chosen from qualitative research and they are specified into a type of interviewing method, after a makeup in structure, wording, order and layout, totally 64 questions are set up and they are composed of: basic information(6), basic health information(10), health awareness(8), medical insurance(8) and healthcare needs(32). 50 example questionnaires had been tested in Chongmin as pilot test. (10 for every person) (The work has been carried out by local student teams; also see Figure 6 and 7)

2.3.3.2 Respondents

Five different rural areas: Jinshan, Qingpu, Fengxian, Nanhui and Songjiang have been chosen as questionnaire areas. 300 questionnaires are sent to each area by team (see Figure 7) and they were back at the second day, so totally 1500 questionnaires were finished.

Table 1 shows the respondents detail of this research, five target groups are separated. In this research, totally 1419 questionnaire are given back and the rate is 94.6%. The highest area is Nanhui and Songjiang (96.3%) and the lowest area is Qingpu (92%).

For the respondent types, farmer gets a highest rate 44.5% and child is least 5.4%, the real number is acceptable according to plan.

2.3.3.3 Question description

Totally 64 questions are designed in this study, and they are divided into five parts:

- Basic personal information (6): Name, gender, age, address, contact phone and Email
- Basic health information (10): like Infectious disease history, impatient history
- Health awareness (8): like "I will trust Village Doctor more if they have advanced product"
- Medical Insurance (8): like "A good medical insurance will let me approach higher quality health care service"

Healthcare Needs (32): like "I prefer to monitoring my body vital signals at home (Temperature, blood pressure)" and more details can be found in table 2. (Because the needs is the prime focus in this article I would provide a table of examples, both closed and open examples)

Most of answers of questions are choices and only a little will be formed by respondents themselves. Commonly five choices are given like "Very agree", "agree", "no sense", "not agree" and "reject"., and the result is imputed into the computer as "5", "4", "3", "2" and "1".

2.3.3.4 Data analysis

Two steps are used to identify and dismiss of error answered questionnaires,

a) Similar comparison: Of 32 questions about healthcare needs, the questionnaire will be ignored if more than 30 answers are same.

b) Complete decision: Of totally 64 questions, the questionnaire will be if ignored if more than 12 questions are skipped.

Area	Respondent type	No of feedback	Area totally	Respondent totally	Plan
	farmer	118		farmer	farmer
	worker	27			
Jin Shan	elderly	30			
	Housing woman	97	288	632	650
	child	16			
	farmer	135		worker	worker
	worker	19			
Qing Pu	elderly	32			
	Housing woman	77	276	125	150
	child	13			
	farmer	127		elderly	elderly
	worker	33			
Feng Xian	elderly	28			
	Housing woman	77	277	148	200
	child	11			
	farmer	134		Housing woman	Housing woman
	worker	21			
Nan Hui	elderly	22			
	Housing woman	94	289	437	400
	child	18			
	farmer	118		child	child
	worker	25			
Song Jiang	elderly	36			
	Housing woman	91	289	77	100
	child	19			

Table 1. Respondents of questionnaires

As a result, 1768 questionnaires are remained for next analysis.

To confirm the healthcare needs, all results of 32 questions are inputted into a 32*1768 matrix (Figure 5):

Where $S = \sum_{j=1}^{1768} Xij$, $Mi = Si/1768$ and $SDi = \sqrt{\frac{\sum_{j=1}^{1768}(Xij-Mi)^2}{1768}}$

M of the statistic means the important level of needs for target group and SD means agreement of the M, and the head ten results of M are showed in table 3.

Q5: Early detection for lung cancer
Q6: Treatment for lung cancer
Q7: Early detection for breast cancer
Q9: Early detection for esophageal cancer
Q14: Blood pressure personal care
Q15: Blood sugar measurement
Q16: Blood sugar personal care
Q27: Improvement for Village healthcare points
Q31: Birth care
Q32: Care for new birth

All M of 32 questions are located between 3.7 and 4.5, which means all above healthcare needs are real and agreed by rural people. (3 is the average line)

Needs	**Needs description**	**Target Group**
Common diseases treatment (4)	Fever, cold, stomach and intestine diseases → Treatment	All
Cancer (6)	Lung cancer(2), breast cancer(2), esophageal cancer, cervical cancer → early detection and treatment	1,2,3,5
Heart Diseases and blood vessel for brain (2)	Immediate treatment and prevention	1,2,3,5
Chronic disease (6)	High blood pressure, high blood sugar and high blood fat → monitoring and personal care	5
Nutrition (1)	Nutrition detection for kids under 1 year old	4
Injury, Poisoning & External Causes (2)	Care and treatment	All
Tuberculosis (3)	Prevention, detection and treatment	All
Diseases of the Respiratory System (2)	Diagnosis and treatment	All
Low cost/safe medical service (3)	Current three types of low cost medical service can't satisfy them	All
Pregnant & Birth (3)	Pregnant care, birth care and mother care for new birth	2,5

1. Farmer; 2. Housing woman; 3.rural worker; 4. Children; 5. Elderly

Table 2. Statistical distribution of respondents

	Mean	SD	Order
Q5: Early detection for lung cancer	4.47	0.63	1
Q6: Treatment for lung cancer	4.29	0.87	2
Q14: Blood pressure personal care	4.25	0.77	3
Q15: Blood sugar measurement	4.19	0.71	4
Q16: Blood sugar personal care	4.17	0.82	5
Q9: Early detection for esophageal cancer	4.03	0.69	6
Q31: Birth care	4.01	0.77	7
Q32: Care for new birth	3.96	0.85	8
Q7: Early detection for breast cancer	3.91	0.93	9
Q27: Improvement for Village healthcare points	3.9	0.82	10

Table 3. The results of statistic, top 10 of approved actual needs

2.3.4 Needs analysis

Through above three stages, a number of user needs from Qualitative Research have been confirmed, which consequently were considered as design objectives. Next we clustered the 32 topics (First of all, these objectives have been listed and concluded into three issues "Chronic diseases", "Cancer" and "Mother and Child". To explain the procedure of needs analysis, "Mother and Child" will be chosen as the example. Secondly, some objectives about "Mother and Child" will be collected as:

1. Pregnant care
2. birth care
3. mother care after new birth

After analyzing local statistic data and videos from field study, we found that more than 70% death of mother and baby happened in the birth process. So birth care was chosen as our major objective for next design steps.

Thirdly, birth care will be focused and sub objectives have been showed:

1. Affordable medical devices
2. Low risk of birth process
3. Safe and clean room environment

Finally, low risk of birth process has been chosen because we found that the problem is still there once 1 and 3 have been improved in a pilot village.

2.3.5 Define preliminary goals and design opportunities

As the last step of user context research, some design opportunities for companies have been submitted as preliminary goals. For example, educational, awareness creation, information and communication enable tools have been considered as design goals. These opportunities will be evaluated by the investor and decide "Go or no go" for next phase (Table 4).

	1	2	3	……	31	32
1	X_{11}	X_{12}	X_{13}	……	X_{131}	X_{132}
2	X_{21}	X_{22}	X_{23}	……	X_{231}	X_{232}
⋮	⋮	⋮	⋮	……	⋮	⋮
1767	X_{i1}	X_{i2}	X_{i3}	……	X_{i31}	X_{i32}
1768	X_{j1}	X_{j2}	X_{j3}	……	X_{j31}	X_{j32}
Sum	S_1	S_2	S_3	……	S_{31}	S_{32}
Mean	M_1	M_2	M_3	……	M_{31}	M_{32}
SD	SD_1	SD_2	SD_3	……	SD_{31}	SD_{32}

Fig. 5. The matrix for data analysis

Needs, Concerns	Directions for solutions	Design innovations
Chronic diseases treatment	Diagnosis and treatment	Educational, awareness creation, ICT enabling tools
Affordable medical cost	Governmental policy	Hybrid Business models
Medical Insurance	Health care policy, financing	ICT enabling tools to reach the poor
Safe food	Food monitoring	Educational, awareness, Packaging Materials, ICT
Safe Living Conditions	Governmental policy, Conditions monitoring & displays	Production Materials, Manufacturing, Ecodesigns advanced technology…
Pregnant & Birthcare	Care	Telemedicine, Medical materials & equipment, Interface, advanced ICT technology…

Table 4. Some design opportunities for rural China healthcare needs

3. Results

In this section, we will discuss what we have learned from the case. And some initial results will be given according to Figure 1.

3.1 Principle: four key words of user needs identification

As an approach to help designers/engineers to understand the designing target group (users) and user needs, it can be helpful to focus in research on four key words

- Who: Who are your users? In healthcare product design, users include patients and medical staffs.

- What: What characters do your users have? User habits and work/life circumstance are always considered as important inputs for product design.
- Where: Where are your users? It should be very clear before a design. Design a product for an American or design for a Chinese is different, especially for their culture.
- When: When will your users benefit from your design? Sometimes particular using time need particular functions, for instance, design for ambulance.

Above four key words should be addressed through the whole process.

3.2 Pre-work of user context research: practice yourself as a user

Once you start a user research, some pre-work is needed. With the key words of four 'W', designers/engineers could write a research proposal to understand users through their experience or special tools such as interview, question and so on. In design practice, before a real user context research, a method called "design trip" (Nigel, 2006) can be used to test your user research proposal. The essential idea of design trip is very simple: you just take a trip through the whole process of using the proposal (it could be your user research plan), making yourself a critically observant user. You may be supervised how much you find out, if you keep yourself enough self-aware and observant. Once this method has been used a few times, more outputs will be received to help you to adapt your proposal and adopt your attitude at the start you had no attitude.

Decide first of all whom your users are and their points of view you are taking: elderly patient, pregnant women, village doctors, etc. You may want to make several mental trips, from different user perspectives. Usually, it is easiest to make a single user's trip, since you may need special permissions, tools or skills before you take more.

Next, decide the limits and variations to mental trips. It seems a good idea to extend the trip into complicated conditions, which provide you more integrated overall solutions for problems you may meet. For example, if you want do a user context research about blood pressure measurement, you may divide a year into different seasons; divide a day into different times and with different weather conditions. The extending of trips will properly bring more problems and indications you can't get from a single user trip.

Now you just have to prepare and conduct the real field trip, recording the actions, impressions, ideas and thoughts. Some tools are often used in the real field trip such as paper poster, video camera or recording pen. Through reviewing the records, some improvements will be achieved, which makes you more confident, relaxed and accepted by user groups.

3.3 User context research process

As one part of product design, user context research also follows the characters of product design, like the process of problem solving and reasoning. Others' research and personal experience is the fundamental for designers to build user context research process. A frequently used process in Tudelft is from Thomas (Thomas, 1961).

In his option, carrying out a user context research project includes five stages:

1. Initial Idea. The initial idea of context research is based on others' research and personal experience in related topic. It means designers can talked with other experienced designers or do literature review in Internet or books to build initial idea about target users.

2. Problem definition. The procedure of problem definition is continuous in the whole user context research process. At the same time, designers should carry out each action with problem such as four "W"s.
3. Data collection. With the problem, some user related data will be collected. The data could be unstructured or structured.
4. Interpretation. Explain the collected data with design words, and find the relationship between user data and product needs.
5. Communication. Document your process, conclude your opinions and present your research results. The evaluation could be done through compare results and initial ideas.

All five steps could be achieved through design tools.

3.4 Data collection tools

Currently, most of tools used for user data collection in product design are originating from social/market science methods, like observation, questionnaire and user scenarios (Heath and Stewart, 2003). These tools are collected and chosen by designers according to local project requirements. Part of frequently-used tools is introduced as follows:

Brainstorm

Brainstorm is the mental process of developing and organizing ideas. Brainstorms often occur as workshops in the above case, and users were often involved into the brainstorms directly. In practice of healthcare design, the participants of brainstorm could be people from medical organizations (hospitals), from government organizations (healthcare policy), industrial companies (product manufactures), education institutes (universities) or even users directly (community). Brainstorm is an important source for user information, especially for those designers who lack of local experiences.

Observation

Observation plays a role in the process of context mapping, and it gives designers first sight scene about users: their life style, their habits and their life environment. The observation provides designers' opportunities to compare outputs from design trips and real feeling in local context, and then improve the shortcomings that previous trip suffered from. (In the case, some added information from rural people in China has been achieved through observation as the beginning)

The results of observation could be recorded through taking notes, photos and video. These records are first hand information for future analysis.

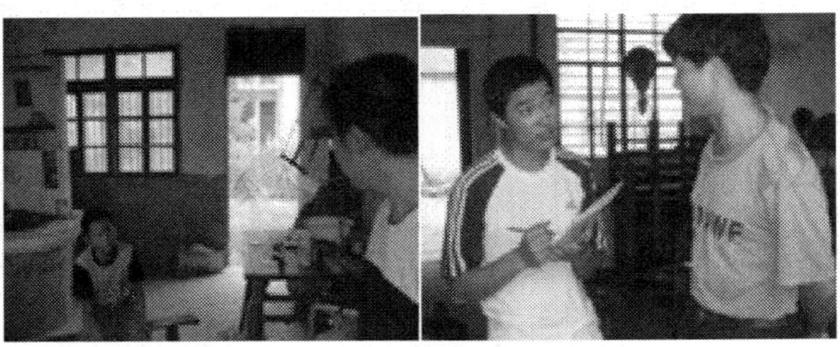

Fig. 6. Interviews in the case (Jiehui and Jennifer, 2007)

Interview

An interview is a conversation between two or more people (the interviewer and the interviewee) where questions are asked by the interviewer to obtain information from the interviewee. Interview is the most important tool in the above case to help designers understand users' thinking. And the aim is to understand "How can user be satisfied?"
The interview could be done through chatting, question and even group discussion. The contents of interviews depends on the interview/ observation set up, compared with observation. (Figure 6: Local students are doing interviews with local users in the case)

Persona

Persona is a tool to record some information. In above case, it has been used to draw the together the varied needs, preferences, wishes and requirements into a "model" of users, in order to guide designers for next step actions. The aim of persona is to construct some "stories" from users' lifestyle into one picture. These stories are user scenarios through observation and interview, and that picture is called persona. The contents of persona are related with design tasks. For example, if you would like to design a solution for blood pressure measurement and your target users are high blood pressure patients, the persona might includes the patient's age, gender, family disease history, the diet and other information that will affect blood pressure.

Questionnaire

A questionnaire is a research tool consisting of a series of questions and other prompts for the purpose of gathering information from respondents. In this topic, the contents of questionnaire may include basic information of stakeholders, social and economic information about users, or the preference on about current solutions. Questionnaire is often used as quantitative method. (Figure 7: Local students are organizing questionnaires with local users in the case)

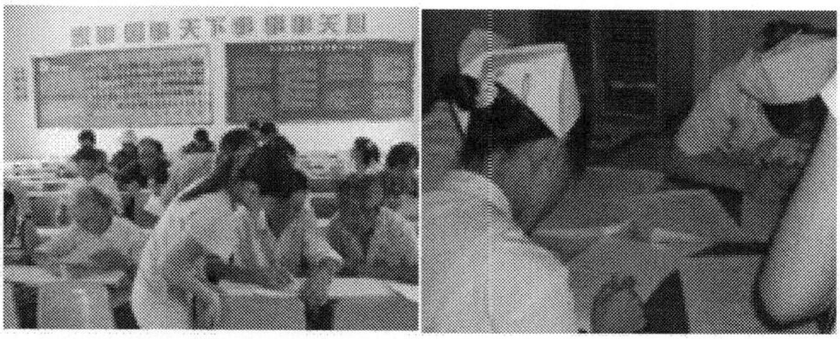

Fig. 7. Interviews in the case (Jiehui and Jennifer, 2007)

3.5 Needs analysis: transform user needs to product needs

The formal start point for the design is the design brief or strategy about new product development. Although it is a very important step in the product planning and development process, it lacks of attentions from product directly. A connect is needed to bridge user needs and product design tasks. This connection is achieved through two steps: preliminary goal definition and clarifying objectives.

3.5.1 Preliminary goal definition

As an important step for the clarification of current situation, user context research answers the question "what is the existing situation". But it is still a distance away from the new solution- what designers would like to generate. In another aspect, when a client, sponsor or company project manager approaches a designer with a product need, further work is needed. The client does not exactly wish to know what kind of product want or what target customer group needs, what kind of functions could be added into their existing products or what kind of artefact improvement is needed to increase customers' purchasing will. Simply speaking, a "problem" needs a "solution".

Therefore, the start point of "solution development" for designers is to define some preliminary goals, although in this step it is quite rare for a designer to give a complete and clear statement of design objectives. The preliminary goal definition can be considered as a desired end. For example, when you find that "High blood pressure is a serious problem for your target group and the reason is they lack of measurement devices and medical staffs in local", an idea on "design a portable, affordable, assessable self-measurement blood pressure device" may appear in your mind.

The Preliminary goal definition should be very logical and the relationship between user needs and preliminary goal should be pointed out directly. In fact, it is feasible to build logic relationship within two steps in healthcare projects. For another example, lung cancer is an important disease in rural India, while the first reason is the indoor pollution. Through user context research in rural Bangalore, the designer team (Master student from TuDelft and designers from Philips) found that the gas from indoor cooking result in pollution and then the design goal is "Design a non-pollution cooking stove for rural India". Lung cancer->indoor pollution ->design new cooking stove is logic.

3.5.2 Clarifying objectives

Once the preliminary goal is defined, the focus of design thinking will be transferred to products. So it is helpful for designers to have a clear statement of design objectives. Clarifying objectives includes three steps:

1. Make a list of design objectives: To achieve the preliminary goal, the first step is preparing a list of design objectives about the "solution" in your mind. The list can be generalized at random as you think or in discussion with the design team.
2. Order the list with different level objectives: As you make a list of objectives, it should become clear that some are high-level objectives and important. In most of time, as a designer you have to chose high-level objectives and forget some low-level objectives because it is difficult to consider every objective equally. For example, in the case of "Design a non-pollution cooking stove for rural India", safety is the highest-level objective. If you want to control the air pollution within a limited scale, new energy technology is necessary, so it means the product cost is higher than original stoves, which are always using woods. (Wood is free in rural India according to our field study) The aim of ordering the objectives is to help designers locate critical innovation direction and the determination might be from design team and even users.
3. Reality of objectives: This is the last step before the real concept design progress. The high-level objectives than can be detailed and implemented into present product markets in this step. The question about objectives now is becoming "How to achieve the high-level objectives". The often used approach is "*drawing a diagrammatic tree*" and finds variables in

the hierarchical diagram. It is not necessary just only a simple tree with the structure of branches, twigs and leaves, which shows the relationship and interconnection among each variable.

3.6 Design opportunities

Design opportunities identification is the last stage of the whole process. After the series of information analysis, some conclusions can be drawn. Some new research activities were added in this stage, such as comparison among existing products in the market.

3.7 Summary of user needs identification for biomedical engineering

This section introduces the procedure for needs identification based on the case, which is as follows:

1. Practice being a user yourself. Imaging you are the target users, and you will be observed, asked questions, and interviewed. What kind of conversation type will be welcomed to you? What kind of questions will be welcomed to you?
2. Identify information source. If you are going to working for an unfamiliar user group, it is a good idea to get some ideas and fundamental information from your local partners. These partners could be industrial companies, educational institutes or nongovernment organizations. You partners will provide you a big picture about users and first sight scenes of their condition. The information is systemic, statistical, but sometimes lacks detail. For biomedical engineering design, two features were found in the case:
    a) Diseases are normally main problems in healthcare issues. (In the case, diseases are also major contexts) In the step of problem definition, diseases are often thought as first element of the needs. It is easy to understand because diseases result in healthcare problems directly. As a result, disease information is often used as the starting of user context research.
    b) Availability is important in healthcare. This differ from other product types, Users' expectation on healthcare is not only about the product, but also healthcare service by medical staff. (Except in the case of self-care) This means designers should extend their attentions from separate users to the whole eco-healthcare system (device-doctor-patient) and context research should meet this need.

3. Qualitative research. Now you will touch with users. First of all, observe user's actions and then you will get both experienced and inexperienced users' valuable insights. Secondly, talk with users, interview them and take notes about the stories you get from conversation. Thirdly, write down these stories and conclude them into different pictures logically and make personas if necessary.
4. Quantitative research. Through qualitative research you have already gained a lot of information about users, sometimes this is structured for your project, but sometimes you have to prove them through quantitative research such as questionnaires. At the same time, it is also helpful to expand your information through quantitative research with different opinions.
5. Needs analysis. You have enough user information, but you should find the relationship between user needs and product needs (solutions). The simplest approach is to compare

user needs and existing solutions through needs analysis. Also two features are found in biomedical engineering:

a) The balance between reliability, durability and affordability should be found. As a basic topic, healthcare is aware by all governments, and there must be existing solutions for every healthcare issue. And as the designers, your tasks are building new innovations, which are better than current ones. In healthcare issue, there are two dominants: improve the reliability or durability through new technology/material, or decrease the device/service cost. Most of time, designers are just looking for the balance of two.

b) Acceptability should also be considered. Here, acceptability is not only for users, but also for healthcare policy maker. The standard about healthcare product/service is higher than many in other domains. For instance: Food and Drug Administration (FDA).

6. Define preliminary goal. The last step of user context research is preliminary goal definition, and it is the start of concept design as well. You should write down your design tasks right now, and they could be completely new products, new functions for existing product etc.

4. Conclusion

Needs identification is the first stage of whole product design, and the aim of it is to understand the insights of target group users. The methodology and process of user context tools are also useful for healthcare issues.

In this paper, a user needs identification project on China rural healthcare design opportunities has been introduced. The research is mainly composed of qualitative research and quantitative research, and the research process is pre-work research → Information source identification → Qualitative research→ Quantitative research → Design opportunities. The healthcare needs were verified through quantitative data analysis. This case shows that the process mentioned is efficient for biomedical engineering design but some adaption work are needed.

As a result, there are six steps in the user context research have been proposed: practice being a user yourself, identify information resources, qualitative research, quantitative research, needs analysis and define preliminary goals. And some tools are used including: brainstorm, interview, questionnaire, experiment and so on. User context research methodology is also suitable for healthcare projects, and this chapter provides a case study about rural China healthcare.

Finally, a special user target group: BoP has been discussed in the paper. Some design features and new challenges about user context research have been introduced. However the research in this issue is still undergoing and more adaption and adoption work are needed to design biomedical engineering (healthcare) devices/systems in the future.

5. Acknowledgement

We would like to thank Msc students Jan Pieter Adriaanse, Jaap Daalhuizen, Jing Zhang, Shijie Shao, Tianlong Shen, and staffs J.C. Diehl, Zhuangzhi Yan, Jun Shi. All of them have given support for the case in China. Also, we would like to thanks Mr. Nalin Wanigasekara, he provided a lot of support in the case.

6. Reference

Carrin G. etc (1999) The reform of rural cooperative medical system in the People's Republic of China: interim experience in 14 pilot counties, *Social Science & Medicine*, pp 961-972, ELSEVIER publisher, ISSN: 0277-9536, UK

Heath M. and Stewart A., (2003), A comparison of online and postal data collection methods in marketing research, Journal of Marketing Intelligence & Planning, Vol. 21, No.2, pp 85-95, Emerald publisher, ISSN: 02634503, Australia.

Hekkert P. and van Dijk M., (2001) Designing from context: Foundations and Applications of the ViP approach, In: *Designing in Context: Proceedings of Design Thinking Research Symposium 5*, DUP Science, ISBN 9789040722719, Delft

Henry W., Wim V. and Joel W., (2006), Open innovation: researching a new paradigm, pp 15- 18, Oxford University Press, ISBN 0199290725, UK

Hoog, W. and Boeijen, A. etc (2008), *Design guide, deign theories and design methodology*, pp 26 - 30, Delft press, ISBN 9789079347076, Delft

Jamie A. and Niels. B., (2007), Serving the world's poor: innovation at the base of the economic pyramid, Journal of Business Strategy, Vol. 28 No. 2, pp. 14-21, Emerald publisher, ISBN: 0275-6668, USA

Jiehui J. and Jennifer F., (2007), Shanghai University club uses technology to fight poverty, *IEEE Engineering in Medical and Biology Magazine*, pp 2-4, EMBC press, ISBN 0739-5175, USA

Jiehui J. and Kandachar P. V., (2008), New market, new challenge, new opportunity (2) -User context research , *Engineering in Medicine and Biology Society, 2008. EMBS 2008. 30th Annual International Conference of the IEEE*, pp 1583-1586, IEEE Express, ISBN: 9781424418145, USA

John T., (1997), Step-by-step QFD, Customer-Driven Product Design, CRC Press, ISBN 1574441108, USA

John W. and Xinming Y., (2006), *Rural Income Volatility and Inequality in China*, NBER working paper series, No 12779, available at http://papers.ssrn.com/sol3/papers.cfm?abstract_id=953202

Kandachar, P.V, and Halme, M., (Editors) (2008). *Sustainability Challenges and Solutions at the Base of the Pyramid: Business, Technology and the Poor*, pp 6-14, Greenleaf Publishing, ISBN 9781906093112, UK

Muller W., (2001) *Order and Meaning in Design*, pp 35-46, G7 books, ISBN 9051896298, Utrecht

National Bureau of Statistics of China (2007), *China Statistical* Yearbook2007,pp 16-20, 85-90 China Statistics Press, ISBN 750375001x, China

Nigel C., (2006), *Engineering Design Methods: Strategies for product design*, pp 60-65 and pp 77-80, Wiley, ISBN 9780470519264, UK

Pahl. G. and Beitz W., (1980), *Engineering Design: A Systematic Approach*, pp 17-21, Springer, ISBN 3540199179, New York

Paul H. K. and Richard C. F., (2008), *Design of Biomedical Devices and Systems*, pp 2-6, CRC Press, ISBN 9781420061796, New York

Prahalad C. K. and Hart, S. L., (2002) Fortune at the Bottom of the Pyramid, The Eradicating Poverty Through Profits, pp304. Wharton School Publishing, ISBN-10: 0-13-187729-1, USA

Robert F. H. and Tomas M., (1998), Innovation, Market Orientation, and Organizational Learning: An Integration and Empirical Examination, The Journal of Marketing, Vol. 62, No. 3 pp. 42-54, Pulished by American Marketing Association, ISSN 00222429, USA

Roozenburg N. etc (2008). *A room with a view*, pp 11-12, Tudelft Press, ISBN 9789079347032, Delft

Roozenburg N. and Eekels (1995), *Product Design: Fundamentals and Methods*, pp.9-16 and pp.75-90, John Wiley & Sons Ltd, ISBN 0471954659, UK

Ronald E. R. and Everett M. R., (1980), Reinvention in the Innovation Process, *Science Communication*, Vol. 1, No. 4, pp. 499-514, SAGE Publication, DOI: 10.1177/107554708000100402

Simon, H., (1969), *The Sciences of the Artificial*, Pp 65-68, MIT Press, ISBN 0262193744, Cambridge, Mass

Tassoul M., (2006) *Creative Facilitation: a Delft Approach*, pp 17-27, Delft press, ISBN 9789071301469, Delft.

Thomas C. and James R., (1995), Marketing research an applied approach, pp 115, McGraw-Hill Companies, ISBN: 0079122523 , USA

Thomas S. K., (1961), *The Function of Measurement in Modern Physical Science*, pp 161-193, The University of Chicago press, ISBN 9780226458069, Chicago

Wiklund, M. E., (1995), *Medical Device and equipment Design-Usability Engineering and Ergonomics. Buffalo* Grove, IL: CRC Press, ISBN 0935184694, USA

Wilson, C. and Wilson P., (2006), *Make Poverty Business: Increase Profits and Reduce Risks by Engaging with the Poor*, Greenleaf Publishing, ISBN-10: 1874719969, UK

5

Biological effects of electromagnetic radiation

Elena Pirogova, Vuk Vojisavljevic and Irena Cosic
Royal Melbourne Institute of Technology
Australia

1. Introduction

There are a considerable number of peer-reviewed publications which show that electromagnetic EMR can result in physiologically beneficial *in vivo, in vitro* and *in situ* biological effects. These bioeffects are already used for therapeutic applications of non-thermal and non-ionizing EMR such as bone repair, nerve stimulation, wound healing, osteoarthritis treatment, electro-acupuncture, tissue regeneration, immune system stimulation, and neuroendocrine modulations.

Pulsed electromagnetic fields, pulsed radio frequency fields, and low frequency sinusoidal waveforms have been shown to promote healing when used as adjunctive therapy for a variety of soft-tissue injuries. It was also shown that specific changes in the field configuration and exposure pattern of low-level EMR can produce highly specific biological responses (Breckenkamp et al., 2003; Kappe and Stadler, 2005; Frochlich, 1984; Jauchem, 2008; Kundi, 2008; Sheppard et al., 2008; Vojisavljevic et al., 2007).

It is widely accepted that electromagnetic pollution is a major environmental factor which is currently not well investigated. The ever-increasing number of mobile phones, base stations, digital mobile communication systems, and other portable devices operating at radio frequencies (RF), motivates the scientific community to better understand the mechanism of interaction between radio/microwave radiation and biological systems. Environmental and occupational health risks are increasingly a focus of public concern. Since all living organisms are exposed to electromagnetic radiation, it is important to establish standards of acceptable exposure levels for a comprehensive range of RF radiation. At present there is no substantiated scientific evidence to indicate adverse health and biological effects produced by RF exposures at levels below national and international safety standards.

Studies on human subjects have shown consistently that there is no evidence that prolonged exposure to weak electric fields results in adverse health effects (Eberhard et al., 2008; ARPANSA, 2008; ICNIRP, 1998). However, the question of whether chronic exposure to weak magnetic fields is equally harmless remains open (Eberhard et al., 2008). Laboratory studies on animals and cell cultures have shown that weak magnetic fields may have effects on several biological processes. For example, they may alter hormone and enzyme levels and the rate of movement of some chemicals through living tissue (ARPANSA, 2008). Although these changes do not appear to constitute a health hazard, they need further investigation particularly of the long term affects, and the possible mechanisms of any effects (ICNIRP, 1998).

Some effects of RF irradiation on biological processes can be reversible and thus, do not impact the health of humans. However, the significance of investigating non-thermal RF biological effects at the molecular level should not be underestimated. Understanding the mechanism of interaction between RF radiation and molecules, determining exposure level and duration (dosimetry protocol) that can result in irreversible changes in biological processes will lead to better understanding of health effects in people due to exposure to RF irradiation.

The effects of RF irradiation on global gene and protein expression in different biological systems have been investigated (Hardell & Sage, 2008) and most studies focused on the mobile phone frequencies (800 MHz -2000 MHz) at a relatively low exposure density (average SAR near 2.0 W/Kg). Based on current literature, it can be summarised that RF exposures can change gene and/or protein expression in certain types of cells, even at intensities lower than the standard recommended exposure levels (Hardell & Sage, 2008). However, the biological consequences of most of the changed genes/proteins are still unclear, and need to be further explored.

Currently the body of knowledge in this area is not sufficient to assess the impact on health due to RF irradiation, considering existing gene and protein expression data. With only a limited number of studies reporting often conflicting results (Hardell & Sage, 2008) the electromagnetic radiation (EMR) research community should pay equal attention to the negative reports as to the positive ones. Not only the positive reports need to be replicated, the negative ones need to be critically assessed and replicated as well (Hardell & Sage, 2008).

One powerful approach to the problem of the unknown effects on proteins of non-thermal RF exposures, is studying the effect of irradiation on protein activity (molecular level of interaction). Proteins are the macromolecules found in a living cell and play a crucial role in almost every biological process. The effects of electromagnetic fields (EMF) at different frequencies of exposure on proteins were analysed within our studies with the aim of understanding the possible mechanisms of interaction between external electromagnetic radiation and biological media.

We focused on enzymes, which are a specific group of proteins crucial in accelerating metabolic reactions in living organisms. In other studies isolated aqueous enzyme solutions were also taken as models to determine if external radiation could influence the selected biological processes (Vojisavljevic et al., 2007; Karu et al., 1999; Vorst et al., 2006; Dutta et al., 1992; Pavicic &Trosic, 1997; Peinnequin et al., 2000). By using isolated enzymes, many of the complexities associated with whole-body irradiation can be eliminated. By undertaking this research we intent to address the issues of biological effects and possible health hazards associated with exposure to RF radiation which are of growing concern to military, industrial and government organizations. We aimed to approach the question of biological effects of low intensity RF exposures in a methodical and quantifiable way.

2. Background

The actual mechanism by which EMFs produce biological effects is under intense study. The ideas of resonant absorption and resonant interactions have been proposed as an explanation for the marked sensitivity of living systems to EMF (Frochlich, 1986; Cosic, 1994; 1997). Evidence suggests that the cell membrane may be one of the primary locations where applied EM fields act. EM forces at the membrane's outer surface could modify ligand-receptor interactions, which in turn would alter the state of large membrane molecules that play a role in controlling the cell's internal processes (ICNIRP, 1998). The electropotential of healthy cells causes a steady flow of ions across the cell membrane which could be disturbed in an unhealthy or damaged cell. Studies have shown that the application of EMR to damaged cells can accelerate the re-establishment of normal potentials, increasing the rate of healing, reducing swelling, and helping to reduce bruising. Faster healing times will provide significant cost savings and improved patient care. The following studies have demonstrated accelerated EMR effects at the cellular and molecular level:

1) Results of several double-blind studies showed that pulsed EMF (PEMF) stimulation promotes cell activation and proliferation by an effect on cell membranes, particularly endothelial cells (Stiller et al., 2006).
3) Extremely Low Frequency (ELF) and RF fields have been applied to accelerate wound healing. Since skin wounds have unique electrical potentials and currents, stimulation of these electrical factors by a variety of EMFs can aid in the healing process by causing dedifferentiation (i.e., conversion to a more primitive form) of the nearby cells followed by accelerated cell proliferation (Teper et al., 2004).
4) PEMF increases the rate of formation of keratinocytes cells in partially healed skin wounds (Vianale et al., 2008).

Light activated changes in protein energy states have been shown to induce or modulate biological processes. For example light-activated excitation of the rhodopsin/ bacteriorhodopsin molecules involved in the hyperpolarisation process of the cell membrane can either generate nerve impulses, ATP synthesis, or light regulated embryogenesis (i.e. seed germination in plants) (Ahma et al., 1993; Karu, 1987; 1999). It has also been suggested that cytochrome C oxidase and certain dehydrogenases may play a key role in the photoreception process, particularly in the near infra-red (NIR) frequency range (Karu 1999). A number of different investigations (Karu, 1987; 1999; Fedoseyeva, 1988) have explored the effects of visible light on cell proliferation and metabolism. Some recent studies into effects of low-intensity non-thermal light irradiation on eukaryotic and prokaryotic cells, both pulsed and continuous, have reported positive results such as accelerated proliferation rate in yeast and mammalian cells after irradiating with a He-Ne laser (Karu, 1987; 1999; Karu et al., 2004) and increased *E. coli* proliferation during argon laser light exposure. An increased proliferation rate has also been observed in various bacterial cultures irradiated by laser light with radiant exposures of 1-50 J/cm^2 at wavelengths of 630 nm and 810 nm (Nussbaum, 2002). The stimulating effect of various light-emitting diodes

(LEDs) and monochromatic light on eukaryotic cells have been documented with pulsed and continuous light exposures. Several studies reported a change in acetylcholinesterase activity of human erythrocytes after low-intensity light radiation at 810 nm (Kujawa et al., 2003)

In our studies we investigated the influence of non-thermal non-ionizing electromagnetic radiation on L-Lactate dehydrogenase enzyme kinetics using the concepts of protein activation outlined in the Resonant Recognition Model (RRM). The RRM approach postulates that selectivity of protein interactions is based on specific resonant electromagnetic interactions (Cosic, 1994; 1997).

Previously (Cosic, 1997; Cosic & Birch, 1994; Cosic, 1989) a relationship between the RRM spectra of some protein groups and their interaction with visible light was established. The RRM theory states that an external EMF at a particular activation frequency would produce resonant effects on protein biological activity. It has been shown that all protein sequences with a common biological function have a common frequency component in the free energy distribution of electrons along the protein backbone. This characteristic frequency was shown to be related to protein biological function (Cosic, 1994; 1997). Furthermore, it was also shown that proteins and their targets share a characteristic frequency. It was postulated that RRM frequencies characterise not only a general function but also a recognition/interaction between the particular proteins and their target at a distance (Cosic & Hearn 1991; 1992). Thus, according to the RRM protein interactions can be viewed as a resonant energy transfer between the interacting molecules (Cosic, 1994; 1997).

Comprehensive computational analysis of different light absorbing proteins using the RRM approach showed that a strong linear correlation exists between the predicted and experimentally determined frequencies corresponding to the absorption of electromagnetic radiation of such proteins (Cosic, 1994). It is inferred that approximate wavelengths in real frequency space can be calculated from the RRM characteristic frequencies for each biologically related group of sequences. These calculations can be used to predict the wavelength of the light irradiation, which might affect the biological activity of exposed proteins (Cosic, 1997). These computational predictions were confirmed by comparison of:

a) Absorption characteristics of light absorbing proteins and their characteristic RRM frequencies (Cosic, 1997; Cosic & Birch, 1994; Cosic et al., 1989).
b) Frequency selective light effects on cell growth and characteristic RRM frequencies of growth factors (Cosic et al., 1989).
c) Activation of enzymes by laser radiation (Biscar, 1976; Vojisavljevic et al., 2007).

All these results indicate that the specificity of protein interaction is based on a resonant electromagnetic energy transfer at the frequency specific for each interaction observed. A linear correlation between the absorption spectra of proteins and their RRM spectra with a regression coefficient of K=201 has been established. Using the RRM postulates, a computationally identified characteristic frequency for a protein functional group can be used to calculate the wavelength of applied irradiation, λ, which assumingly would activate this protein sequence and modify its bioactivity (Cosic et al., 1989):

$$\lambda=201/f_{RRM}$$

In our study we utilised this relationship to calculate the frequencies/wavelengths that might modulate the bioactivity of the selected LDH enzyme. Its activation using the external EMR was investigated experimentally. The influence of visible light, infra-red and low level microwaves and their modulating effects on enzyme kinetics were evaluated.

Study	Exposure	Frequency	Effects
(Dutta et al., 1991)	0.3-8.0V/m	147 MHz (modulated with 16 Hz)	Exposures to modulated RF radiation with different powers produce different effects on Accetilholesterase activity
(Pavicic & Trosic, 2008)	0.3-8.0V/m	864 MHz; 935 MHz	RF irradiation significantly affected cell proliferation kinetics
(French et al. 1997)	200-400 V/m	835 MHz	The EMF at 835 MHz and power densities similar to the exposures emitted by mobile phones can alter cell morphology and inhibit the proliferation of Astrocytoma cells.
Peinnequin et al. 2000	137.3 V/m	2.45 GHz	RF interacts either with Fas pathway between receptor and caspase-3 activation or with membrane proteins
(Tian-Yong Zhao, 2007)	Mobile phone	900 MHz - 1800 MHz	Exposure to cell phone RF radiation emissions can up-regulate the specific intermediaries of apoptotic pathways of neurons.
(Fesenko et al., 1995)	86 V/m	42.2 MHz	The data suggest that the effects of the field on the ion channels are mediated, at least partially, by changes in the solution properties.
(Porcellia et al. 1997)	High Power	10.2 GHz	Conformational changes of S-adenosylhomocysteine hydrolase.
(Byus et al. 1984)	10mW/cm^2	450 MHz (modulated 60 Hz)	Large reduction in histone kinase activity in lymphocytes.

Table 1. Biological effects of low power radiofrequency irradiation

Doubt remains about the existence of non-thermal biological effects. Non-thermal biological effects are measurable changes in biological systems that may or may not be associated with adverse health effects. Thirty years ago, Frohlich suggested that extremely weak microwave signals may act as a trigger for certain bioeffects (Frohlich, 1986). For example, non-thermal effects such as: calcium ion efflux; changes in blood-brain barrier permeability; changes in melatonin level; and alterations in EEG signals have been observed at low-intensity modulated RF fields Little is known about the molecular mechanisms involved in putative non-thermal effects. One hypothesis is that RF radiation can induce dipole oscillations in a protein active site and thus can alter its function (Kape &Stadler, 2005). This hypothesis accords well with observed increased permeability of aqueous protein solutions measured using dielectric spectroscopy at the frequency range of 10 MHz - 1000 MHz (Dutta et al., 1992).

The use of radiofrequency (RF) sources increased dramatically in the last century particularly with the introduction of radio, television, mobile communication and other specific applications in medicine and industry. Although the level of radiation from these RF sources is well below exposure levels where thermal effects are induced in biological systems, there is still intense debate about the impact of RF radiation on human health. Two types of effects can be ascribed to RF fields, i.e. thermal and non-thermal. The heating effect of radio waves is already well-known and documented. The thermal effects are related to the heat generated by the absorption of RF energy by the water medium or by organic complex systems (Vorst et al., 2006). It has been known for many years that exposure to very high levels of RF radiation can be harmful due to the ability of RF energy to rapidly heat biological tissue (Vorst et al., 2006).

The first studies into possible non-thermal biological effects were carried out using various commercial/industrial RF apparatuses working at their particular frequencies and powers of radiation (Duta et al., 1992, Vorst et al., 2006). Researchers have had difficulty reproducing the results of these studies and have not been able to determine the reasons for this inconsistency. Note that only selected frequency exposures emitted by radiofrequency equipment (microwave ovens, radars or mobile phones) have been tested on selected cells and proteins (Table 1) whereas this study has covered a comprehensive range.

3. Experimental study

3.1 Effects of visible light and infrared radiation on enzyme activity

In this study we demonstrated that visible light and infrared (IR) radiation at specific frequencies in the range of 550 nm - 850 nm and 1140 nm - 1200 nm respectively can modulate enzyme activity (Vojisavljevic et al., 2007; Pirogova et al., 2008).

Dehydrogenase enzymes catalyse a variety of oxidation-reduction reactions within the cells. Aiming to avoid any ambiguities and inconsistencies in interpretation of the experimental findings, the enzyme example, LDH (EC1.1.1.27, rabbit muscle), has been selected on the basis its commercial availability, simplicity of the enzymes assay, and the possibility of measuring its bioactivity using the standard well accepted procedure, i.e. Continuous Spectrophotometric Rate Determination. LDH catalyses the inter-conversion of the l-lactate into pyruvate with the nicotin amide adenine dinucleotide (NAD+) acting as a coenzyme. The suitability of the LDH enzyme for this reaction is attributed to the absorption characteristics of the NADH (Nicotinamide Adenine Dinucleotide, Reduced form). NADH is able to absorb light at 340 nm in contradict to the NAD (Nicotinamide Adenine Dinucleotide Nicotinamide Adenine Dinucleotide, Oxidised form), which is inactive at this frequency. Due to the different optical characteristics of the NADH and NAD we are able to optically asses if the reaction Pyruvate → Lactate in the presence of the LDH as an accelerator has occurred and then determine the amount of the reactants. The reaction rate depends on the concentration of the enzyme and substrate.

As a source of near IR and visible light we used a SPEX 270M monochromator with a wavelength range of 400-890 nm and a resolution of 0.1 nm. For measurement of absorbance of the analysed enzyme solutions we will use an Ocean Optics USB2000 spectrometer coupled to a CCD array which can detect in the 190-870 nm range. Software control automatically monitors and saves the absorption coefficient at the required wavelength every 30 sec.

Enzyme activity measurement

The assay contained the following components: 3.00 ml reaction mix includes 10 mM sodium phosphate, (SIGMA, St Louis, MO USA) 0.12 mM -NADH, disodium salt (ROCHE, Roche Diagnostics GmbH Nonnenwald 2 DE-82377 Penzberg GERMANY) reduced form, 2.3 mM pyruvate,(BioWhittaker™ Cambrex Bio Science Walkersville, MD USA) 0.033% (w/v) of bovine serum albumin (SIGMA, St Louis, MO USA) and 0.05 units of L-lactic dehydrogenase (ROCHE, Roche Diagnostics GmbH Indianapolis In, USA).

The LDH kinetics was measured by the continuous monitoring of the NADH absorption at 340 nm. The activity of the enzyme examples is determined by the rate of substrate utilization during the enzyme-catalysed reaction. The temperature was controlled during the enzyme solution irradiation as well as during the activity measurement procedures. Enzyme concentration was determined by the extinction coefficient. For each irradiated sample we measured the absorption spectra for 10 min by recording the solution's absorption values every 30 sec as follows:

$$A_{\lambda} = -\log_{10}\left(\frac{S_{\lambda} - D_{\lambda}}{R_{\lambda} - D_{\lambda}}\right)$$

where S_{λ} is the sample intensity at wavelength λ defined as an intensity of incident light that passes the cuvette with the sample, D_{λ} is the dark intensity at wavelength λ, or intensity measured on the surface of the CCD detector (spectrometer) when the light source is switched off. R is the reference intensity at the wavelength λ. The activity rate was determined by calculating the gradient of $A_{\lambda}(t)$.

It was observed that during the first 10 min the increase of the absorbance is a linear process and can be calculated as a value of the gradient of the line representing the relation between the absorbance and time. For each wavelength of light radiation we undertook 3-5 control experiments to measure the activity of non-radiated protein solutions. With the aim at eliminating the effect of all possible artefacts we repeated our measurements with the irradiated enzyme example at the particular wavelengths of light that correspond to the resonant effects. Also we have randomised an order of measurements (596nm, 844nm, 724nm etc.) to eliminate a possible modification of the enzyme or substrate during the experimental procedure. The results obtained were analysed and the enzymatic activity of non-radiated solutions was compared to the activity of the irradiated samples (calculation of the P value). To evaluate a significance of differences between the mean values of the activity of irradiated and non-irradiated samples, we used an independent two-sided T-test.

3.2 Effects of low level microwaves on enzyme activity

In the next study we investigated the effects of low level RF irradiation on LDH enzymatic activity. The activity of LDH was calculated from absorption curves using the "gradient methods" (Vojisavljevic et al., 2007). The enzyme solutions were exposed to ultra high frequency (UHF) electromagnetic radiation using a TC-5062A UHF TEM Cell, TESCOM Ltd (TC-5060 Operating Manual). The frequencies of applied radiation were in the range 400 MHz - 975 MHz and enzyme activity was monitored (by measuring optical density of the LDH solution) at steps of 25 MHz.

For each frequency of irradiation the effect was measured for the following electrical fields: 0.02135 V/m, 0.06754 V/m 0.21358 V/m 0.675 V/m and 2.136 V/m (0.0000012 W/m^2, 0.000012 W/m^2, 0.00012 W/m^2, 0.0012 W/m^2, and 0.012 W/m^2 respectively). Measurements were repeated 3-8 times depending on their standard deviations, irradiating frequency and electrical field values.

4. Results and Discussion

4.1. Visible light irradiation

In order to computationally predict the activation frequency/wavelength of light irradiation that could produce significant effects on LDH function, a database of 176-LDH protein sequences was established and analysed using the RRM approach. All protein sequences have been taken from SWISSPROT database. Accordingly to their different structural origins and functions the selected LDH sequences were divided onto 4 sub-groups: LDH_A, LDH_B, LDH_C and bacterial LDH. The cross spectral functions were calculated for each of these groups and are shown in Figure 1a,b,c,d.

The characteristic frequencies of the LDH enzymes were identified at the following prominent frequencies: **0.1688, 0.332 ± 0.08 and 0.242 ± 0.08**, which correspond to the light radiation with a wavelength of **1190 nm, 605 nm ± 10 nm and 830 nm ± 12 nm** respectively. The RRM frequencies **0.332 ± 0.08 and 0.242 ± 0.08** are particularly prominent in the LDHB cross-spectral function. While for the LDH_A, LDH_C and bacterial LDH amplitude ratio of the peaks at the frequencies **0.332 ± 0.08 and 0.242 ± 0.08** are significantly smaller (Fig.1).

Based on the characteristic frequencies determined for the whole dehydrogenase functional group, we have calculated the wavelength of irradiation, $\lambda=201/f_{RRM}$ which assumingly would activate dehydrogenase sequences and modify their bioactivity. Thus, the wavelengths of the electromagnetic exposure required for dehydrogenase enzymes activation would be at **1191± 15 nm and 846±15 nm.**

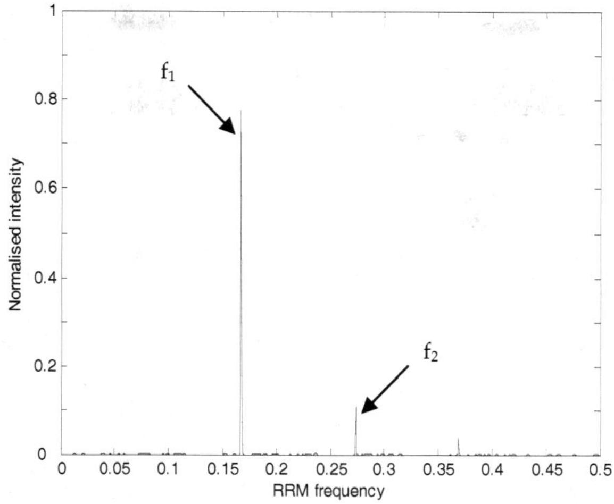
f1
f2
Normalised intensity
0
0.2
0.4
0.6
0.8
1
0 0.05 0.1 0.15 0.2 0.25 0.3 0.35 0.4 0.45 0.5
RRM frequency

(a)

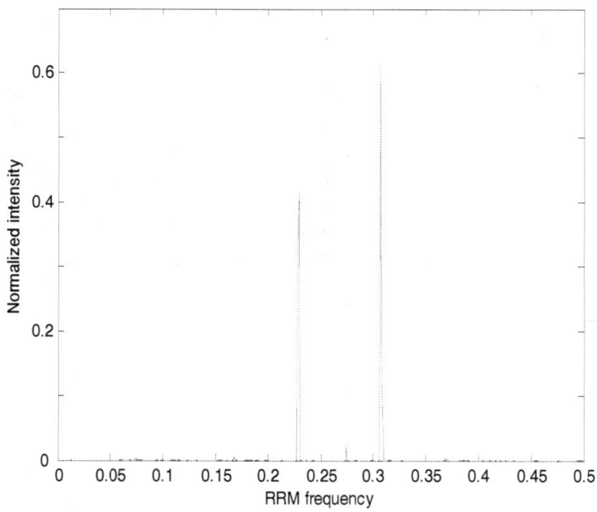
Normalized intensity
0
0.2
0.4
0.6
0 0.05 0.1 0.15 0.2 0.25 0.3 0.35 0.4 0.45 0.5
RRM frequency

(b)

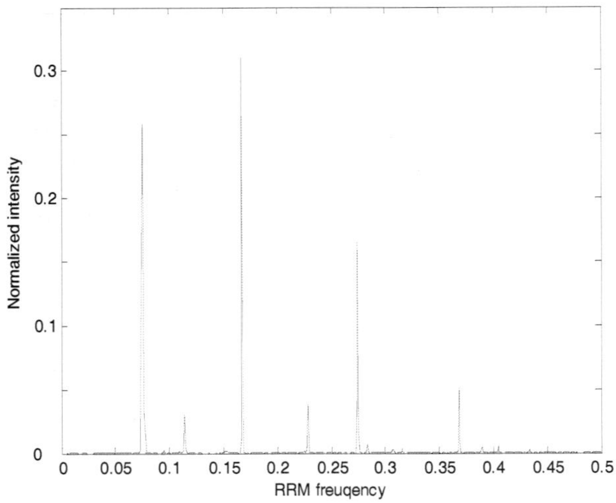

(c)

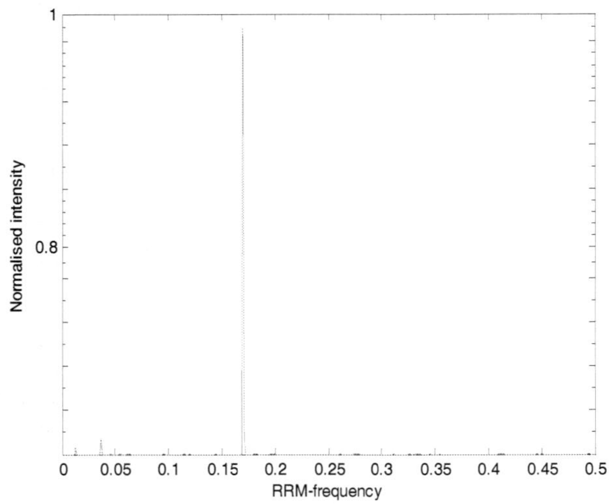

(d)

Fig. 1. Multiple cross spectral function of (a) LDH_A sequences, (b) LDH_B sequences, (c) LDH_C sequences and (d) LDH_bacterial. The x axis represents the relative RRM frequency and corresponding wavelength of the electromagnetic radiation. The y axis represents the normalized intensity of the multiple cross spectral function in the RRM spectra.

Therefore, we investigated the effects of visible light in the range of 550 nm - 850 nm and infra-red ranging from 1140 nm to 1200 nm on the LDH kinetics (Vojisavljevic et al., 2007; Pirogova et al., 2008).

Data were collected and presented in Figure 2. The effects of light exposures on the L-LDH activity are measured as the rate of change of the NADH concentration per second. There is the evident increase in the L-LDH activity after irradiation by visible light at the particular wavelengths: 829 nm and 595 nm (Figure 2). The enzyme solutions were irradiated for 15 min. The enzyme activity measured immediately after irradiation at 829 nm is 0.025 ± 0.001 and at 595 nm is 0.025 ± 0.001 respectively.

However, there is no significant difference in activity observed between LDH example, which was radiated by light of other wavelengths, and activity of the control non-radiated solutions. In comparison to the non-radiated LDH solutions that have average rate of 0.022 with a standard deviation of $\pm$ 0.0015, the results obtained demonstrate the increase of LDH activity in order of 11.9% ($P < 0.001$) at 596 nm and 12.67% ($P < 0.001$) at 829 nm respectively.

To evaluate how significant is the difference between the mean values of the activity of irradiated and non-irradiated samples, we have used an independent two-sided T-test. This value is much higher than the value of the variability caused by the variations in concentrations of the LDH, NADH and pyruvate that were determined within the control experiment with the non-irradiated solutions. It is important to note, the increase of biological activity achieved upon radiation by light of the particular wavelengths at 596 nm and 829 nm has been already reported in literature.

Study of the effect of burn healing in non-diabetic rats produced by LED light at 596 nm was published (Al-Watban & Andres, 2003). Also light radiation at 829 nm is close to the 810 nm that was proved to be effective for bacteria's growth rate. In particular, the low-level laser at 830 nm has produced the effects in control of the painful stomatitis in patients with hand-foot (Toida et al., 2003).

Summarising the results of our study we have to point out that the computationally predicted activation frequencies of the LDH enzymes using the RRM approach closely correspond to our experimental data and findings of other researchers showing the maximum change in the LDH activity after irradiation at 596 nm and 829 nm.

Hence, the results reveal that this specific biological process can be modulated by irradiation with the defined frequencies strongly supporting the main concept of the RRM methodology. Moreover, if we observe the increase of the LDH activity at 550-900 nm wavelength range, it is expected that much stronger effect in protein activation would be obtained if we could perform the experiment with the predicted by the RRM characteristic frequency $f=0.1680$ (λ=1156nm) that correspond to the common dehydrogenase activity. Such study would be the next step of our research of protein interactions with the EMF.

4.2 Infra-red radiation

Measurement of the NADH absorbance

1. We have diluted the stock coenzyme solution with the 0.003 M potassium phosphate assay buffer.

2. Using the properly diluted coenzyme solution, we have measured the NDAH absorbance after irradiation at 1140 - 1200 nm with the interval of 2-5 nm.

3. The spectrophotometer was set to 100% transmittance (zero absorbance) at each wavelength using 0.003 M K_2HPO_4 assay buffer blank. The results reveled that NADH concentration corresponds to the maximum absorbance of 1.6 at 340 nm. Fig. 3 shows how NADH sample absorbance is affected by the applied radiation of the defined wavelength.

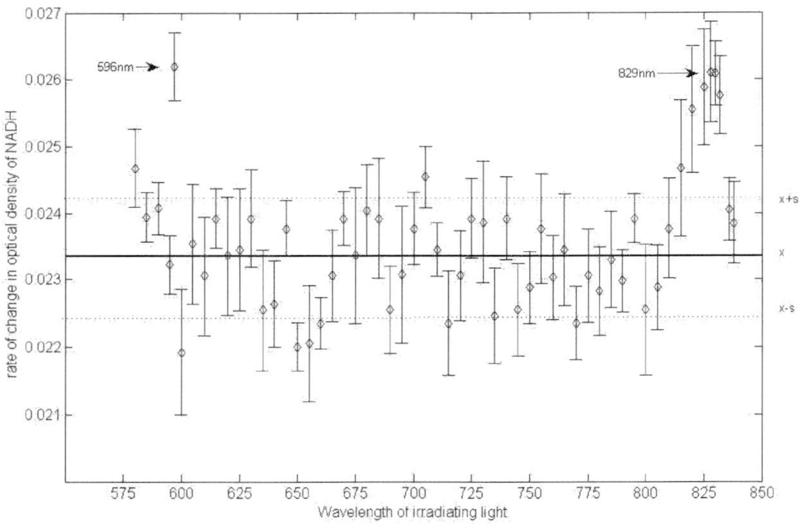

Fig. 2. The activity of the LDH is measured after irradiation of the LDH with different wavelengths of light.. The ordinate represents the rate of change in optical density of NADH per minute. By Beer-Lambert low the optical density is proportional to the concentration of absorbing molecule or NADH. Thus, the rate of change represents practically the rate of change of the NADH concentration per unit of time, or activity of the LDH. Horizontal bold line represents an average (x) for the non-irradiated samples. Horizontal dashed lines (x+s; x-s) values distant for one standard deviation (s) up and bellow from average value

The experiments were performed at room temperature 27°C (Temperature controller Quantum Northwest). The cuvettes were filled with 0.3ml of the LDH samples. The samples were previously irradiated with the light of different wavelengths (1140-1200 nm) for 600 sec. These irradiated samples were added then to the already prepared solution of NADH and pyruvate. The optical density of NADH was measured at 340nm foe each irradiating wavelength. The results obtained have revealed the change of the NADH absorbance under the influence of irradiated LDH.

From Fig. 3, we can observe that maximum optical density of the NADH is achieved at the wavelengths **1192 and 1200 nm (f_1=0.1688±0.004)** as was predicted by the RRM as the possible activation frequency of the dehydrogenase enzymes. Hence, the results suggest that this specific biological process can be modulated by irradiation with defined frequencies strongly supporting the main concept of the RRM methodology. The possibility to computationally calculate the frequencies with the following use of IR and visible light to produce the desired biological mutations and alterations in proteins would benefit the development of new biomaterials, non-invasive treatments and advanced technologies.

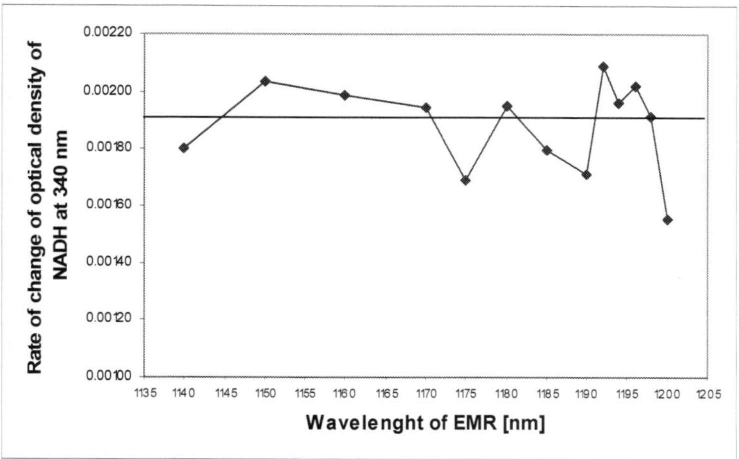

Fig. 3 Gradient of change in the NADH absorbance

4.3 Low level microwave radiation

In this study, the LDH samples were exposed to low level RF fields in the range of 400 MHz-1000 MHz. As a source of microwave radiation we will use a TC-5062A UHF TEM Cell (100 kHz - 3GHz), TESCOM Ltd. Through the input port, an external signal is applied to generate a predictable field inside the TEM Cell. A GTEM camera will be used to expose the enzyme solution samples. The GTEM can be calibrated using a broadband electric field probe to determine the electric field produced at the sample position inside the GTEM for a given input power. The field values provided for 10 dBm (10 mW) input to the power levels applied can be scaled using the following equation (TC-5060 Operating Manual):

$$E_1 = E_0\sqrt{\frac{P_1}{10mW}} \quad (1)$$

Where E_1 is the exposure field of the sample, E_0 is the calibration field we found using a test power of 10 mW, and P_1 is the test power we used in our exposure.

The proposed exposure technique enables us to maintain the control (non-radiated) and exposed enzymes at similar temperatures, and to accurately monitor the specific absorption rate (SAR, mW/g) and temperature of the studied aqueous enzyme solutions. The estimated uncertainty in the generated field is ± 30%.

Procedure and data collection

1. To measure the absorption coefficients of the studied enzyme samples we used an Ocean Optics USB2000 spectrometer. Sampling rate for absorption coefficient at 340 nm was set at 1 sec.
2. The experimental solutions were prepared according to the assay description provided by Sigma-Aldrich.
3. The temperature was controlled by the Temperature controller (Quantum Northwest).
4. The enzyme solutions were exposed/sham exposed to ultra high frequency (UHF) electromagnetic radiation. The electromagnetic field (EMF) is generated by the certified Transversal Electromagnetic mode GTEM-cell TC 5061A with a signal generator, ROHDE&SCHWARZ Signal Generator SMX. The EMF inside of the test volume is proportional to the input voltage and inversely proportional to the cell height. Therefore, the electrical field generated at the test point inside the TC-5061A can be calculated as (TC-5060 Operating Manual):

$$E = \frac{signal\ level\ [V]}{dis.\ from\ top\ [M]} \tag{2}$$

   Magnetic field produces by the GTEM-cell is orthogonal and proportional to electric field. Their relation is described by (TC-5060 Operating Manual):

$$magnetic \quad field(A/m) = \frac{Electric \quad field(V/m)}{377(Ohm)} \tag{3}$$

Although, we cannot distinguish which field is more responsible for non-thermal effects, we suggest that one of the main effects, i.e. change in protein's hydration is induced by applied electrical field.

5. The cuvettes were filled with the sample and kept at 22 cm distance from the top of the camera. The exposure duration was 240 sec.
6. After exposure the optical density of the NADH was recorded continuously for the next 5 minutes with the step of 1 sec. The control cuvettes were also kept under the same experimental conditions inside the camera with the signal generator being in the switched off mode (sham exposed).
7. The activity of the enzyme samples was calculated from the absorption curves using the gradient methods.
8. The frequencies of the applied radiofrequency irradiation were in the range of 400 MHz up to 1800 MHz with step of 25 MHz.

9. For each frequency of radiation the effect was measured for the following electrical fields: 0.02135 V/m, 0.06754 V/m 0.21358 V/m 0.675 V/m and 2.136 V/m (0.0000012 W/m^2, 0.000012 W/m^2, 0.00012 W/m^2, 0.0012 W/m^2, and 0.012 W/m^2 respectively).
10. The measurements were repeated 3-8 times depending on their standard deviations, irradiating frequency and electrical field values.

Data analysis

The data obtained were collected and analysed. The significance of the data was analysed using a single factor ANOVA analysis. For each frequency and power we tested H_0 hypothesis that variability among the irradiated and non-irradiated samples represents a random error. For the hypothesis being tested we set α=0.05.

The results obtained provide sufficient data for summarising on the influence of applied non-thermal radiation on the studied biological process. In particular, the results showed that biological activity of the LDH enzyme increased by 5%-10% using low power microwaves at 500-525 MHz for electric fields of 0.021-2.14 V/m. We also showed that 900 MHz irradiation increased LDH bioactivity for electric fields in the range of 0.021 V/m-0.068 V/m and decreased activity if the field was stronger than 0.67 V/m. We observed a slight inhibiting effect on LDH activity at the frequencies of 650 MHz (0.214 V/m); 700 MHz (0.68-2.14 V/m) and for 875-925 MHz (0.68-2.14 V/m), when LDH activity was decreased by 2%-15%. In particular, we observed the maximal increase in LDH activity, induced by the microwave radiation, at two particular frequencies (Figure 4).

In summary, biological activity increased and decreased as follows:

- increased - at 500 MHz and electric field of 0.021 ($p< 0.17$), 0.068 ($p< 0.056$), 0.213 ($p< 0.038$), 0.675V/m ($p< 0.023$), 2.14V/m ($p< 0.021$) (Figure 4).
- increased - at 900 MHz and electric field ranging from 0.021V/m ($p<0.032$) to 0.0675V/m ($p<0.024$) (Figure 4).

The outcomes of this study show that low intensity level microwaves of particular frequencies can induce changes in enzyme bioactivity and thus, affect the specific biological process involving the LDH enzyme. This important finding requires more comprehensive investigation with different enzyme examples and a wider frequency range (not just frequencies emitted by common RF devices) in order to better understand the effects of non-thermal RF radiation on proteins. The outcomes of this study will eliminate uncertainties in the present state of knowledge on the effects of radiofrequency radiation which are of concern to national and international regulatory and other health agencies.

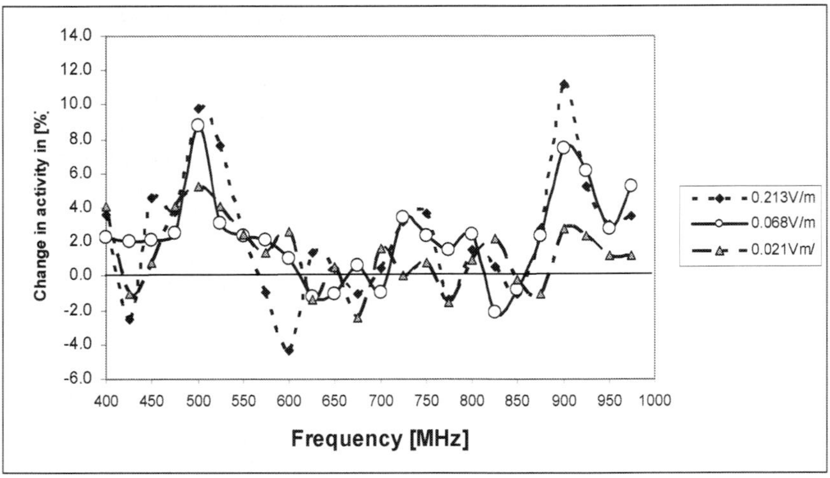

Fig. 4. Radiofrequency effects on LDH activity, calculated as relative rate of change of optical density of NADH in an irradiated sample to the rate of change in a non-irradiated sample, measured for electrical fields of 0.021V/m, 0.068V/m and 0.213V/m.

5. Conclusion

Our research presents an attempt to shed a new light on possible deeper physical grounds underlying the process of protein interactions. To elucidate the possible mechanism of influence of the EMF on proteins we have conducted a series of *in vitro* experiments where L-Lactate dehydrogenase was irradiated by visible light of different wavelengths ranging from 550 nm up to 900 nm, infrared exposures at 1140-1200 nm. These ranges of applied EMR were determined by the RRM. The computational results revealed that the RRM frequencies corresponding to the dehydrogenase enzymes activation are at f_1=0.1688±0.004 and less prominent at f_2=0.2392±0.004 (corresponding to 1191±15 nm and 846±15 nm respectively) can be directly related to the resonances in electron differential scattering cross section of these macromolecules.

The results obtained have shown the sensitivity of the reaction rate depends on the frequency of the visible light, albeit a low-intensity visible light has energy incomparable to the characteristics energies of electron excitations. Our experimental results are in a close agreement with the characteristic wavelengths corresponding to the activation of LDH enzyme predicted computationally within the RRM. Based on similarity between the RRM spectra calculated and the LDH activity spectra obtained experimentally we conclude that the distribution of the electron-ion potentials along the whole peptide chain could have a crucial impact on the interactive process between visible light and enzymes. The presented methodology may allow the generalization of the main advantage of the RRM in the case when the space structure of macromolecules is taken into account in a more realistic way. Based on the RRM spectral characteristic we can calculate the wavelength of the electromagnetic energy that can be used to modulate protein activity, hence giving rise to an innovative efficient methodology to program, predict, design and modify proteins and their bioactivity.

In addition, we studied the effects of low level microwaves ranging from 400 MHz up to 975 MHz on the L-Lactate Dehydrogenase enzymatic activity. It was shown that extremely low level ultra high frequency irradiation with the electric field strength of 5-0.05 V/m can alter enzyme activity. The results of this study revealed that the biological function of the studied LDH enzyme can be increased by 10% using the low power microwaves at 500 MHz (0.02 V/m-2.1 V/m) and 900 MHz (0.021-0.21 V/m). Based on these results we can conclude that enzyme (and possibly other proteins) activity can be modulated by the specific frequencies of low power microwave radiation.

This finding may explain some non-thermal effect of microwaves on biomolecules and lead to a whole range of possibilities of controlled modulation of protein activity, which could benefit the development of new biomaterials, non-invasive treatments and advanced technologies. This could have major implications in drug design, medicine, agriculture, pharmacology and biotechnology. This finding could contribute towards development of a novel microwave technology for cancer diagnosis/therapy, treatment of metabolic diseases, and bacterial infections.

6. References

Ahme, M., Cashmore A.R. (1993). HY4 Gene of A. Thaliana Encodes a Protein with Characteristics of Blue-light Photoreceptor, *Nature*, 366:162-166.

Al-Watban, F.A.H. & Andres, B.L. (2003). Polychromatic LED Therapy in Burn Healing of Non-diabetic and Diabetic Rats, *Journal of Clinical Laser Medicine & Surgery*, V. 21(5): 249-258.

ARPANSA Australian Radiation Protection and Nuclear Safety Agency (in press) (2008) "Maximum Exposure Levels to Radiofrequency Fields - 3 kHz to 300 GHz, Annex 3: Epidemiological studies of exposure to radiofrequencies and human health, Sydney.

Biscar, G. (1976). Photon Enzyme Activation, *Bull. Math. Biology*, 38, pp. 29-38, 1976.

Breckenkamp, J., Berg, G., Blettner, M. (2003). Biological effects on human health due to radiofrequency/microwave exposure: a synopsis of cohort studies, *Radiat Environ Biophys*, Vol. 42, pp.141–154.

Byus, C.V., Lundak, R. L., Fletche, R. M., Adey, W. R. (1984). Altenation in Protein kinease activity following exposure of cultured human lymphocites to modulated microwave fields, *Bioelectromagnetics*, vol 5, no 3, pp. 341-351.

Cosic, I. (1994). Macromolecular Bioactivity: Is it Resonant Interaction between Macromolecules?-Theory and Applications,. on IEEE Transactions *Biomedical Engineering*, 41:1101-1114.

Cosic, I., Hearn, M.T.W. (1991). Hot spot amino acid distribution in Ha-ras oncogene product p21: Relationship to Guanine binding site. *Journal of Molecular Recognition*, vol. 4, pp 57-62

Cosic, I. & Hearn, M.T.W. (1992). Studies on protein-DNA interactions using the resonant recognition model: Application to repressors and transforming proteins. *Eur. J. Biochem*, 205, pp.613-619

Cosic, I. & Birch, S. (1994). Photoreceptors Having Similar Structure but Different Absorptions Can be Distinguished using the Resonant Recognition Model, Proceeding IEEE EMBS , 16: 265-266.

Cosic, I, Vojisavljevic, V. Pavlovic, M. 1989. The Relationship of the Resonant Recognition Model to effects of Low-intensity Light on Cell Growth, *International Journal of Radiation Biology*, 56: 179-191.

Cosic, I. (1997). *The Resonant Recognition Model of Macromolecular Bioactivity: Theory and Applications*, Basel, Birkhauser Verlag.

Dutta, S.K., Das, K., Ghosh, B., Blackman, C.F. (1992). Dose dependence of acetylcholinesterase activity in neuroblastoma cells exposed to modulated radio-frequency electromagnetic radiation, *Bioelectromagnetics* 13:317-322

Eberhardt, J.L. Persson, B.R. Brun, A.E. Salford, L.G. Malmgren L.O. (2008). Blood-brain barrier permeability and nerve cell damage in rat brain 14 and 28 days after exposure to microwaves from GSM mobile phones, *Electromagn Biol Med.*, Vol. 27(3), pp. 215-29.

Hardell, L. & Sage, C. (2008). Biological effects from electromagnetic field exposure and public exposure standards, *Biomedicine and Pharmacotherapy*, Vol. 62, Issue 2, pp. 104-109.

Fedoseyeva, G.E., Karu, T.I., Lyapunova, T.S., Pomoshnikova, N.A., Meissel, M.N. (1988). The Activation of Yeast Metabolism with He-Ne Laser Radiations-II. Activity of Enzymes of Oxidative and Phosphorous Metabolism, *Lassers in the Life Sciences*, 2(2):147-154.

Fesenko, E.E., Geletyuk, V.I., Kazachenko, V.N., Chemeris, N.K. (1995). Preliminary microwave irradiation of water solutions changes their channel-modifying activity, *FEBS Lett.* 366, pp. 49-52,.

Frochlich, H. (1984). IEEE Trans Microwave Theory Technology, Vol. 26, pp. 613-617.

Frohlich, H. (1986). Coherent excitation in active biological systems, *ModernBioelectrochemistry*, F. Gutmann, & H. Keyzer, eds., New York: Plenum, pp. 241-261.

ICNIRP Guidelines for limiting exposure to time varying electric, magnetic and electromagnetic fields (up to 300 GHz), *Health Physics* 1998, Vol. 74, pp. 494-522.

Jauchem, J.R. (2008) Effects of low-level radio-frequency (3 kHz to 300 GHz) energy on human cardiovascular, reproductive, immune, and other systems: A review of the recent literature, *Int. Journal of Hygiene and Environmental Health*, Vol. 211, Issue 1-2, pp. 1-29

Kappe, C.O. & Stadler, A. (2005). *Microwaves in Organic and Medical Chemistry*, Wiley-VCH, Vol. 25, pp. 16-25.

Karu, T. (1987). Photobiological fundamentals of low-power laser therapy, *IEEE Journal of Quantum Electronics*, *QE-23*: 1703-1717.

Karu, T. (1999). Primary and Secondary Mechanisms of Actions of Visible to Near-IR Radiation on Cells, *Photochemistry and Photobiology*, 49:1-17.

Karu. T.I., Pyatibrat, L.V., Kalendo, G.S. (2004). Photobiological modulation of cell attachment via cytochrome c oxidaze, *Photochemical and Photobiological Science*. 3(2): 211-216.

Kujawa, J., Zavodnik, L.; Zavodnik, I., (2003). Low-Intensity Near-Infrared Laser Radiation-Induced Changes of Acetylcholinesterase Activity of Human Erythrocytes. Journal of *Clinical Laser Medicine Surgery*. 21 (6):351–355.

Kundi, M. (2009). The Controversy about a Possible Relationship between Mobile Phone Use and Cancer. *Environmental health perspectives* 117(3):316-24

Nussbaum, E.L., Lilge, L., Mazzulli, T. (2002). Effects of 630-, 660-, 810-, and 905-nm laser irradiation delivering radiant exposure of 1-50 J/cm2 on three species of bacteria in vitro, *Journal of clinical laser medicine & surgery*, 20(6), pp. 325-33.

Pavicic, I. & Trosic, I. (2008). Impact of 864 MHz or 935 MHz radiofrequency microwave radiation on the basic growth parameters of V79 cell line *Acta Biol Hung*. 59(1):67-76.

Peinnequin, A., Piriou, A., Mathieu, J., Dabouis, V., Sebbah, C., Malabiau, R., Debouzy, J.C. (2000). Non-thermal effects of continuous 2.45 GHz microwave on Fas-induced apoptosis in human Jurkat T-cell line, *Bioelectrochemistry* 51, 157-161 .

Pirogova, E. Cosic, I. Vojisavljevic, V. Fang, (2008). Use of infrared and visible light radiation as modulator of protein activity, *Estonian Journal of Engineering*, Vol. 14, No. 2, 107-123.

Porcellia, M., Cacciapuoti, G., Fusco, S., Massa, R., D'Ambrosio, G., Bertoldo, V., De Resa, M., Zappia, V., (1997). Non-thermal effects of microwaves on proteins: thermophilic enzymes as model system, *FEBS* letters , vol. 402, pp. 102-106,

Sheppard, A.R., Swicord, M.L., Balzano Q. (2008). Quantitative evaluations of mechanisms of radiofrequency interactions with biological molecules and processes, *Health Phys.*; Vol. 95(4), pp. 365-96.

Stiller, M.J., Pak, G.H. Shupak, J.L., Thaler S., Kenny, C., Jondreau, L. (2006). A portable pulsed electromagnetic field (PEMF) device to enhance healing of recalcitrant venous ulcers: a double-blind, placebo-controlled clinical trial, *British Journal of Dermatology*, Vol, 127 Issue 2, pp.147-154

TC-5060 UHF TEM Cell Operating Manuel Tescom Co, Pty.

Tepper, O.M., Callaghan, J., Chang, E.I., Galiano, R.D., Bhatt, K.A., Baharestani, S., Gan J., Simon, B., Hopper, R.A., Levine J.P., Gurtner, G.C. (2004). Electromagnetic fields increase in vitro and in vivo angiogenesis through endothelial release of FGF-2 *The FASEB Journal*. 2004;18:1231-1233

Tian-Yong Zhao, Shi-Ping Zou, Pamela E. Knapp, (2007). Exposure to cell phone radiation up-regulates apoptosis genes in primary cultures of neurons and astrocytes, *Neuroscience Letters*, 412, 34–38.

Toida M; Watanabe F; Kazumi Goto K; Shibata T. 2005. Usefulness of Low-Level Laser for Control of Painful Stomatitis in Patients with Hand-Foot-and-Mouth Disease, *Journal of Clinical Laser Medicine&Surgery*. 21 (6): 363–367.

Vojisavljevic, V., Pirogova, E., Cosic, I. (2007). The effect of Electromagnetic Radiation (550nm-850nm) on l-Lactate Dehydrogenase Kinetics, *Int. Journal of Radiation Biology*, Vol. 83(4), pp. 221-230.

Vorst, V., Rosen, A., Kotsuka. (2006). *RF/Microwave Interaction with Biological Tissue*. Wiley-Interscience, pp. 90-105.

6

Synchrotron Radiation Microangiography for Investigation of Metabolic Syndrome in Rat Model

Keiji Umetani[1], Kazuhito Fukushima[2] and Kazuro Sugimura[3]
[1]*Research & Utilization Division, Japan Synchrotron Radiation Research Institute*
[2]*Research Institute, National Cardiovascular Center*
[3]*Department of Radiology, Kobe University School of Medicine*
Japan

1. Introduction

Imaging research for preclinical in-vivo small animal studies has pursued development of high spatial resolution scanners to reveal fine details in rats, mice, and rabbits since the mid-1990s because drugs can be tested more easily in animals than in humans (Service, 1999; Ritman, 2002). Laboratory animal imaging plays a decisive role in drug discovery and in elucidating the mechanisms of disease. In terms of basic laboratory investigations using CT, positron emission tomography, magnetic resonance imaging, optical imaging, and ultrasound, preclinical laboratory animal imaging modalities are becoming valuable research tools for investigating biology and disease (Colby & Morenko, 2004).

Medical imaging using synchrotron radiation has been utilized as a safe intravenous angiography technique since the end of the 1970s. This safe intravenous angiography technique is useful in place of conventional selective coronary arteriography. Research groups in several synchrotron radiation facilities have improved imaging systems for human studies (Rubenstein et al., 1986; Dix et al., 2003). In addition to intravenous coronary angiography, an intra-arterial high-resolution angiography system with spatial resolution of 20 μm was developed at the Photon Factory (Tsukuba, Japan) for use in laboratory animal studies (Mori et al., 1996).

Subsequently, a new microangiography system with spatial resolution as high as 10 μm was developed at SPring-8 using an X-ray direct-conversion type detector incorporating an X-ray SATICON pickup tube. The imaging system has been used at the BL20B2 beamline for depiction of tumor-derived angiogenic vessels in a rabbit model of cancer (Umetani et al., 2003) and microvascular reactivity in transgenic mice (Yamashita et al., 2002). The beamline instrumentation, incorporating X-ray optical and imaging devices, provides synchrotron radiation users with a high-flux monochromatic X-ray beam for imaging experiments. The imaging system has been improved with respect to spatial resolution and exposure time (shutter speed) at another beamline, the BL28B2 beamline, to obtain sequential, sharp, blur-free images of hearts (Iwasaki et al., 2007; Umetani et al., 2008) and brains (Kidoguchi et al., 2006; Morishita et al., 2006) in rats and mice.

For conventional microangiography, an X-ray generator with a small focal spot has been employed using an X-ray direct-conversion type VIDICON camera as a two-dimensional high-resolution detector (Sada et al., 1985; Shirai et al., 1999). However, the X-ray generator system has limited capability for displaying in vivo images of blood vessels smaller than 50-μm diameter because images cannot be magnified without blurring as a result of its focal-spot dimensions. The only X-ray source is a synchrotron that can produce small blood vessel images with diameters of less than 50 μm.

Metabolic syndrome refers to a clustering of cardiovascular disease risk factors including obesity, insulin resistance, unhealthy lipid levels, and hypertension (Grundy et al., 2004). Patients exhibiting this syndrome are known to be at higher risk of cardiovascular disease, and insulin resistance confers increased risk for type 2 diabetes mellitus. Hypertension and diabetes can cause damage to the inner walls of arteries. We investigated the characteristics of vascular endothelial function in coronary arteries of rats using a microangiography technique for visualizing vascular diameter changes produced by vasoactive agents. Synchrotron radiation imaging can generate high-resolution and high-speed images with spatial resolution in the micrometer range. For this study of a rat heart under Langendorff perfusion, coronary microangiography was performed with spatial resolution of 6 μm and exposure time of 2 ms. Using rat models of hypertension and diabetes, we performed radiographical evaluation of changes in small coronary arteries by clearly depicting vasodilatation of coronary arteries under the influence of vasoactive agents: acetylcholine, adenosine triphosphate, and sodium nitroprusside (Umetani et al., 2004).

2. Imaging system

Experimental arrangements at the BL28B2 beamline for biomedical imaging using monochromatic synchrotron radiation X-rays are presented in Fig. 1. Coronary and cerebral microangiographic imaging was conducted at the BL28B2 (Kidoguchi et al., 2006; Morishita et al., 2006; Iwasaki et al., 2007; Umetani et al., 2008) because this beamline, which uses a single <111> silicon crystal monochromator, produces higher flux X-rays than those at the BL20B2, which uses a double <311> crystal monochromator.

A useful source of synchrotron radiation is a storage ring, which uses bending magnets to maintain an electron beam at relativistic speeds in a closed trajectory for many hours. By bending the path of electrons at relativistic speeds, X-rays are emitted at each bending magnet in a direction that is tangential to the beam trajectory, as portrayed in Fig. 1. Synchrotron radiation generated by bending magnets produces a fan-shaped beam and has a broad and continuous spectrum from infrared to the X-ray region. The single crystal monochromator selects a single energy of synchrotron radiation. Consequently, X-rays with a small energy bandwidth are used for imaging. The monochromatic X-ray energy was adjusted by the monochromator to 33.2 keV just above the iodine K-edge energy to produce the highest contrast image of the iodine contrast agent.

An X-ray imaging system must have a high shutter speed (short exposure time) to produce sharp and blur-free images of objects. For high-speed imaging, we developed an X-ray shutter system using a moving-coil galvanometer-based optical scanner to produce pulsed monochromatic X-rays. The shutter is situated between the monochromator and the object in Fig. 1. An optical scanner is a high-accuracy mirror-positioning motor for laser optics. Figure 2 shows that after an optical mirror was removed from the galvanometer-based scanner, a rotating X-ray chopper was attached to the center shaft of the scanner. Twin tantalum blades on each side of the chopper move in a seesaw-like manner, synchronizing timing with the synchronous signals of the video camera. By about 9° rotation of the chopper, the shutter opens or closes a route for the X-ray beam. The exposure time per image was finally adjusted to 2–4 ms using the shutter (Umetani et al., 2004).

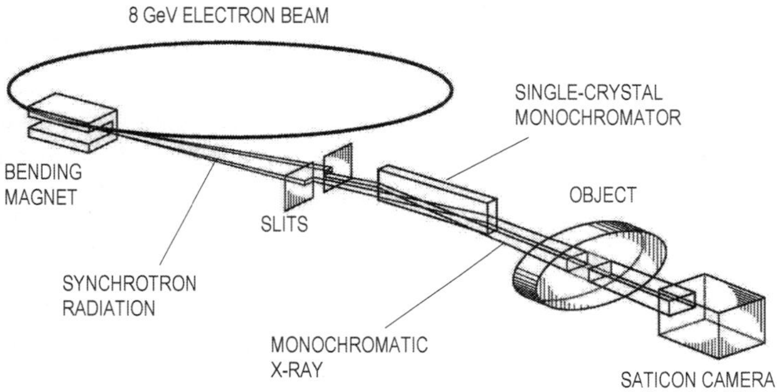

Fig. 1. Experimental arrangement for synchrotron radiation microangiographic imaging.

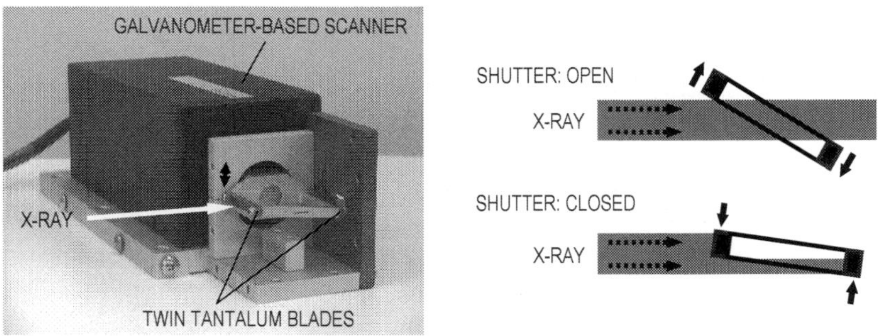

Fig. 2. Photograph of the X-ray shutter (left) and illustration of the chopper action (right).

Pulsed monochromatic X-rays transmitted through the object are detected using the X-ray direct-conversion type detector depicted in Fig. 3, which incorporates the X-ray SATICON pickup tube. The camera system comprises a camera head incorporating the X-ray SATICON pickup tube and a camera control unit with an analog-to-digital converter for digital signal output. The X-ray direct-conversion type SATICON tube consists of a photoconductive target layer of amorphous selenium. Absorbed X-rays in the photoconductive layer of the tube are converted directly into electron-hole pairs. Charge carriers generated by X-rays are transported across the photoconductive layer by an electric field. Then, a charge-density pattern is formed on the photoconductive layer surface. To produce a video signal, a scanning beam of low-velocity electrons reads out the electrostatic image on the surface.

This X-ray SATICON camera for biomedical imaging has resolution of 1050 scanning lines. It can record images at a maximum rate of 30 frame/s. Sequential images were obtained with an input field of view of 4.5 mm × 4.5 mm. By synchronizing the timing with the camera's synchronous pulse signals, image signals can be converted into a digital format and stored in a frame memory with a format of 1024 × 1024 pixels and 10-bit resolution. An equivalent pixel size projected onto the input window was 4.5 μm for a 1024 × 1024-pixel format.

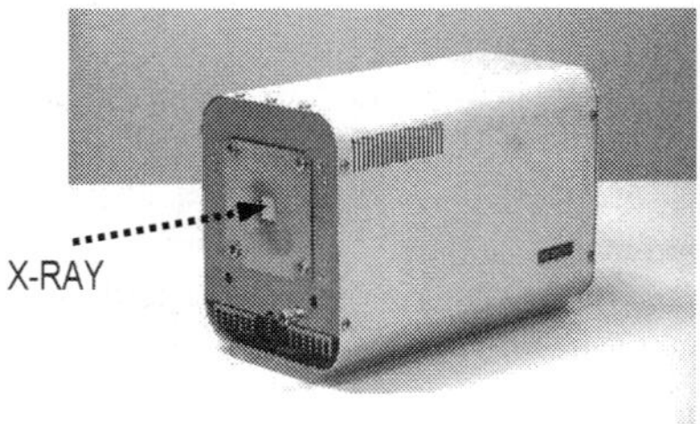

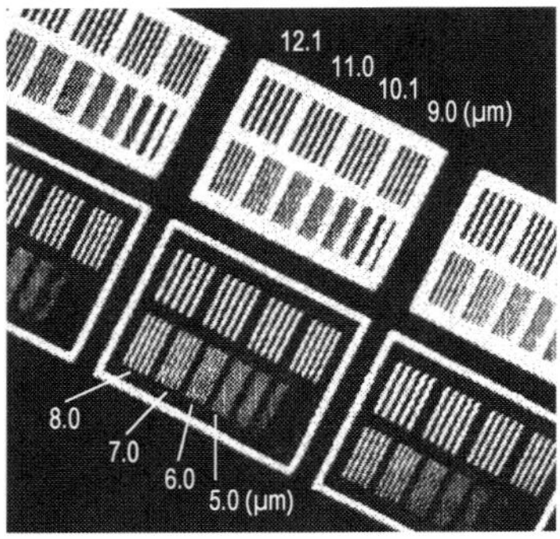

Fig. 3. Photograph of the X-ray SATICON camera (left) and zoomed image of the central area of the 5-μm-thick chart. Numerical values show bar widths (right).

The input field of view of the X-ray SATICON camera was adjusted to 9.5 mm × 9.5 mm for depiction of tumor-derived angiogenic vessels in a rabbit model of cancer (Umetani et al., 2003). In coronary microangiography, the detector's input field of view was reduced to 4.5 mm × 4.5 mm for higher spatial resolution imaging. Performance of the direct-conversion type detector was evaluated by taking images of a custom-designed gold resolution chart. The chart thickness was 5 μm; the bar pattern widths were 5.0–12.1 μm. An X-ray image of the chart with micrometer-scale bar patterns was obtained in the zoom-imaging mode of the detector with the 4.5 mm × 4.5 mm field of view at an X-ray energy of 20.0 keV. Figure 3 (right) presents an image of the 5-μm-thick chart in which the 6.0-μm-wide bars are visible. The limiting spatial resolution is between 5.0 and 6.0 μm in the zoom imaging mode. The 6.0 μm bar width is comparable to the capillary blood vessels' size. Images of the capillaries are obtainable using an X-ray energy of 33.2 keV just above the iodine K-edge energy, which produces the highest contrast image of the iodine contrast agent if capillaries are opacified using a high-density contrast agent. In reality, however, the contrast agent is diluted substantially in the blood flow.

The distance between the source in the bending magnet and the detector is about 46 m. A nearly parallel X-ray beam was used for imaging without image blur because of the small X-ray source and the extremely long source-to-object distance. The storage ring was operated at 8 GeV electron beam energy; the beam current was 100 mA. Monochromatic X-ray energy was adjusted to 33.2 keV using the monochromator. The X-ray flux at the object position was ca. 1×10^{10} photon/mm^2/s in imaging experiments.

3. Angiographic Imaging

3.1 Animal experiments

Acetylcholine, adenosine triphosphate, and sodium nitroprusside are vasoactive agents inducing endothelium-dependent vasodilatation through the release of endogenous nitric oxide, a nitro vasodilator. We conducted an experimental study of microangiography in isolated perfused rat hearts to evaluate the vascular response for vasoactive agents by measuring internal diameters of small blood vessels on the baseline and under stress of vasoactive agents in rat models of hypertension and diabetes.

Wistar rats weighing about 300 g were used for imaging. The rats were anesthetized with sodium pentobarbital, after which heparin, an anticoagulant, was administered intraperitoneally. After an abdominal incision was made, the heart was excised. The isolated rat heart was mounted on a steel cannula, secured with a suture, as portrayed in Fig. 4, and perfused with oxygenated perfusion fluid (a modified Krebs–Henseleit buffer 95%O_2 + 5%CO_2 warmed to 37°C). Perfusion fluid was directed into blood vessels and perfused through the entire mass of the organ.

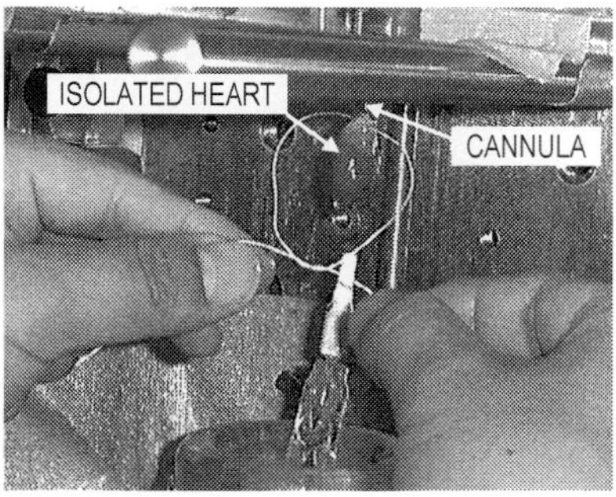

Fig. 4. Isolated perfused rat heart. The aorta was secured to the cannula with a suture.

In the isolated rat heart, contractile function and regular heart rhythm returned within a few seconds. Maximum function was established in several minutes. Arterioles in coronary arteries were visualized by injection of iodine contrast agent into the ascending aorta. The volume of the non-ionic contrast agent used for imaging was 0.4 ml per injection at a rate of 0.2 ml/s. First, baseline angiography was performed; then the contrast agent was washed out from the isolated heart using perfusion with normal perfusate for 10 min. Next, the perfusate was changed to one containing a vasoactive agent; microangiography was performed a second time after 10 min. Microangiography was performed similarly a third and a fourth time with other agents.

Microangiographic images were obtained sequentially at a rate of 30 frame/s and at an X-ray energy of 33.2 keV just above the iodine K-edge energy in the zoom-imaging mode of the detector with the 4.5 mm × 4.5 mm field of view. For the imaging experiment, an X-ray shutter using a galvanometer-based scanner was used; the exposure time per image was adjusted to 2 ms. Images were stored in the digital-image acquisition system at 10-bit resolution and 1024 × 1024-pixel format. During the total imaging time of 1.67 s, 50 frames were acquired. All animal experiments conformed to the SPring-8 Guide for Care and Use of Laboratory Animals.

3.2 Results

The SATICON camera's field of view (4.5 mm × 4.5 mm) is limited to dimensions smaller than a rat's heart. An angiographic image produced by combining nine separate photographs presented in Fig. 5 was created to show the angiographic anatomy of all vessels in the rat heart: the left anterior descending artery (LAD), the left circumflex coronary artery (LCX), and the right coronary artery (RCA). Angiographic imaging was repeated nine times for the nine imaging regions in a normal rat heart. Each image in Fig. 5 was selected from each angiographic sequence at the same cardiac phase. Consequently, the composite image was formed using nine diastole phase images because the heart ventricles are relaxed and the heart wall motion is slow in the diastole phase.

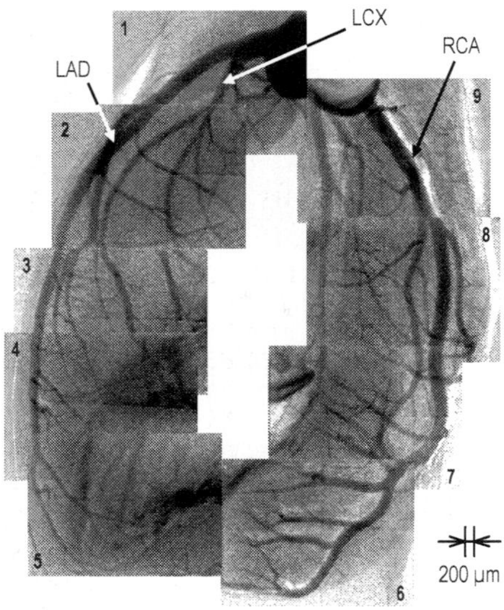

Fig. 5. Composite image of the rat coronary arteries showing the angiographic anatomy of all vessels in a rat heart. The image shows the left anterior descending artery (LAD), the left circumflex coronary artery (LCX), and the right coronary artery (RCA).

The composite whole heart image can exhibit the most suitable region for radiographical evaluation. For this study, the sixth region was selected for evaluation of diameter changes in small coronary arteries. The region includes a few of the right coronary arteries near the cardiac apex. This condition is useful to isolate individual vessels for quantitative analyses of the vessel dimensions.

Figure 6 shows representative coronary artery images of one heart cycle in a normal rat heart corresponding to the sixth region in Fig. 5. The detector's X-ray field of view was 4.5 mm × 4.5 mm in the zoom imaging mode, but the images show the area of 4.5 mm × 3.2 mm after image trimming. The interval of consecutive images was 33.3 ms; one heart cycle time was 200 ms, corresponding to a heart rate of 300 per minute. Black arrows indicate the direction of the heart wall motion at the diastole and systole phases. The second image in Fig. 6 shows the mid-systole phase in a cardiac cycle. The fourth and fifth images indicate the mid-diastole phase. Compared with the scale bars of 100 μm spacing in the first image, small blood vessels of less than 50 μm diameter were displayed in images. We have succeeded in establishing a new microangiographic technique to visualize rat coronary arteries with high spatial resolution in real time.

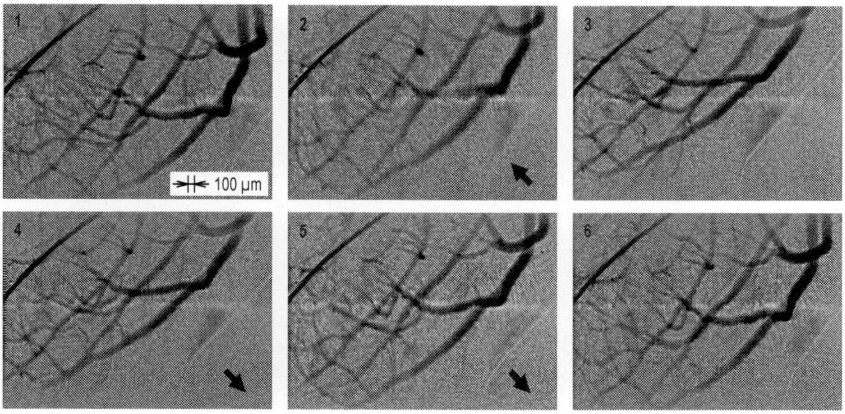

Fig. 6. Sequential images of the right coronary arteries collectively depicting one heart cycle. The interval is 33.3 ms in consecutive images. Black arrows indicate the direction of the heart wall motion.

We directly investigated the effects of hypertension and diabetes on the response of small arteries to drugs. Then, we demonstrated vessel dilation by drug manipulation because the drugs used for this study are known to induce vessel dilation. Figure 7 portrays three sets of right coronary artery images showing the effects of drug manipulation in normal (left column), hypertensive (center column), and diabetic (right column) rat hearts. Each image shows an area of 4.5 mm × 4.5 mm, which is the same as the detector's field of view. In each column, the first images in the top are the baseline angiogram, the second ones depict responses of coronary arteries under the influence of acetylcholine, the third ones depict the influence of adenosine triphosphate, and the fourth ones depict the influence of sodium nitroprusside. These images portray typical diameter changes or no change of small coronary arteries in response to vasoactive agents. In each column, four pairs of white arrows indicate the same coronary arteries with vessel diameters of less than 200 μm.

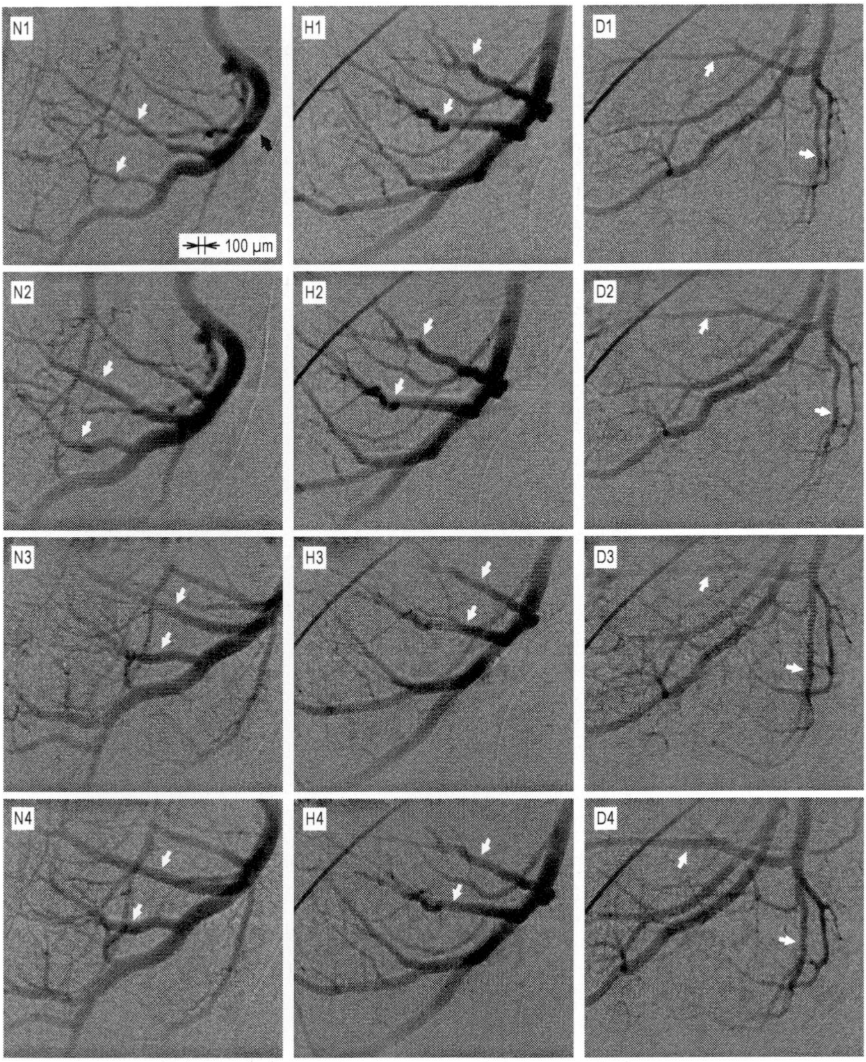

Fig. 7. Three sets of right coronary artery images showing the effects of drug manipulation in normal (N1–N4), hypertensive (H1–H4), and diabetic (D1–D4) rat hearts: (N1, H1 and D1) baseline, (N2, H2 and D2) acetylcholine stress, (N3, H3 and D3) adenosine triphosphate stress, and (N4, H4 and D4) sodium nitroprusside stress.

Small arteries of less than 200 μm diameter are called resistance vessels. The vascular resistance regulates the blood flow by changing the vessel diameter. Only small arteries have a blood flow regulation function. In the normal rat, vasodilatation, indicated by white arrows in the left column of Fig. 7, was observed in small arteries of less than approximately 200 μm diameter, whereas major trunk vessels (black arrow in Fig. 7(N1)), from which small arteries branch directly, showed almost no change of internal diameter caused by vasoactive agents. The existence of regulation function is determined by the diameter of individual vessels. Third-order branches of coronary arteries are visible in Fig. 7 (N2–N4). Furthermore, new arterial branches are visible in Fig. 7 (N3 and N4). Diameters of these new branches are 20–30 μm. On the other hand, in the hypertensive rat, the four images in Fig. 7 (H1–H4) exhibit no change in vascular caliber (white arrows) over time. Moreover, in the rat with diabetes, the second image in Fig. 7 (D2) shows no change of diameter in acetylcholine stress but the third and fourth images in Fig. 7 (D3 and D4) show vascular response to adenosine triphosphate and sodium nitroprusside stress. New arterial branches with diameters of 20–30 μm are also visible in Fig. 7 (D3 and D4).

4. Discussion

We specifically examined the small arteries (white arrows) that branch off directly from the major trunk (black arrow in N1) in the normal rat image in Fig. 7. Diameters of the arteries (N2–N4) indicated by white arrows were increased by almost two times through dilation compared to the baseline arteries (N1). Furthermore, the apparent increase in the number of small vessels with diameters of less than 50 μm was observed (N3 and N4) because the vasoactive agents might increase the diameter not only of intermediate-size vessels, but also of invisible small blood vessels to visible sizes. Comparison with the scale bars of 100 μm spacing shows that these small arteries have diameters of 20-30 μm. On the other hand, diameters of the arteries larger than 200 μm showed no diameter change. Vessel dilation of the coronary arteries depends greatly on the vascular size. Only small arteries with diameters less than 200 μm have a dilation function. We established a new microangiographic technique to visualize diameter changes and the apparent increase in the number of small vessels in rat coronary arteries with high spatial resolution in real time. The present imaging system enables the direct evaluation of vasodilatation caused by acetylcholine, adenosine triphosphate, and sodium nitroprusside stress.

For the hypertensive rat heart shown in the center column of Fig. 7, no artery exhibited a change of diameter. The images do not display a vascular response to the three vasoactive agents; the results showed that the vasoactive-agent-induced relaxation was considerably impaired. Hypertension can damage the arteries' inner walls. The results reveal the mechanism and effect of disease: vessel dilation of the arteries might be specifically impaired in hypertension. Impairment of vessel dilation function might result in cardiovascular diseases.

For the heart of the rat with diabetes shown in the right column of Fig. 7, the images do not exhibit vascular response to acetylcholine stress but show a response to adenosine triphosphate and sodium nitroprusside stress. However, rates of increase in vessel diameter and in the number of small vessels in dilation compared to the baseline angiogram were smaller than those in the normal rat. We were able to visualize variations in the response among the three vasoactive agents. Acetylcholine-induced relaxation was impaired significantly by dysfunction of the inner walls of arteries, although marked impairment was not observed in adenosine triphosphate and sodium nitroprusside stress. This imaging system can visualize the severity of relaxation impairment directly.

Hypertension and diabetes can cause the inner walls' dysfunction. The synchrotron radiation microangiography system was suitable to investigate characteristics of vascular endothelial function in coronary arteries of rats by taking high-resolution, real-time images. The present system offers the potential of direct investigation into the mechanisms of vascular dysfunctions and is useful to evaluate the severity of damage to arterial inner walls resulting from hypertension and diabetes.

5. Conclusion

Microangiographic imaging with spatial resolution in the micrometer range and at an exposure time of 2 ms was conducted using the combination of the high-speed shutter, the direct-conversion detector, and the nearly parallel X-ray beam provided at SPring-8. Small cardiac blood vessels of less than 50-μm diameter were visualized at heart rates of around 300 per minute in isolated perfused rat hearts. Furthermore, the apparent increase in the number of small vessels with diameters of 20–30 μm was observed after the vasoactive agents increased the diameter not only of intermediate-size vessels, but also that of the invisible small blood vessels to visible sizes. This synchrotron radiation imaging system is a useful tool for depicting large and small coronary arteries in fast-moving hearts and for quantifying actual changes in their diameter caused by vasoactive agents.

Isolated perfused organs provide excellent test-beds for undertaking carefully controlled dose-response studies. Furthermore, these measurements can be made in the absence of confounding effects of other organs. The present imaging system is useful for precise study not only of vascular response, but also of endothelial and smooth muscle function in small blood vessels of less than 50 μm diameter in an isolated perfused heart. Particularly in rat models of metabolic syndrome, the relaxation in response to vasoactive agents can be impaired in coronary arteries compared to normal rats. This angiographic technique will be beneficial for evaluating vascular endothelial dysfunction attributable to metabolic syndrome. Aside from isolated perfused organs, this system offers the potential to investigate mechanisms of vascular dysfunctions directly in any vascular bed (Shirai et al., 2009).

An X-ray imaging system must have a high shutter speed to produce sharp and blur-free images of objects. After the present experiments using the galvanometer-based X-ray shutter system, we developed a rotating-disk X-ray shutter for higher speed imaging. The shutter consists of two disks with radial slots rotating about an axis that is parallel to the X-ray beam. The radial slot width can be changed to adjust the duration of X-ray pulses according to the rotation of one disk with another one. The disks also rotate to match the timing with synchronous signals of the video camera. Using this new shutter system, we have been performing a new line of imaging experiments to investigate the mechanisms of vascular dysfunctions in various vascular beds (Kidoguchi et al., 2006; Morishita et al., 2006; Iwasaki et al., 2007; Shirai et al., 2009).

The authors would like to thank Mr. Tadaaki Hirai and Mr. Toshiaki Kawai of Hamamatsu Photonics K.K. for development of the X-ray SATICON tube. The authors also thank Mr. Sadao Takahashi of Hitachi Denshi Techno-System, Ltd. and Mr. Norio Iwanaga of Zenisu Keisoku Inc. for development of the camera and frame memory system. Synchrotron radiation experiments were performed at the SPring-8 BL28B2 beamline with the approval of the Japan Synchrotron Radiation Research Institute (Acceptance Nos. 2004A0128, 2005A0104, 2006A1493, 2006B1093, and 2007B1052).

6. References

Colby, L. A. & Morenko, B. J. (2004). Clinical considerations in rodent bioimaging, *Comp Med*, 54, 6, pp. 623–630

Dix, W. -R.; Kupper, W.; Dill, T.; Hamm, C. W.; Job, H.; Lohmann, M.; Reime, B. & Ventura, R. (2003). Comparison of intravenous coronary angiography using synchrotron radiation with selective coronary angiography, *J Synchrotron Rad*, 10, pp. 219–227

Grundy, S. M.; Brewer, Jr, H. B.; Cleeman, J. I.; Smith, Jr, S. C. & Lenfant, C. (2004). Definition of metabolic syndrome, Circulation, 109, pp. 433–438

Iwasaki, H.; Fukushima, K.; Kawamoto, A.; Umetani, K.; Oyamada, A.; Hayashi, S.; Matsumoto, T.; Ishikawa, M.; Shibata, T.; Nishimura, H.; Hirai, H.; Mifune, Y.; Horii, M.; Sugimura, K.; Suehiro, S. & Asahara, T. (2007). Synchrotron radiation coronary microangiography for morphometric and physiological evaluation of myocardial neovascularization induced by endothelial progenitor cell transplantation, *Arterioscler Thromb Vasc Biol*, 27, 6, pp. 1326–1333

Kidoguchi, K.; Tamaki, M.; Mizobe, T.; Koyama, J.; Kondoh, T.; Kohmura, E.; Sakurai, T.; Yokono, K., & Umetani, K. (2006). In vivo X-ray angiography in the mouse brain using synchrotron radiation, *Stroke*, 37, 7, pp. 1856–1861

Mori, H.; Hyodo, K.; Tanaka, E.; Uddin-Mohammed, M.; Yamakawa, A.; Shinozaki, Y.; Nakazawa, H.; Tanaka, Y.; Sekka, T.; Iwata, Y.; Handa, S.; Umetani, K.; Ueki, H.; Yokoyama, T.; Tanioka, K.; Kubota, M.; Hosaka, H.; Ishikawa, N. & Ando, M. (1996). Small-vessel radiography in situ with monochromatic synchrotron radiation, *Radiology*, 201, pp. 173–177

Morishita, A.; Kondoh, T.; Sakurai, T.; Ikeda, M.; Bhattacharjee, A. K.; Nakajima, S., Kohmura, E.; Yokono, K. & Umetani, K. (2006). Quantification of distension in rat cerebral perforating arteries, *NeuroReport*, 17, pp. 1549–1553

Ritman, E. L. (2002). Molecular imaging in small animals—roles for micro-CT, *J Cell Biochem Supp*, 39, pp. 116–124.

Rubenstein, E.; Hofstadter, R.; Zeman, H. D.; Thompson, A. C.; Otis, J. N.; Brown, G. S.; Giacomini, J. C.; Gordon, H. J.; Kernoff, R. S.; Harrison, D. C. & Thomlinson, W. (1986). Transvenous coronary angiography in human using synchrotron radiation, *Proc Natl Acad Sci USA*, 83, pp. 9724–9728

Sada, K.; Shirai, M. & Ninomiya, I. (1985), X-ray TV system for measuring microcirculation in small pulmonary vessels, *J Appl Physiol*, 59, pp. 1013–1018

Shirai, M.; Ikeda, S.; Min, K. -Y.; Shimouchi, A.; Kawaguchi, T. & Ninomiya, I. (1999). Segmental difference in vasodilatation due to basal NO release in in vivo cat pulmonary vessels, *Respir Physiol*, 116, pp. 159–169

Shirai, M.; Schwenke, D. O.; Eppel, G. A.; Evans, R. G.; Edgley, A. J.; Tsuchimochi, H.; Umetani, K. & Pearson, J. T. (2009). Synchrotron-based angiography for investigation of the regulation of vasomotor function in the microcirculation in vivo, *Clin Exp Pharmacol Physiol*, 36, pp. 107–116

Service, R. F. (1999). Scanners get a fix on lab animals, *Science*, 286, pp. 2261–2263

Umetani, K.; Yamashita, T.; Maehara, N.; Tokiya, R.; Imai, S. & Kajihara, Y. (2003). Small-field angiographic imaging of tumor blood vessels in rabbit auricle using X-ray SATICON camera and synchrotron radiation, *Proceedings of 25th Annual International IEEE EMBS Conference*, Cancún, September 17-21, pp. 978–981

Umetani, K.; Fukushima, K. & Sugimura, K. (2004). Synchrotron radiation microangiography for observation of vasodilatation using X-ray SATICON, *the Journal of the Institute of Image Information and Television Engineers*, 58, 3, pp. 344-351 (in Japanese)

Umetani, K.; Fukushima, K. & Sugimura, K. (2008). Microangiography system for investigation of metabolic syndrome in rat model using synchrotron radiation, *Proceedings of 30th Annual International IEEE EMBS Conference*, Vancouver, August 20-24, pp. 2693-2696

Yamashita, T.; Kawashima, S.; Ozaki, M.; Namiki, M.; Shinohara, M.; Inoue, N.; Hirata, K.; Umetani, K. & Yokoyama, M. (2002). In vivo angiographic detection of vascular lesions in apolipoprotein e-knockout mice using a synchrotron radiation microangiography system, *Circ J*, 66, pp. 1057-1059

7

Wireless Power Technology for Biomedical Implants

Anthony N. Laskovski, Tharaka Dissanayake and Mehmet R. Yuce
The University of Newcastle
Australia

1. Introduction

Biomedical Implants require a clean and medically safe source of energy to perform their operations. Early implants such as pacemakers sourced their power from small lithium ion batteries. While this solution allows for the operation of the implantable device without a wire connecting the internal and external circuitry, limited battery life causes the impracticality, health risks and expense of operating on patients for the mere purpose of replacing the battery.

A significant development in the supply of power to implantable devices is the use of inductive coupling to charge an implantable rechargeable battery. The concept may be understood by considering two windings of a weakly coupled transformer, where the core is in fact a large air gap as shown in Fig. 1. The primary winding is the transmission coil, and the secondary winding is the receiving coil. Numerous applications have been developed along this wireless battery charging idea, varying in size, frequency and coil structure (Li & Bashirullah, 2007; Lim et al., 2005).

The concept of wireless battery charging has been extended to the idea of supplying power only wirelessly, where implanted batteries are not used at all. Real-time powering systems save a considerable amount of implant space; however they require the constant supply of wireless energy to the implant.

Wireless power transfer has generally been implemented in the kHz to MHz range, and the transfer of energy becomes less efficient as the frequency of transmission increases (Vaillancourt et al. 1997). In addition to making circuit elements smaller, this naturally makes the design of highly efficient transmission circuits a point of interest.

The use of wireless power technology in implantable devices led to a more flexible range of applications which were not otherwise possible; retinal prosthesis being one such example.

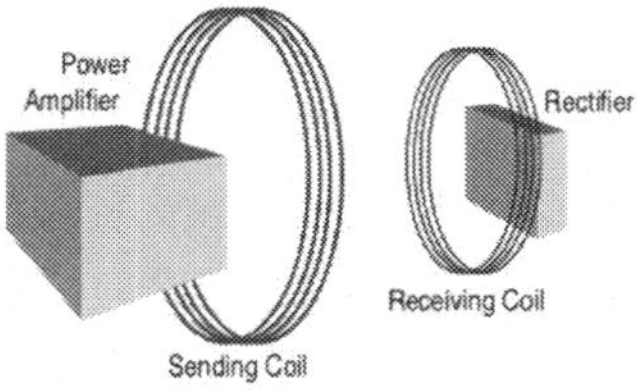

Fig. 1. A general block diagram showing the flow of power to an implantable device.

Implanted devices generally consist of power and data receiving-coils. The power signal is generally rectified and used to store energy or directly supply the implant's electronic blocks. The data signal is demodulated and supplied to an implanted processor, which turns the information into a form understood by an actuator, which stimulates the body as required.

Medical prosthesis generally involves sending a signal to a transducer in order to conduct a particular function, which the body cannot perform. Fig. 2 shows a general block diagram of a prosthetic device, where information is processed and sent to the implant wirelessly. It is further processed and sent to the organ being stimulated. An example of prosthesis is muscular stimulation, where a signal is sent from an electronic device directly to muscle fibres to stimulate muscles in cases where the nervous system fails to do so. Another example of prosthesis is the Bionic Eye.

Telemetry involves using an implant used to monitor a particular parameter in the body, such as temperature, blood pressure, or other parameters which electronic transducers have been designed for. Implanted telemetry units generally comprise blocks similar to those used in prosthesis units. Fig. 3 shows a block diagram of a telemetry device, where information is sensed, digitised, modulated and wirelessly transmitted to an external device.

The supply of power to both prosthetic and telemetric implants involves similar principles. An oscillating unit produces the desired transmission frequency, a power amplifier, power transmission coils and rectifiers.

2. Switched Power Amplifiers

The supply of wireless power to biomedical implants begins with power amplifiers, which supply energy to an antenna or coil at a particular frequency. As the size of implants decreases so does the available space for receiving antennas. This leads to shorter wavelength antennas and lower size constraints for coils, which increases the frequency of power transmission. Higher transmission frequencies place a particular focus on utilising power amplifiers, which operate efficiently at these levels. Switched power amplifiers have been a popular choice to drive inductive power links for implantable electronics due to their ability to minimise losses at higher frequencies. Three types of such amplifier configurations will be discussed in this section.

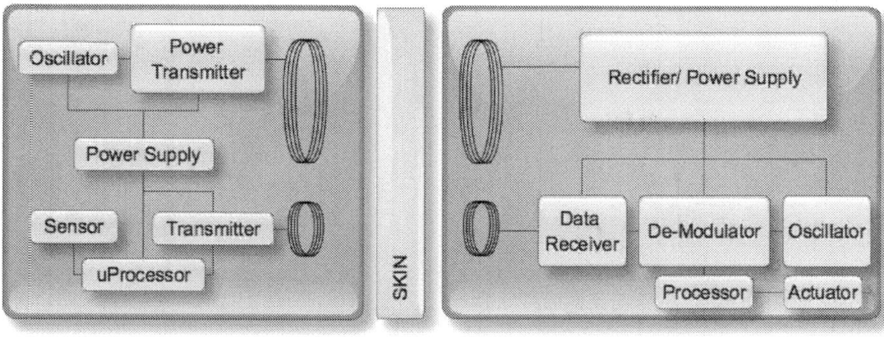

Fig. 2. A block diagram of a prosthesis system, where the external element is on the left and the internal element on the right.

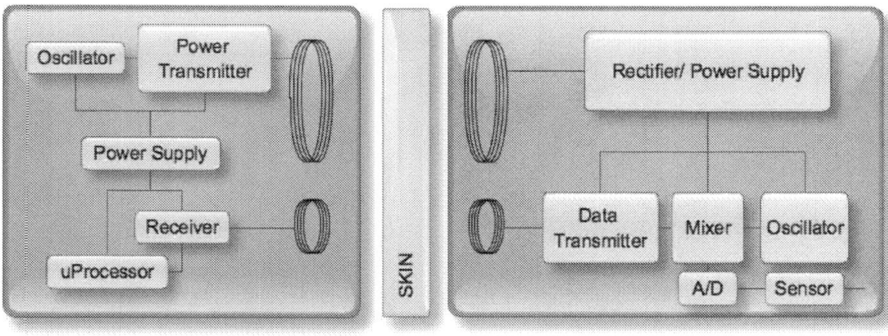

Fig. 3. A block diagram of a telemetry system, where the external element is on the left and the internal element on the right.

2.1 Class-D Amplifier

The Class-D amplifier consists of an inverter, which switches two transistors on and off alternatively to generate a theoretically square wave. The output of the inverter is connected to a series RLC network as shown in Fig. 4, which is resonant at the fundamental frequency of the square-wave, producing a sinusoidal signal at this frequency. The gain of the amplifier is given by (1) as a function of R, L, C elements shown in Fig. 4. The theoretical efficiency of the Class-D amplifier is 100%, which assumes that all circuit elements are ideal.

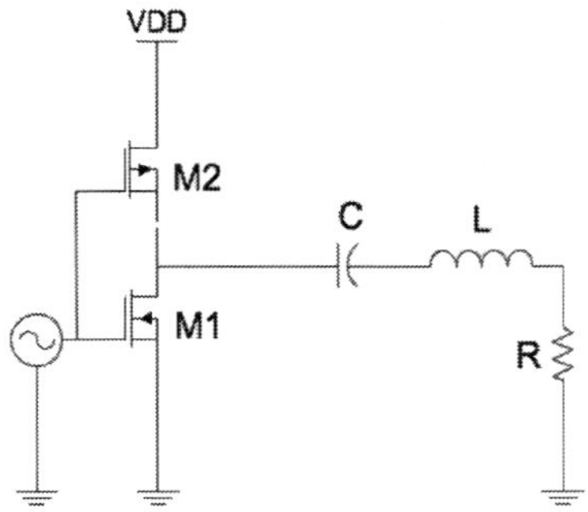

Fig. 4. Class-D power amplifier

$$\frac{v_{out}}{v_{in}} = \frac{s\frac{R}{L}}{s^2 + s\frac{R}{L} + \frac{1}{LC}} \tag{1}$$

In reality, circuit elements are not ideal and several losses have been analysed with a focus on parasitic drain-source capacitance in each of the transistors, which becomes significant in higher frequency RF designs (El-Hamamsy, 1994).

The drain-source capacitance, C_{ds} actually introduces a capacitor where an otherwise open circuit should ideally exist and at high frequencies, typical capacitor values are in the order of pico Farads. This means that parasitic capacitance C_{ds} becomes a significant circuit element, which allows the dissipation of energy during switching cycles thus decreasing the amplifier's efficiency.

2.2 Class-E Amplifier

The Class-E amplifier, shown in Fig. 5 is a circuit designed for high frequency applications, making its application suitable as a power transmitter for biomedical implants (Troyk, 1992). It comprises a capacitor C_1 across the transistor terminals, which absorbs the transistor's parasitic capacitance and forms a key component of the circuit's high efficiency operation at high frequencies by shaping the voltage across its terminals in a particular way.

The principle of the class-E amplifier's high efficiency operation lies in the shape of the voltage across C_1, which is shown in Fig. 6. Parameters for the amplifier are chosen such that the voltage at this point is zero when the transistor is switched on such that no stored energy is dissipated from the capacitor. The voltage is shaped such that the rate of change of voltage (dv_{c1}/dt) across this point is also zero (Sokal,N.O. & Sokal A., 1975; Kazimierczuk, M., 1986; Sokal, N.O., 2000). This feature enables robustness to phase or frequency irregularities in practice.

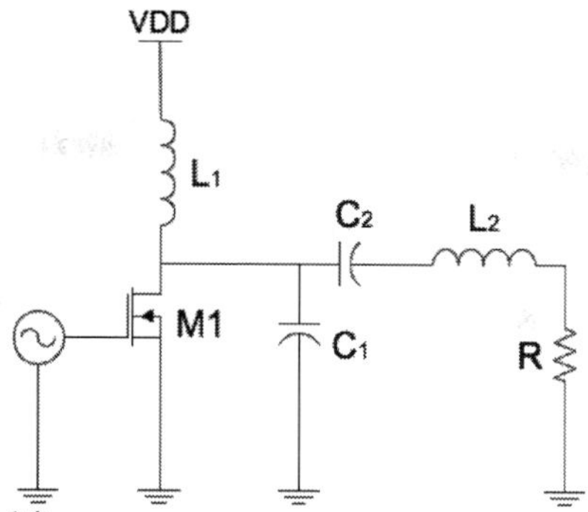

Fig. 5. Class-E power amplifier

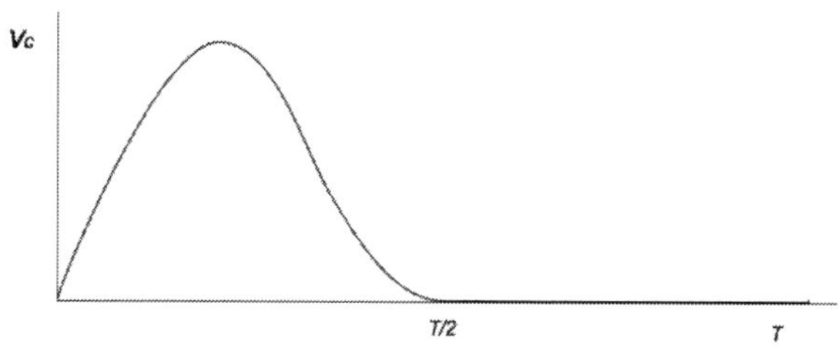

Fig. 6. Voltage across C_1 for one period.

Analysing the amplifier in the frequency domain is an elegant way to model the performance of the circuit. The small signal model corresponding to the Class-E amplifier is shown in Fig. 7. It is possible to interpret the input signal supplied to the class-E amplifier as a series of alternating step inputs, as shown in Fig. 8. The voltage signal supplied to the gate of the transistor (base if it is a BJT) is translated to a step increase in the current flowing through the drain. This means that parameters such as resonant frequency ω and damping factor ζ may be used to optimise the response of the class-E amplifier upon a step increase or decrease in the current. The impedance seen by the current source of Fig. 7 is expressed by (2).

$$Z_L = sL_c \parallel r_o \parallel \frac{1}{s(C_1 + C_{ds})} \parallel \left(\frac{1}{sC_2} + sL_2 + R \right) \tag{2}$$

$$Z_L = \frac{s^2 L_2 C_2 + sRC_2 + 1}{s^3 L_2 (C_1 + C_{ds}) C_2 + s^2 \left[\frac{L_2 C_2}{r_o} + R(C_1 + C_{ds}) C_2 \right] + s \left[\frac{RC_2}{r_o} + (C_1 + C_{ds}) + \frac{L_2 C_2}{L_1} + C_2 \right] + \left[\frac{1}{r_o} + \frac{RC_2}{L_1} \right] + \frac{1}{sL_1}} \tag{3}$$

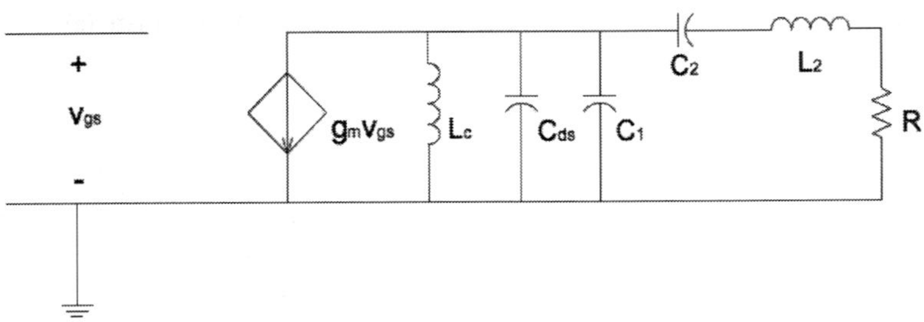

Fig. 7. Small signal model of a class-E power amplifier

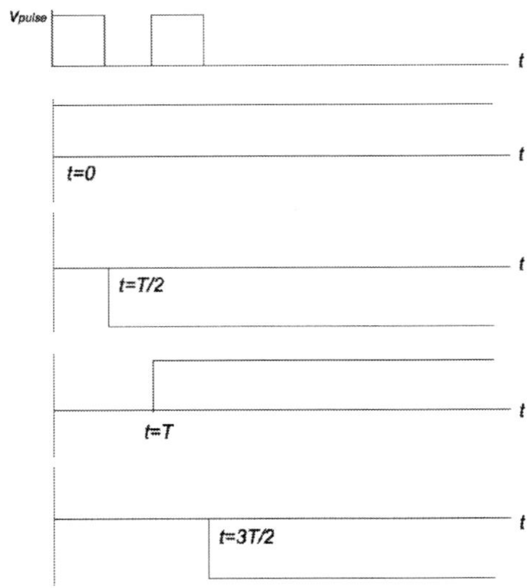

Fig. 8. A clock signal split up into several time-displaced step inputs

The expression for the voltage across C_1, called v_{in}, is determined by multiplying the impedance Z_L by a step input of *1/s*, as shown in (4).

$$v_{in} = \frac{1}{s} Z_L \tag{4}$$

The output voltage of the circuit is considered to be the voltage across the resistance R, and obtaining an expression for the output voltage is as simple as applying a voltage divider as shown in (5).

$$v_{out} = \frac{R}{R + sL_2 + \frac{1}{sC_2}} v_{in} \tag{5}$$

Substituting the expression for Z_L obtained from (3) into (4) and then (5) allows the determination of the transfer function (6).

$$\frac{v_{out}}{v_{in}} = \frac{s^2 RC_2 g_m}{s^4 L_2 (C_1 + C_{ds}) C_2 + s^3 \left[\frac{L_2 C_2}{r_o} + R(C_1 + C_{ds}) C_2 \right] + s^2 \left[\frac{RC_2}{r_o} + (C_1 + C_{ds}) + \frac{L_2 C_2}{L_1} + C_2 \right] + s \left[\frac{1}{r_o} + \frac{RC_2}{L_1} \right] + \frac{1}{L_1}} \quad (6)$$

The conditions that allow for the maximum transfer of power occur when the denominator of (6) is minimal, that is when the *j*-component is zero. Using the relationship $s=j\omega$ the expression (7) shows the resonant frequency with respect to circuit parameters.

$$\omega_n = \sqrt{\frac{\frac{1}{r_o} + \frac{RC_2}{L_1}}{\frac{L_2 C_2}{r_o} + R(C_1 + C_{ds})C_2}} \quad (7)$$

If the parasitic elements of r_o and C_{ds} are approximated to very large and very small values respectively, the transfer function in (6) will become:

$$\frac{v_{out}}{v_{in}} = \frac{RC_2 g_m}{s^2 L_2 C_1 C_2 + sRC_1 C_2 + (C_1 + C_2)} \quad (8)$$

Since (8) is a second order transfer function, the resonant frequency ω_n and damping factor ζ are determined to be:

$$\omega_n = \sqrt{\frac{1}{L_2 C_1 \| C_2}} \quad (9)$$

$$\zeta = \frac{R}{2} \sqrt{\frac{C_1 \| C_2}{L_2}} \quad (10)$$

These two parameters are useful tools to analyse the points at which zero switching occurs. Parameters are chosen such that the resonant frequency ω_n matches that of the input signal, and the damping factor ζ is used to control the point at which zero switching occurs.

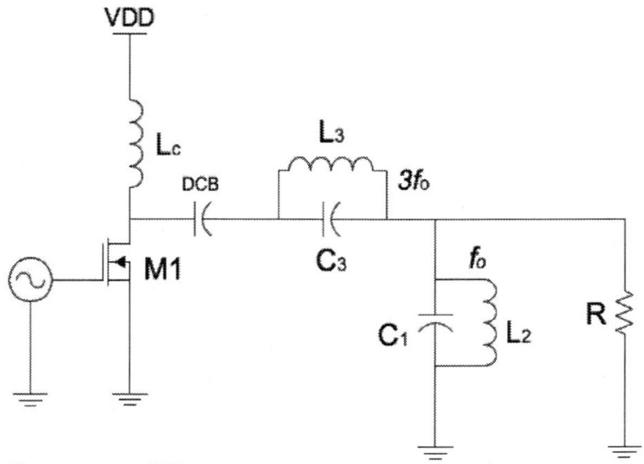

Fig. 9. The class-F power amplifier

2.3 Class-F Amplifier

The class-F amplifier, like its class-E counterpart, includes a transistor and a choke inductor. It differs from the class-E amplifier by its load network, which includes multiple resonating circuits that resonate at frequencies in the harmonic spectrum of the driving signal, which is supplied to the amplifier's input. Like its class-D counterpart, the amplifier does not account for the parasitic capacitance across the transistor's terminals, making it less commonly used as a wireless power transmitter compared to the class-E.

3. Coils and Energy Transfer

Wireless power is most commonly transferred with inductive links, which comprise primary and secondary coils that operate together as a weakly coupled transformer (Yang et al., 2007). The structure of each coil determines several factors in the coil's ability to inductively transfer power. It is important to consider the way in which different coil structures produce different field patterns. Aspects which influence the transfer of power with inductive coils involve coil size, separation, shape and performance at different orientations.

It is more efficient to transmit wireless power at lower frequencies (Vaillancourt et al. 1997), and as the complexity of implants is increasing, data rates are required to keep up with the increased sophistication. Wang et al. (2006) proposed the advantages of biomedical implants operating in dual frequency bands for sending power and data, and the dual-band concept has been extended upon in subsequent research. The optimal orientation of power and data coils were determined to be orthogonal, based on interference and spatial restrictions (Silay et al., 2008).

3.1 Spiral Coils

Biomedical implants mostly employ traditional wire-wound cylindrical inductors for the power transmitting and receiving coils. Zeirhofer & Hochmair (1996) investigated the enhancement of magnetic coupling between coils using a geometric approach. It is concluded that coupling is enhanced when turns of the coil are distributed across the radii rather than concentrating them at the outer radius of the inductors. Printed spiral coils are therefore worthwhile investigating for use in biomedical implants.

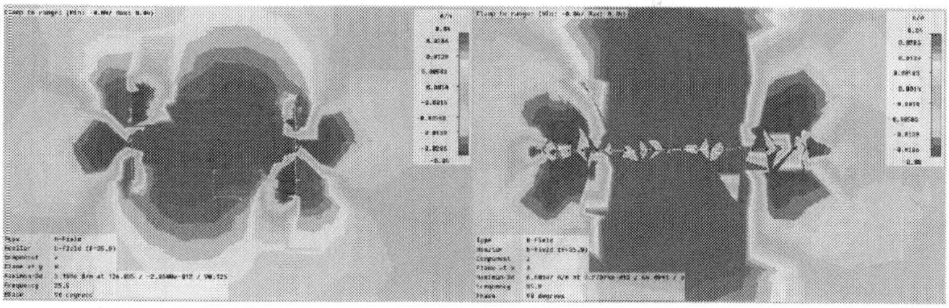

(a) (b)

Fig. 10. A comparison of flux patterns for two similarly sized coils simulated in CST. (a)The coil on the left is a cylindrical helix coil, while the one on the right (b) is an Archimedean planar spiral.

Spiral coils are not always suitable for biomedical implants. Implementing a spiral coil for retinal prosthesis for example (Wang et al. 2006) may not be desirable from an aesthetic or psychological perspective. Similarly, if a large number of turns are required, the equivalent spiral coil would be much larger.

3.2 Spiral Coil Arrays

Research in this field has focused mainly on optimising certain orientations of primary and secondary coils, from finding optimal coupling factors to space-efficient packaging. In situations such as pre-clinical monitoring, the issues related to wireless power transfer to implanted devices become more difficult to manage, mainly due to random and variable movement by the subject of the experiments.

A common pre-clinical scenario involves an enclosure in which the subject is free to move. Zimmerman et al. (2006) investigated the optimisation of wireless power transfer in such a situation, monitoring the overall transfer efficiency by varying transmission frequency and the number of turns on the secondary coil, which was 1cm from the primary coil. The system produced 3V at 1.3mA in the implant itself, accounting for a tilting angle of 60^{0}. The primary coil was a cylindrical wire-wound coil, wrapped around the circumference of the base of the enclosure.

Fig. 10 shows the difference in field patterns between two similarly sized coils in the order of 100mm x 100mm, one a cylindrically wire-wound coil and the other, a planar Archimedean spiral as simulated by advanced electromagnetic simulation software from

Computer Simulation Technologies (CST™). The green areas in the colour plot show zero magnetic field intensity. The spiral coil produces a stronger field for a similar size, which makes it a clear point of interest to investigate for a power transfer scenario in an enclosure. The planar profile of the coil is also less intrusive. If a single power transmission coil is implemented on the base of an enclosure as a spiral, it is interesting to consider the fact that the magnetic field produced by the coil will not be uniform. In fact, it varies greatly within the spatial limits of the spiral, as shown in Fig. 12 (a) and (b). Note that there are permanent "blind spots" within which the secondary coil will not be able to receive any energy.

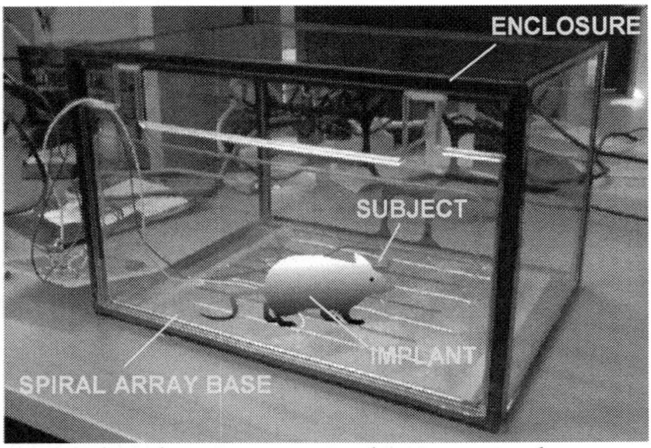

Fig. 11. A sample pre-clinical testing scenario showing an enclosure, n array of spirals connected in series and parallel and a subject.

This leads to the idea of producing an array of several small coils, connected in series or parallel networks, depending on the desired array's impedance. Fig. 12(b) shows a simulation conducted in an identical scenario and scale to that of Fig. 12(a) . It is evident that there are smaller and less powerful neutral areas, appearing green, while having more distributed and more intense zones. This idea was extended to a simulation of 20 coils connected in an array. Fig. 13 shows that the z-component of the magnetic field level on the surface of the base had very few neutral green zones.

The behaviour of the spiral array should be investigated further, by experimenting with materials of different dielectric constants, eventually introducing non-live tissue such as raw meat, with the aim to resemble its performance in an implanted environment. Fig. 13 shows the system concept of collecting data from an implant in a mouse roaming on the spiral array base. The orientation of the mouse varies and simulations are required to understand the coupling between the spiral array base and the implanted coil.

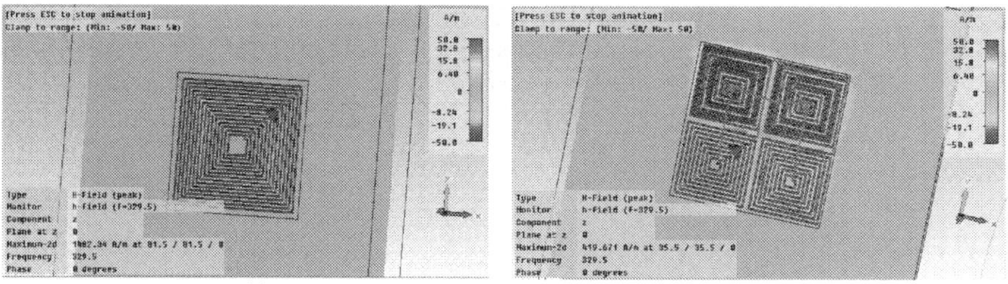

(a) (b)

Fig. 12. A comparison between two scenarios simulated in CST. (a) The magnetic field pattern of the z-vector on the plane of the spiral. (b) Four spirals covering the same area as (a).

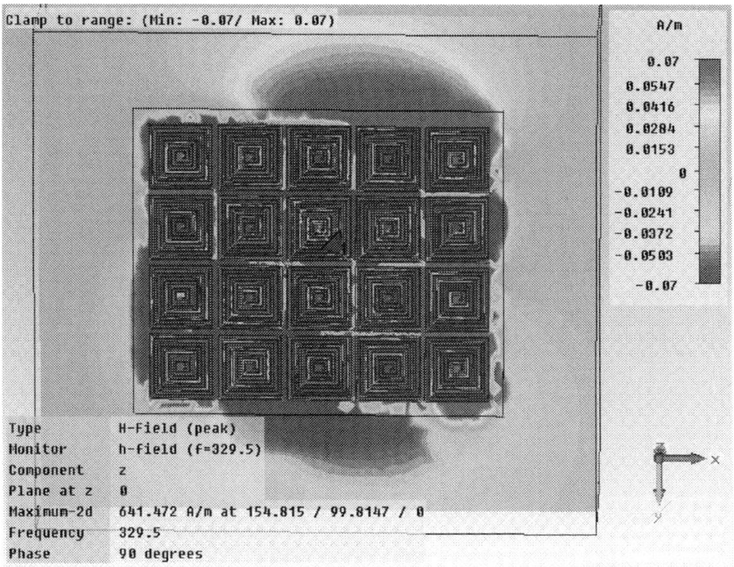

Fig. 13. A simulation conducted on CST to determine the magnetic field patterns of an array of 20 spiral coils.

4. Rectification

Rectification is an important element of wireless power transfer, in that it is vital to capture and utilise the power received at the secondary coils of the implant. In higher power non-biomedical applications, rectification is a straightforward task. Diode bridges and voltage regulating units such as the ones shown in Fig. 14(a)-(b) are typical examples. However, implementing this at higher frequencies with lower power levels is difficult. The first obstacle is the diode, which is the basic building block of any rectifier. It has an immediate voltage drop ranging from 0.1 to 0.7V, depending on the type of diode, meaning that it is favourable to use less number of diodes in most medical inductive power transfer applications (Li & Bashirullah, 2007; Chaimanonart & Young, 2006; Zimmerman et al., 2006). The highest frequencies used to transfer power inductively are in the order of MHz, and most designs simply send more power to compensate for the forward voltage drop of the rectification diodes (Sauer et al., 2005).

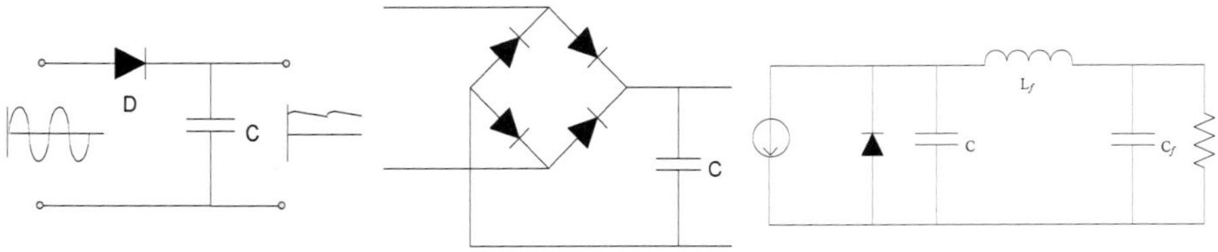

(a) (b) (c)

Fig. 14. (a) Half-wave diode rectifier. (b) Full-wave bridge rectifier. (c) Class-E rectifier (Kazimierczuk, 1989).

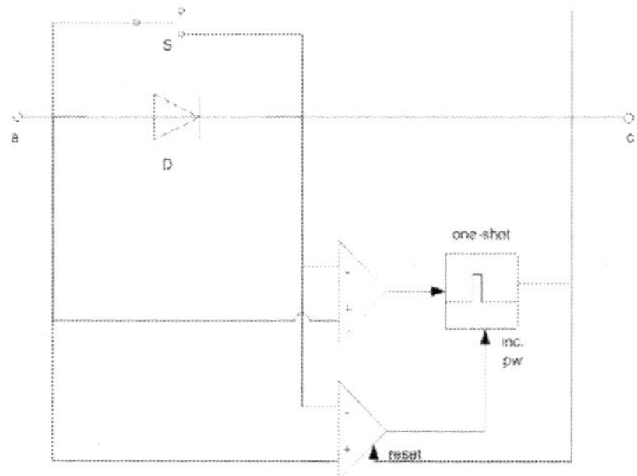

Fig. 15 An active diode presented by Lehmann & Moghe (2005)

The Class-E rectifier, shown in Fig. 14(c), has the potential to work well at high frequencies in implantable devices. It is designed for high efficiency operation at high frequencies due to its zero switching properties. It is mostly used in DC/DC converters (Kazimierczuk & Jozwik, 1989; Reatti et al., 1993), and despite not having been implemented in biomedical applications, it is an attractive circuit for use in implantable electronics.

A concept introduced by Lehmann & Moghe (2005) aims to remove the voltage drop on a rectifier all together by using comparators to sense the initiation of the diode's forward-bias, then sending a one-shot pulse to a switch, allowing the energy to bypass the diode and supply the load, as shown in Fig. 15. The concept has been tested with an input voltage at 5 MHz and the target implant supply voltage at 3V with variable loads of 2kΩ and 10kΩ. The results from these investigations show up to a 70% increase in received power compared with an on-chip passive rectifier.

5. Conclusion

This chapter has presented an overview of current techniques in the field of wireless power transfer technology for biomedical implants, including the types and theory behind switch mode power amplifiers, techniques in transmitting between two coils, and the types of rectification employed in implantable devices. System optimization can be achieved in all three sections. Class-E power amplifiers provide a robust and highly efficient means to transmit power to implantable devices due to their zero voltage and voltage derivative switching. The magnetic coupling between the primary and secondary coils can be analysed using full wave simulators. This enables one to achieve optimized coil designs after taking tissue properties and device orientation into account. The arraying technique of primary coils has shown promising results in eliminating blind spots. Several interesting solutions are developing for the rectification of received power to implants, including creative ways of avoiding voltage drops across diodes, which are a fundamental element of rectification.

6. References

Chaimanonart, N.; Young, D. (2006). Remote rf powering system for wireless mems strain sensors. *Sensors Journal, IEEE.* Vol.6, No. 2 (April 2006) page numbers (484-489).

El-Hamamsy, S.-A, (1994). Design of high-efficiency rf class-d power amplifier. *Power Electronics, IEEE Transactions on,* Vol. 9, No. 3, (May, 1994) page numbers (297-308).

Kazimierczuk, M. (1986). Class E tuned power amplifier with nonsinusoidal output voltage. *Solid state Circuits, IEEE Journal of,* Vol. 21, No. 4 (August 1986) page numbers (575-581)

Kazimierczuk, M. & Jozwik, J. (1989). Resonant dc/dc converter with class-e inverter and class-e rectifier. *Industrial Electronics, IEEE Transactions on.* Vol. 36, No. 4, (November 1989) page numbers (468-478)

Lehmann, T. & Moghe, Y. (2005). On-chip active power rectifiers for biomedical applications. *Circuits and systems, 2005. ISCAS 2005. IEEE International Symposium on.* pp. 732-735, ISSN 0-7803-8834-8/05, Kobe, Japan, May 2005.

Li, P. & Bashirullah, R. (2007) A wireless power interface for rechargeable battery operated medical implants. *Circuits and Systems II: express Briefs, IEEE Transactions on [see also Circuits and Systems II: Analog and Digital Signal Processing, IEEE Transactions on],* Vol. 54, No. 10, (October, 2007) page numbers (912-916).

Lim, H.; Yoon, C.; Lee, I.; Park, B.; Song B. & Cho, J. (2005). Implementation of a transcutaneous charger for fully implantable middle ear hearing device. *IEEE-EMBS 2005. 27th Annual International Conference on the Engineering in medicine and Biology Society, 2005.* pp. 6813-6816 ISSN 0-7803-8740-6, Shanghai, China, September 2005.

Raab, F. H., (2002) Power amplifiers and transmitters for RF and microwave. *Microwave theory and techniques, IEEE Transactions on,* Vol. 50, No. 3, (March, 2002) page numbers (814-826)

Realti, A.; Kazimierczuk, M. & Redl, R. (1993). Class e full-wave low dv/dt rectifier. *Circuits and Systems I: Fundamental theory and Applications,* Vol. 40, No. 2, page numbers (73-85), ISSN 1057-7122/92

Sauer, C.; Stancevic, M.; Cauwenberghs, G. & Thakor, N. (2005). Power harvesting and telemetry in cmos for implanted devices. *Circuits and Systems I: Regular Papers, IEEE Transactions on [Circuits and Systems I: Fundamental Theory and Applications, IEEE Transactions on].* Vol. 54, No. 12, (December 2005) ISSN 1057-7122.

Silay, K.M.; Dehollain, C. & Declerq, M. (2008). Orthogonally oriented coils for minimization of cross-coupling in cortical implants. *Biomedical Circuits and Systems Conference, 2008. BioCAS 2008, IEEE.* pp. 109-112, ISSN 978-1-4244-2879-3/08, Baltimore, USA, November 2008.

Simons, R. N.; Hall & Miranda, F. A. (2004). Spiral Chip Implantable radiator and printed Loop external receptor for RF telemetry in bio-sensor systems. *IEEE Radio and Wireless Conference, 2004.* pp. 203-206, ISSN 0-7803-8451-2/04.

Sokal, N.O. (2000) Class-E switching-mode high efficiency tuned rf/microwave power amplifier: improved design equations. *Microwave Symposium Digest, IEEE MTT-S International.* Vol. 2 (2000) pages (779-782), ISSN 0-7803-5697

Sokal, N.O. & Sokal, A. (1975) Class E- A new class of high-efficiency tuned single-ended switching power amplifiers. *Solid State Circuits, IEEE Journal of,* Vol.10 No. 3 (June 1975) pages (168-176)

Troyk, P. & Schwan, M. (1992). Closed-loop class e transcutaneous power and data link for microimplants. *Biomedical Engineering, IEEE Transactions on,* Vol. 39, No.6, (June 1992) page numbers (589-599)

Tsukamoto, H., (2007). Hermetically sealed lithium rechargeable batteries for high reliability applications: medical, aerospace and other specialties. *Battery Conference on Applications and Advances, 2002. The seventeenth Annual* pp.129-134, ISSN 0-7803-7132-1, Long Beach, California, January 2002, Los Angeles, California

Vaillancourt, P.; Djemouai, A.; Harvey, J.; & Sawan, M. (1997). EM radiation behaviour upon biological tissues in a radio-frequency power transfer link for a cortical visual implant. *Engineering in Medicine and biologicy Society, 1997. Proceedings of the 19th International Conference of the IEEE.* pp. 2499-2502, ISSN 0-7803-4262-3, Chicago, USA, November 1997.

Wang, G.; Liu, W.; Sivaprakasam, M.; Zhou, M.; Weiland, J.D. & Humayun, M.S. (2006). A dual Band wireless Power and Data Telemetry for Retinal prosthesis. *Proceedings of the 28th IEEE EMBS Annual International Conference.* pp. 4392-4395, ISSN 1-4244-0033-3/06, New York City, USA, August-September 2006.

Wang, G.; Liu, W.; Sivaprakasam, M. & Kendir, A. (2005). Design and analysis of an adaptive transcutaneous power telemetry for biomedical implants. *IEEE Transactions on circuits and systems-I: Regular Papers.* Vol. 52, No. 10 (October, 2005) page numbers (2109-2117), ISSN 1057-7122.

Yang, Z.; Liu, W.; & Basham, E. (2007) Inductor Modelling in Wireless Links for Implantable Electronics. *IEEE Transactions on Magnetics.* Vol. 43 No. 10 (October, 2007) page numbers (3851-3860) ISSN 0018-9464.

Zeirhofer, C.M. & hochmair, E.S. (1996). Geometric approach for coupling enhancement of magnetically coupled coils. *Biomedical Engineering, IEEE Transactions on.* Vol. 43, No. 7, (July 1996), page numbers (708-714)

Zimmerman, M. D.; Chaimanonart, N. & Young, D.J. (2006) In vivo rf powering for advanced biological research. *28th Annual Conference of the IEEE, Engineering in Medicine and Biology Society.* pp. 2506-2509. ISSN 1-4244-0033-3/06, New York City, USA, August-September 2006.

8

Assessment of the shadow caused by the human body on the personal RF dosimeters reading in multipath environments

Alfonso Bahillo[*,**], Rubén M. Lorenzo*, Santiago Mazuelas[**],
Patricia Fernández* and Evaristo J. Abril*
[**]*CEDETEL (Centre for the Development of Telecommunications)*
**University of Valladolid*
Spain

1. Introduction

Over the last decades, the environmental levels of electromagnetic emissions have increased due to the exponential growth rate of radio frequency (RF) systems. This fact is the cause of the concerns expressed by some members of the public about the safety of exposure to RF radiation from wireless communication devices, with particular reference to cellular phone handsets. As a consequence, several national and international organizations have set limits for human exposure to RF fields. These include the IEEE C95.1 standard (IEEE C95.1-2005, 2006) and the recommendations of the National Council on Radiation Protection and Measurements (NCRP) (NCRP, 1986), the International Commission on Non-Ionizing Radiation Protection (ICNIRP) (ICNIRP, 1999) and the National Radiation Protection Board (NRPB) in the United Kingdom (NRPB, 1993). The different standards vary somewhat in their exposure limits and in other particulars. However, at frequencies used for common wireless communication systems, these different guidelines are broadly similar. To date, despite a considerable amount of speculation, the only health effect from RF radiation identified by the scientific community has been related to an increase in body temperature. The levels of RF exposure from base stations and local wireless networks are so below the recommended limits in those guidelines that temperature increases are insignificant and they do not affect human health. An open issue for the scientific community is the possibility of long-term non-thermal effects of RF fields from which the importance of RF exposure assessment emerges.

Electromagnetic dosimetry which attempts to evaluate the interaction between electromagnetic waves and biological tissues is primarily used for the evaluation of human exposures. It has become common for exposure situations to be characterized by a mixture of spectral contributions from different services, while exposures to single frequencies are rare. This is the particular case of frequency selective dosimeters, which can measure different frequency bands while identifying the contribution of each service. Current personal dosimeters are inherently measuring devices for free field since they are calibrated

in free space. In (Blas et al. 2007), it has been shown that personal dosimeters used to assess exposure to RF electric fields were subject to potential errors associated with perturbations of the fields caused by the presence of the human body. In a common worst-case scenario, when the dosimeter is in a shadow area generated by the presence of the human body, an underestimation up to 30 dB of the E-field level could occur. In (Blas et al. 2007), only waves impinging on the human front have been considered. Because of diffractions and reflections, the RF signal could impinge on the human body with different directions of arrival (DoA) and at a given location, the RF signal is the sum of various waves having different amplitudes and DoAs. Therefore, the goal of this chapter is to help in the task of assessing the human exposure by analyzing the local interaction behavior of the dosimeter with an anatomical model of the human body (Spitzer, et al. 1996) bearing in mind the multiple waves that impinges on the body with different amplitudes and DoAs in a multipath environment and at different frequencies.
As a first approach, the potential errors associated with perturbations of the fields by the presence of the human body have been evaluated taking into account that only the main E-field contribution impinges on the human body with a certain DoA and at different frequencies (Bahillo et al. 2008b). This has been made bearing in mind a single bounce multipath in addition to the direct path between the transmitter and the human body as the dominant mode of propagation. Once the effect of the E-field perturbation around the human body has been evaluated for each DoA and frequency, multiple E-field contributions impinging on the human body at the same time with different amplitudes and DoAs will be analyzed according to the different mean azimuth power distributions taking place in different multipath environments (Bahillo et al. 2008a). Due to the particular public concerns about cellular phones, this chapter focuses the analysis on the Global System for Mobile Communications frequency band (GSM-900MHz).
Computer simulations give a detailed description of the surface E-field on the human body. Nowadays, the finite-difference time-domain (FDTD) method (Taflove, 2005) is the most used technique in dosimetry studies. This algorithm is currently the most acceptable choice when a digital anatomical model of a human body has to be analyzed. Therefore, numerical simulations have been performed with the FDTD method in order to analyze the interaction between a plane wave and the whole human body in a stable situation. Forasmuch as the FDTD method is not computationally efficient to study scattering problems involving large areas such as the urban environments, the ray-tracing technique is used for the computation of the power distribution with respect to the azimuth angle averaged over a distance corresponding to 6 minutes walk, in order to evaluate the average human exposure in an urban environment.

2. Methods and Model

2.1 Numerical Methods of Analysis

In dosimetry studies, the FDTD method is currently the most acceptable choice if a digital anatomical model of a human body is going to be analyzed. Forasmuch as the FDTD method is not computationally efficient to study scattering problems involving large regions, such as urban environments, the ray-tracing technique is used for the evaluation of the azimuth angle power distribution averaged over a distance corresponding to 6 minutes walk in an urban environment. Therefore, numerical simulations are performed with the

FDTD method to evaluate the interaction between the E-field and the human body, while the ray-tracing technique is used to perform the azimuth angle power distribution. As the FDTD method and the ray-tracing technique are well known and they are described in detail in (Taflove, 2005) and (Glassner, 1991) respectively, only a brief outline of the implementation used is described in this chapter. Due to the huge memory and computational time requirements needed, mainly by the FDTD method but also by the ray-tracing technique, a server with a 64-bit architecture and 16GB RAM is used to be able to tackle, in a reasonable time, the simulation model and areas.

As a first step, the FDTD method is used to study the exposure of an anatomical model of the human body according to different DoAs. A monochromatic plane wave with vertical polarization is used as excitation source. To calculate the spatial distribution of the E-field around the human body, the impulse response of the system is evaluated in the frequency domain. A narrow Gaussian pulse is considered which if it is narrow enough it would be a good approximation to an impulse. Keeping in mind the computational resources limitation, the sampling nodes must be taken to ensure that a suitable representation of the human body is made. On the other hand, a good rule of thumb is to take at least 10 points per wavelength (Taflove, 2005). To accomplish these two objectives, the grid computation cell has dimensions 2mm × 2mm × 2mm resulting a good accuracy for the FDTD simulations, where the tissue in each node is assigned permittivity and conductivity values according to the frequency (Gabriel, 1996). As E-field is shared out at each half spatial increment, a three-dimensional E-field is obtained every $\Delta x = 4$ mm. Once the spatial increment size is chosen, and in order to avoid numerical instabilities, the time step is fixed to $\Delta t = \Delta x/2c$ which satisfies the well-known Courant condition of scheme stability (Kunz, 1993). In order to avoid the E-field to be reflected in the limits of the computational volume, 15-layers of uniaxial perfectly matched layer (UPML) absorbing boundary conditions have been used. In addition, a total/scatterd field formulation is chosen to minimize the load on the absorbing boundary conditions and to avoid any interaction between the incident propagation wave and the absorbing boundary conditions (Sullivan, 2000).

As a second step, the two-dimensional ray tracing technique is used to evaluate the mean azimuth power distribution of the E-field in urban environments, starting from an omnidirectional base-station antenna and taking into account wall reflections and corner diffraction present in the environment. For microcellular studies wall transmission is often ignored. The ray-tracing technique is based on geometrical optics and it has been modeled with only third-order reflections and first-order diffractions. In the microcellular environment less than 50% of the incident power is reflected by the walls and even less power is diffracted by the corners. The mean azimuth power distribution is evaluated by using the "ray-launching" approach, having characterized each wall through its permittivity and conductivity values, and having used the well-known reflection and diffraction coefficients (Balanis, 1989).

2.2 Model Description of the Human Body

To study the interaction of the radiated E-field with an exposed subject, a full 3D human body with 2mm resolution has been used for simulation purposes (see left hand of Fig. 1). This model has been obtained from tissue-classified version of the "Visible Human Project" developed at Brooks Air Force base Laboratories and sponsored by the National Library of Medicine (NLM) in the USA. The original model has 1 mm resolution, it is based on anatomical slices from a male cadaver (1.80m tall and 90kg mass, adult male, aged 38) and it has been downsampled to obtain a final resolution of 2 mm. The whole human body was included inside the computational domain. The body model has a total of 31 different types of tissues/organs, for the electrical characterization of the tissues at the frequencies considered the data reported in (Gabriel, 1996) has been used.

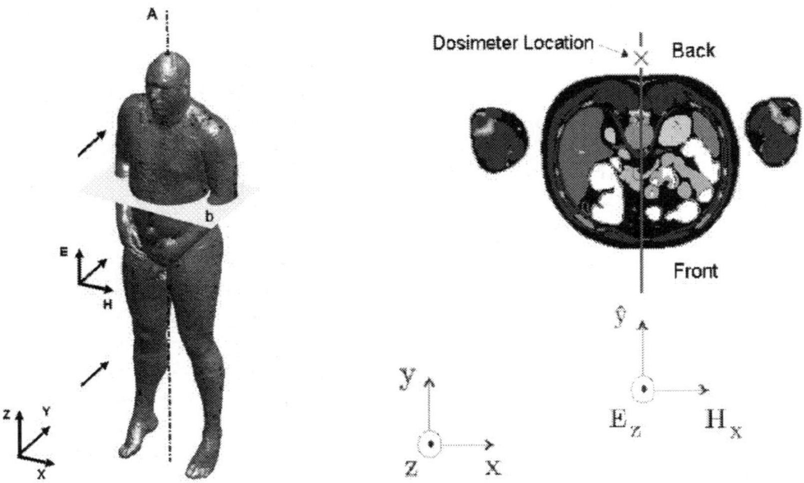

Fig. 1. Left hand, 3D human body computational volume, where *A* is the rotation axis. Right hand, outcome visualization plane, cross-section of the anatomical human body through plane *b* (approximately 2/3 body height).

In the computational volume, Y = 0 is the illumination plane while Z = 120 cm (approximately 2/3 body height) is the outcome visualization plane (see right hand of Fig. 1). The wavefront travels toward positive values of axis Y at each time step. Inside the FDTD computational domain, the presence of the human body in dosimeter reading is only considered. In order to have more control over the E-field behavior around the human body, the alteration of the pattern of the plane wave propagation has been analyzed by means of its DoA variations at different frequencies. The DoA is modified every 10 degrees from 0 to 180 degrees in azimuth. Instead of modifying the wavefront phase which illuminates the human body model, the human model has been rotated upon itself. In this way, the different scenarios have been shown as far as the DoA changes are concerned.

3. Simulation Results

3.1 RF Exposure of the Human Model at Different DoAs and Frequencies

This section presents an analysis of the surface E-field on the human body model when it is illuminated by a plane wave at different DoAs (from 0 to 180 every 10 degrees in azimuth) and frequencies (FM-100 MHz, GSM-900 MHz and DCS-1800 MHz) based on the FDTD simulations. Fig. 2 shows the simulation results. These results represent the spatial variability of the E-Field when it is compared with the incident wave through an imaginary line. The characteristics of this line are the following ones: it is parallel to the ground and it goes approximately through the central part of the stomach of a human (2/3 body height and 1/2 body width). The assumption which states that the plane wave arrives horizontally is valid since the following topic is fulfilled, the distance between the human body and the RF source is larger than the difference between the height of the RF source and the scatters around the human body, for more details see (Petrus, 2002).

In Fig. 2 different scenarios are shown, where the human body is illuminated by a plane wave at different frequencies and from different azimuthal angles. The simulation results fit well with the experimental measurements reported by (Blas, 2007) at FM-100 and GSM-900 bands when the DoA of the plane wave is 0 degrees in azimuth. In order for the dosimeter not to bother the human or interfere with his movements, it is assumed that the person has the dosimeter fixed to his back (five centimeters from it) approximately 2/3 body height, although from Fig. 2 other distances could be analyzed. Due to the relative orientation of the human body with regard to the plane wave DoA, the dosimeter could be located either within the maximum shadow zone, within the peak or in an intermediate case of the stationary wavefront which takes place when the plane wave impinges on the human body. In addition to the previous work in (Blas, 2007), simulations in DCS-1800 band are also included.

The first interesting issue is that due to the arrival angle uncertainty, there are differences in dosimeter readings up to 35dB in DCS-1800, 25dB in GSM-900 and 12dB in FM-100 bands due to the human body presence, in these two opposite scenarios, when the plane wave impinges on the human body to the front or to the back. On the other hand, as frequency increases and due to the shorter wavelength, the E-field has more difficulties in penetrating the human body. Consequently, most of the E-field behind the body comes from its going around it, not from going through it. As a result, the higher the frequency, the higher the attenuation in the region shaded by the human body. In the DCS-1800 and GSM-900 bands, it is worth pointing out that the standing wave ratio when the DoA is 180 degrees is much higher than the one when the DoA is 0 degrees, because the energy has more difficulties in going around the human body when impinging on the back than when impinging on the front, because the body front is more rounded than the body back.

3.2 Mean Azimuth Power Distribution in Urban Environments

In a multipath scenario, such as the urban environment, the human exposure is characterized by several waves impinging on the human body with different amplitudes and DoAs. Exposure guidelines, such as those published by (ICNIRP, 1999), require exposures to be averaged over 6 minutes to be compared with their basic restrictions. By using the two-dimensional ray-tracing technique, according to that time-averaging of exposure, the mean azimuth power distribution has been computed over two different routes of a distance of 300 m each, corresponding to a human walking of 50 m/minute for 6 minutes. The routes have been simulated by using a map of a neighbourhood of the Valladolid city center, Spain (see Fig. 3). A circle (0.25 m radius) acting as a human model, the same urban environment and the same position for the omnidirectional transmitter have been considered in all the scenarios simulated. Fig. 4 shows the mean azimuth power distribution for the two different routes, which have different line-of-sight (LOS) percentage, route A with 35% LOS and route B with 21 % LOS.

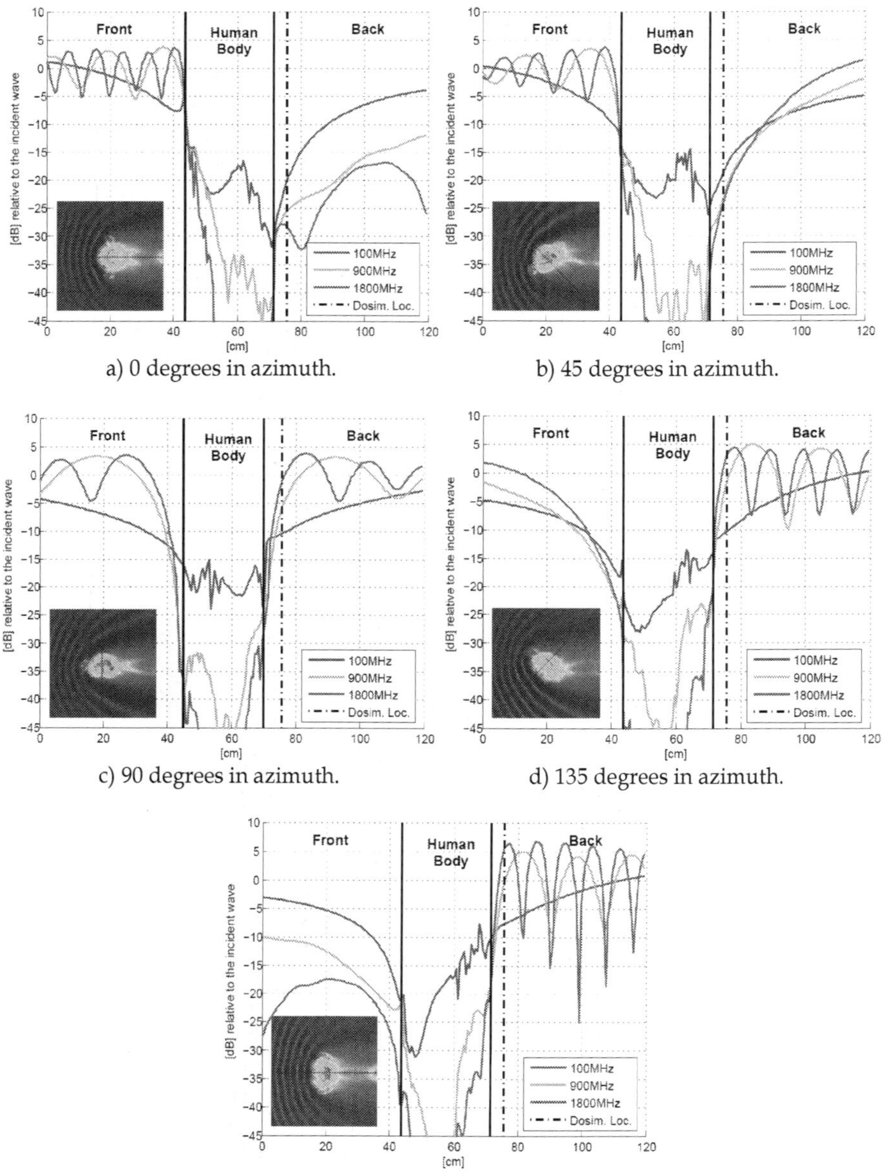

a) 0 degrees in azimuth.

b) 45 degrees in azimuth.

c) 90 degrees in azimuth.

d) 135 degrees in azimuth.

e) 180 degrees in azimuth.

Fig. 2. Spatial variability of the E-field due to the presence of the human body. Rotating the model around *A* axis at FM-100 MHz, GSM-900 MHz and DCS-1800 MHz bands.

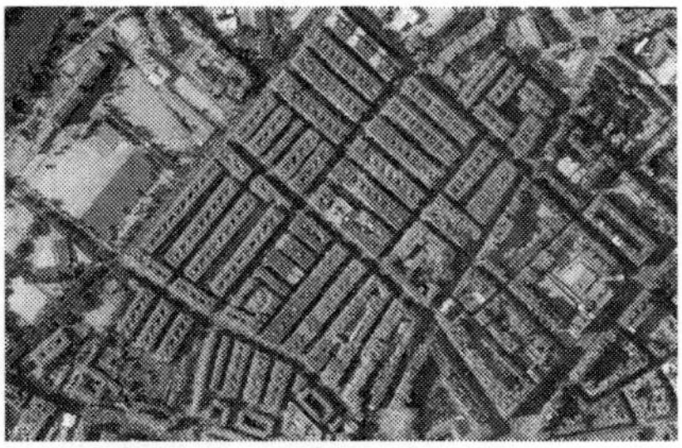

a) Valladolid city neighbourhood satellite view (by Google).

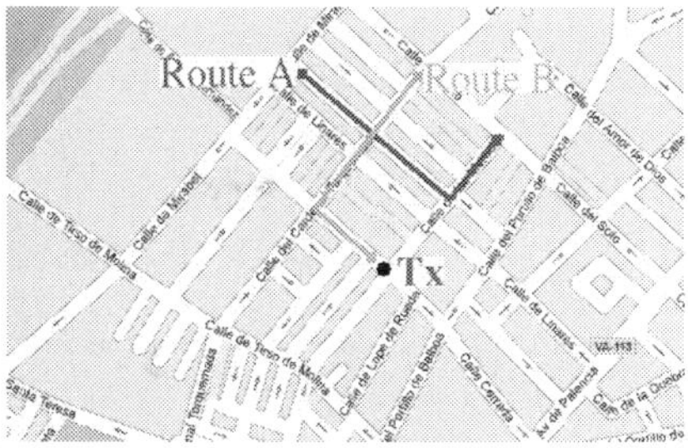

b) Valladolid city neighbourhood map view (by Google).

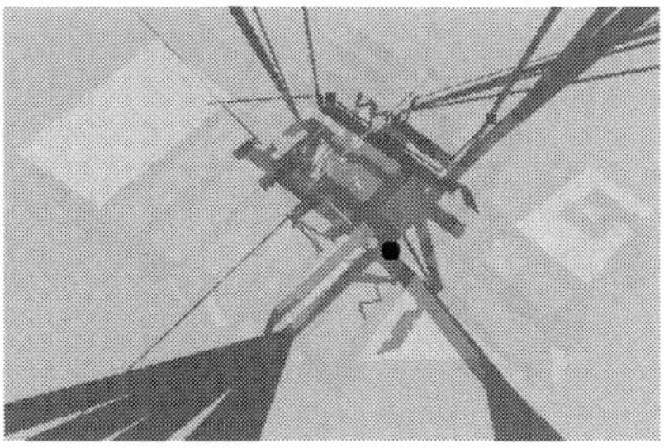

c) Ray-tracer view.

Fig. 3. Ray-tracer simulation results in the Valladolid city neighbourhood.

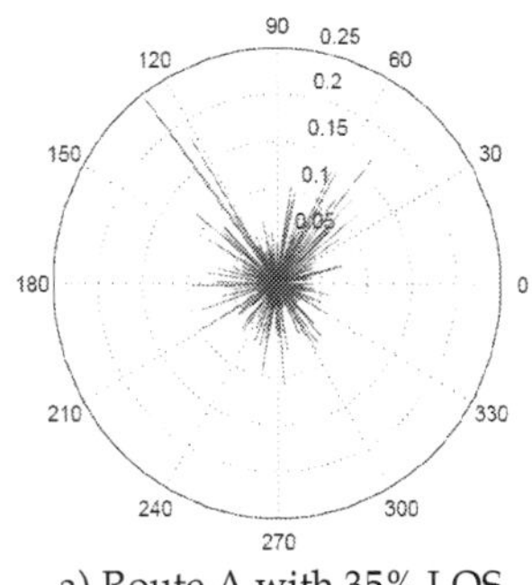

a) Route A with 35% LOS.

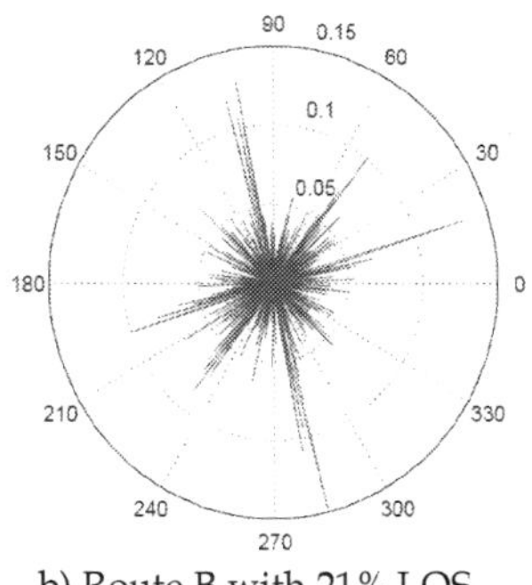

b) Route B with 21% LOS.

Fig. 4. Mean azimuth power distribution.

4. Discussion

In this section the effect of the E-field perturbation around the human body is going to be evaluated for each DoA and frequency taking into account that only the main E-field contribution impinges on the human body. Afterwards, multiple E-field contributions impinging on the human body at the same time with different amplitudes and DoAs are going to be analyzed according to the different mean azimuth power distributions which take place in different urban environments. In this case, due to the particular public concerns about the cellular phones, this section focuses on the frequency GSM-900 MHz.

4.1 Main E-field contribution

If a LOS path exists between the transmitter and the human body and a single bounce multipath is the dominant mode of propagation (in addition to the direct path), the multipath components will be tightly clustered in angle about the direct path component. For an urban microcell environment, it was found that the average angle spread was 9.4 degrees (Liberti, 1996). But, DoA variations of ±5 degrees do not change significantly the surface E-field pattern in the potential location of the dosimeter, near the human body. Under these assumptions, only the main RF azimuthal contribution would be considered. As seen in Fig. 2, the resulting shadow, solely due to the human body presence, can cause high differences in the dosimeter reading because of the DoA uncertainty of the main RF contribution, due to the relative position between the transmitter and the human body. For this reason, in order to better estimate the surface E-field behavior around the human body, it is necessary to gather information of the individual simulation results for each DoA by using an azimuthal angle with a certain probability to simulate different scenarios based on the main RF contribution. The symmetry of right and left human body is assumed.

In the first scenario, suppose that all the DoA are equally likely which takes place when the person is walking randomly in locations free from scatters or scatters have a uniform angular distribution around the subject. In the second scenario, the DoA 0 and 180 degrees are more likely than the others. This scenario takes place when the RF source is located away from a narrow street in the direction of the human front or human back equally likely. Therefore, the most probable movement of the person is the straight line. The third scenario is an intermediate situation where the street is wider than the one in the second scenario. Therefore, the person can follow other directions different from the straight line with the same probability. Table 1 presents the probability of the main contribution of the RF source of impinging with a certain DoA in these three scenarios.

	0°	45°	90°	135°	180°
Uni	0.125	2 x 0.125	2 x 0.125	2 x 0.125	0.125
NS	0.4	2 x 0.05	2 x 0	2 x 0.05	0.4
WS	0.2	2 x 0.125	2 x 0.05	2 x 0.125	0.2

Table 1. Probability of the DoA of the main E-field contribution. Uni, uniform; NS, narrow street; WS, wide street.

Fig. 5. shows the simulation results. It represents the spatial variability of the E-field compared to the incident wave caused by the presence of the human body in three different scenarios, uniform (Uni), narrow street (NS) and wide street (WS) illumination. As it can be seen in Fig. 5, five centimeters from the human back, where the dosimeter would be located, the E-field strength is similar in the three scenarios at each frequency, -13 dB with a variation of ±1 dB in FM band, -6 dB with a variation of ±1 dB in GSM-900 band and -3 dB with a variation of ±1 dB in DCS-1800 band. While a few centimeters from the potential location of the dosimeter, the E-field variation is higher. In the FM-100 band the E-field has a variation up to 2 dB, in GSM-900 up to 12 dB and in DCS-1800 up to 16 dB.

As shown in Fig. 5, under the assumption that body front and body back illumination are equally likely, the variations of the surface E-field on the body taken either from the front or from the back are the following ones: five centimeters from the body front, the E-field is approximately 2 dB higher than the E-field on the back at FM-100 and GSM-900 and 3 dB lower at DCS-1800 bands. This cannot be applied when differences of illumination probabilities occur between body front and body back.

From the results presented in Fig. 5, it can be conclude that if the dosimeter is used as a system for the assessment of personal exposures in epidemiological studies, on average, the dosimeter reading is always lower than the E-field when the human is not present.

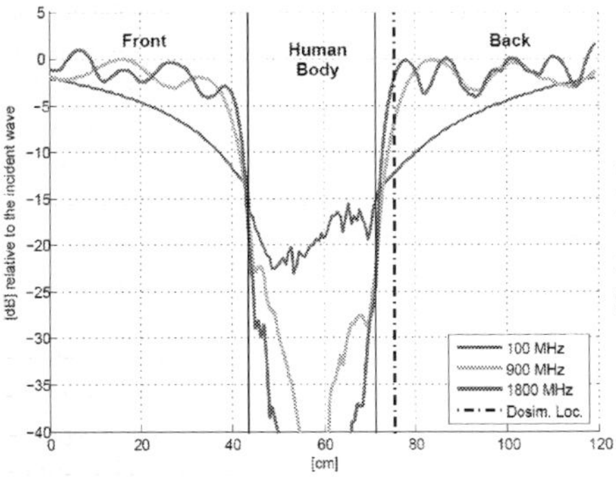

a) Uniform illumination.

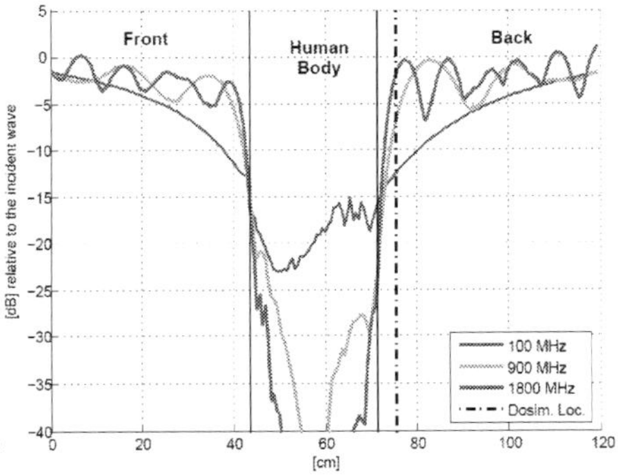

b) Narrow street illumination.

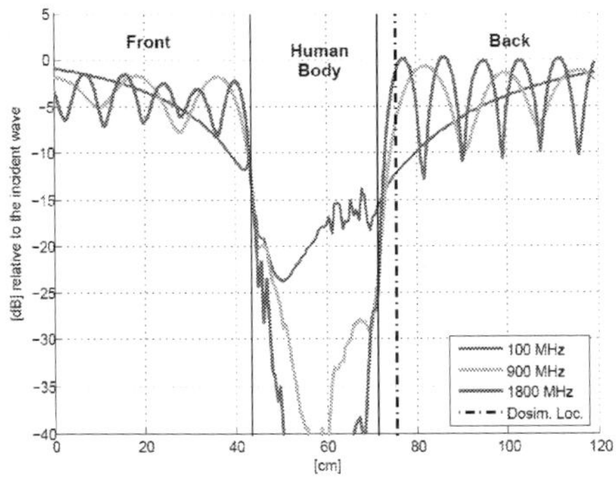

e) Wide street illumination.

Fig. 5. Spatial variability of the E-field compared to the incident wave at FM-100 MHz, GSM-900 MHz and DCS-1800 MHz bands in three different scenarios.

4.2 Multiple E-field contributions

It is natural to assume that when a mobile user moves randomly in any environment, the incident waves can arise from any azimuthal direction with equal probability. As a consequence, the uniform distribution is a justified assumption for the azimuth power distribution averaged over a random route. To better estimate the surface E-field behavior around the human body in an urban environment, four different mean azimuth power distributions have been considered, uniform distribution, routes A and B inside the neighborhood of the city of Valladolid, and the mean azimuth power distribution obtained by measurements (Kimmo, 2002) in an urban microcell in the city of Helsinki, Finland.
In simulations, the human body model is not illuminated with plane waves arising from different DoAs at the same time, but a weighted average of the individual simulation results from the different DoAs have been done. The weight of each DoA has been obtained from the mean azimuth power distribution results shown in Fig. 4 and it has been normalized to the total incident power. As a result, the different individual DoAs simulation results have been added constructively. Therefore, an upper bound is fixed under which the dosimeter reading could be found.

Fig. 6 shows the upper bound of the spatial variability of the E-field according to the four scenarios presented in this section. As it can be seen in this figure, five centimeters from the human back, where the dosimeter would be located, the E-field strength is similar for the four mean azimuth power distributions that have been considered. The dosimeter in that position would read an E-field value between -5 dB and -7.5 dB at GSM-900 band. Therefore, the E-field strength is underestimated even in a multipath scenario, where the dosimeter is not always located in the shadow region. A few centimeters from the potential location of the dosimeter the E-field variation is higher, in the GSM-900 band the E-field has a variation up to 6 dB.

As it can be inferred from the results presented in Fig.6, if a body-worn dosimeter is used as a system for the assessment of personal exposures in epidemiological studies, on average, the dosimeter reading is at least 5 dB lower than the E-field when the human is not present.
Despite of the power distribution in azimuth, no straightforward assumption can be justified for the elevation angle. It was found (Lee, 1973) that for most of the streets, field measurements of mobile radio signals have shown that signal arrival is concentrated in elevation angles lower than 16 degrees along the horizontal level. Therefore, the shadowing effect has to be analyzed also with respect to changes in elevation angles.

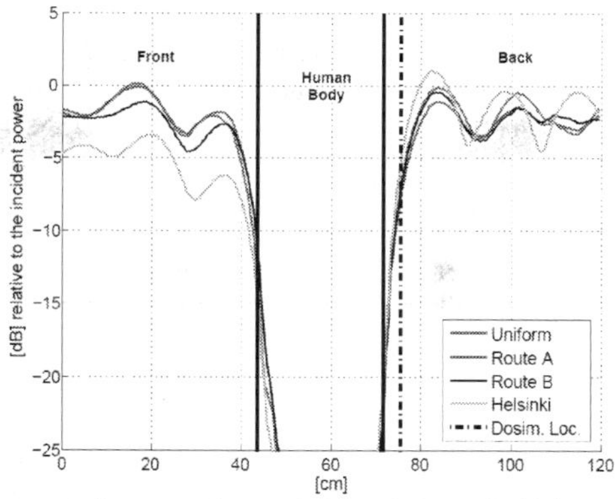

Fig. 6. Weighted average of the spatial variability of the E-field for the four different mean azimuth distributions at GSM-900 band.

5. Conclusions

Assuming that the dosimeter is fixed to the human body back at waist level, the first interesting issue is that due to the uncertainty in the angle of arrival of the E-field, there are differences in dosimeter readings up to 35 dB at DCS-1800 band, 25 dB at GSM-900 band and 12 dB at FM-100 band caused by the human body presence, in these two opposite scenarios, when the plane wave impinges on the human body to the front or to the back. On the other hand, as frequency increases and due to the shorter wavelength, the E-field has more difficulties in penetrating the human body, consequently most of the E-field behind the body comes from its going around it, not from going through it. As a result, the higher the frequency, the higher the attenuation in the area shaded by the human body. Therefore, the dosimeter reading is generally lower than the E-field strength when the human is not present. Even in a multipath scenario, where the dosimeter is not always in the shaded area, the E-field level is underestimated because, as it will be shown in this chapter, despite the differences among all the multipath scenarios analyzed, in the place where the dosimeter would be located, the variations in E-field strength are similar but always lower than the E-field when the human is not present. Therefore, understanding and predicting in which way the presence of the human body alters the plane wave propagation is a fundamental aspect when a dosimeter is used for the assessment of personal exposure in an urban environment.

6. References

IEEE C95.1-2005 (2006). *IEEE standard for safety levels with respect to human exposure to radio frequency electromagnetic fields, 3 KHz to 300 GHz,* IEEE, ISBN: 0738148342, New York.

NCRP (1986) *Biological effects and exposure criteria for radio frequency electromagnetic fields,* National Council on Radiation Protection and Measurements, ISBN: 0913392804, Washington D.C.

ICNIRP (1999) *Guidelines on limiting exposure to non-ionizing radiation,* International Commission on Non-Ionizing Radiation Protection, ISBN: 3-9804789-6-3, Germany.

NRPB (1993) *Board statement on restrictions on human exposure to static and time-varying electromagnetic fields and radiation,* Chilton Oxon NRPB, ISN: 859513661, UK.

Blas, J., Lago, F., Fernández, P., Lorenzo, R. M. and Abril, E. J. (2007). Potential exposure assessment errors associated with body-worn RF dosimeters. *Bioelectromagnetics,* No. 28, (July 2007) 573-576.

Bahillo, A., Blas, J., Fernández, P., Mazuelas, S., Viñuela, A., Lorenzo, R. M., and Abril, E. J. (2008a). E-Field errors associated with RF dosimeters for RF human exposure assessment in urban environments. *Proceedings of 30th annual international conference of Engineering in Medicine and Biology,* pp. 2821-2824, ISBN: 978-1-4244-1814-5, Vancouver, BC, August 2008, IEEE EMBS.

Bahillo, A., Blas, J., Fernández, P., Lorenzo, R. M., Mazuelas, S. and Abril, E. J. (2008b). E-Field assessment errors associated with RF dosimeters for different angles of arrival. *Radiation Protection Dosimetry,* No. 132(1), (October 2008) 51-56.

Spitzer, V., Ackeman, M. J., Scherzinger, A. L. and Whitlock, D. (1996). The visible human male: a technical report, *J. Am. Med. Inform. Assoc.,* No. 2, (April 1996) 118-130.

Taflove, A. (2005). *Computational electrodynamics: The Finite-Difference Time-Domain method,* Artech House; 3rd edition, ISBN: 1-58053-076-1, Norwood, MA.

Glassner, A. S. (1991). *An Introduction to Ray Tracing,* Academic Press, Harcourt Brace Jovanovich Publishers, ISBN: 0-12-286160-4, Cambridge, UK.

Balanis, C. A. (1989). *Advanced Engineering Electromagnetics,* John Wiley & Sons Inc., ISBN: 0-47-162194-3, New York.

Gabriel, C., (1996). Compilation of the dielectric properties of body tissues at RF and microwave frequencies. *Brooks Air Force, Brooks AFB, TX,* Tech. Rep. AL/OE-TR-1996-0037, 1996.

Kunz, K. S., and Luebbers, R. J. (1993). *The Finite Difference Time Domain Method for Electromagnetics,* CRC-Press, ISBN: 0-84-938657-8.

Sullivan, D. M. (2000). *Electromagnetic simulation using the FDTD method.* Wiley-IEEE Press, ISBN: 0-7803-4747-1, NewYork.

Petrus, P., Reed, J. H., and Rappaport, T. S. (2002). Geometrical-based statistical macrocell channel model for mobile environments. *IEEE Trans. on Communications,* No. 50, (2002) 495-502.

Kimmo, K., Sulonen, K., Laitinen, H., Kivekäs, O., Krogerus, J., and Vainikainen, P. (2002). Angular Power Distribution and Mean Effective Gain of Mobile Antenna in Different Propagation Environments. *IEEE Trans. on Vehicular Technology,* No. 51, (September 2002) 823-838.

Sacks, Z. S., Kingsland, D. M., Lee, R., and Lee, J.-F. (1995). A perfectly matched anisotropic absorber for use as an absorbing boundary condition. *IEEE Trans. On Antennas Propagation,* No. 43, (1995) 1460-1463.

Liberti, J. C., and Rappaport, T.S. (1996). Analysis of CDMA cellular radio systems employing adaptive antennas in multipath environments. *Proceedings of 46th international conference of Vehicular Technology, Mobile Technology for the Human Raceapos,* pp. 1076-1080, April 1996, IEEE VTC.

Lee, W., and Brandt, R. H., (1973). The elevation angle of mobile radio signal arrival. *IEEE Trans. On Communications,* Vol. COM-21, (1973) 1194-1197.

9

Monitoring drowsiness on-line using a single encephalographic channel

Antoine Picot, Sylvie Charbonnier and Alice Caplier
Gipsa-Lab, Grenoble University
France

1. Introduction

Drowsiness is the transition state between awakening and sleep during which a decrease of vigilance is generally observed. This can be a serious problem for tasks that need a sustained attention, such as driving. According to a report of the American National Highway Safety Traffic Administration (Royal, 2002) driver drowsiness is annually responsible for about 56,000 crashes which is the reason why more and more researches have been developed to build automatic detectors of this dangerous state.

Both behavioural and physiological modifications occur during drowsiness. Reaction time is slower, vigilance is reduced and information processing is less efficient, which can generate abnormal driving. Moreover, as drowsiness is the transition between awakening and sleep, it induces an increase of the number and the duration of blinks and yawns. Changes in cerebral activity also happen and can be observed thanks to electroencephalography.

Researches on driver state monitoring has begun about thirty years ago and are still very active. The driver state monitoring systems can be classified into three kinds of system: those focusing on the vehicle behaviour, those focusing on the driver physical behaviour and those focusing on the driver physiological behaviour.

The first systems developed were the ones using sensors monitoring the vehicle behaviour (O'Hanlon & Kelley, 1974, Klein et al., 1980). The main features studied are the steering wheel movements, the lateral position of the car on the road, the standard deviation of lateral position (SDLP) and the time to line crossing (TLC). The purpose is to detect an abnormal behaviour of the car, due to the driver drowsiness. The problems encountered by this kind of methods are that the features used depend on the shape of the road and how one drives, which may change a lot from one driver to another (Renner & Mehring, 1997).

To overcome these problems, researches have focused on systems using sensors monitoring drivers' awareness. One widespread technique to monitor the driver state is the use of a video camera. Indeed, a lot of information can be extracted from the driver face to monitor fatigue such as gaze, frequency and duration of eye blinking and yawning or percentage of eyelid closure. A lot of examples using camera to monitor the driver state can be found in the literature (Grace et al., 1998; Ji & Yang, 2001; Vural et al., 2007).

These kinds of systems focus on the drivers' visual attention. Face, mouth and eye tracking algorithms are used to detect the face. Once the face, the eyes and the mouth are located, it is easy to detect eye blinking or yawning and calculate their frequency and duration. Frequency and duration of yawning or eye blinking too high indicate a decrease of attention. The gaze can be calculated with the eyes and the face position (Smith et al., 2003) or using a stereoscopic camera (Ji et al., 2004). Then, it allows the driver to be warned when he is not looking at the road.

However, many differences can be observed between drivers, which makes it hard to monitor fatigue with only one feature (Karrer et al, 2004). An interesting way of merging the different features (eye blinking, yawning, gaze...) is used by Ji et al. (Ji et al., 2006). They use probabilistic networks which allow all features to contribute to the decision of the level of attention. Moreover, external factors (weather, hour of the day, etc...) can contribute in these networks to determine the level of attention.

However, video features are not the best indicators of drowsiness. According to Dinges (Dinges, 1995), the best indicators of fatigue are the physiological indicators. The electroencephalogram (EEG) and the electro-oculogram (EOG) are mainly used to study drowsiness. Yet, several researches have focused on other physiological indicators such as the electrocardiogram (ECG) to monitor drivers' heart rate (Törnros at al., 2000) or the drivers' temperature (Quanten et al., 2006).

The EOG is the measurement of the resting potential of the retina. It gives an accurate measurement of eyes movements. Many features can be extracted from this information such as eyelid opening and closing parameters, blinks frequency, blinks amplitude, blinks duration... According to Galley et al. (Galley et al., 2004), EOG is a relevant measure to monitor fatigue since some extracted features are really sensitive to drowsiness. One of the most efficient features extracted is the PERCLOS (PERcentage of eyelid CLOSure). This feature has been defined by Wierwille (Wierwille et al., 1994). It is the percentage of eyelid closure over the time. Knippling (Knippling, 1998) showed that PERCLOS is a good indicator of drowsiness that increases with fatigue.

Electroencephalography measures the electrical activity of the brain from electrodes placed over the scalp. Drowsiness appears into the EEG spectrum by an increase of activity in the frequency bands [8-12]Hz (alpha band) and [4-8]Hz (theta band) predominantly in the parietal and central regions of the brain. In the same time, a decrease of activity in the band [12-26]Hz (beta activity) can also be observed, as beta activity increases with cognitive tasks and active concentration. This has been shown in several studies (Santamaria & Chiapa, 1987; Akerstedt & Gillberg, 1990; Kay et al., 1994). EEG is so efficient in detecting drowsiness that it is often used as a reference indicator. In this case, the reference is built by expert doctors who visually observe the proportion of alpha and theta activity on a short-time window as in (Muzet et al., 2003). The analysis is done off-line and is time consuming.

In order to make the analysis of drowsiness in an automatic way, the EEG power spectrum can be computed using Fast Fourier Transform or using wavelets Transform but none of these techniques seems better than the other. The number of EEG channels used to monitor drowsiness fluctuates from a few to about thirty. The advantage of using a large number of EEG channels is to obtain spatial information on how the EEG energy is shifting from one frequency band to another (Makeig et al., 1996; Lin et al., 2005b). However, using only a few EEG channels is faster and easier to compute.

The features obtained from EEG can be used in many ways. Several studies proposed to monitor some ratios between different EEG power bands. De Waard and Brookhuis (De Waard & Brookhuis, 1991) suggest to monitor the ratio between the alpha activity and the theta activity on the beta activity [(alpha+theta)/beta] which increases with driver drowsiness. Drowsiness decision can be made using EEG features used as inputs to a classifier. Ben Khalifa et al. (Ben Khalifa et al., 2004) used a connexionist method to detect drowsiness. They proposed to use a single parieto-occipital channel (P4-O2) to avoid ocular frontal artefacts. Relative power in the [1- 23]Hz band is computed using a short term fast Fourier transformation and divided in twenty three sub-bands of 1Hz. These features are then used as entries in a linear vector quantization (LVQ) neural network to detect artefacted states and in a self organizing map (SOM) neural network to classify states into two states: awake and drowsy. Lin et al. (Lin et al., 2005a) applied Principal Component Analysis (PCA) on the whole spectrum of a 2-channels EEG. A fast Fourier transform is then computed on the principal component to extract the power in 10 EEG bands from 1 to 40Hz. These features are used for training a linear regression model which estimates the driving performance, i.e. the deviation between the car and the centre of the road, assuming that driving performances are correlated with driver's alertness. They also used the two principal components obtained using an independent component analysis (ICA) on a 33-channels EEG instead using a PCA on a 2-channels EEG with their linear regression model to improve their estimation of driving performance. Most recently, Rosipal et al. (Rosipal et al., 2007) used hidden Gaussian mixture model to monitor drowsiness. A hierarchical Gaussian mixture model (hGMM) with two mixture components at the lower hierarchical level is used. Each mixture models the data density distribution of one of the two drowsiness cornerstones/classes represented by 4-second long EEG segments with low and high drowsiness levels. The spectral content of each EEG segment is transferred into a compact form of autoregressive model coefficients. Their study is performed on a large number of drivers.

However, even if some on-line techniques exist, they seem hard to implement: they either need to be trained on numerous data previously recorded on a driver or they require a large number of EEG channels. Yet, the fact that EEG is used as a drowsiness reference by expert doctors in physiological studies proves the utility of an on-line driver drowsiness detection system using EEG.

In this paper, we propose to develop a system to detect driver drowsiness that uses as few EEG channels as possible that works on-line and that does not need to be trained. Indeed, it seems that a relatively simple drowsiness detection system for drivers would be easier to implement in a car.

The method proposed is described in section 2. The results obtained on a significant database of 40 EEG recordings from 20 drowsy drivers are shown and discussed in section 3. Finally, conclusions and perspectives are presented.

2. Drowsiness detection method

After a short presentation on EEG and how drowsiness appears in EEG, the drowsiness detection method is presented step by step.

2.1 EEG and drowsiness

An electroencephalogram is a measurement of the electrical activity of the brain from electrodes placed on the scalp (Blinowska & Durka, 2006), according to the international 10-20 system shown in fig. 1.

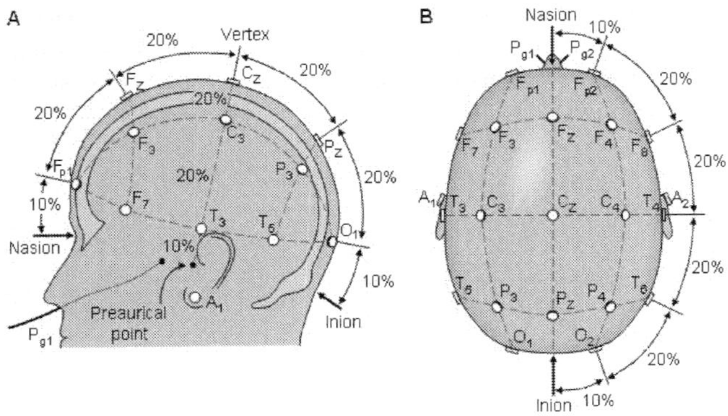

Fig. 1. 10-20 system

EEG is described in term of rhythmic activity and transients. The rhythmic activity is divided into frequency bands: delta (δ) activity ([0.5-4]Hz), theta (θ) activity ([4-8]Hz), alpha (α) activity ([8-12]Hz), beta (β) activity ([12-26]Hz) and gamma (γ) activity (over 26Hz). Most of the time, only the range [1-30]Hz is used because activity below or above this range is likely to be artefactual (under standard clinical recording techniques).
Drowsiness is characterized by an increase of alpha and theta activities, predominantly in the parietal (P) and central (C) regions of the brain, and a slowdown of blinks and eye movements (Akerstedt & Gillberg, 1990; Kay et al., 1994; Muzet et al., 2003). Even if different scales of drowsiness classification exist, none of them are standardized and there are no standardized rules to differentiate the levels of drowsiness (as the Rechtschaffen and Kales rules (Rechtschaffen & Kales, 1968) for the study of sleep). This may be due to the quite recent interest on drowsiness compared to the sleep analysis and the difficulty to collect drowsiness data.

Objective sleepiness score	α and θ cumulative duration	Blinks and eye movements
0	Negligible	Normal
1	Less than 5s	Normal
2	Less than 5s or Less than 10s	Slow Normal
3	Less than 10s or More than 10s	Slow Normal
4	More than 10s	Slow

Table 1. OSS Criteria

There are two kinds of scales: subjective sleepiness scales like the Karolinska Sleepiness Scale (KSS) (Akerstedt & Gillberg, 1990) which allows drivers to directly evaluate their own drowsiness and Objective Sleepiness Scales (OSS) which is used by expert doctors to evaluate drivers' drowsiness after driving. The OSS used in this study is the five levels scale from 0 (awake) to 4 (very drowsy) developed by Muzet (Muzet et al., 2003). Decisions are made every 20s and depend on the length of alpha and theta bursts as well as on the speed of eyes movements and blinks. The different criteria are presented in table 1. This scale is used by doctors to make decisions.

2.2 Method Principle

The purpose is to design a drowsiness detection algorithm which can work on-line, inspired by the OSS. The overview of the detection method is shown in fig. 2. First the EEG power spectrum is computed using a Short Time Fourier Transform (STFT) to calculate the relative power into the different EEG bands every second. Then, the relative power of the alpha band is median filtered using a sliding window to reject abnormal values. A Means Comparison Test (MCT) is computed at last to compare the energy to a reference level, learnt at the beginning of the recording while the patient is not supposed to be drowsy. MCT is normalized. A common threshold of detection can be proposed taking into account the acceptable level of false alarms and validated using experiments which has been presented in (Picot et al., 2008). Concomitantly, a Variances Comparison Test (VCT) is computed on the raw EEG data to detect high amplitude artefacts. Information on the occurrence of artefacts can be used as an index of reliability on the "drowsy decision".

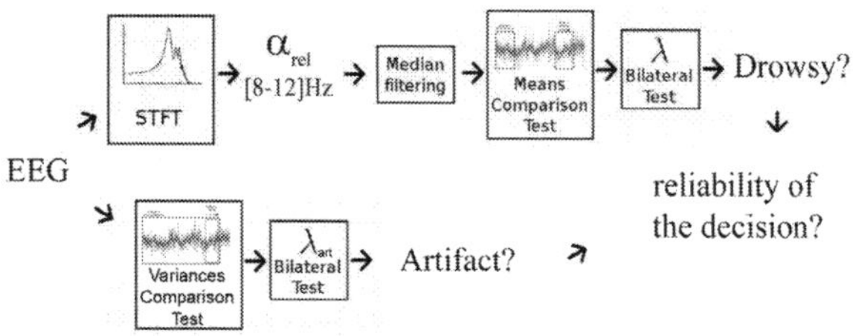

Fig. 2. Drowsiness detection method

2.2.1 EEG Power Spectrum

The EEG power spectrum is computed using a Short Time Fourier Transform (STFT). The power spectrum is computed every second on a window of two seconds using Welch's periodogram method (Welch, 1967). The overlapping window between the previous and next value is 1 second. Then, the relative powers in each band are calculated as the ratio of the power in one band and the power of the whole EEG spectrum. Only the range [1-30]Hz is used because activity below or above this range is likely to be artefactual. For example the α relative power is calculated as follows:

$$\alpha_{relative\_power} = \frac{\alpha_{power}}{EEG_{power}} \tag{1}$$

The relative power in the bands α ([8-12]Hz) , θ ([4-8]Hz) and β([12-26]Hz) are named α_{rel}, θ_{rel} and β_{rel} respectively.

2.2.2 Median filtering

Median filtering is used to smooth the α_{rel} signal and to reject abnormal values. The median is the value separating the higher half of a population from the lower half. Compared to the mean, the median is known for its robustness towards outliers, as far as the number of outliers is lower than half the length of the population. Here, the median of the relative powers is calculated every second, before performing MCT, using a sliding window of 10s.

2.2.3 Means Comparison Test

The method of MCT is inspired by Ragot (Ragot et al., 1990) and is applied on the relative powers in the alpha band. A moving window is compared to a fixed reference window as shown in fig. 3.

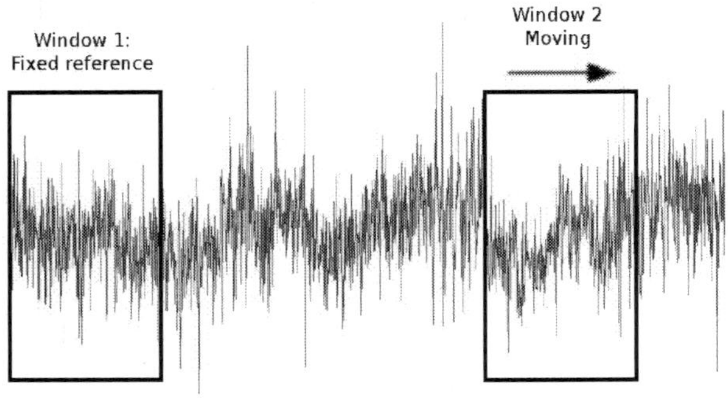

Fig. 3. Illustration of the windows for the MCT

The classical MCT has quite restrictive conditions due to the fact that the theoretical variances are unknown. Let us consider two independent populations of length n_1 and n_2, whose means are $\bar{x}_1$ and $\bar{x}_2$ and whose variances are s_1^2 and s_2^2. Then, the variable:

$$t = \frac{\bar{x}_1 - \bar{x}_2}{\sqrt{\frac{n_1 s_1^2 + n_2 s_2^2}{n_1 + n_2 - 2}\left(\frac{1}{n_1} + \frac{1}{n_2}\right)}} \qquad (2)$$

follows a $n_1 + n_2 - 2$ liberty degrees Student law. The equality of the two means can be tested by a bilateral test with a confidence threshold λ: $-t_{1-\lambda/2} < t < t_{1-\lambda/2}$.

If the two populations have the same length n (i.e. $n_1=n_2=n$) and their theoretical variances are equal, (2) can be formulated as:

$$t = \frac{\bar{x}_1 - \bar{x}_2}{\sqrt{\frac{s_1^2 + s_2^2}{n}}} \qquad (3)$$

So, the variable t follows a n-1 liberty degrees Student law.
Moreover, if the populations are large enough, i.e. if n_1 and n_2 are equal or greater than 20, the test is performed with the variable:

$$u = \frac{\bar{x}_1 - \bar{x}_2}{\sqrt{\frac{s_1^2}{n_1} + \frac{s_2^2}{n_2}}} \tag{4}$$

which then follows a centred reduced normal law. The means equality is then tested by a bilateral test with a confidence threshold λ: $-u_{1-\lambda/2} < u < u_{1-\lambda/2}$. Furthermore, the theoretical variances equality is no longer necessary.
Here, the test is computed on the relative power signals calculated every second. The reference, calculated from the fixed window, is calculated at the beginning of a recording with the assumption that, before driving, the driver is not drowsy. The mean value calculated during this period provides a reference for the not drowsy stage. The mean values calculated on line are compared to this "not drowsy" reference value. The length of the fixed reference window is n_1=60s and the one of the moving window is n_2=30s, so n_1 and n_2 are greater than 20 as α_{rel} is calculated every second. Hence, the formula (4) can be used. The threshold λ fixes the percentage of false alarms expected. The higher the threshold, the lower the percentage of false alarms. In this study, λ is empirically chosen and discussed in section 3.

2.3 Artefact detection

An artefact is an electric perturbation of the EEG signal due to patient movements or measurement problems. Artefacts pollute the whole EEG band and it is quite impossible to extract reliable EEG information when an artefact occurs. There are several types of artefacts. They may be due to ocular movements, face muscles movements or measurement devices problems such as electrode unstuck.
The proposed solution to detect high-amplitude artefacts corresponding to electrode unstuck is to apply a Variances Comparison Test (VCT) on the EEG. Artefact values are around mV whereas EEG signal values are around µV. High-amplitude artefacts pollute the whole EEG band as shown in the red box on the spectrogram in fig. 4.
The method of VCT is inspired by Ragot (Ragot et al., 1990) and is directly applied on the raw EEG. The principle is the same than the MCT: the variance of a moving window is compared to the variance of a reference window. Let us consider two independent populations with normal distributions. Their lengths are n_1 and n_2 and their experimental variances are s_1^2 and s_2^2. Then, the variable:

$$F = \frac{s_1^2}{s_2^2} \tag{5}$$

follows a Fisher law with $k_1=n_1-1$ and $k_2=n_2-1$ liberty degrees. The variances equality is then tested by a bilateral test with a confidence threshold λ_{art}: $F_{\lambda art/2} < F < F_{1-\lambda art/2}$.

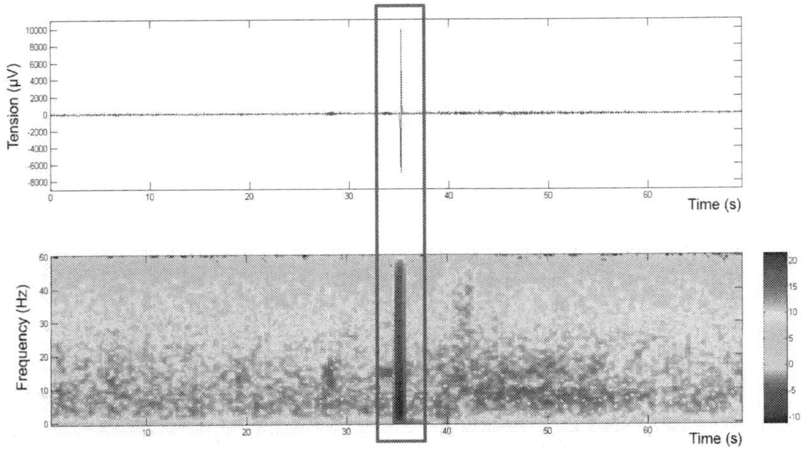

Fig. 4. Example showing a high-amplitude artefact

Here, the test is computed on the raw EEG data every 10s. A moving window is compared to a fixed reference window as shown in fig. 3. The reference variance is calculated on an artefact-free time window lasting one minute, chosen at the beginning of the recording,. Then, a moving window of 10s is compared to this reference every 10s. The threshold λ_{art} is empirically chosen and discussed in section 3.
The goal is to detect the artefact, not to reject it. As the system is working on a minimal number of EEG channels, it is not possible to recover lost EEG information of the artefact since missing information cannot be found somewhere else. Nevertheless, detecting the occurrence of an artefact provides information on the signal quality: whenever an artefact is detected, the concomitant relative power extracted from EEG should not be used to evaluate drowsiness.

2.4 Method relevance

The whole algorithm can be applied on-line. However, the sliding window of 10s used for median filtering induces a delay of 5s and the sliding window of 30s used for the MCT induces a delay of 15s. The artefact detection is computed in parallel with a sliding window of 10s which induces a delay of 5s. So, the decision provided by the algorithm is delayed by 20s from the signals recording. This latency in the decision will be taken into account when comparing the results to the expert's decisions.
The general purpose of this algorithm is the detection of drowsiness. The MCT detects α bursts, which are indicators of drowsiness as seen in section 1. The reference is calculated on a fixed window chosen at the beginning of the signal, supposing that the driver is completely awake when he starts driving. So, the mean calculated on the moving window is compared to a wakefulness reference. If the bilateral test is higher than the threshold, the driver is then considered as drowsy, otherwise he is considered as awake. Fig. 6 shows how the signal is processed in the detection system. First the relative power in the α band (b) of

the EEG (a) is calculated. Then, it is smoothed by median filtering (c). A MCT is performed (d) on the filtered signal and is thresholded to make the decision awake or drowsy (e).

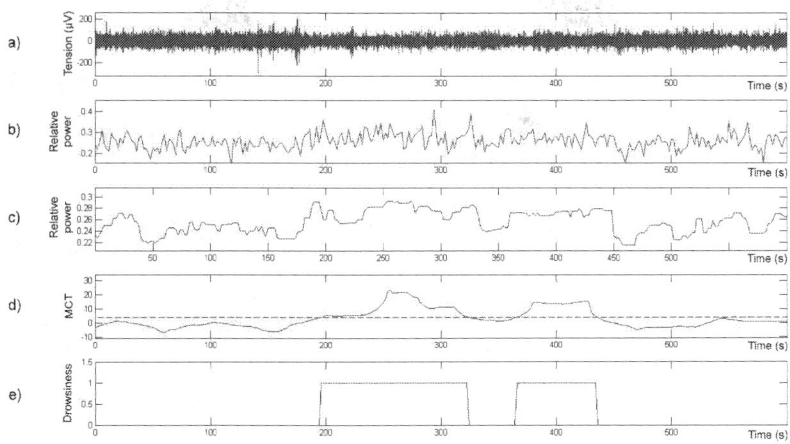

Fig. 6. Signal processing from EEG to drowsiness detection

High-amplitude artefacts pollute the EEG signals and generate isolated high abnormal values on the whole EEG band of the power spectrum. A median filter is used to smooth the α relative power signal and to reject abnormal isolated values to avoid false detection. Moreover, a VCT is calculated on the raw EEG signal to detect the occurrence of high-amplitude artefacts polluting the whole EEG band. The detection of these high-amplitude artefacts does not allow rejecting them but provides information on the quality of signal around this point. It means that if artefacts are found on a part of the signal, decisions on drowsiness in this part tend to be less reliable than if not.

The point with detecting α bursts in EEG signal is the difficulty to define a common threshold for all drivers because of the large inter-individual differences (Karrer et al., 2004). Here, the level of α_{rel} power in the "awake" state is learned on each driver from the reference window. Moreover, the output of MCT is a variable following a centred reduced normal law. So, the threshold used in the bilateral test has statistical meaning and is the same for all drivers.

In the same way, as the output of the VCT is a variable following a Fisher distribution, the threshold used to detect high-amplitude artefacts has a statistical meaning and is the same for all drivers.

3. Results and discussion

3.1 Database

The database used for the evaluation of the method has been provided by the CEPA (Centre d'Etudes de Physiologie Appliquée) from Strasbourg (France) using the driving simulator

PAVCAS ("Poste d'Analyse de la Vigilance en Conduite Automobile Simulée"). PAVCAS is a moving base driving simulator composed of a mobile base with four liberty degrees (vertical and longitudinal movements, swaying and pitching) and a real-time interactive visualization unit. The visualisation unit reproduces very well the driving conditions on a freeway by day or night. Images are shown on five screens in front of the vehicle and are arranged in semicircle.
The database is composed of forty recordings from twenty subjects. Each subject was recorded while driving for 90 minutes, a first time perfectly rested and a second time suffering from sleep deprivation (the subject had slept 4 hours only) in diurnal conditions. The database is thus composed of 60 hours of driving data. Each recording includes four EEG channels (left frontal (F3), central (C3), parietal (P3) and occipital (O1)), one EOG channel and a video of the driver's face. Objective sleepiness was evaluated on each recording by an expert doctor using the scale described in section I. Data acquisition of physiological signals was performed at 250Hz.

3.2 Technical validation

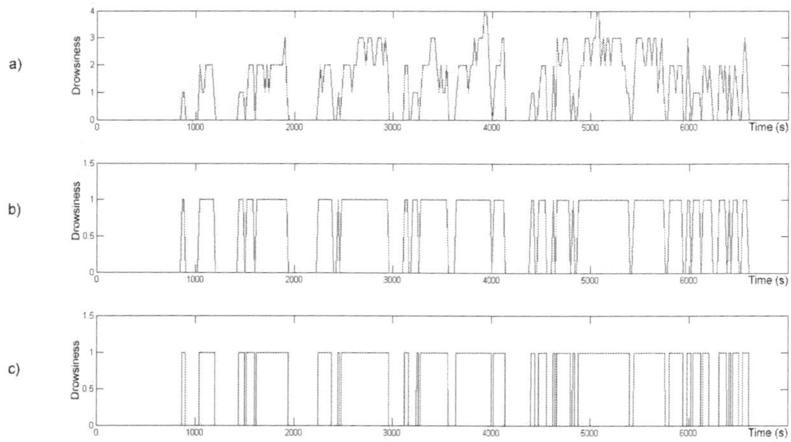

Fig. 9. Comparison between expert decision (a and b) and system decision (c)

The method proposed in this chapter provides a binary decision [awake; drowsy] while the database has been manually labelled using five levels. Moreover, the expert classified non overlapping intervals of 20s (epochs) while the automatic system makes a decision every second. To compare our results with the expert's decision, the following validation technique was used. The five expert decision levels were converted into a binary decision by considering as drowsy any decision superior or equal to 1 in the expert's scale as shown in fig. 9. This figure shows the expert decision on a five levels scale (a) and on a binary scale (b) and the drowsiness detection obtained using our system (c).

Furthermore, each 20s epoch classified by the expert was directly compared to the system decision: if during the 20s interval, the system classifies at least 1s as "drowsy", then the decision for the epoch was "drowsy". Else it was "awake".
Epochs were then compared one by one and classified according to the table of confusion 2.

		Expert decision: awake	Expert decision: drowsy
Automatic decision	awake	True Negative (TN)	False Negative (FN)
	drowsy	False Positives (FP)	True Positive (TP)

Table 2. Table of confusion

The true positive rate (TP_{rate}) or detection rate is the ratio between the number of true "drowsy" automatic decisions and the number of "drowsy" expert decisions. The false positive rate (FP_{rate}) is the ratio between the number of false "drowsy" automatic decisions and the number of "awake" expert decisions. They are calculated according to (6) and (7).

$$TP_{rate} = \frac{TP}{TP + FN} \quad (6)$$

$$FP_{rate} = \frac{FP}{FP + TN} \quad (7)$$

The results are displayed as Receiver Operating Characteristic (ROC) curves (Hanley & McNeil, 1982), plotting TP_{rate} in function of FP_{rate}. The purpose is to have the highest TP_{rate} with the lowest FP_{rate}.

3.3 Results using alpha relative power

3.3.1 Results without artefact detection

The drowsiness detection algorithm was applied on the whole database, with a decision threshold λ (defined in section 2.4) varying from 1.5 to 5, on each of the four EEG channels. The results presented in fig. 10 are those obtained when the MCT is applied on the alpha relative power without considering artefact detection. "Star" markers correspond to the P3 channel, "circle" markers to the F3 channel, "square" markers to the C3 channel and "triangle" markers to the O1 channel. The head at the bottom right of Fig.10 reminds the reader of the position of each channel. For each channel, the results represented with the markers the further on the right corresponds to the smallest λ and those with the markers the further on the left to the biggest λ. It is coherent: increasing λ diminishes the FP_{rate} while decreasing the TP_{rate}.

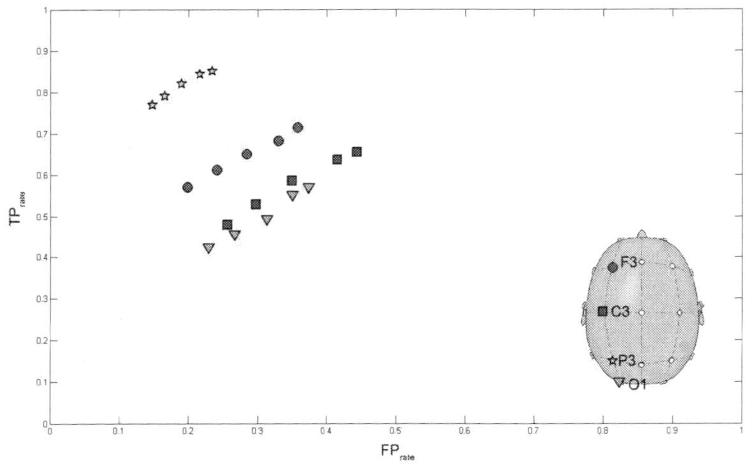

Fig. 10. Results obtained using different EEG channels

It is obvious from fig. 10 that the results are better when the P3 parietal channel is used, which is in concordance with results from the literature: drowsiness is characterized by an increase of α activity predominately in the parietal region of the brain. Indeed, results obtained with EEG recorded by C3, F3 or O1 are only slightly better than those that would be obtained with a random classifier. In the following sections, only the results obtained on P3 channel are shown.

The optimal result on P3 are TP_{rate}=82,1% and TP_{rate}=19,2% with λ=3. However changing the threshold does degrade the performances (TP_{rate}=85,1% and TP_{rate}=23,5% with λ=1,5 and TP_{rate}=76,9% and TP_{rate}=14,8% with λ=5), which proves that the method is not sensitive to the threshold value.

3.3.2 Results with artefact detection

An example of artefact detection is shown on fig. 11. The first signal (a) is the EEG raw data. The signal (b) is the result of the VCT. The dotted line corresponds to the threshold λ_{art}=6. The last signal (c) shows the result of the artefact detection (dotted line): when "zero" no high amplitude artefact is detected and when "one", an artefact is detected. The dotted line boxes underline high-amplitude artefacts.

First, this example shows that the detected artefacts correspond to high-amplitude electric perturbations of the EEG signal. As high-amplitude artefacts have not been evaluated by an expert on the dataset, it is not possible to quantify the performances of the artefact detection method. Nevertheless, a visual check of all the recordings shows that all the apparent high-amplitude artefacts have been detected. Fig. 12 shows the number of artefacts detected in the database (total number and corresponding percentage on the database) in function of the value of the threshold λ_{art} (used for artefact detection).

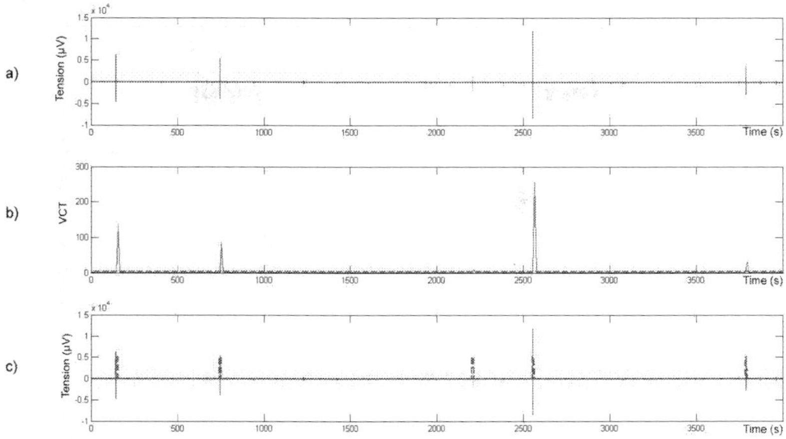

Fig. 11. Example of high amplitude artefact detection

It can be seen in fig. 12 that if the threshold is too small (λ_{art}<5), detection is really sensitive and a lot of points are rejected. Visually, this means a lot of false alarms. When increasing λ_{art}, the number of artefacts detected decreases quickly till λ_{art}=6, which visually seems an appropriate threshold. Indeed, for this threshold value, all the visible high-amplitude artefacts are detected without false alarms. At this point, one can see that high-amplitude artefacts represent only a small part of the dataset: about 2%.

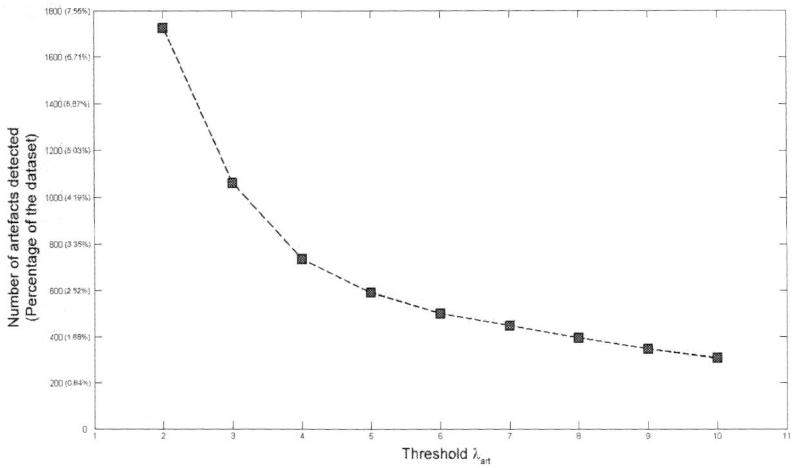

Fig. 12. Number of artefact detected in function of λ_{art}

Results obtained when no decision is made if artefacts are detected are displayed in fig. 13 with "circle" markers. The threshold used for the artefact detection is λ_{art} =6. "square" markers represent the results obtained without considering the artefact detection.

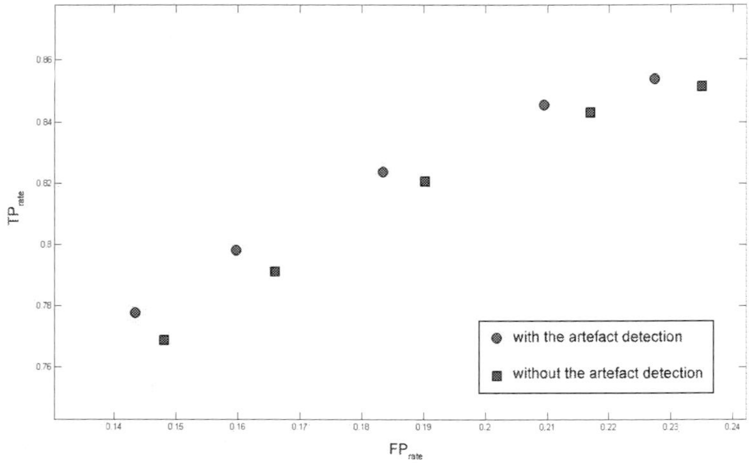

Fig. 13. ROC curve for drowsiness detection when artefact detection is used

It is obvious in fig. 13 that results are slightly improved: TP_{rate} is a bit increased while FP_{rate} is a bit decreased. Using the threshold λ=3, results increase from TP_{rate}=82,1% and FP_{rate}=19,2% to TP_{rate}=82,4% and FP_{rate}=18,3%. So, artefact detection decreases the number of false decisions. The fact that results are only slightly increased can be explained by the fact that high-amplitude artefacts represent about 2% only of the dataset.
Artefact detection will be taken into account in the following sections.

3.4 Results using other features than alpha relative power

Results presented in section 3.3 are now compared to results obtained with other features proposed in the literature. The results are displayed in fig. 14. Results from section 3.3, obtained using MCT on the median filtered α_{rel} signal, are represented by "star" markers. "Square" and "circle" markers represent results obtained using MCT and median filtering respectively on θ_{rel} and β_{rel} signals. Note that β activity increases with cognitive tasks and active concentration, so drowsiness is characterized by a decrease of the β activity. So, the detection algorithm using β as the main feature consider the driver as "drowsy" when the output of the MCT is lower than the threshold -λ (varying from -5 to -1). "Triangle" markers correspond to results obtained with the combined signals $\alpha_{rel} | \theta_{rel}$. Decisions are made independently on α_{rel} and on θ_{rel} and then merged with a logical OR. The optimum threshold λ=3 was used for α_{rel}. Displayed results are obtained with a threshold varying from 1,5 to 5 for θ_{rel} detection. The idea to use both α_{rel} and θ_{rel} is inspired by table 1, where it is assumed that drowsiness is characterized by an increase of the activity in one of the two frequency bands α and θ. "Hexagram" markers represent the $(\alpha+\theta)/\beta$ feature. This feature has been suggested by De Waard and Brookhuis (De Waard & Brookhuis, 1991). As α and θ activity are supposed to increase with drowsiness whereas β activity is supposed to decrease, this feature should be increasing with drowsiness. In this case, MCT is computed on the sum of the signals α_{rel} and θ_{rel} divided by the β_{rel} signal and only one threshold is used to make the decision.

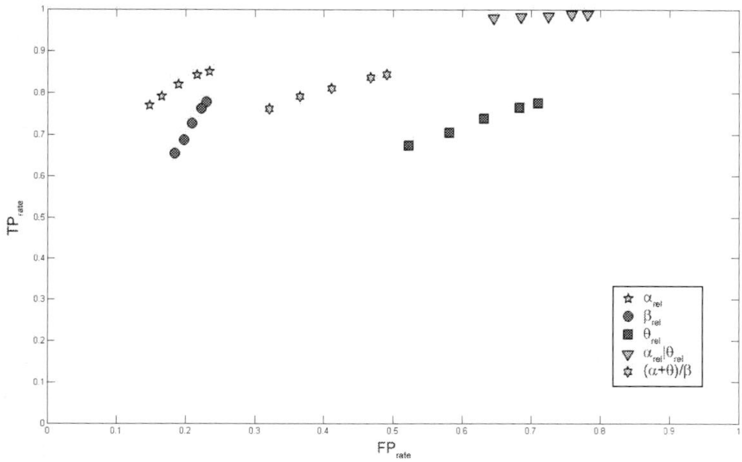

Fig. 14. ROC curves using different features for drowsiness detection

The best results are obtained with the drowsiness detection algorithm applied on the α_{rel} signal (TP_{rate}=82,4%, FP_{rate}=18,3%). Since the algorithm was tested with the same threshold on data recorded from 20 different persons, this tends to show that the method can be applied on different persons without adapting the tuning parameter.

The results obtained with $\alpha_{rel} | \theta_{rel}$ show that θ_{rel} is not relevant to detect drowsiness since the number of false positive increases tremendously when this information is added. This is confirmed by the results obtained with θ_{rel} only. The $(\alpha+\theta)/\beta$ ratio and β_{rel} give correct results (TP_{rate}=76,2% and TP_{rate}=32,1% for $(\alpha+\theta)/\beta$ and TP_{rate}=75,9% and TP_{rate}=24,1% for β_{rel}) but worse than the results obtained with the α_{rel} information only.

Now, if we compare the results obtained with the literature, the results obtained are as good as those found when using a trained algorithm. Lin et al. (Lin et al., 2005a) proposed to monitor driving performance, i.e. the capacity to maintain the car in the middle of the road computing a linear regression model on a 2-channels EEG. They obtained a correlation of r=0,88 between their model and the driving performances when the model is trained and tested on the same session. The correlation decreases to r=0,7 when trained and tested on different sessions. So, this method needs to be tuned for each driver as the model estimated for one driver does not work so well on another. Lin et al. increase these results using ICA on a 33-channel EEG (Lin et al., 2005a) to compute their linear regression model and obtain a correlation of r=0,88 between their estimation and the driving performances on the testing session. Nevertheless, this model needs to be trained on a large amount of data and has been tested on five drivers only. Ben Khalifa et al. (Ben Khalifa et al., 2004) obtained 92% of true drowsiness detections by training a neural network on a the EEG spectrum of the P4-O2 channel but this result is obtained on the training set and decreases to 76% of true detections on the validation set. Moreover, these results are obtained on a set of only four drivers. At least, Rosipal et al. (Rosipal et al., 2007) obtained about 77% of true detections of drowsiness states by using hGMM on the spectral content of EEG transferred into a compact form of autoregressive model coefficients. This study has been performed on a large number of drivers and needs a period of training.

The advantage of the method proposed in this paper is that it does not need to be trained or adapted. The same threshold can be used for all drivers. Moreover, as the method has been tested on huge dataset, the results can be considered significant.

3.5 Results merging alpha and beta relative powers

From the previous section, the best results are obtained when α_{rel} or β_{rel} are used as features, which naturally gives the idea to merge these two features to increase the decision reliability The technique used to merge α_{rel} and b_{rel} is fuzzy logic, which is based on the theory of fuzzy sets developed by Zadeh (Zadeh, 1965). Let us consider $\mu_{Dr}(\alpha_{rel})$ and $\mu_{Dr}(\beta_{rel})$, the membership functions, which represent the membership degree of α_{rel} and β_{rel}, independently considered, to the "drowsy" state. The purpose is to make a decision $Dr(\alpha_{rel}, \beta_{rel})$ using both $\mu_{Dr}(\alpha_{rel})$ and $\mu_{Dr}(\beta_{rel})$,. The driver is considered to be drowsy if both the decision made using α_{rel} and the decision made using β_{rel} is "drowsy". This is expressed thanks to the t-norm product as follows:

$$\mathrm{Dr}(\alpha_{\mathrm{rel}}, \beta_{\mathrm{rel}}) = \frac{\mu_{\mathrm{Dr}}(\alpha_{\mathrm{rel}})\mu_{\mathrm{Dr}}(\beta_{\mathrm{rel}})}{\mu_{\mathrm{Dr}}(\alpha_{\mathrm{rel}})\mu_{\mathrm{Dr}}(\beta_{\mathrm{rel}}) + \mu_{\mathrm{Aw}}(\alpha_{\mathrm{rel}})\mu_{\mathrm{Aw}}(\beta_{\mathrm{rel}})} \tag{8}$$

Note that $\mu_{Aw}(.)$ is the membership function of the "awake" state and is the complementary of $\mu_{Dr}(.)$. The denominator is used here to normalize $Dr(\alpha_{rel},\beta_{rel})$ between 0 and 1.

One has to define the membership function $\mu_{Dr}(\alpha_{rel})$ and $\mu_{Dr}(\beta_{rel})$. A study of the probability of being drowsy in function of the MCT's threshold λ on α_{rel} and β_{rel}, $P(dr\,|\,\alpha_{rel})$ and $P(dr\,|\,\text{-}\beta_{rel})$, is displayed in fig. 15. The "square" markers line displays the experimental $P(dr\,|\,\alpha_{rel})$ and the "circle" markers line displays the experimental $P(dr\,|\,\text{-}\beta_{rel})$. Probabilities are calculated as the percentage of true drowsiness detections obtained on periods when the relative power is over λ.

The membership function μ_{Dr} (α_{rel}) and μ_{Dr} (β_{rel}) are then designed from the results presented in fig. 15. As α_{rel} and β_{rel} have a very similar behaviour, the same membership is used for α_{rel} and β_{rel}. This membership function is presented in fig. 16.

The driver is considered as "drowsy" when $Dr(\alpha_{rel},\beta_{rel})$ is larger than 0.5 The results obtained with this method are shown in fig. 17 with the "circle" markers. They are compared to the results obtained using the MCT on α_{rel} only ("square" markers).

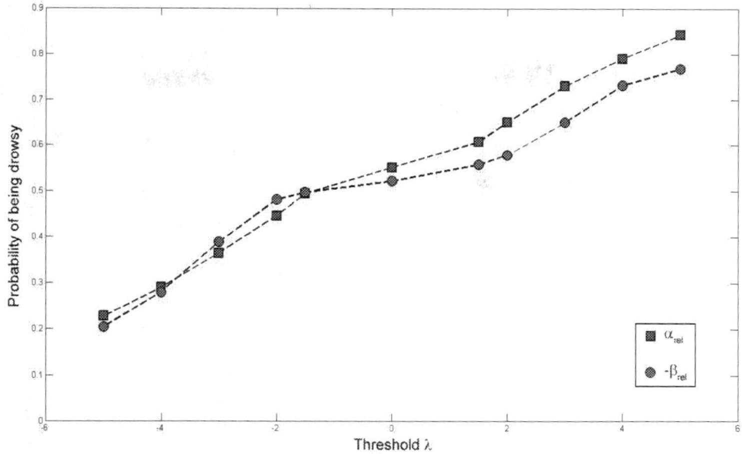

Fig. 15. Experimental probabilities of being drowsy in function of threshold λ

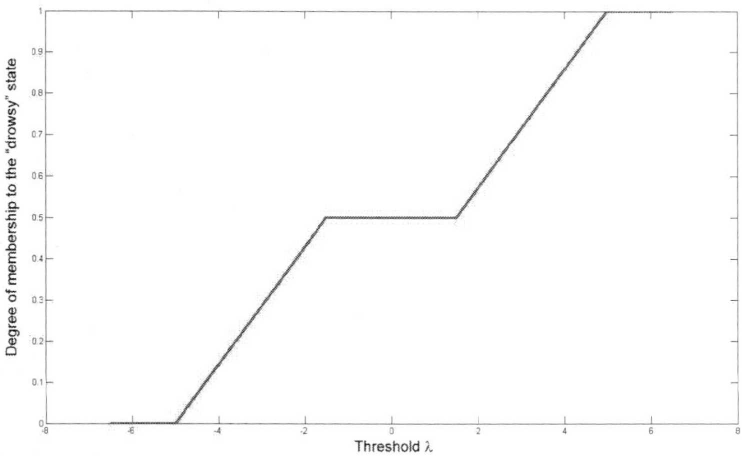

Fig. 16. Membership function in function of threshold λ

Results are improved using this fuzzy logic approach since FP_{rate} is increased and FP_{rate} is decreased. The results obtained with this method are TP_{rate}=84,6% and FP_{rate}=17,9% (TP_{rate}=82,4% and FP_{rate}=18,3% with λ=3 when using only α_{rel} information). This means that the β_{rel} information is relevant to detect drowsiness when combined with α_{rel}. Moreover, compared to the method proposed in section 3.5, there is no need to select an appropriate detection threshold for α_{rel} and β_{rel}. The fuzzy approach increased the detection reliability.

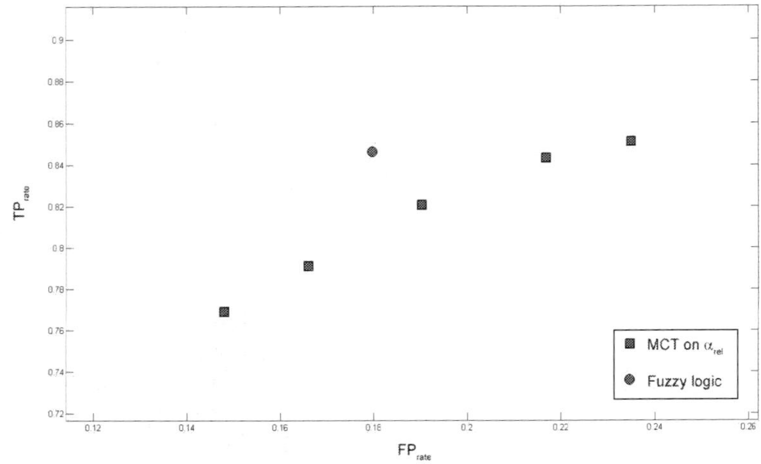

Fig. 17. Performances obtained using α_{rel}, β_{rel} and (α_{rel}, β_{rel}) merged with fuzzy logic

4. Conclusion

An algorithm to detect on line drivers' drowsiness from a P3 EEG channel has been presented in this paper. This algorithm is based on a means comparison test (MCT) applied on the EEG relative power calculated in the alpha band and in the beta band. The results of the MCT test are then merged using fuzzy logic. The algorithm can operate on-line with a short delay and does not need to be tuned. Performances obtained on a large data set recorded from 20 different drivers are 84,6% of true detection and 17,9% of false detection using the parietal EEG channel only. A high-amplitude artefact detection system has been developed and combined to the drowsiness detector. It enables periods of time when the EEG signal is unreliable to be detected on line. No decision is made by the drowsiness detector while the artefact detector classifies the EEG signal as unreliable. The artefact detector is tuned by a single threshold whose value is independent of the driver.
The next step of this work is to add an "eye blinks and yawn" detection system thanks to a high frame rate camera and to merge the decisions to obtain a highly reliable automatic drowsiness detector. Fuzzy logic could be a first step to merge this information.

5. Acknowledgements

The authors are grateful to the Centre d'Etudes de Physiologie Appliquée (CEPA) in Strasbourg (FR) for providing the data and their help, as well as the Laboratoire d'Automatique, de Mécanique, et d'Informatique industrielles et Humaines (LAMIH) in Valenciennes (FR).

6. References

Akerstedt, T. and Gillberg, M. (1990). Subjective and objective sleepiness in the active individual. *International Journal of Neuroscience*, Vol. 52, pp. 29–37

Ben Khalifa, K., Bédoui, M., Dogui, M., and Alexandre, F. (2004). Alertness states classification by SOM and LVQ neural networks. *International Journal of Information Technology*, Vol. 4, pp. 228–231

Blinowska, K. and Durka, P. (2006). Electroencephalography(EEG), In: *Wiley Encyclopedia of Biomedical Engineering*, Ed. Metin Akay, Wyley

DeWaard, D. and Brookhuis, K. (1991). Assessing driver status: a demonstration experiment on the road. *Accident Analysis and Prevention*, Vol. 23, No. 4, pp. 297–307

Dinges, D. (1995). An overview of sleepiness and accidents. *Journal of sleep research*, Vol. 4, No. 2, pp. 4–14

Galley, N., Schleicher, R., and Galley, L. (2004). Blink parameter as indicators of driver's sleepiness - possibilities and limitations. *Vision in Vehicles*, Vol. 10, pp. 189–196

Grace, R., Byrne, V.E., Bierman, D.M., Legrand, J.-M., Gricourt, D., Davis, B.K., Staszewski, J.J., Carnahan, B. (1998). A drowsy driver detection system for heavy vehicles, *Proc. of the 17th Digital Avionics Systems Conference*, Vol. 2, pp. I36/1-I36/8

Hanley, J. and McNeil, B. (1982). The meaning and use of the area under a receiver operating characteristic (roc) curve. *Radiology*, Vol. 143, No. 1, pp. 29–36

Ji, Q., Lan, P., and Looney, C. (2006). A probabilistic framework for modeling and real-time monitoring human fatigue. *IEEE Transactions on systems, man, and cybernetics - Part A: Systems and humans*, Vol. 36, No. 5, pp. 862–875

Ji, Q. and Yang, X. (2001). Real time visual cues extraction for monitoring driver vigilance. *Proc. of International Workshop on Computer Vision Systems*, pp. 107–124

Ji, Q., Zhu, Z., and Lan, P. (2004). Real time non-intrusive monitoring and prediction of driver fatigue. *IEEE Transport Vehicle Technology*, Vol. 53, No. 4, pp. 1052–1068

Karrer, K., Vohringer-Kuhnt, T., Baumgarten, T., and Briest, S. (2004). The role of individual differences in driver fatigue prediction. *The third International Conference on Traffic and Transportation Psychology*

Kay, A., Trinder, J., Bowes, G., , and Kim, Y. (1994). Changes in airway resistance during sleep onset. *Journal of Applied Physiology*, Vol. 76, pp. 1600–1607

Klein, R., Allen, R., and Miller, J. (1980). Relationship between truck ride quality and safety of operations: methodology development. Technical Report DOT HS 805 494, Systems Technology, Inc., Hawthorne, CA

Knippling, R. (1998). Perclos: A valid psychophysiological measure of alertness as assessed by psychomotor vigilance. Technical Report FHWA-MCRT-98-006, Federal Highway Administration

Lin, C., Wu, R., Liang, S., Chao, W., Chen, Y., and Jung, T. (2005a). Eeg-based drowsiness estimation for safety driving using independent component analysis. *IEEE Transactions on Circuits and Systems*, Vol. 52, No. 12, pp. 2726–2738

Lin, C.-T., Wu, R.-C., Jung, T.-P., Liang, S.-F., and Huang, T.-Y. (2005b). Estimating driving performance based on eeg spectrum analysis. *EURASIP Journal on Applied Signal Processing*, Vol. 19, pp. 3165–3174

Makeig, S., Bell, A., Jung, T.-P., and Sejnowski, T. (1996). Independent component analysis of electroencephalographic data. *Advances in Neural Information Processing Systems*, Vol. 8, pp. 145–151

Muzet, A., Pébayle, T., Langrognet, J., and Otmani, S. (2003). Awake pilot study no.2: Testing steering grip sensor measures. Technical Report IST-2000-28062, CEPA

O'Hanlon, F. and Kelley, G. (1974). A psychophysiological evaluation of devices for preventing lane drift and run-off-road accidents. Technical Report 1736-F, Federal Highway Administration

Picot, A., Charbonnier, S. and Caplier, A. (2008). On-line automatic detection of driver drowsiness using a single EEG channel. *30th Conference of the IEEE Engineering in Medicine and Biology Society*, pp. 3864-3867.

Quanten, S., Valck, E. D., Cluydts, R., and Berckmans, D. (2006). Thermoregulatory changes at driver sleepiness. *International Journal of Vehicle Design*, Vol. 42, pp. 87–100.

Ragot, J., Darouach, M., Maquin, D., and Bloch, G. (1990). *Validation de données et diagnostic.* Ed. Hermès, Traité des nouvelles technologies

Rechtschaffen, A. and Kales, A. (1968). *A Manual of Standardized Terminology, Techniques and Scoring System for Sleep Stages of Human Subject.* National Institute of Health Publication, Washington DC, us government printing office edition

Renner, G. and Mehring, S. (1997). Lane departure and drowsiness - two major accident causes - one safety system. Technical report, Transport Research Laboratory

Rosipal, R., Peters, B., Kecklund, G., Akerstedt, T., Gruber, G., Woertz, M., Anderer, P. and Dorffner, G. (2007). EEG-Based Drivers' Drowsiness Monitoring Using a Hierarchical Gaussian Mixture Model, *Hum. Comp. Interaction*, Vol. 16, pp. 294-303

Royal, D. (2002). National survey of distracted and drowsy driving attitudes and behavior. Technical Report DOT HS 809 566, National Highway Traffic Safety Administration

Santamaria, J. and Chiappa, K. H. (1987). The EEG of Drowsiness in normal Adults. Journal of clinical Neurophysiology, Vol. 4, No. 4, pp. 327-382.

Smith, P., Shah, M., and Lobo, N. D. V. (2003). Determining driver visual attention with one camera. *IEEE Trans. on intelligent transportation systems*, Vol. 4, No. 4, pp. 205–218

Törnros, J., Peters, B., and Östlund, J. (2000). Heart rate measures as drowsiness indicators. Technical report, Swedish National Road and Transport Research Institute

Vural, E., Cetin, M., Ercil, A., Littlewort, G., .Bartlett, M. and Movellan, J., (2007). Drowsy driver detection through facial movement analysis, *Proc. ICCV*, pp. 6-18.

Welch, P. (1967). The use of fast fourier transform for the estimation of power spectra: A method based on time averaging over short, modified periodograms. *IEEE Trans. Audio & Electroacoust.*, Vol. 15, pp. 70–73

Wierwille, W., Ellworth, L., Wreggit, S., Fairbanks, R., and Kim, C. (1994). Research on vehicle-based driver status/performance monitoring. Technical report, NHTSA

Zadeh, L. (1965). "Fuzzy sets". *Information and Control*, Vol. 8, No. 3, pp. 338-353

The merits of artificial proprioception, with applications in biofeedback gait rehabilitation concepts and movement disorder characterization

Robert LeMoyne[1], Cristian Coroian[1], Timothy Mastroianni[2], Pawel Opalinski[3], Michael Cozza[4], and Warren Grundfest[1]
1. UCLA
USA
2. Cognition Engineering
USA
3. Google
USA
4. Converge Robotics Corporation
USA

1. Introduction

The advance of wireless accelerometer technology has become increasingly integrated with respect to biomedical applications. With the amalgamation of wireless technology and MEMS applications, the synthesis of wireless accelerometer technology has yielded the biomedical/ neuroengineering artificial equivalent of proprioception. The merits of artificial proprioception are addressed in tandem with recent and novel applications incorporating wireless accelerometers as an artificial form of proprioception. Recent and novel applications span concepts such as virtual proprioception, a real-time biofeedback system for gait rehabilitation; gait analysis and quantification; quantification of Parkinson's disease status; and reflex characterization. The steady evolution of accelerometers has enabled the permeation of the technology from initial conceptualization to recent integration of the technology for biomedical applications (Saunders et al., 1953; Culhane et al., 2005; LeMoyne et al., 2008c).

Accelerometers were initially proposed for the quantification of movement characteristics during the 1950's; but the supporting technologies for developing robust accelerometer applications were not sufficiently evolved (Saunders et al., 1953; Culhane et al., 2005). During this era accelerometers were actually characterized as too expensive, unreliable, and cumbersome, which could perturb the actual nature of human movement (Culhane et al., 2005). Throughout the decade of the 1990's the accelerometer technology space obtained the capability for movement quantification. Essentially lateral technologies, such as airbag release systems for the automotive industry, provided the basis for the evolution of the accelerometer technology space. Successive developments of accelerometer devices demonstrated high levels of quality and reliability, while attributed with high volume capacity and low-cost production. The implications are that current accelerometer systems are capable for clinical applications, such as the characterization and quantification of human movement (Culhane et al., 2005; LeMoyne et al., 2008c).

The current technology status for accelerometer systems provides the capability for quantitative evaluation of locomotion and movement disorder with greater autonomy of application (Culhane et al., 2005; LeMoyne et al., 2008c). Sensors are extremely useful for movement analysis, such as gait, in both clinical rehabilitation applications and biomedical research, as provided by accelerometer technology (Wong et al., 2007). With micromachining technology, accelerometers produce a signal capable of measuring acceleration, representing both dynamic movement and static gravity. A general strategy for developing an accelerometer is to utilize a mass capable of producing a signal representative of the acceleration based on the deflection of the mass (Culhane et al., 2005).

The evolving technology applications for accelerometer devices provide the fundamentals for expanding the functionality of accelerometer systems as wearable proprioception applications. Accelerometer components provide the spatial representation imperative for the inertial navigation system of robotic applications, which is analogous to a proprioceptive system in humans. Spatial representation of proprioception for human beings is enabled through afferent systems, such as Golgi tendon organs and muscle spindles (Bekey, 2005).

The application of accelerometers as a wearable form of proprioception has an exceptional utility. A wearable accelerometer system can record and store the resultant accelerometer signal (LeMoyne et al., 2009a; LeMoyne et al., 2009b; LeMoyne et al., 2009c; LeMoyne et al., 2009d). The afferent proprioception of a human experience may be difficult to recall over an extended period of time and possibly especially difficult for a patient to communicate to a clinician. In contrast, wearable accelerometers are capable of providing artificial proprioception, which can be efficiently stored in a database and post-processed for potential diagnostic interpretation (LeMoyne et al., 2009a; LeMoyne et al., 2009b; LeMoyne et al., 2009c; LeMoyne et al., 2009d). The paradigm of wearable and wireless accelerometer systems providing artificial proprioception enables the foundation for current and unique applications.

Four novel applications utilizing wearable and wireless accelerometer devices as a form of artificial proprioception are quantification of Parkinson's disease status, reflex quantification and characterization, gait analysis quantification and classification, and virtual proprioception. Virtual proprioception is a real-time biofeedback application suitable for gait rehabilitation, especially for hemiparetic subjects. In essence the virtual proprioception system enables a subject to engage in real-time adjustment of gait disparities. Two wearable and wireless accelerometers are mounted to an anatomical anchor on each leg. The acceleration waveforms of both the affected and unaffected leg are provided to the subject. With the disparity of acceleration waveforms presented, the subject can modify gait during real-time of the gait cycle so that both legs are closer to parity of the acceleration waveforms as gait cycle continues (LeMoyne et al., 2008e; LeMoyne et al., 2008f).

Gait analysis quantification and classification incorporates wearable and wireless accelerometers with expanded application autonomy. Current applications of the system have been applied to a home-based setting and the outdoor environment. The value of the system is autonomy of the application beyond clinical confines. The concept is even relevant to situations for which the patient and clinician reside at distant locations. Subsequent post-processing techniques can characterize the current status and quality of gait for a subject (LeMoyne et al., 2009b; LeMoyne et al., 2009d).

Reflex quantification incorporating wireless accelerometers provides unique insight as to the neurological status of a subject. In essence the application is an extension from current methods for evaluating deep tendon reflexes as an integral aspect of the traditional neurological examination. As a form of artificial proprioception, the reflex response is characterized as a three dimensional acceleration waveform. With a tandem wireless accelerometer positioned to a potential energy derived reflex hammer evoking the reflex, the latency can also be derived given the temporal disparity of the tandem accelerometer acceleration waveforms. The wireless reflex quantification system enables a unique strategy for evaluating central nervous system and peripheral nervous system status, potentially reducing strain on critical economic resources (LeMoyne et al., 2008a; LeMoyne et al., 2008h; LeMoyne et al., 2009c).

Artificial proprioception through the application of wireless accelerometers also provides insight and autonomy for the assessment of Parkinson's disease status. Traditional evaluation for the response of a patient with respect to therapy strategy is performed by a clinician, tasked with the endeavor of qualitatively examining the patient and applying the findings to an ordinal scale (www.mdvu.org; LeMoyne et al., 2008c). Presumably the clinical assessment is conducted during an appointment, not continuously evaluated in the autonomous environment of the patient. In contrast the application of wireless accelerometry as a form of wearable proprioception may enable continual tracking for the Parkinson's disease status in the autonomous environment of the patient. The application of wireless accelerometers enables the opportunity for long-term data reduction and advanced insight as to the efficacy of treatment strategy (LeMoyne et al., 2009a).

The applications for virtual proprioception, gait analysis, reflex quantification, and Parkinson's disease status classification demonstrate the present and future capabilities that artificial proprioception has for advancing biomedical engineering and the medical industry. Artificial proprioception is attributed as wearable and equipped with the capability to store and convey information through wireless transmission. The integration of artificial proprioception can potentially advance clinical acuity and perceptivity as to the status of a patient with movement disorder, while reducing rampant strain on the medical economy. Gait rehabilitation biofeedback concepts, such as virtual proprioception, can be amenable to homebound environments. The diagnostic capabilities of wireless gait analysis and Parkinson's disease classification through wireless accelerometer devices are amenable to autonomous home settings. Wireless accelerometer reflex quantification systems may provide advanced acuity and perceptivity for clinicians with respect to the neurological status of a patient, while alleviating strain on medical resources, such as electrodiagnostic evaluation (LeMoyne et al., 2008a; LeMoyne et al., 2008e; LeMoyne et al., 2008f; LeMoyne et al., 2008h; LeMoyne et al., 2009a; LeMoyne et al., 2009b; LeMoyne et al., 2009c; LeMoyne et al., 2009d).

Fundamental demand for artificial proprioception through wireless accelerometers is initially illustrated through the consideration of people with trauma to the central nervous system undergoing motor control therapy, such as gait rehabilitation, possibly in tandem having a disparity in proprioceptive afferent representation, respective of both limbs. Ordinal scales, which are currently standard for clinical evaluations, are subject to controversy, especially in consideration of the qualitative basis for deriving the ordinal scale value. In particular ordinal scales lack the capacity to fully address the temporal nature of the movement characteristics being evaluated (LeMoyne et al., 2008c). With the accelerometer technology recently evolving to a sufficient capacity for biomedical applications, initial applications of accelerometer systems, such as activity monitors, are addressed. Other standard technologies for characterizing gait are contrasted to previous and current accelerometer gait analysis applications; and the successful test and evaluation results of the accelerometer systems pertaining to gait are considered.

2. Natural biological inspired proprioception contrasted to artificial proprioception

A contrast of the proprioceptive afferent sensory receptors relative to artificial proprioception establishes the fundamental utility of artificial proprioception. Proprioception is defined as the afferent representation for the spatial position of the body (Nolte & Sundsten, 2002; Seeley et al., 2003). Two proprioceptive afferent sensory receptors are selected for contrast: the muscle spindle and Golgi tendon organ (Kandel et al., 2000; Nolte & Sundsten, 2002; Seeley et al., 2003).

The muscles spindle is a predominant proprioceptive afferent, enabled with the ability to ascertain muscle length status. Consideration of the muscle spindle requires defining the disparity between the intrafusal and extrafusal class of muscles fiber. "Fusus" is Latin for spindle. Therefore intrafusal muscle fiber is within the muscle spindle, and extrafusal is outside of the muscle spindle. Intrafusal and extrafusal fibers are attached to each other (Nolte & Sundsten, 2002). The muscle spindles are parallel to their respective muscle fibers (Clark et al., 2008). Intrafusal fibers representing the muscle spindles are classified by two distinct types: nuclear bag fibers and nuclear chain fibers (Nolte & Sundsten, 2002).

Further consideration of the nuclear bag fibers establishes two disparate subclasses: the static nuclear bag fibers and dynamic nuclear bag fibers. The type 1a afferent fibers innervate all three forms of intrafusal fibers: nuclear chain fibers, static nuclear bag fibers, and dynamic nuclear bag fibers. Type 2 afferent fibers innervate static nuclear bag and nuclear chain fibers. The disparity in terms of afferent innervation enables the muscle spindle to measure two distinct types of muscle stretch characteristics (Kandel et al., 2000).

The muscle spindle is equipped with the ability to convey information pertinent to both muscle length rate of change and length status. The dynamic nuclear bag fibers innervated by the type 1a nerve fiber contribute to acquiring rate of muscle length change. The nuclear chain and static nuclear bag fibers are capable of conveying the steady state status of the muscle length and are innervated by both type 1a and type 2 afferent fibers (Kandel et al., 2000).

The Golgi tendon organ also provides afferent feedback, with respect to spatial representation of the body. In contrast to the muscle spindle, the Golgi tendon organ is aligned in series to the relevant muscle fiber. The Golgi tendon organ is innervated by 1b afferent fibers, which are activated in response to muscle contraction inducing tension on the pertinent tendon (Kandel et al., 2000; Nolte & Sundsten, 2002).

In contrast to biological (natural) proprioception, artificial proprioception using accelerometry enables a recordable modality for movement status. The accelerometer derives an accelerometer signal through a representative mass (Culhane et al., 2005; LeMoyne et al., 2008c). With the introduction of wireless technology, artificial proprioception has been synthesized into a fully wearable system through the incorporation of small wireless accelerometers. In the event of disparity of proprioceptive representation for affected and unaffected legs during hemiparetic gait, artificial proprioception can inform the user of the limb disparity during locomotion and also the efficacy of real-time compensatory strategies. Gait, reflex, and Parkinson's disease status can be characterized and stored on a database using artificial proprioception, and acquired data can be post-processed (LeMoyne et al., 2008a; LeMoyne et al., 2008e; LeMoyne et al., 2008f; LeMoyne et al., 2008h; LeMoyne et al., 2009a; LeMoyne et al., 2009b; LeMoyne et al., 2009c; LeMoyne et al., 2009d).

3. Ordinal scale classification of movement quality

Clinicians can apply ordinal scales as a strategy to classify their findings during an examination. The clinician is tasked with the goal of selecting a relevant ordinal parameter with an associated subjective qualitative definition. In consideration of a reflex evaluation during an examination, the clinician may rate the reflex response of a subject as 2+ representing normal reflex, 3+ representing brisker than normal reflex, and 1+ representing diminished relative to normal reflex. The ordinal reflex scale described above includes a 0 and 4+ ordinal component to classify the extreme bounds of the reflex response (Bickley & Szilagyi, 2003). Notably, the above reflex scale is highly dependent on the clinician's interpretation of 'normal' along with the interpretation of delineating acuity for the ordinal scale values.

There are other types of reflex scales, such as the broader Mayo Clinic scale. The Mayo Clinic scale is based on a 9 point ordinal interpretation. The clinician may classify an above normal reflex as +1 classified as brisk and +2 classified as very brisk (Manschot et al., 1998). Likewise the 9 point scale is extremely dependent on the clinician's interpretation and differentiation between the qualitative classification of 'brisk' and 'very brisk'. Another concern is the comparability and compatibility of multiple scales with a different number of ordinal classifying components. Two clinicians with preference for disparate scales may even be prone to prescribing disparate therapy protocols.

Ordinal scales are applied to other movement classification scenarios. Mobility can be classified through the incorporation of the modified Rivermead Mobility Index (Lennon & Johnson, 2000). Parkinson's disease status is characterized through the Unified Parkinson's Disease Rating Scale (www.mdvu.org).

Another issue of the ordinal scale method is the need for a clinician to conduct the evaluation. Parkinson's disease is neurodegenerative in nature (Kandel et al., 2000). The degenerative cycle can possibly persist between clinical appointments, for which the frequency of appointments may be correlated to the ability to modify therapy strategy in coherence with the potentially variant severity of the degenerative cycle. Essentially a prolonged duration between clinical appointments may lack the timely feedback with respect to the progressively degenerative cycle. However, for instance daily clinical appointments for tracking the status of the neurodegenerative disease might impart a rampant strain on limited medical resources.

The controversy of the accuracy of ordinal scale evaluation methods is demonstrated in consideration of reflex quantification. Litvan assessed the reliability of the five point ordinal NINDS Myotatic Reflex Scale. The results obtained substantial to near perfect reliability for intraobservers and moderate to substantial reliability for interobservers (Litvan et al., 1996). The findings of Manschot contradict the findings of Litvan. Manschot investigated the reliability of the five point NINDS scale and the nine point Mayo Clinic scale. In consideration of both scales interobserver agreement was bound by a fair level of agreement (Manschot et al., 1998). Further investigation by Stam shows an extensive level of interobserver disagreement while using the nine component Mayo Clinic scale. The study discovered that for 28% of the examination neurologists disagreed by a minimum of two ordinal scale units. For 45% of the reflex pairs there was disagreement as to the existence of asymmetry (Stam & van Crevel, 1990).

Artificial proprioception institutes a paradigm shift from the traditional ordinal scale evaluation technique. With the selection of defined anatomical anchors, the application of accelerometers can reliably characterize movement attributes (Kavanagh et al., 2006; Saremi et al., 2006). A wireless three dimensional accelerometer node can be positioned at a specified anatomical location, acquiring an acceleration derived bio-signal. The acquired acceleration signal can be post-processed for computing significant quantification parameters for augmented classification.

4. Evolution of accelerometer technology for biomedical applications

Accelerometer technology has progressively evolved respective of biomedical applications. Current technology innovations enable the application of wireless accelerometers, which are highly portable and even wearable. The synthesis of the wireless accelerometer technology space has resulted in the biomedical/ neuroengineering equivalent of biological derived proprioception termed artificial proprioception (LeMoyne et al., 2008c).

Technology applications for accelerometer systems have been applied to fields correlated with locomotion, such as the quantification of movement status (Bouten et al., 1997;

Uiterwaal et al., 1998; Zhang et al., 2003). A device developed by Aminian termed Physilog integrated accelerometers, successfully demonstrating the capability of measuring physical activity (Aminian et al. 1999). Applications using accelerometers have been developed for characterizing physical activity status for children (Busser et al. 1997; Hoos et al., 2004). Accelerometer devices incorporating classification techniques have reliably ascertained posture and activity status (Fahrenberg et al., 1997; Lyons et al., 2005).

Given the inherent autonomy of accelerometer synthesized devices, the spatial-temporal relationships of specific aspects of the body during gait cycle has been acquired (Moe-Nilssen, 1998; Menz et al., 2003a). Accelerometer systems have characterized important gait parameters: velocity, stride frequency, and gait symmetry (Auvinet et al., 2002; Menz et al. 2003b). Accelerometer systems have been evaluated as feedback modalities for augmenting functional neuromuscular stimulation (Willemsen et al., 1991; Veltink & Franken, 1996). Given the light weight and portable qualities of accelerometers, triaxial accelerometers have been placed on the trunk and head to contrast gait strategy for young and elderly people (Menz et al., 2003b; Kavanagh et al., 2004). The research endeavors further establish the relevance of accelerometer systems for the quantification of locomotion and movement characteristics, especially enabled given their minimally intrusive nature and attributes.

4.1 Research validation of accelerometers for gait quantification

Testing and evaluation of accelerometers is imperative for the validation of applications involving the quantification of movement characteristics. A subclass of general movement status is relevant to gait. The validation and confirmation for the efficacy of accelerometers to evaluate locomotion has been conducted with the evolving accelerometer technology space, with applications using uniaxial, integrated biaxial, and wireless triaxial accelerometers (Mayagoitia et al., 2002; Kavanagh et al., 2006; Saremi et al., 2006; LeMoyne et al., 2009d). The process for validating the ability of accelerometers to quantify gait has been established through the contrast to standard gait analysis systems, such as optical motion analysis (Mayagoitia et al., 2002).

4.2 Body mounted sensors incorporating uniaxial accelerometers

Mayagoita developed a body mounted sensor device, which integrated uniaxial accelerometers. The body mounted sensor system was represented with a series of uniaxial accelerometers operating in tandem, which was contrasted to the Vicon® system for optical motion analysis. The body mounted system incorporating uniaxial accelerometers yielded similar results in contrast to the Vicon® optical motion analysis system. Mayagoita envisions future applications, which instill portable data-logger systems for enhanced operational autonomy (Mayagoitia et al., 2002).

4.3 Biaxial accelerometer applications for gait analysis

As accelerometer technology is continuously evolving, the logical procession of the technology space would be from uniaxial to biaxial to triaxial accelerometer applications. The ultimate would be the evolution of a wireless triaxial accelerometer node (LeMoyne et al., 2008c). Subsequent research involving biaxial accelerometer technology also advances the application through the use of highly specified anatomical mounting positions for the accelerometer devices (Kavanagh et al., 2006; Saremi et al., 2006).

4.4 Biaxial accelerometers with portable microprocessor

Saremi evaluated an accelerometer based system termed the Intelligent Device for Energy Expenditure and Activity (IDEEA) created by MiniSun for the capacity to evaluate gait parameters. The device integrated five biaxial accelerometers mounted at highly specified anatomical positions. One accelerometer node was mounted 4cm below the sternum top. The other four accelerometers were allocated in pairs of two for both legs: under the medial forefoot and the anterior aspect of the thigh. With respect to the medial forefoot, further anatomical specification defined the position as below the 4th metatarsal head by a distance of 2cm. The anterior aspect of the thigh was further classified as the midpoint in terms of the distance between the anterior superior iliac spine and the knee. The selection of the anatomical mounting points for the accelerometer nodes enabled the acquisition of data relevant to the sagittal plane. The sampling rate for the accelerometer components was established at 32Hz (Saremi et al., 2006). The fundamental objective of the MiniSun IDEEA device was to measure the energy expenditure for physical activity in a more autonomous application relative to the laboratory environment (Zhang et al. 2003; Zhang et al., 2004). The IDEEA device represents the integration of multiple accelerometers with the capacity to obtain spatiotemporal data relevant to gait. The IDEEA system is applicable in both community and clinical settings (Saremi et al., 2006).

The accuracy of the IDEEA device was compared to multiple traditional systems for gait analysis, such as EMG, a footswitch device, and a video gait analysis system using infrared markers. The investigation amended a triaxial accelerometer positioned on the thigh as contrast to the biaxial accelerometers of the MiniSun device. Relative to the MiniSun biaxial accelerometers, the triaxial accelerometers mounted to the thigh produced nearly identical waveforms. No statistically significant difference was ascertained for the parameters acquired from the footswitch device in comparison to the MiniSun device. The temporal aspect of gait parameters familiar to clinicians, such as EMG bursts, hip, knee, and ankle joint angle were characterized through the MiniSun device. The MiniSun accelerometer system demonstrated a high test to retest reliability. The reliable acquisition of leg acceleration waveforms during gait cycle could augment therapist insight in consideration of patient rehabilitation (Saremi et al., 2006).

4.5 Tandem biaxial accelerometers with wireless connectivity from processor box to PC

Another study evaluating the reliability of an integrated biaxial accelerometer system was conducted by Kavanagh. The accelerometer system involved four nodes consisting of two biaxial accelerometers positioned orthogonally. The accelerometer nodes were wired by shielded cable to a processor box mounted to the waist of the subject. The subcomponents of the processor box were a power regulation system, microprocessor, Bluetooth system enabling wireless connectivity, and two AAA batteries. With the Bluetooth component, the system could transmit wireless information to a local PC (Kavanagh et al., 2006).

The objective of the research was to ascertain the reliability of the gait analysis system using accelerometers in consideration of intra/inter-examiner and stride to stride reliability. Four well defined anatomical positions were selected for the mounting of the accelerometer nodes: the C7 and L3 spinous process, 3cm proximal to the lateral malleolus, and the occipital pole of the skull. The study ascertained comparable reliability for intra/inter-examiner evaluations and for individual stride to stride reliability. The conclusion was the accelerometer node reapplication errors for the same or different examiner were minimal. The research implicates the reliability of accelerometer systems for the quantification of gait (Kavanagh et al., 2006).

The investigations by Saremi and Kavanagh have a significant implication. With the use of highly specified anatomical mounting points for the accelerometers, such as the L3 spinous process or 4cm below the sternum top, reliable data could be acquired (Kavanagh et al., 2006; Saremi et al., 2006). Essentially such highly specified anatomical anchor positions are suitable for a clinician with a considerable degree of anatomical specialization, rather than a subject applying and wearing the accelerometer systems in an autonomous and personalized environment.

Wearable proprioception is represented by even more autonomous applications, such as wireless three dimensional accelerometer nodes. Since the concept is envisioned for the operation by the actual subject in a fully autonomous setting, more simplified and robust anatomical mounting positions are considered. For gait related applications, such as virtual proprioception and gait quantification, the anatomical mounting points are the lateral malleolus and lateral epicondyle of the femur, secured by an elastic band. These two mounting positions can be readily identified as above and adjacent to the ankle joint and the top of the knee joint (LeMoyne et al., 2008e; LeMoyne et al., 2008f; LeMoyne et al., 2009b; LeMoyne et al., 2009d). Reflex quantification has also advocated the mounting position adjacent to the lateral malleolus, also described as the lateral aspect of the leg to the medial malleolus, which is essentially the ankle joint (LeMoyne et al., 2008a; LeMoyne et al., 2008h). With respect to the quantification of Parkinson's disease, the anatomical position is the dorsum of the hand, secured through a flexible strap and readily identifiable as the top of the hand (LeMoyne et al., 2009a).

4.6 Accelerometer systems for Parkinson's disease evaluation

Accelerometer systems have enabled the potential for automated and quantitative evaluation of Parkinson's disease motor status uniquely specified for an individual patient in an effectively autonomous environment while conducting daily activities. The accelerometer device was amalgamated with a neural network algorithm for classifying 'on' and 'off' Parkinson's disease states. Information acquired from the signal of the accelerometers was transmitted to a data-logger also mounted to the subject. The research study ascertained a high level of specificity for classifying the disparity between the 'on' and 'off' states for Parkinson's disease subjects based on the capabilities of the accelerometer system and associated algorithm. The advancement of accelerometer systems providing automated and quantified evaluation under autonomous conditions for Parkinson's disease status can potentially lead to individually optimized medication strategy and quantified measurement for the efficacy of novel therapy strategies (Keijsers et al., 2006).

The synthesis of an accelerometer system with neural networks was applied to classify the attributes of Levodopa-induced dyskinesia for subjects with Parkinson's disease. Given the findings of the research, the integrated system, equipped with accelerometers as the sensor and neural networks as the algorithm, was demonstrated as a means for classifying severity of Levodopa-induced dyskinesia. Future concepts based on the study would address the attributes of Levodopa-induced dyskinesia spanning the complete dose cycle (Keijsers et al., 2000). The system also could quantify the temporal feature for Parkinson's disease progression.

For patients with advanced pathologies, the establishment of a prudent drug therapy strategy may be obfuscated with both positive and negative outcomes. Accelerometers have been introduced for studies to evaluate the efficacy of drug therapy for patients with both dementia and Parkinson's disease. The medication could potentially improve cognitive function while amplifying tremor characteristics. The incorporation of accelerometers enables an advancement of diagnostic acuity, especially in light of conflicting effects from the presumptive therapy strategy (Gurevich et al., 2006).

With accelerometer data quantifying the characteristics of tremor, the efficacy of drug therapy can be analyzed through the incorporation of advanced numerical methods. Spectral analysis has been applied to the elucidation of accelerometer data derived tremor attributes. Research integrating the processing of the accelerometer signal through spectral analysis has been applied for ascertaining the efficacy of medication strategies for reducing tremor (Schrag et al., 1999).

Another unique application of accelerometer technology is as a feedback modality for deep brain stimulation efficacy. In a study involving patients with Parkinson's disease or essential tremor, accelerometers were used to quantify the effectiveness of deep brain stimulation. The study ascertained a significant improvement in tremor attributes with the stimulator in the 'on' mode (Obwegeser et al., 2001). Other research incorporated accelerometers for the determination that deep brain stimulation induces improved motor function characteristics (Kumru et al., 2004).

4.7 Integrated wireless three dimensional accelerometer systems for gait analysis

A wireless accelerometer system consisting of integrated subcomponents was produced and evaluated by Lee. A footswitch device was operated in tandem with the wireless accelerometer system, serving as a standard contrast for the acquisition of temporal parameters for gait. A triaxial accelerometer subsystem was integrated with the wireless accelerometer system, and the data was sampled at 61Hz. Other aspects of the integrated device were a battery powered subsystem and subsystem for conveying data wireless to a local PC, with a maximum operating range of 15 meters. The system mass was 50 grams. The attributes of the integrated wireless accelerometer system enabled mounting of the device at the lateral aspect of the ankle. Both ankles were mounted with an integrated wireless accelerometer system. The research by Lee confirms the temporal parameter correlation acquired from the footswitch device and the accelerometer system using integrated components for achieving wireless capability (Lee et al., 2007).

4.8 Wearable shoe integrated wireless gait quantification system integrating multiple biaxial accelerometers

A gait analysis device termed GaitShoe integrates multiple devices for quantification of locomotion attributes into a wearable system by integrating the components of the GaitShoe into a typical shoe. The shoe effectively represents the mounting point for the anatomical position, greatly reducing the need for even basic knowledge of anatomy. The GaitShoe device consists of multiple gait analysis sensors: pressure sensors, electric field height sensors, force sensors, bend sensors, gyroscopes, and accelerometers. Multiple biaxial accelerometers are integrated into the GaitShoe application. Acquired gait quantification data is conveyed from the GaitShoe through wireless transmission (Bamberg et al. 2008).

The GaitShoe device and integrated wireless accelerometer application by Lee represent evolutions of gait analysis and quantification. Wearable artificial proprioception further evolves the technology space for the more global application of movement analysis and quantification, for which the topic of locomotion is a subset. Wearable artificial proprioception is demonstrated by a fully integral wireless three dimensional accelerometer node, such as the G-Link® Wireless Accelerometer Node (www.microstrain.com).

In contrast to the device developed by Lee, the G-Link® Wireless Accelerometer Node is equipped with signal strength for wireless transmission spanning a range of 70 meters (www.microstrain.com). Even with a wireless range of 4-5 times the range for the system developed by Lee, the G-Link® Wireless Accelerometer Node has a mass of 46 grams, which is about 10% less than the system mass for the device composed by Lee. Also the G-Link® Wireless Accelerometer is powered by a rechargeable system as opposed to a battery, which would presumably need periodic replacement (www.microstrain.com; Lee et al., 2007).

The GaitShoe introduces a unique concept for evaluating gait, through the integration of multiple sensors into the wearable application of a shoe. However inherent limitations may exist with the incorporation of 6 sensor components, such as requirements for packaging the sensors and providing sufficient power. With the integration of the sensor apparatus, the integrated device has a volume on the scale of the actual shoe (Bamberg et al. 2008). The GaitShoe apparatus has a mass 6-7 times greater than the G-Link® Wireless Accelerometer Node. The GaitShoe provides accelerometer data through biaxial accelerometers, as opposed to the G-Link® Wireless Accelerometer Node that utilizes triaxial accelerometers (www.microstrain.com; Bamberg et al. 2008). The mounting of gait quantification sensors to a wearable shoe application may limit perceptivity as to locomotion quality and status, since the spatial temporal aspects of the foot during gait cycle are the result of a triple joint system represented by the ankle, knee, and hip joint.

4.9 Wireless three dimensional accelerometers and future technology

As demonstrated by the previous research, accelerometer technology has become increasingly integrated for applications of movement quantification, such as gait. As illustrated in figure 1, the accelerometer technology has progressed from uniaxial to biaxial to triaxial accelerometers with volumetric packaging decreasing with advances in miniaturization as a function of year (www.enablingmnt.com; LeMoyne et al., 2008c).

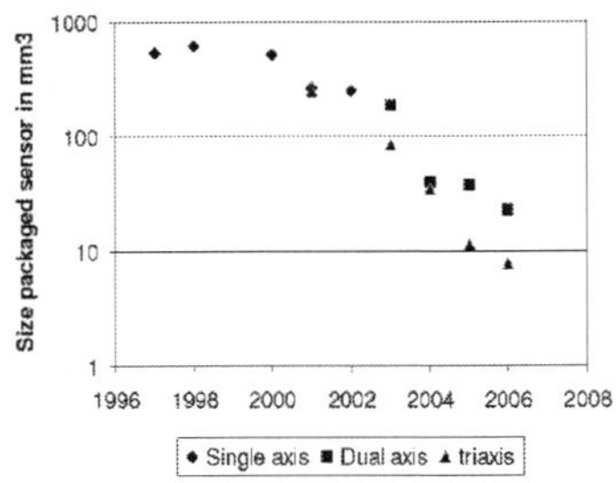

Fig. 1. Evolution trend progress for accelerometer miniaturization versus year (www.enablingmnt.com; LeMoyne et al., 2008c)

Multiple technologies support and affect the evolution of accelerometer systems (Culhane et al., 2005; LeMoyne et al., 2008c). Evolution of microelectronics based on the principle of Moore's Law establishes a basis for the advance of accelerometer technology. Moore's Law asserts that with respect to a chip the number of transistors doubles roughly within a two year duration. Basically Moore's Law implicates cost reduction with expanding performance (www.intel.com). The trend defined by Moore's Law should also pertain to advances in performance and decrease in cost for accelerometer technology.

4.10 Wireless accelerometers for artificial proprioception

The implementation of wireless technology has further advanced accelerometer systems (www.microstrain.com; www.sparkfun.com; Jafari et al., 2005; LeMoyne et al., 2008c). Wireless accelerometer systems provide expanded autonomy for the characterization of movement disorder and gait analysis (Lee et al., 2007; Bamberg et al. 2008; LeMoyne et al., 2008a; LeMoyne et al., 2008c; LeMoyne et al., 2008e; LeMoyne et al., 2008f; LeMoyne et al., 2008h; LeMoyne et al., 2009a; LeMoyne et al., 2009b; LeMoyne et al., 2009d). In essence a compact, lightweight, and minimally intrusive wireless accelerometer provides an artificial type of proprioception.

The utility of a wireless accelerometer node functioning as artificial proprioception has numerous benefits to the biomedical field. While a non-intrusive wireless accelerometer node can measure human movement such as reflex response and latency, Parkinson's disease tremor, and gait quality; the quantified measurements can also be stored on a database of a local PC (Lee et al., 2007; Bamberg et al. 2008; LeMoyne et al., 2008a; LeMoyne et al., 2008c; LeMoyne et al., 2008e; LeMoyne et al., 2008f; LeMoyne et al., 2008h; LeMoyne et al., 2009a; LeMoyne et al., 2009b; LeMoyne et al., 2009d). Downloading the resultant measurements of artificial proprioception through a wireless accelerometer node enables the implementation of subsequent post-processing algorithms and tracking of status progression.

The G-Link® Wireless Accelerometer Node currently represents the state of the art for artificial proprioception. The device is capable of sampling data at a rate of 2048Hz in a wireless activated data-logger mode, using tandem wireless accelerometer nodes. The sampling rate for the G-Link® Wireless Accelerometer Node, using tandem activated accelerometers, may be set to alternative sampling rates, such as 512Hz, according to the discretion of the operator and the research scenario requirements (www.microstrain.com).

Subsequently the wireless technology has been integrated into sensors, such as accelerometers (www.microstrain.com; www.sparkfun.com; Jafari et al., 2005). Advances in wireless technology may substantially benefit the accelerometer technology space, such as greater autonomy for research applications (LeMoyne et al., 2008c). The next logical step for the advancement of the technology is for the development of fully wireless and portable three dimensional accelerometer sensors.

The G-Link® Wireless Accelerometer Node represents the frontier of the wireless three dimensional accelerometer technology space with features such as a real-time streaming rate of up to 4kHz and wireless activated data-logger mode with 2MB of data storage capacity (www.microstrain.com). The variable sampling rates for the G-Link® Wireless Accelerometer Node provide flexibility in light of the Nyquist rate, which the is the minimum sampling rate required to prevent aliasing. Aliasing is known as the scenario, for which sampling disparate continuous signals becomes indistinguishable. Aliasing can be avoided through defining a sampling rate greater than the Nyquist rate, which is twice the maximum bandwidth frequency of the signal (www.vias.org).

The gait analysis study conducted by Saremi incorporated a sampling rate of 32Hz (Saremi et al., 2006). During the study by Lyons a sampling rate of 50Hz was considered to exceed the Nyquist criterion applicable to mobility data (Lyons et al., 2005). The G-Link® Wireless Accelerometer Node is certainly capable of exceeding the above sampling rates. Another advantage of the G-Link® Wireless Accelerometer Node is the sampling rate can be modulated at the discretion of the researchers. For instance the 2048Hz sampling rate may be reduced to 512Hz, which would reduce the data size of the sampling event by a factor of four (www.microstrain.com).

There are many other advantages for the G-Link® Wireless Accelerometer Node. The device is powered by rechargeable batteries integrated into the node, negating the need for battery replacement. The wireless accelerometers have a wireless transmission range of 70 meters. If the potential for a break in wireless signal continuity exists, the nodes can utilize a wireless activated data-logger mode. The G-Link® Wireless Accelerometer Node can store up to 2MB of data in the data-logger mode, and data can be downloaded to a PC by wireless transmission. G-Link® Wireless Accelerometer Nodes have a mass of 46 grams (www.microstrain.com). These attributes make the wireless accelerometer technology ideal for applications in reflex response and latency quantification, Parkinson's disease tremor evaluation, gait analysis, and real-time biofeedback of hemiparetic gait disparity (LeMoyne et al., 2008c; LeMoyne et al., 2008e; LeMoyne et al., 2008f; LeMoyne et al., 2008h; LeMoyne et al., 2009a; LeMoyne et al., 2009b; LeMoyne et al., 2009c; LeMoyne et al., 2009d).

5. Applications for artificial proprioception

Wireless three dimensional accelerometers have demonstrated the ability to serve as an artificial form of proprioception. There are numerous biomedical applications for which wireless three dimensional accelerometers are relevant. Recent research has been successfully applied to aspects of the classification and quantification of movement characteristics, such as the evaluation of tendon reflex, Parkinson's disease status, gait analysis, and virtual proprioception, which is a real-time biofeedback system for gait rehabilitation (LeMoyne et al., 2008e; LeMoyne et al., 2008f; LeMoyne et al., 2008h; LeMoyne et al., 2009a; LeMoyne et al., 2009b; LeMoyne et al., 2009c; LeMoyne et al., 2009d).

5.1. Reflex quantification using wireless accelerometer system as artificial proprioception

The tendon reflex, such as the patellar tendon reflex, is a standard aspect of a typical neurological examination (Kandel et al., 2000; Bickley & Szilagyi, 2003). The tendon reflex can provide insight as to the status of both central and peripheral nervous system function and possible trauma (Bickley & Szilagyi, 2003). Ordinal scales have been developed for evaluating reflex response, for which some researchers assert the validity of the ordinal scale system (Litvan et al., 1996). However, other studies contradict the validity of ordinal scale systems (Stam & van Crevel, 1990; Manschot et al., 1998). One notable aspect of the ordinal scale system is the lack of temporal parameters to characterize the temporal aspect of the reflex response (Stam & van Crevel, 1990; Litvan et al., 1996; Manschot et al., 1998). The tendon reflex can also indicate latency (Frijns et al., 1997; Voerman et al., 2005). The reflex loop may provide a less resource intensive first screen alternative to electrodiagnostic evaluation. The appropriateness of electrodiagnostic evaluation has been demonstrated as a subject of controversy (Mondelli et al., 1998; Podnar et al., 2005; Cocito et al., 2006). An alternative solution could be provided through a reflex quantification system.

Some reflex quantification systems have emphasized quantification of response, such as a load cell tethered to the ankle by a cable using an instrumented hammer; a strain gauge system measuring reflex response using a manual sweep triggered hammer for input; and EMG measurement of response while evoking the reflex with a motorized component (Van de Crommert et al. 1996; Faist et al. 1999; Pagliaro & Zamparo, 1999; Cozens et al., 2000; Lebiedowska & Fisk, 2003). Other systems have synchronized the reflex input and reflex response aspects of the reflex quantification system, deriving the effective latency as the temporal disparity between input and reflex response signals. Synchronized reflex quantification systems without the requirement of EMG have incorporated instrumented reflex hammers synchronized with a wired accelerometer; an instrumented hammer with a torque sensor locked in a defined position; and a motorized reflex hammer input functioning in tandem with a strain gauge sensor measuring response (Koceja & Kamen, 1988; Kamen & Koceja, 1989; Zhang et al. 2000; Mamizuka et al., 2007). Such strategies for quantifying tendon reflexes are noteworthy of credit; however the proposed wireless accelerometer reflex quantification system enables advances in terms of portability, flexibility, ease of use, scalability, and functional robustness. The proposed wireless accelerometer reflex quantification system has been progressively evolved over the course of three evolutionary cycles, with a modified third generation system applied to an artificial reflex configuration (LeMoyne et al., 2005b; LeMoyne & Jafari 2006a; LeMoyne et al., 2007b; LeMoyne et al., 2008a; LeMoyne et al., 2008g; LeMoyne et al., 2008h; LeMoyne et al., 2009c).

5.1.1 Wireless accelerometer reflex quantification device (first generation)

The initial concept of wireless reflex quantification, conceptualized and developed in 2005, consisted of two global system requirements: quantification of reflex response and reflex input for the patellar tendon (LeMoyne, 2005a; LeMoyne et al., 2005b; LeMoyne & Jafari 2006a). Eventually the system was evolved to successfully quantify both patellar tendon reflex input, reflex response, and reflex latency (LeMoyne et al., 2007b; LeMoyne et al., 2008a; LeMoyne et al., 2008h). Further confirmation of the wireless accelerometer reflex quantification system was obtained through the use of an artificial reflex device, which also demonstrated a high degree of accuracy and reliability (LeMoyne et al., 2008g; LeMoyne et al., 2009c).

The first generation wireless quantified reflex system was envisioned in 2005, and demonstrated the ability to contrast disparity of reflex response for a hemiparetic affected/unaffected leg in comparison to a nominal neurology control, through a wireless two dimensional accelerometer device. The prime objective of the first generation wireless quantified reflex system was to demonstrate the capacity of the system to objectively quantify the disparity of hemiparetic reflexes, contrasting affected leg to unaffected leg. The numerical algorithm strategy used for the application was the ratio of time averaged acceleration for affected versus unaffected leg (LeMoyne et al., 2005b).

The first generation wireless reflex system consisted of a Mednode two dimensional wireless accelerometer mounted near the ankle and coplanar to the sagittal plane for the reflex response of the subject. The signal of the Mednode wireless accelerometer was transmitted to a local PC for later post-processing of the data. The reflex input evoking the patellar tendon reflex was based on a hinged device with a reflex hammer attached to the moment arm, enabling consistent potential energy derived reflex input. The results indicated a significant disparity for the hemiparetic subject with an affected to unaffected leg patellar tendon reflex ratio of 1.5; in contrast the ratio was effectively parity at 1.0 for the nominal neurology subject (LeMoyne et al., 2005b).

5.1.2 Wireless accelerometer reflex quantification device (second generation)

The test and evaluation of the first generation wireless accelerometer reflex quantification system established the evolutionary insight for the second generation wireless accelerometer reflex quantification system developed in 2006. A more application robust three dimensional wireless accelerometer Mednode was integrated into the system, with the acquired data conveyed wirelessly to a local PC for post-processing. The reflex input component has evolved by developing a potential energy derived swing arm mounted to the reflex hammer incorporating aluminum parts with adjustable knobs for expanded simplicity of operation (LeMoyne & Jafari, 2006a; LeMoyne & Jafari, 2006b; LeMoyne et al., 2008a). Similar to the research of Kavanagh and Saremi, an anatomical mounting point was selected for optimizing accuracy for multiple evaluations (Kavanagh et al., 2006; Saremi et al., 2006). The anatomical location selected was the above the lateral malleolus, which is also the lateral aspect of the leg in consideration of the medial malleolus (LeMoyne & Jafari, 2006a; LeMoyne & Jafari, 2006b; LeMoyne et al., 2008a).

Given the expanded capacity of the second generation wireless accelerometer reflex quantification system to evoke the patellar tendon reflex with specified potential energy settings, multiple potential energy increments were incorporated. Three subjects comprised the test and evaluation experiment; consisting of one chronic hemiparetic and two subjects without any neurological traumas. The experiment was comprised of three sets of six reflex input settings (45, 30, 15, 15, 30, and 45 degrees) for each leg. Each set was conducted on a different day, obtaining 108 measurements. The objective of the test and evaluation of the second generation wireless accelerometer reflex quantification system was to provide proof of concept from an engineering perspective, ascertaining the accuracy and reliability of the system for quantifying the patellar tendon reflex (LeMoyne & Jafari, 2006a; LeMoyne & Jafari, 2006b; LeMoyne et al., 2008a).

Of the 108 measurements acquired by the second generation wireless accelerometer reflex quantification system, 107 of the measurements were bound by a 10% relative variation, with respect to the amplitude of the quantified reflex response. Only one measurement exceeded this 10% bound requiring a bound of 15%. The test and evaluation of the second generation reflex system using three dimensional accelerometers implicates a considerable level of reproducibility and accuracy (LeMoyne & Jafari, 2006a; LeMoyne & Jafari, 2006b; LeMoyne et al., 2008a).

5.1.3 Wireless accelerometer reflex quantification device (third generation)

The third generation wireless accelerometer reflex quantification system further evolves the application by integrating two tandem activated wireless accelerometers. Testing and evaluation was commenced during 2007. The primary modification for the third generation system was the incorporation of the G-Link® Wireless Accelerometer Node (LeMoyne et al. 2007b; LeMoyne et al., 2008h).

The G-Link® Wireless Accelerometer Node advanced the capacity of the wireless accelerometer reflex quantification system. The wireless accelerometers were capable of conveying a real-time data stream with a sampling rate of 100Hz. Two G-Link® Wireless Accelerometer Nodes were capable of tandem activation with a temporally synchronized data stream. The real-time data stream was subsequently conveyed to a local PC for post-processing (www.microstrain.com).

Tandem and synchronized operation of two accelerometer nodes enables event detection based on the temporal disparity of both acceleration waveforms. One wireless accelerometer was mounted to the swing arm of the third generation reflex quantification system, with the respective acceleration waveform indicating reflex hammer strike initiating the reflex loop. The other tandem and synchronized wireless accelerometer was mounted to the lateral malleolus, indicating the reflex response acceleration waveform. With both wireless accelerometers functioning in synchronicity and activated in tandem, the temporal disparity between the acceleration waveforms can derive latency of the reflex loop. The objective of the test and evaluation of the third generation wireless accelerometer reflex quantification system was to accurately and reliably acquire both quantified reflex response and latency of the patellar tendon reflex (LeMoyne et al. 2007b; LeMoyne et al., 2008h).

The following experimental protocol was used for the test and evaluation of the third generation wireless reflex quantification system:

1. Mount the wireless three dimensional accelerometer using an elastic band adjacent and above the lateral malleolus.
2. Aim the reflex hammer for evoking the patellar tendon reflex at the level of the tibial tubercle.
3. Retract the swing arm to a 30 degree setting relative to gravity vector.
4. Release the swing arm.
5. Save the acquired data from the wireless three dimensional MEMS accelerometers (LeMoyne et al., 2008h).
6. Delay evoking the next patellar tendon reflex by one minute (Cozens et al., 2000; LeMoyne et al., 2008h).
7. Repeat the protocol (LeMoyne et al., 2008h).

The test and evaluation experiment was comprised of the unaffected leg of a chronic hemiplegic (subject 1) and a subject without any neurological injuries (subject 2), using the leg on the same side as the preferred arm. Twenty measurements were obtained per subject. The experiment was intended to illustrate engineering proof of concept (LeMoyne et al., 2008h).

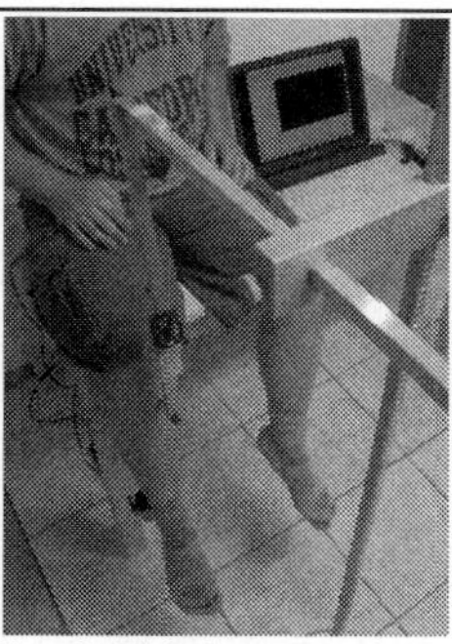

Fig. 2. Third generation wireless accelerometer reflex quantification device

Table 1. Quantified reflex parameters

Reflex parameter	Subject 1	Subject 2
Reflex latency mean (msec)	95.5	154.5
Reflex latency standard deviation (msec)	6.863	9.987
Coefficient of variation	0.07186	0.06464
Maximum reflex response mean (g's)	1.024	1.017
Maximum reflex response standard deviation (g's)	0.00446	0.00870
Coefficient of variation	0.00436	0.00855
Minimum reflex response mean (g's)	0.8825	0.9495
Minimum reflex response standard deviation (g's)	0.01243	0.00927
Coefficient of variation	0.01408	0.00976

(LeMoyne et al., 2008h)

The third generation wireless accelerometer reflex quantification system is illustrated in figure 2. The quantified reflex parameters are displayed in table 1. The resultant parameters, such as maximum reflex response, minimum reflex response, and latency, demonstrated consistent accuracy and reliability. The sample size of 20 measurements was bound with a confidence level of 95%, according to a 5% margin of error relative to the mean, respective of both subjects. All reflex parameters were considered for the determination of the bounding confidence level. Based on the quantified measurements, the sample size may be reduced to 10, with a 90% confidence level and a 5% margin of error relative to the mean (LeMoyne et al., 2008h).

The findings of the research implicate the third generation reflex quantification system is capable of ascertaining quantified reflex response, both minimum and maximum, and latency with a considerable accuracy and reliability. Based on the results of the third generation wireless accelerometer reflex quantification system test and evaluation, clinical trials are warranted for the establishment of reproducibility for the device to acquire patellar tendon reflex parameters (LeMoyne et al. 2007b; LeMoyne et al., 2008h). The evaluation of an artificial reflex system could also further validate the reflex quantification system incorporating wireless three dimensional accelerometers.

5.1.4 Wireless accelerometer reflex quantification device using artificial reflex

The tendon reflex is inherently variable, as the functionality is based on the inherently variable neurological system (Kandel et al., 2000; Bickley & Szilagyi, 2003; Seeley et al., 2003). An artificial reflex system, developed and evaluated from 2007 to 2008, was evaluated using the current third generation wireless accelerometer reflex quantification device. The artificial reflex system uses mechanically derived reflex response from stored potential energy of a rubber band and mechanically derived latency from a trigger subsystem incorporating a cam. The third generation reflex system was modified, with the G-Link® Wireless Accelerometer Node configuration set to a wireless activated data-logger mode with a sampling rate of 2048Hz, which provided a more user-convenient methodology for acquiring measurement samples (LeMoyne et al., 2009c). As anticipated, the modified third generation wireless accelerometer reflex quantification system obtained pertinent reflex parameters, such as maximum and minimum reflex response and latency (LeMoyne et al., 2008g; LeMoyne et al., 2009c). Based on a sample of 15 measurements, all significant reflex parameters were sufficient bound with a 96% confidence level using a 4% margin of error about the mean; implicating a considerable degree of accuracy and reliability (LeMoyne et al., 2009c).

5.2 Wireless accelerometer system for quantifying Parkinson's disease attributes

Parkinson's disease is classified as a movement disorder affecting about one million people in the United States, while predominantly occurring after an age of 55 years (Kandel et al., 2000; Seeley et al., 2003). A typical attribute of Parkinson's disease is a four to five per second resting tremor (Kandel et al., 2000; Bickley & Szilagyi, 2003). Two therapy strategies with variable dosage allocations are drug therapy and deep brain stimulation (Kandel et al., 2000; Nolte & Sundsten, 2002; Volkmann et al., 2006). Drug therapy efficacy eventually diminishes over time, and adverse side effects can precipitate (Kandel et al., 2000; Nolte & Sundsten, 2002). Accelerometers have been demonstrated for quantifying the efficacy of drug therapy, deep brain stimulation parameter settings, and classifying temporal oscillations of the disease severity (Schrag et al., 1999; N. L. Keijsers et al., 2000; Obwegeser et al., 2001; Kumru et al., 2004; Gurevich et al., 2006; N. L. Keijsers et al., 2006). A wireless three dimensional accelerometer, serving as an artificial form of proprioception, is the next evolution for the integration of accelerometer technology quantification of Parkinson's disease tremor.

Wireless accelerometer systems were initially proposed as a feedback modality for deep brain stimulation of Parkinson's disease subjects as of 2007 (LeMoyne, 2007a; LeMoyne et al., 2008b). Subsequent evaluation involved G-Link® Wireless Accelerometer Nodes for quantifying a simulated tremor in contrast to a static control. Both accelerometers were set to a sampling rate of 2048Hz using the data-logging mode with wireless activation (LeMoyne et al., 2009a).

The conceptual evaluation of the G-Link® Wireless Accelerometer Node capacity for quantifying Parkinson's disease tremor involved a simulated hand tremor. One wireless accelerometer was secured to the dorsum of the hand through a flexible strap, and the other wireless accelerometer was placed in a static location. Five trials were conducted during the evaluation, and the data samples were analyzed over one second increments. The time averaged acceleration was calculated using a trapezoid method. The quantified data for both simulated tremor and static control were both sufficiently bound using a 90% confidence level and a 10% margin of error respective of the mean. The Parkinson's disease quantification system involving a wireless accelerometer is illustrated in figure 3. The simulated tremor and static control are characterized in figures 4 and 5 (LeMoyne et al., 2009a).

The fundamental utility of the wireless accelerometer system for evaluating Parkinson's disease is based on the opportunity to characterize disease status and progression in a relatively autonomous environment, such as a home setting. The measurements could provide a database and effective baseline for tracking therapy efficacy and variation over a 24 hour cycle. Advances in data processing techniques may enable the opportunity of possible continuous tracking (LeMoyne et al., 2009a).

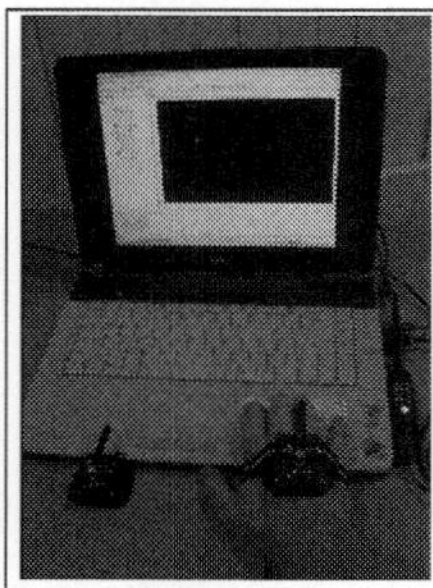

Fig. 3. Wireless accelerometer system for quantifying Parkinson's disease (LeMoyne et al., 2009a)

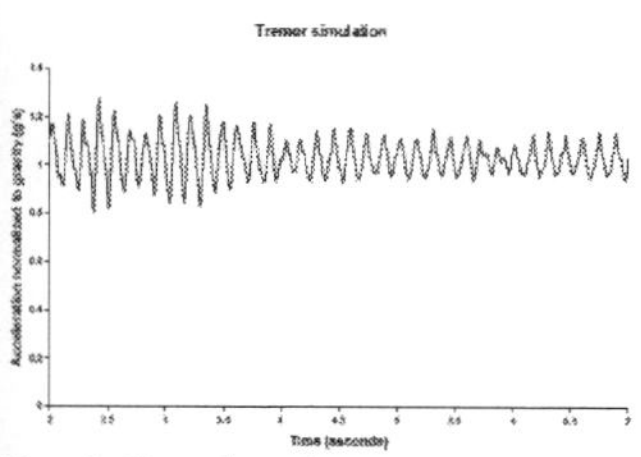

Fig. 4. Simulated tremor acceleration signal

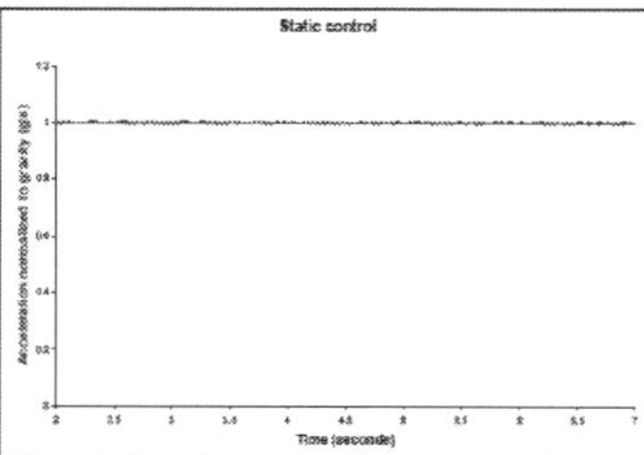

Fig. 5. Static control acceleration signal

5.3 Wireless three dimensional accelerometer device for quantifying gait

The incorporation of wireless and wearable accelerometer systems enables a considerable expansion for the autonomy of gait analysis, permitting both outdoor and indoor gait analysis and quantification beyond clinical confines (LeMoyne et al., 2009b; LeMoyne et al.,

2009d). Standard gait evaluation technologies consist of devices, such as EMG systems, electrogoniometers, metabolic energy expenditure systems, ground reaction force analyzers, foot switch stride analyzers, and optical motion analysis systems (Mayagoitia et al., 2002; Dobkin, 2003; LeMoyne et al., 2008c). Relative to traditional gait analysis technologies, effectively wearable and wireless accelerometers offer advanced utility, such as autonomy of application, portability, minimal intrusion on gait cycle, ease of operation, and operation beyond the setting of a gait analysis laboratory (LeMoyne et al., 2008c; LeMoyne et al., 2009b; LeMoyne et al., 2009d). The evolution of accelerometer devices for analyzing the gait cycle has steadily progressed from uniaxial to biaxial to triaxial accelerometers (Mayagoitia et al., 2002; Kavanagh et al., 2006; Saremi et al., 2006; LeMoyne et al., 2008c). Initial experimentation of novel wireless gait analysis systems integrating three axis accelerometers and multiple two axis accelerometer systems have been conducted (Lee et al., 2007; Bamberg et al. 2008). As previously discussed, the G-Link® Wireless Accelerometer Node offers an advance in utility of wearable and wireless three dimensional accelerometer systems for gait analysis and quantification in contrast to the integrated wireless accelerometers (www.microstrain.com; LeMoyne et al., 2008c).

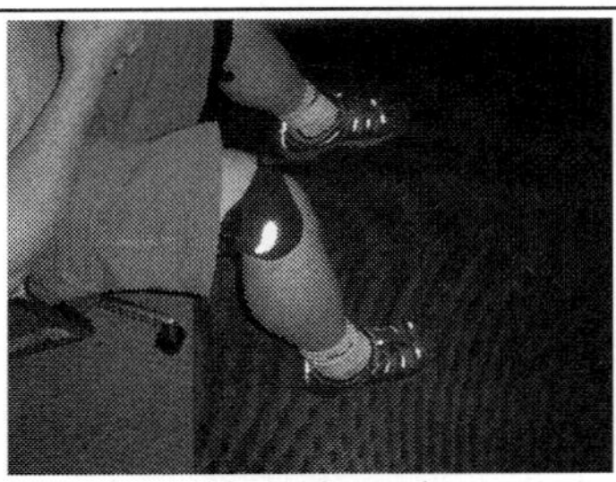

Fig. 6. Wearable and wireless accelerometer device mounted at lateral epicondyle adjacent to the knee joint

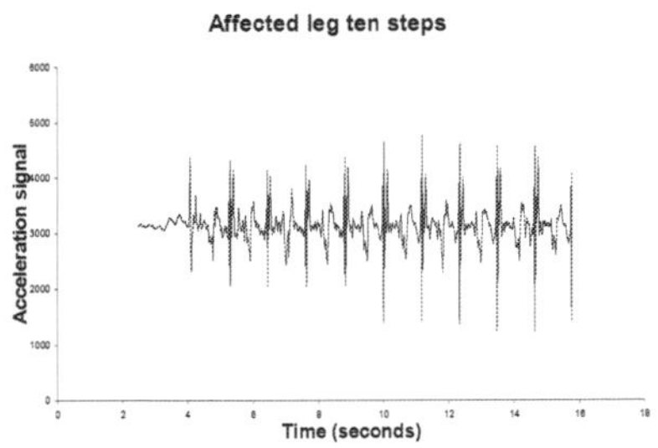

Fig. 7. Acceleration waveform of affected leg during gait cycle

Table 2. Stance to stance time averaged acceleration ratio with 100 milliseconds bound about the stance component removed (affected leg/ unaffected leg)

Trial	Stance to stance time averaged acceleration ratio with 100 milliseconds bound about the stance component removed (affected leg/ unaffected leg)
1	0.79
2	0.94
3	0.73

(LeMoyne et al., 2009d)

The functional utility of the G-Link® Wireless Accelerometer Node was demonstrated with respect to two disparate experiments, both conducted in 2008: a gait evaluation of a chronic hemiparetic while walking on an outdoors sidewalk and a gait evaluation of a chronic hemiparetic while walking through the hallway of a house (LeMoyne et al., 2009b; LeMoyne et al., 2009d). Previous research has established the utility of well defined anatomical mounting points for the accelerometer nodes (Kavanagh et al., 2006; Saremi et al., 2006). With respect to the outdoor gait analysis, the anatomical mounting position was the readily identifiable lateral epicondyle next to the knee joint (LeMoyne et al., 2009d). For the indoor homebound gait analysis the anatomical mounting position was selected as above the lateral malleolus adjacent to the ankle joint (LeMoyne et al., 2009b). For both experiments the G-Link® Wireless Accelerometer Nodes were set to a sampling rate of 2048Hz, while using the wireless activated data-logger mode; acquired gait cycle data was subsequently transmitted wireless to a local PC for post-processing (LeMoyne et al., 2009b; LeMoyne et al., 2009d).

The first experiment was the outdoors application of the wearable and wireless three dimensional accelerometer gait quantification system. The chronic hemiparetic subject was instructed to walk on a sidewalk for three trials with ten steps per leg, with the G-Link® Wireless Accelerometer Nodes activated by wireless transmission, recording in data-logger mode, and subsequently downloading the acquired data by wireless transmission to a local PC for data processing. Figure 6 characterizes the mounting of the wearable and wireless accelerometer device at the lateral epicondyle adjacent to the knee joint; and figure 7 illustrates a characteristic acceleration waveform (LeMoyne et al., 2009d).

Subsequent analysis involved calculating the stance to stance time averaged acceleration ratio (affected leg/ unaffected leg), using a trapezoid method to compute the respective integrals. A 100 millisecond bound about the stance aspect of the gait cycle was removed, in order to focus attention toward the swing aspect of gait. As indicated with table 2 an apparent and quantified affected to unaffected leg disparity was ascertained. Based on the acceleration waveform time averaged acceleration ratio, the unaffected leg was bound with a 95% confidence level using 5% margin of error about the mean with respect to all trials. For the affected leg trial 1 was bound by a 95% confidence level using a 5% margin of error about the mean, but trial 2 and 3 diminished to a 90% confidence level using a 10% margin of error about the mean (LeMoyne et al., 2009d).

The subsequent application of a wearable and wireless three dimensional gait analysis system focused on analyzing and quantifying gait cycle in a homebound setting. The subject, a chronic hemiparetic, was instructed to walk through the hallway of a home environment. Three trials were acquired using four complete step cycles. The application in the home setting involved mounting the wireless accelerometers to the lateral malleolus adjacent to the ankle joint as illustrated in figure 8 (LeMoyne et al., 2009b).

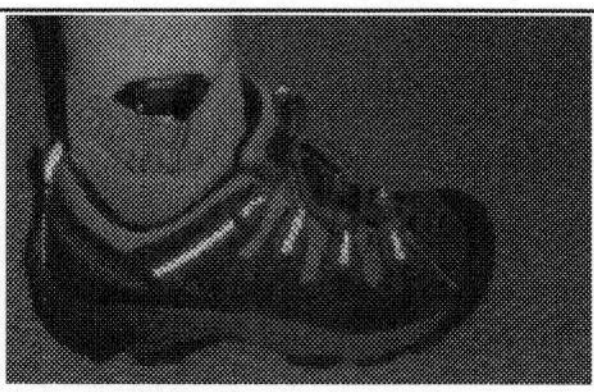

Fig. 8. Wireless accelerometer mounted to the lateral malleolus (LeMoyne et al., 2009b)

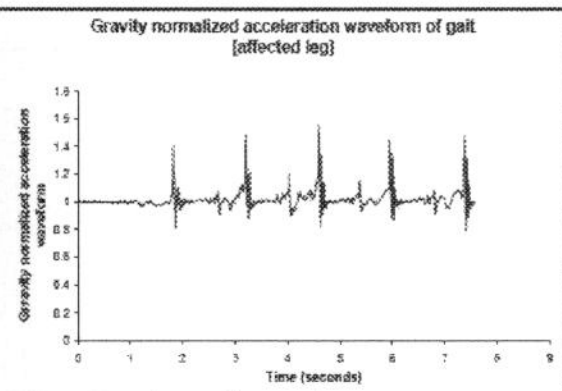

Fig. 9. Acceleration waveform affected leg

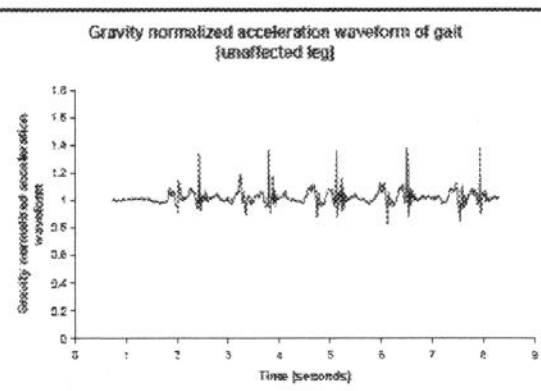

Fig. 10. Acceleration waveform unaffected leg

Figure 9 and 10 characterize the disparate acceleration waveforms respective of the affected and unaffected leg during gait. Visual inspection of the acceleration waveforms for affected and unaffected leg warranted the separation of stance and swing aspects of the gait cycle. The stance cycle component was bound to a 0.20 second duration, with the remaining temporal allocation of the gait cycle allocated to swing. The temporal disparity between stance to stance was highly consistent, with 1.32 seconds for the affected leg with a standard deviation of 0.06 seconds and 1.31 seconds with a standard deviation of 0.06 seconds for the unaffected leg. The stance to stance temporal aspects of gait cycle were bound with a 95% confidence level using a 5% margin of error about the mean. The time averaged acceleration ratio of the affected leg divided by unaffected leg was calculated for the stance aspect of gait cycle yielding 2.23 with a 0.30 standard deviation. The remaining swing aspect of the gait cycle produced a time averaged acceleration ratio of 0.71 with a standard deviation of 0.11 for affect leg per unaffected leg. The respective stance and swing aspect time averaged acceleration ratios were bound with a 90% confidence level incorporating a 10% margin of error about the mean (LeMoyne et al., 2009b).

The previous applications in outdoors and homebound environments for wireless accelerometer gait analysis and quantification underscore the flexible and autonomous nature of the device. Essentially a patient could be evaluated by a therapist from a remote distance. The gait cycle acceleration waveforms could be stored in a database for monitoring the status of therapy, while augmenting the acuity of the therapy strategy and respective efficacy (LeMoyne et al., 2009b; LeMoyne et al., 2009d).

5.4 Virtual proprioception real-time artificial proprioception biofeedback for gait rehabilitation

Virtual proprioception is envisioned to provide an alternative modality for the progressively strained resources encompassing neurorehabilitation, with the attributes to evolve to an autonomous gait rehabilitation system. The concept of virtual proprioception is envisioned to provide real-time biofeedback respective of gait disparity characteristics. The device is particularly envisioned for hemiparetic gait rehabilitation. Two systems incorporating virtual proprioception are currently presented. The first version of virtual proprioception conceptualized as of 2005 and developed in 2007, which focuses on real-time acceleration waveform disparity while incorporating G-Link® Wireless Accelerometer Nodes, is presented (LeMoyne, 2005a; LeMoyne et al., 2008f). The second version of virtual proprioception developed in 2008, which provides auditory feedback based on the quantified disparity of stance to stance time averaged acceleration ratio of affected per unaffected leg using wireless three dimensional accelerometers from a system termed the Wireless Health package, is addressed (LeMoyne et al., 2008e). Virtual proprioception especially offers the capacity to advance gait-related neurorehabilitation for patients with traumatic brain injury.

Locomotion is inherently regulated through the influence of subcortical, cortical, and interneuronal networks. Traumatic brain injury can impair the quality of locomotion, resulting in diminished muscle activation, hypertonicity, muscle coactivation, and leg length disparity. With these features, compensatory strategies can develop, such as circumduction and vaulting from the foot of the stance leg, given the inherent attributes hemiparetic gait

(Dobkin, 2003). Trauma to the central nervous system can lead to decrements in proprioceptive feedback acuity (Dietz, 2002). Virtual proprioception provides a wearable form of artificial proprioception, which as demonstrated through preliminary test and evaluation may circumvent decrements to gait caused by traumatic brain injury (LeMoyne et al., 2008e; LeMoyne et al., 2008f).

Biofeedback applications for rehabilitation, such as the rehabilitation of gait, have been soundly established (Huang et al., 2006). EMG biofeedback has been demonstrated for rehabilitation of hemiparetic gait (Aiello et al., 2005). The accelerometer system of the MiniSun IDEEA device has illustrated that acceleration waveforms are temporally representative of EMG waveforms (Saremi et al., 2006).

The first version of virtual proprioception emphasizes the real-time modification of the affected leg acceleration waveform to acquire near parity with the unaffected leg acceleration waveform. Virtual proprioception emphasized the following system-level parameters: minimization of accelerometers, an easily wearable application, and real-time feedback with minimal distraction to the subject. As illustrated in figure 11, the anatomical mounting point for the first evolution of virtual proprioception was the lateral epicondyle of the femur adjacent to the knee joint (LeMoyne et al., 2008f). The second version of virtual proprioception also selected the lateral epicondyle of the femur adjacent to the knee joint as the mounting position (LeMoyne et al., 2008e).

The operation of the first version of virtual proprioception involved an assistant walking in tandem while holding the laptop PC receiving real-time acceleration waveform graphic data with a sampling rate of 100Hz. The user of virtual proprioception, a chronic hemiplegic subject, would follow the assistant while observing the laptop PC monitor screen. During the 'off' status, the subject would observe the screen without any modification of gait. During the 'on' status for virtual proprioception, the subject would attempt to modify the gait pattern of the affected leg acceleration waveform to relative parity of the real-time acceleration waveform for the unaffected leg (LeMoyne et al., 2008f).

The following experimental protocol, involving three trials, was applied to the first evolution of virtual proprioception:

1. Secure the wireless accelerometers to the lateral epicondyle of each leg with an elastic band.
2. Initiate the real-time data stream of the wireless accelerometers to the laptop PC.
3. Walk 10 steps per leg while observing the affected and unaffected leg acceleration waveform disparity ('off' mode).
4. For next 10 steps per leg focus on the disparity of the acceleration waveforms. Adjust the affected leg acceleration waveform to correspond in parity with the unaffected leg acceleration waveform ('on' mode).
(LeMoyne et al., 2008f)

The first generation prototype version of virtual proprioception consisted of two G-Link® Wireless Accelerometer Nodes mounted with elastic knee bands to each leg. The laptop PC was equipped with wireless connectivity to the wireless accelerometers, while visually conveying real-time wireless accelerometer signals. The portable and autonomous attributes of the first generation virtual proprioception system enabled effectively natural gait cycle, with minimal intrusion. The objective of the first generation virtual proprioception system was to provide the capacity for real-time modification of hemiparetic gait, using real-time biofeedback of acceleration waveforms from wireless accelerometers (LeMoyne et al., 2008f).

The waveforms of the wireless accelerometer signals were analyzed after completion of the experimental protocol. The stance to stance time averaged acceleration ratio of the affected leg divided by unaffected leg was calculated. The trapezoid method was incorporated to calculate the integral of the time averaged acceleration. The gravity aspect of the signal was removed from the time averaged integrated acceleration signal. Transient aspects of the gait cycle measurements were removed, and measurements which involved discontinuity of the wireless signal were removed (LeMoyne et al., 2008f).

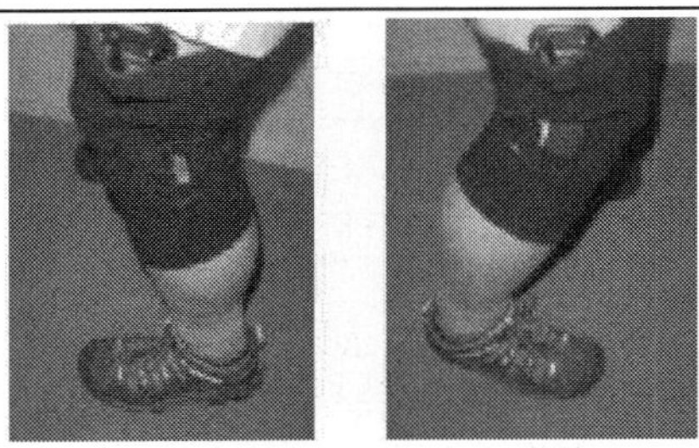

Fig. 11. The wireless three dimensional accelerometers secured to the lateral epicondyle with an elastic band

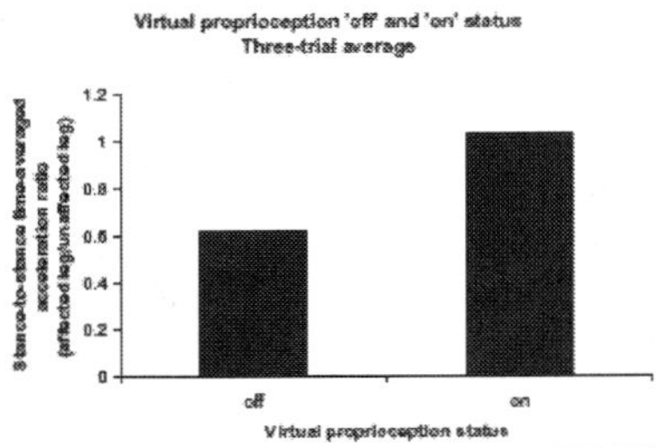

Fig. 12. Three-trial average of chronic hemiplegic, during gait cycle with 'off' and 'on' status of virtual proprioception

(LeMoyne et al., 2008f)

All three trials were characterized by a notable and quantified improvement in the gait, which is summarized in the three trial global averaging of figure 12. The global averaging of all three trials resulted in a stance to stance time averaged acceleration ratio of 0.615 during the 'off' mode and 1.029 during the 'on' mode. The relative variation of the stance to stance time averaged acceleration ratios were bound by a 15% relative variation respective of the mean, implicating the accuracy of the system even while adjusting to the device and incorporating a new real-time biofeedback induced gait strategy. The 'off' mode consists of walking without using the first generation virtual proprioception system for biofeedback modification of gait cycle disparity. During the 'on' mode the first generation virtual proprioception system is used as a biofeedback method for adjusting gait cycle to near parity during real-time operation. In consideration of the initial results for the first generation virtual proprioception device, further research and evolution of this highly novel real-time biofeedback system for modifying gait is warranted. Further research should be extended into evaluating the virtual proprioception concept using other learning modalities, such as auditory feedback (LeMoyne et al., 2008f).

The second generation virtual proprioception system incorporated auditory feedback to inform the subject of the quantified comparison of affected to unaffected leg and efficacy of real-time gait modification strategies. As an alternative to the G-Link® Wireless Accelerometer Nodes, comparable wireless three dimensional accelerometers that support the Wireless Health package affiliated with the research laboratory of Dr. Kaiser of the UCLA Electrical Engineering Department were incorporated. The selected accelerometer package resembles the inherent features of the G-Link® Wireless Accelerometer Node, in consideration of data sampling capacity, portability, and minimal intrusion respective of the gait cycle (LeMoyne et al., 2008e).

The second generation virtual proprioception system utilizing wireless accelerometers incorporating the Wireless Health package is uniquely equipped with a software analysis program enabling a real-time step detection algorithm. The step detection algorithm employs peak detection to ascertain the status of stance initiation. Peak initiation and termination are acquired upon the acceleration signal exceeding a prescribed threshold bound and subsequent threshold bound respectively. The algorithm implements a temporal threshold to prevent a single step from being counted multiple times. A Riemann summation numerical method is applied to calculate the time averaged acceleration integral (LeMoyne et al., 2008e). The offset is removed from the acceleration signal, which is obtained through a three dimensional application of Pythagorean's theorem (LeMoyne et al., 2008e; LeMoyne et al., 2008f). The Riemann sum numerical technique has been contrasted as accurate in comparison to the trapezoid method for the virtual proprioception application (LeMoyne et al., 2008d). The moving average of the time averaged acceleration integrals for ten steps was obtained for both affected and unaffected leg. The ratio of affected divided by unaffected leg, based on time averaged acceleration integrals, was calculated. The Wireless Health package enables all computations to be determined in real-time. The second generation virtual proprioception system was amenable for an assistant to provide auditory biofeedback respective of the affected per unaffected leg ratio of the time averaged acceleration waveform integrals. The assistant could provide the subject with quantified information of the real-time status comparison of affected and unaffected leg during gait cycle (LeMoyne et al., 2008e).

Preliminary testing and evaluation of the second generation virtual proprioception system was applied to one chronic hemiparetic subject. During gait cycle the subject was provided with verbal auditory feedback from the assistant operating the second generation virtual proprioception system, pertaining to the real-time computed time averaged acceleration signal integral ratio of affected divided by unaffected leg. With the auditory biofeedback of gait status, the subject would modify gait pattern with the objective of achieving an effectively parity ratio (LeMoyne et al., 2008e). The experimental protocol of the second generation system was similar to the first generation virtual proprioception experimental protocol. The predominant disparity was the incorporation of real-time quantified auditory feedback, as opposed to real-time visual evaluation of the respective acceleration waveforms (LeMoyne et al., 2008e; LeMoyne et al., 2008f). Five trials were conducted. The wireless accelerometers were mounted above the lateral epicondyle of the femur using an elastic band, as illustrated in figure 13. With the Wireless Health package active, the subject would walk approximately 75 feet during 'off' mode without biofeedback from virtual proprioception. Subsequently, for the next 75 feet the subject would walk using the 'on' mode of virtual proprioception, while adjusting gait in real-time according to the verbal feedback respective of the affected per unaffected leg ten step moving averaged time averaged acceleration integral ratio. The goal of the subject was to modify gait in real-time to achieve a near parity ratio (LeMoyne et al., 2008e).

As illustrated in trial 5 according to figure 14, the chronic hemiparetic subject while using virtual proprioception demonstrated the capacity to modify gait cycle to a near parity ratio of affected per unaffected leg. Figure 15 summarizes the comprehensive efficacy of virtual proprioception with a global averaging of all five trials, respective of the 'off' and 'on' status for the second generation of virtual proprioception. Statistical analysis of the test and evaluation was considered. During the 'off' status for virtual proprioception, the global mean for the affected per unaffected leg ratio was 79.38 with a standard deviation of 3.83. By contrast, during the 'on' status using virtual proprioception, the ratio of affected per unaffected leg achieved near parity status with a global mean of 103.75 and a standard deviation of 10.65. Full parity of the ratio would be achieved with a value of 100.00. The 'off' status affected per unaffected leg ratio for the virtual proprioception device application was bound with a 95% confidence level using a 5% margin of error about the mean. During 'on' status for virtual proprioception the affected per unaffected leg ratio was bound with a 90% confidence level using a 10% margin or error about the mean. The disparity in confidence level implicates the intrinsic variability while adapting to a new gait strategy during the real-time application of the second generation of virtual proprioception (LeMoyne et al., 2008e).

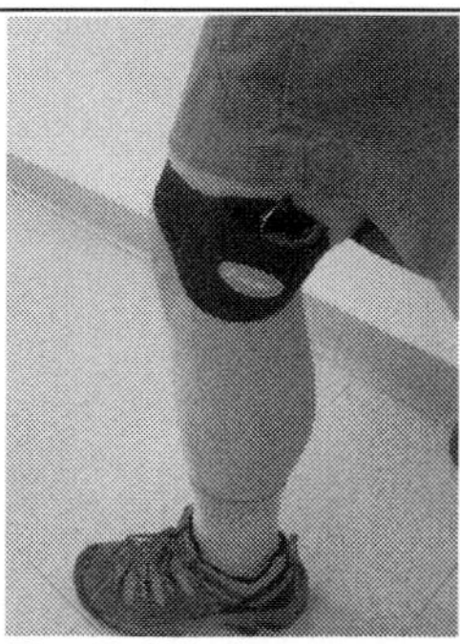

Fig. 13. Wireless accelerometer for virtual proprioception (LeMoyne et al., 2008e)

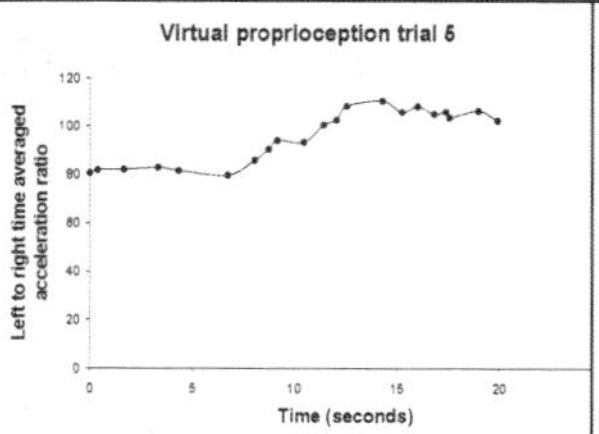

Fig. 14. Virtual proprioception trial 5 results for affected (left) leg relative to unaffected (right) leg

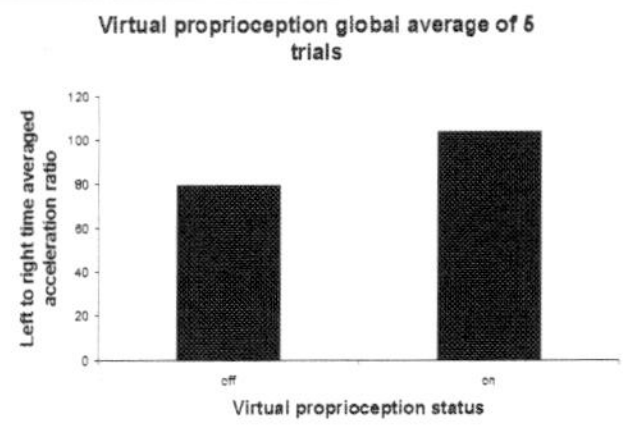

Fig. 15. Virtual proprioception five trial global average for affected (left) leg relative to unaffected (right) leg

6. Conclusion

As demonstrated throughout the chapter the merits of artificial proprioception have been advocated in consideration of the progressive advance of wireless accelerometer technology. Current wireless accelerometer technology has provided the foundation for the biomedical/ neuroengineering artificial equivalent of proprioception. The application of wireless accelerometers representing artificial proprioception has enabled the quantification of movement attributes, such as reflex, Parkinson's disease tremor, and gait. Artificial proprioception has also been demonstrated as a biofeedback application for real-time gait rehabilitation termed virtual proprioception.

The virtual proprioception system has been evolved over the course of two generations. The first generation incorporating visualization of the real-time status of both affected and unaffected leg acceleration waveforms for biofeedback; and the second generation utilizing auditory feedback of the real-time ten step moving average affected per unaffected leg time averaged acceleration integral ratio (LeMoyne et al., 2008e; LeMoyne et al., 2008f). Gait quantification and analysis has been demonstrated in autonomous settings, such as outdoors on a sidewalk and the hallway of a home setting, while selecting anatomical mounting positions such as the lateral epicondyle of the femur and the lateral malleolus (LeMoyne et al., 2009b; LeMoyne et al., 2009d). By mounting a wireless accelerometer to the dorsum of the hand for evaluating hand tremor, a concept intended for quantifying and classifying Parkinson's disease status has been developed (LeMoyne et al., 2009a). The quantification of reflex parameters, such as response and latency, has been demonstrated through a third generation device and novel artificial reflex system (LeMoyne et al., 2008h; LeMoyne et al., 2009c).

With the progressive development of foundational technologies for artificial proprioception, represented by wireless accelerometers, there is the potential for considerable evolution for future applications. Future generational systems incorporating artificial proprioception are anticipated to alleviate strain on medical resources, while also potentially advancing therapy and treatment strategies. Progress in fields, such as the software and robotics industry, will likely augment the implementation of artificial proprioception applications.

7. Future concepts

In tandem with multiple technology applications, the wireless accelerometer is anticipated to likewise evolve, in consideration of miniaturization, data storage capacity, wireless transmission strength, and robust software development. Virtual proprioception has the potential to expand to multiple biofeedback modalities, such as advances in visual, auditory, and eventually haptic/tactile sensation biofeedback. Refinements in software should enable improvements in step detection algorithms and improved strategies for learning alternative gait strategies. Another tangent application would be for improved proprioceptive feedback, monitoring, and learning techniques for prosthetic limbs. Future evolutions of virtual proprioception may significantly advance gait rehabilitation and ameliorate strain on medical resources.

A similar application is gait monitoring through wireless accelerometers functioning as artificial proprioception. Essentially the gait status of a patient may be recorded and analyzed for recovery status or disease progression in an effectively autonomous environment. Wireless accelerometer monitoring of gait status can be conducted with the therapist at a location remote to the patient. The incorporation of wireless accelerometer systems for quantifying locomotion enables advanced post-processing numerical techniques, such as spectral analysis; potentially initiating novel approaches for therapy strategies. Incorporating the progressive status of gait quality in a database could advance the evaluation of therapy strategy efficacy.

Database status tracking may be especially useful for a progressive neurodegenerative disease, such as Parkinson's disease. The status of a Parkinson's disease patient could be monitored through wireless accelerometers over durations in excess of 24 hours. Continual monitoring could augment drug therapy dose allocation and efficacy assessment. Improvements in wireless transmission strength, such as conveying the accelerometer signal to a wireless phone for subsequent transmission to a database, could provide significant advances in application autonomy. Similar to wireless accelerometers providing the basis for biofeedback with virtual proprioception, wireless accelerometers could provide feedback insight for deep brain stimulation parameter settings. Wireless accelerometer feedback could provide the basis for temporally optimal deep brain stimulation parameters with the integration of multi-disciplinary design optimization algorithms.

Wireless accelerometer systems for reflex quantification could advance the evaluation of central and peripheral nervous system trauma. The application has been developed with the intent to alleviate the growing strain on medical resources. Advances in machine learning classification techniques may further augment the impact of the wireless accelerometer reflex quantification system. Future advances envision the integration of machine learning and wireless accelerometer applications, such as reflex quantification for trauma and disease status classification.

Machine learning incorporates development of software programs, which improve with experience at a specific task, such as the classification of a phenomenon. Machine learning has been envisioned for optimizing treatment efficacy for medical issues (Mitchell, 1997). For example, machine learning algorithms have been applied for predicting pneumonia attributed mortality of hospital patients (Cooper et al. 1997). Machine learning intrinsically utilizes multiple disciplines, such as artificial intelligence, neurobiology, and control theory. Speech recognition software can be derived from machine learning, while incorporating learning methods such as neural networks (Mitchell, 1997).

Speech recognition has been successfully tested and evaluated in robust applications. Effectively speech recognition techniques incorporate analysis of acoustic waveforms (Englund, 2004). Similar to the attributes of an acoustic waveform, human movement may be recognized through the use of a wireless accelerometer representing artificial proprioception to derive an acceleration waveform. The testing and evaluation of activity classification using the frequency domain of the acceleration waveform has been demonstrated (Chung et al., 2008). Machine learning classification techniques in consideration of the derived acceleration waveform may augment the status evaluation of reflexes; Parkinson's disease; and gait diagnostic and treatment methods. Machine learning applications respective of virtual proprioception may advance and optimize near autonomous rehabilitation strategies.

The concept of artificial proprioception utilizing wireless accelerometers emphasizes a non-invasive approach for acquiring movement status characteristics. A machine learning algorithm with a tandem philosophy would be advantageous. During 2003 at Carnegie Mellon University a machine learning software program called HiLoClient demonstrated the ability to ascertain classification status while incorporating non-invasive methods. The HiLoClient software actually enabled researchers to detect, classify, and extrapolate the data statistically turning patterns into predictions from seemingly random generated data (Mastroianni, 2003).

Progress relevant to technology applications incorporating artificial proprioception will likely be augmented through tandem advances in the fields of the robotics industry and feedback control theory. The field of robotics incorporates a hierarchical control architecture, generally consisting of high, intermediate, and low level control. In general biological control systems and robotic control systems are representative of similar control system structures. The hierarchical nature of human locomotion provides a relevant example, with the high level representing descending commands from the brain. The central pattern generator may be applied to represent the intermediate level of control; and the lower level of control could encompass proprioceptors, such as muscle spindles and Golgi tendon organs. Respective of this control architecture, reflexes provide an important feedback control system (Bekey, 2005).

Progress in the fields of robotics and feedback control theory will likely advance biomedical applications of artificial proprioception, such as the characterization of reflexes and gait. The tandem technology evolutions are envisioned to provide substantial improvement in prosthetic applications. Alternative strategies and concepts incorporating robotics and feedback control theory should advance virtual proprioception biofeedback applications for augmented rehabilitation methods.

8. References

Aiello, E.; Gates, D.; Patritti, B.; Cairns, K.; Meister, M.; Clancy, E. & Bonato, P. (2005). Visual EMG biofeedback to improve ankle function in hemiparetic gait, *Proc. 27th Int. Conf. IEEE EMBS*, pp. 7703-7706, Shanghai, China, Sep., 2005

Aminian, K.; Robert, P.; Buchser, E.; Rutschmann, B.; Hayoz, D. & Depairon, M. (1999). Physical activity monitoring based on accelerometry: validation and comparison with video observation. *Med. Biol. Eng. Comput.*, Vol. 37, No. 3, (May, 1999) 304–308

Auvinet, B.; Berrut, G.; Touzard, C.; Moutel, L.; Collet, N.; Chaleil, D. & Barrey, E. (2002). Reference data for normal subjects obtained with an accelerometric device. *Gait Posture*, Vol. 16, No. 2, (Oct., 2002) 124–134

Bamberg, S.; Benbasat, A.; Scarborough, D.; Krebs, D. & Paradiso, J. (2008). Gait analysis using a shoe-integrated wireless sensor system. *IEEE Trans. Inf. Technol. Biomed.*, Vol. 12, No. 4, (Jul., 2008) 413-423

Bekey, G. (2005). *Autonomous Robots: From Biological Inspiration to Implementation and Control*, MIT Press, Cambridge, MA

Bickley, L. & Szilagyi, P. (2003). *Bates' Guide to Physical Examination and History Taking, 8th ed.*, Lippincott Williams and Wilkins, Philadelphia, PA

Bouten, C.; Koekkoek, K.; Verduin, M.; Kodde, R. & Janssen, J. (1997). A triaxial accelerometer and portable data processing unit for the assessment of daily physical activity. *IEEE Trans. Biomed. Eng.*, Vol. 44, No. 3, (Mar., 1997) 136–147

Busser, H.; Ott, J.; van Lummel, R.; Uiterwaal, M. & Blank, R. (1997). Ambulatory monitoring of children's activities. *Med. Eng. Phys.*, Vol. 19, No. 5, (Jul., 1997) 440–445

Chung, W.; Purwar, A. & Sharma, A. (2008). Frequency domain approach for activity classification using accelerometer, *Proc. 30th. Int. Conf. IEEE EMBS*, pp. 1120-1123, Vancouver, Canada, Aug., 2008

Clark, M.; Lucett, S. & Corn, R. (2008). *NASM Essentials of Personal Fitness Training, 3rd ed.*, Lippincott Williams and Wilkins, Philadelphia, PA

Cocito, D.; Tavella, A.; Ciaramitaro, P.; Costa, P.; Poglio, F. ; Paolasso, I.; Duranda, E.; Cossa, F. & Bergamasco, B. (2006). A further critical evaluation of requests for electrodiagnostic examinations. *Neurol. Sci.*, Vol. 26, No. 6, (Feb., 2006) 419–422

Cooper, G.; Aliferis, C.; Ambrosino, R.; Aronis, J.; Buchanan, B.; Caruana, R.; Fine, M.; Glymour, C.; Gordon, G.; Hanusa, B.; Janosky, J.; Meek, C.; Mitchell, T.; Richardson, T. & Spirtes, P. (1997). An evaluation of machine-learning methods for predicting pneumonia mortality. *Artif. Intell. Med.*, Vol. 9, No. 2, (Feb., 1997) 107-138

Cozens, J.;. Miller, S.; Chambers, I. & Mendelow, A. (2000). Monitoring of head injury by myotatic reflex evaluation. *J. Neurol. Neurosurg. Psychiatry*, Vol. 68, No. 5, (May, 2000) 581-588

Culhane, K.; O'Connor, M.; Lyons, D. & Lyons, G. (2005). Accelerometers in rehabilitation medicine for older adults. *Age Ageing*, Vol. 34, No. 6, (Nov., 2005), 556–560

Dietz, V. (2002). Proprioception and locomotor disorders. *Nat. Rev. Neurosci.*, Vol. 3, No. 10, (Oct., 2002) 781-790

Dobkin, B. (2003). *The Clinical Science of Neurologic Rehabilitation, 2nd ed.*, Oxford University Press, New York

Englund, C. (2004). Speech recognition in the JAS 39 Gripen aircraft - adaptation to speech at different G-loads, Royal Institute of Technology, Master Thesis in Speech Technology, Stockholm, Sweden, Mar., 2004

Fahrenberg, J.; Foerster, F.; Smeja, M. & Muller, W. (1997). Assessment of posture and motion by multichannel piezoresistive accelerometer recordings. *Psychophysiology*, Vol. 34, No. 5, (Sep., 1997) 607–612

Faist, M.; Ertel, M.; Berger, W. & Dietz, V. (1999). Impaired modulation of quadriceps tendon jerk reflex during spastic gait: differences between spinal and cerebral lesions. *Brain*, Vol. 122, No. 3, (Mar., 1999) 567–579

Frijns, C.; Laman, D.; van Duijn, M. & van Duijn, H. (1997). Normal values of patellar and ankle tendon reflex latencies. *Clin. Neurol. Neurosurg.*, Vol. 99 No. 1, (Feb., 1997) 31-36

Gurevich, T.; Shabtai, H.; Korczyn, A.; Simon, E. & Giladi, N. (2006). Effect of rivastigmine on tremor in patients with Parkinson's disease and dementia. *Mov. Disord.*, Vol. 21, No. 10, (Oct., 2006) 1663–1666

Hoos, M.; Kuipers, H.; Gerver, W. & Westerterp, K. (2004). Physical activity pattern of children assessed by triaxial accelerometry. *Eur. J. Clin. Nutr.*, Vol. 58, No. 10, (Oct., 2004) 1425–1428

Huang, H.; Wolf, S. & He, J. (2006). Recent developments in biofeedback for neuromotor rehabilitation. *J. Neuroeng. Rehabil.*, Vol. 3, No. 11, (Jun., 2006) 1-12

Jafari, R.; Encarnacao, A.; Zahoory, A.; Dabiri, F.; Noshadi, H. & Sarrafzadeh, M. (2005). Wireless sensor networks for health monitoring, *Proc. 2nd ACM/IEEE Int. Conf. on Mobile and Ubiquitous Systems (MobiQuitous)*, pp. 479–481, San Diego, CA, Jul., 2005.

Kamen, G. & Koceja, D. (1989). Contralateral influences on patellar tendon reflexes in young and old adults. *Neurobiol. Aging*, Vol. 10, No. 4, (Jul.-Aug., 1989) 311-315

Kandel, E.; Schwartz, J. & Jessell, T. (2000). *Principles of Neural Science, 4th ed.*, McGraw-Hill, New York

Kavanagh, J.; Barrett, R. & Morrison, S. (2004). Upper body accelerations during walking in healthy young and elderly men. *Gait Posture*, Vol. 20, No. 3, (Dec., 2004) 291–298

Kavanagh, J.; Morrison, S.; James, D. & Barrett, R. (2006). Reliability of segmental accelerations measured using a new wireless gait analysis system. *J. Biomech.*, Vol. 39, No. 15, (2006) 2863–2872

Keijsers, N.; Horstink, M.; van Hilten, J.; Hoff, J. & Gielen, C. (2000). Detection and assessment of the severity of Levodopa-induced dyskinesia in patients with Parkinson's disease by neural networks. *Mov. Disord.*, Vol. 15, No. 6, (Nov., 2000) 1104–1111

Keijsers, N.; Horstink, M. & Gielen, S. (2006). Ambulatory motor assessment in Parkinson's disease. *Mov. Disord.*, Vol. 21, No. 1, (Jan., 2006) 34–44

Koceja, D. & Kamen, G. (1988). Conditioned patellar tendon reflexes in sprint- and endurance-trained athletes. *Med. Sci. Sports Exerc.*, Vol. 20, No. 2, (Apr., 1988) 172-177

Kumru, H.; Summerfield, C.; Valldeoriola, F. & Valls-Solé, J. (2004). Effects of subthalamic nucleus stimulation on characteristics of EMG activity underlying reaction time in Parkinson's disease. *Mov. Disord.*, Vol. 19, No. 1, (Jan., 2004) 94–100

Lebiedowska, M. & Fisk, J. (2003). Quantitative evaluation of reflex and voluntary activity in children with spasticity. *Arch. Phys. Med. Rehabil.*, Vol. 84, No. 6, (Jun., 2003) 828-837

Lee, J.; Cho, S.; Lee, J.; Lee, K. & Yang, H. (2007). Wearable accelerometer system for measuring the temporal parameters of gait, *Proc. 29th. Int. Conf. IEEE EMBS*, pp. 483-486, Lyon, France, Aug., 2007

LeMoyne, R. (2005a). UCLA communication, UCLA, NeuroEngineering, Jun., 2005a

LeMoyne, R.; Jafari, R. & Jea, D. (2005b). Fully quantified evaluation of myotatic stretch reflex, *35th Society for Neuroscience Annual Meeting*, Washington, D.C., Nov., 2005b

LeMoyne, R. & Jafari, R. (2006a). Quantified deep tendon reflex device, *36th Society for Neuroscience Annual Meeting*, Atlanta, GA, Oct., 2006a

LeMoyne, R. & Jafari, R. (2006b). Quantified deep tendon reflex device, second generation, *15th International Conference on Mechanics in Medicine and Biology*, Singapore, Dec., 2006b

LeMoyne, R. (2007a). Gradient optimized neuromodulation for Parkinson's disease, *12th Annual Research Conference on Aging (UCLA Center on Aging)*, Los Angeles, CA, Jun., 2007a

LeMoyne, R.; Dabiri, F.; Coroian, C.; Mastroianni, T. & Grundfest, W. (2007b). Quantified deep tendon reflex device for assessing response and latency, *37th Society for Neuroscience Annual Meeting*, San Diego, CA, Nov., 2007b

LeMoyne, R.; Dabiri, F. & Jafari, R. (2008a). Quantified deep tendon reflex device, second generation. *J. Mech. Med. Biol.*, Vol. 8, No. 1, (Mar., 2008a) 75-85

LeMoyne, R.; Coroian, C. & Mastroianni, T. (2008b). 3D wireless accelerometer characterization of Parkinson's disease status, *Plasticity and Repair in Neurodegenerative Disorders*, Lake Arrowhead, CA, May, 2008b

LeMoyne, R.; Coroian, C.; Mastroianni, T. & Grundfest, W. (2008c). Accelerometers for quantification of gait and movement disorders: a perspective review. *J. Mech. Med. Biol.*, Vol. 8, No. 2, (Jun., 2008c) 137–152

LeMoyne, R.; Coroian, C. & Mastroianni, T. (2008d). Virtual proprioception using Riemann sum method, *16th International Conference on Mechanics in Medicine and Biology*, Pittsburgh, PA, Jul., 2008d

LeMoyne, R.; Coroian, C.; Mastroianni, T.; Wu, W.; Grundfest, W. & Kaiser, W. (2008e). Virtual proprioception with real-time step detection and processing, *Proc. 30th. Int. Conf. IEEE EMBS*, pp. 4238-4241, Vancouver, Canada, Aug., 2008e

LeMoyne, R.; Coroian, C.; Mastroianni, T. & Grundfest, W. (2008f). Virtual proprioception. *J. Mech. Med. Biol.*, Vol. 8, No. 3, (Sep., 2008f) 317–338

LeMoyne, R.; Coroian, C.; Mastroianni, T. & Grundfest, W. (2008g). Quantified deep tendon reflex device for evaluating response and latency using an artificial reflex device, *38th Society for Neuroscience Annual Meeting*, Washington, D.C., Nov., 2008g

LeMoyne, R.; Coroian, C.; Mastroianni, T. & Grundfest, W. (2008h). Quantified deep tendon reflex device for response and latency, third generation. *J. Mech. Med. Biol.*, Vol. 8, No. 4, (Dec., 2008h) 491–506

LeMoyne, R.; Coroian, C. & Mastroianni, T. (2009a). Quantification of Parkinson's disease characteristics using wireless accelerometers, *Proc. IEEE/ICME International Conference on Complex Medical Engineering (CME2009)*, pp. 1-5, Tempe, AZ, Apr., 2009a

LeMoyne, R.; Coroian, C. & Mastroianni, T. (2009b). Wireless accelerometer system for quantifying gait, *Proc. IEEE/ICME International Conference on Complex Medical Engineering (CME2009)*, pp. 1-4, Tempe, AZ, Apr., 2009b

LeMoyne, R.; Coroian, C. & Mastroianni, T. (2009c). Evaluation of a wireless three dimensional MEMS accelerometer reflex quantification device using an artificial reflex system, *Proc. IEEE/ICME International Conference on Complex Medical Engineering (CME2009)*, pp. 1-5, Tempe, AZ, Apr., 2009c

LeMoyne, R.; Coroian, C.; Mastroianni, T. & Grundfest, W. (2009d). Wireless accelerometer assessment of gait for quantified disparity of hemiparetic locomotion. *J. Mech. Med. Biol.*, Vol. 9, No. 3, (Sep., 2009d) 329-343

Lennon, S. & Johnson, L. (2000). The modified Rivermead Mobility Index: validity and reliability. *Disabil. Rehabil.*, Vol. 22, No. 18, (Dec., 2000) 833–839

Litvan, I.; Mangone, C.; Werden, W.; Bueri, J.; Estol, C.; Garcea, D.; Rey, R.; Sica, R.; Hallett, M. & Bartko, J. (1996). Reliability of the NINDS Myotatic Reflex Scale. *Neurology*, Vol. 47, No. 4, (Oct., 1996) 969-972

Lyons, G.; Culhane, K.; Hilton, D.; Grace, P. & Lyons, D. (2005). A description of an accelerometer-based mobility monitoring technique. *Med. Eng. Phys.*, Vol. 27, No. 6, (Jul., 2005) 497–504

Mamizuka, N.; Sakane, M.; Kaneoka, K.; Hori, N. & Ochiai, N. (2007). Kinematic quantitation of the patellar tendon reflex using a tri-axial accelerometer. *J. Biomech.*, Vol. 40, No. 9, (2007) 2107-2111

Manschot, S.; van Passel, L.; Buskens, E.; Algra, A. & van Gijn, J. (1998). Mayo and NINDS scales for assessment of tendon reflexes: between observer agreement and implications for communication. *J. Neurol. Neurosurg. Psychiatry,* Vol. 64, No. 2, (Feb., 1998) 253-255

Mastroianni, T. (2003). Application of machine learning using object recognition in computer vision for detecting and extrapolating patterns, Computational Analyses of Brain Imaging Psychology, (Just, M. & Mitchell, T.), Carnegie Mellon University, Apr., 2003

Mayagoitia, R.; Nene, A. & Veltink, P. (2002). Accelerometer and rate gyroscope measurement of kinematics: an inexpensive alternative to optical motion analysis systems. *J. Biomech.,* Vol. 35, No. 4, (Apr., 2002) 537-542

Menz, H.; Lord, S. & Fitzpatrick, R. (2003a). Acceleration patterns of the head and pelvis when walking on level and irregular surfaces. *Gait Posture,* Vol. 18, No. 1, (Aug., 2003a) 35–46

Menz, H.; Lord, S. & Fitzpatrick, R. (2003b). Age-related differences in walking stability. *Age Ageing,* Vol. 32, No. 2, (Mar., 2003b) 137–142

Mitchell, T. (1997). *Machine Learning,* McGraw-Hill, New York

Moe-Nilssen, R. (1998). A new method for evaluating motor control in gait under real-life environmental conditions. Part 2: gait analysis. *Clin. Biomech,* Vol. 13, No. 4-5, (1998) 328–335

Mondelli, M.; Giacchi, M.; & Federico, A. (1998). Requests for electromyography from general practitioners and specialists: critical evaluation. *Ital. J. Neurol. Sci.,* Vol. 19, No. 4, (Aug., 1998) 195-203

Nolte, J. & Sundsten, J. (2002). *The Human Brain: An Introduction to Its Functional Anatomy, 5th ed.,* Mosby, St. Louis, MO

Obwegeser, A.; Uitti, R.; Witte, R.; Lucas, J.; Turk, M. & Wharen, R. (2001). Quantitative and qualitative outcome measures after thalamic deep brain stimulation to treat disabling tremors. *Neurosurgery,* Vol. 48, No. 2, (Feb., 2001) 274–281

Podnar, S. (2005). Critical reappraisal of referrals to electromyography and nerve conduction studies. *Eur. J. Neurol.,* Vol. 12, No. 2, (Feb., 2005) 150-155

Pagliaro, P. & Zamparo, P. (1999). Quantitative evaluation of the stretch reflex before and after hydro kinesy therapy in patients affected by spastic paresis. *J. Electromyogr. Kinesiol.,* Vol. 9, No. 2, (Apr., 1999) 141–148

Saremi, K.; Marehbian, J.; Yan, X.; Regnaux, J.; Elashoff, R.; Bussel, B. & Dobkin, B. (2006). Reliability and validity of bilateral thigh and foot accelerometry measures of walking in healthy and hemiparetic subjects. *Neurorehabil. Neural Repair,* Vol. 20, No. 2, (Jun., 2006) 297-305

Saunders, J.; Inman, V. & Eberhart, H. (1953). The major determinants in normal and pathological gait. *J. Bone Joint Surg. Am.,* Vol. 35A, No. 3, (Jul., 1953), 543–558

Schrag, A.; Schelosky, L.; Scholz, U. & Poewe, W. (1999). Reduction of Parkinsonian signs in patients with Parkinson's disease by dopaminergic versus anticholinergic single-dose challenges. *Mov. Disord.,* Vol. 14, No. 2, (Mar., 1999) 252–255

Seeley, R.; Stephens, T. & Tate, P. (2003). *Anatomy and Physiology, 6th ed.,* McGraw-Hill, Boston, MA

Stam, J. & van Crevel, H. (1990). Reliability of the clinical and electromyographic examination of tendon reflexes. *J. Neurol.,* Vol. 237, No. 7, (Nov., 1990) 427-431

Uiterwaal, M.; Glerum, E.; Busser, H. & van Lummel, R. (1998). Ambulatory monitoring of physical activity in working situations, a validation study. *J. Med. Eng. Technol.*, Vol. 22, No. 4, (Jul.-Aug., 1998) 168-172

Van de Crommert, H.; Faist, M.; Berger, W. & Duysens, J. (1996). Biceps femoris tendon jerk reflexes are enhanced at the end of the swing phase in humans. *Brain Res.*, Vol. 734, No. 1-2, (Sep., 1996) 341-344

Veltink, P. & Franken, H. (1996). Detection of knee unlock during stance by accelerometry. *IEEE Trans. Rehabil. Eng.*, Vol. 4, No. 4, (Dec., 1996) 395-402

Voerman, G.; Gregoric, M. & Hermens, H. (2005). Neurophysiological methods for the assessment of spasticity: the Hoffmann reflex, the tendon reflex, and the stretch reflex. *Disabil. Rehabil.*, Vol. 27, No. 1-2, (Jan., 2005) 33-68

Volkmann, J.; Moro, E. & Pahwa, R. (2006). Basic algorithms for the programming of deep brain stimulation in Parkinson's disease. *Mov. Disord.*, Vol. 21, No. S14, (Jun., 2006) S284–S289

Willemsen, A.; Frigo, C. & Boom, H. (1991). Lower extremity angle measurement with accelerometers—error and sensitivity analysis. *IEEE Trans. Biomed. Eng.*, Vol. 38, No. 12, (Dec., 1991) 1186-1193

Wong, W.; Wong, M. & Lo, K. (2007). Clinical applications of sensors for human posture and movement analysis: a review. *Prosthet. Orthot. Int.*, Vol. 31, No. 1, (Mar., 2007) 62-75

www.enablingmnt.com/MEMS_sensors_evolution_and_trends_-_Henne_van_Heeren_Jan2007.pdf

www.intel.com

www.mdvu.org/library/ratingscales/pd/updrs.pdf

www.microstrain.com/g-link.aspx

www.sparkfun.com/commerce/categories.php

www.vias.org/simulations/simusoft_nykvist.html

Zhang, L.; Wang, G.; Nishida, T.; Xu, D.; Sliwa, J. & Rymer, W. (2000). Hyperactive tendon reflexes in spastic multiple sclerosis: measures and mechanisms of action. *Arch. Phys. Med. Rehabil.*, Vol. 81, No. 7, (Jul., 2000) 901-909

Zhang, K.; Werner, P.; Sun, M.; Pi-Sunyer, F. & Boozer, C. (2003). Measurement of human daily physical activity. *Obes. Res.*, Vol. 11, No. 1, (Jan., 2003) 33–40

Zhang, K.; Pi-Sunyer, F. & Boozer, C. (2004). Improving energy expenditure estimation for physical activity. *Med. Sci. Sports Exerc.*, Vol. 36, No. 5, (May, 2004) 883-889

Robust and Optimal Blood-Glucose Control in Diabetes Using Linear Parameter Varying paradigms

Levente Kovács* and Balázs Kulcsár**
*Dept. of Control Engineering and Information Technology,
Budapest University of Technology and Economics, Hungary.
**Delft Centre for Systems and Control
Delft University of Technology, Netherlands.

1. Introduction

The normal blood glucose concentration level in the human body varies in a narrow range (70 - 110 ml/dL). If for some reasons the human body is unable to control the normal glucose-insulin interaction (e.g. the glucose concentration level is constantly out of the above mentioned range), diabetes is diagnosed. The phenomena can be explained by several causes, most important ones are stress, obesity, malnutrition and lack of exercise.

The consequences of diabetes are mostly long-term; among others, diabetes increases the risk of cardiovascular diseases, neuropathy and retinopathy (Fonyo & Ligeti, 2008). Consequently, diabetes mellitus is a serious metabolic disease, which should be artificially regulated. This metabolic disorder was lethal until 1921 when Frederick G. Banting and Charles B. Best discovered the insulin. Nowadays the life quality of diabetic patients can be enhanced though the disease is still lifelong.

The newest statistics of the World Health Organization (WHO) predate an increase of adult diabetes population from 4% (in 2000, meaning 171 million people) to 5,4% (366 million worldwide) by the year 2030 (Wild et al., 2004). This warns that diabetes could be the "disease of the future", especially in the developing countries (due to stress and unhealthy lifestyle).

Type I (also known as insulin dependent diabetes mellitus (IDDM)) is one of the four classified types of this disease (Type II, gestational diabetes and other types, like genetic deflections are the other three categories of diabetes), and is characterized by complete pancreatic β-cell insufficiency (Fonyo & Ligeti, 2008). As a result, the only treatment of Type I diabetic patients is based on insulin injection (subcutaneous or intravenous), usually administered in an open-loop manner.

Due to the alarming facts of diabetes, the scientific community proposed to improve the treatment of diabetes by investigating the applicability of an external controller. In many biomedical systems, external controller provides the necessary input, because the human body could not ensure it. The outer control might be partially or fully automated. The self-

regulation has several strict requirements, but once it has been designed it permits not only to facilitate the patient's life suffering from the disease, but also to optimize (if necessary) the amount of the used dosage.
However, blood-glucose control is one of the most difficult control problems to be solved in biomedical engineering. One of the main reasons is that patients are extremely diverse in their dynamics and in addition their characteristics are time varying. Due to the inexistence of an outer control loop, replacing the partially or totally deficient blood-glucose-control system of the human body, patients are regulating their glucose level manually. Based on the measured glucose levels (obtained from extracted blood samples), they often decide on their own what is the necessary insulin dosage to be injected. Although this process is supervised by doctors (diabetologists), mishandled situations often appear. Hyper- (deviation over the basal glucose level) and hypoglycaemia (deviation under the basal glucose level) are both dangerous cases, but on short term the latter is more dangerous, leading for example to coma.
Starting from the 1960s lot of researchers have investigated the problem of the glucose-insulin interaction and control. The closed-loop glucose regulation, as it was several times formulated (Parker et al., 2000), (Hernjak & Doyle, 2005), (Ruiz-Velazques et al., 2004), requires three components:

- glucose sensor;
- insulin pump;
- a control algorithm, which based on the glucose measurements, is able to determine the necessary insulin dosage.

1.1 Modelling diabetes mellitus

To design an appropriate control, an adequate model is necessary. The mathematical model of a biological system, developed to investigate the physiological process underling a recorded response, always requires a trade off between the mathematical and the physiological guided choices. In the last decades several models appeared for Type I diabetes patients (Chee & Tyrone, 2007).
The mostly used and also the simplest one proved to be the minimal model of Bergman (Bergman et al., 1979) for Type I diabetes patients under intensive care, and its extension, the three-state minimal model (Bergman et al., 1981).
However, the simplicity of the model proved to be its disadvantage too, as it is very sensitive to parameters variance, the plasma insulin concentration must be known as a function of time and in its formulation a lot of components of the glucose-insulin interaction were neglected. Therefore, extensions of this minimal model have been proposed (Hipszer, 2001), (Dalla Man et al., 2002), (Benett & Gourley, 2003), (Lin et al., 2004), (Fernandez et al., 2004), (Morris et al., 2004), (de Gaetano & Arino, 2000), (Chbat & Roy, 2005), (Van Herpe et al., 2006) trying to capture the changes in patient dynamics of the glucose-insulin interaction, particularly with respect to insulin sensitivity or the time delay between the injection and absorption. Other approximations proposed extensions based on the meal composition (Roy & Parker, 2006a), (Roy & Parker, 2006b), (Dalla Man et al., 2006a) , (Dalla Man et al., 2006b).
Beside the Bergman-model other more general, but more complicated models appeared in the literature (Cobelli et al., 1982), (Sorensen, 1985), (Tomaseth et al., 1996), (Hovorka et al., 2002), (Fabietti et al., 2006).

1.2 The Sorensen-model

The most complex diabetic model proved to be the 19th order Sorensen-model (Sorensen, 1985) (the current work focuses on a modification of it, developed by (Parker et al., 2000)), which is based on the earlier model of (Guyton et al., 1978). Even if the Sorensen-model describes in a very exact way the human blood glucose dynamics, due to its complexity it was rarely used in research problems.

The model was created with a great simplification: glucose and insulin subsystems are disconnected in the basal post absorptive state, which can be fulfilled with no pancreatic insulin secretion. Nomenclature and equations can be found in the Appendix of the current book chapter.

The Sorensen-model can be divided in six compartments (brain, heart and lungs, liver, gut, kidney, periphery), and its compartmental representation is illustrated by Fig. 1.

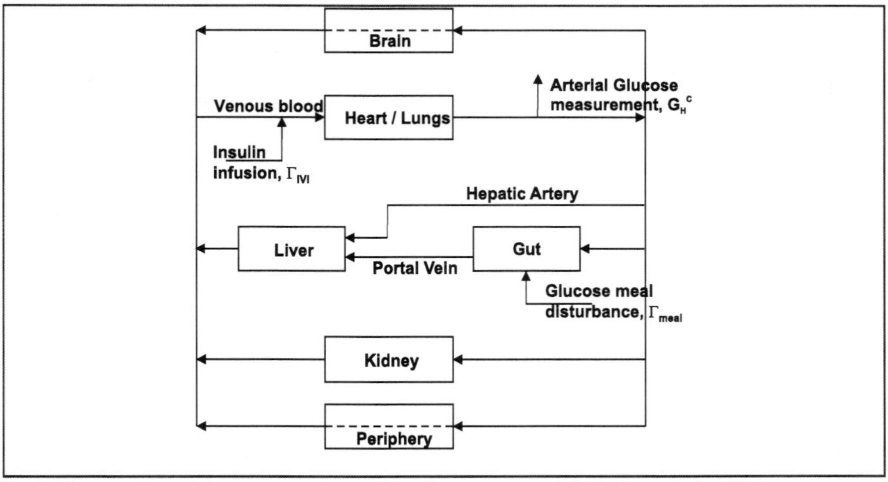

Fig. 1. Compartmental representation of the Sorensen model (Parker et al., 2000).

Transportation is realized with blood circulation assuming that glucose and insulin concentrations of the blood flow leaving the compartment are equal to the concentrations of the compartment. The compartments can be divided into capillary and tissue subcompartments, since glucose and insulin from the blood flow entering the compartment are either utilized or transported by diffusion. In compartments with small time constant or with no absorption the division into subcompartments is unnecessary.

1.3 Control of diabetes mellitus

Regarding the applied control strategies for diabetes mellitus, the palette is very wide (Parker et al., 2001).

Starting from classical control strategies (PID control (Chee et al., 2003), cascade control (Ortis-Vargas & Puebla, 2006)), to soft-computing techniques (fuzzy methods (Ibbini, 2006), neural networks (Mougiakakou et al., 2006), neuro-fuzzy methods (Dazzi et al., 2001)), adaptive (Lin et al., 2004), model predictive (MPC) (Hernjak & Doyle, 2005), (Hovorka et al.,

2004), or even robust H_∞ control were already applied (Parker et al., 2000), (Ruiz-Velazques et al., 2004), (Kovacs et al., 2006), (Kovacs & Palancz, 2007), (Kovacs et al., 2008).
Most of the applied control methods were focused on the Bergman minimal model (and so the applicability of the designed controllers was limited due to excessive sensitivity of the model parameters). On the other hand, for the Sorensen-model, only linear control methods were applied (H_∞ (Parker et al., 2000), (Ruiz-Velazques et al., 2004), MPC (Parker et al., 1999)). An acceptable compromise between the model's complexity and the developed control algorithm could be the parametrically varying system description (Shamma & Athans, 1991), identification (Lee, 1997), optimal control (Wu et al., 2000), (Balas, 2002) and diagnosis (Kulcsar, 2005).

1.4 The aim of the current work

The main contribution of the present work is to give a possible solution for nonlinear and optimal automated glucose control synthesis.
Considering the high-complexity nonlinear Sorensen-model a nonlinear model-based methodology, the LPV (Linear Parameter Varying) technique is used to develop open-loop model and robust controller design based on H_∞ concepts. The results are continuously compared with those obtained by (Parker et al., 2000) where a linear model based robust control algorithm was used (see section 1.5).
The validity of the Sorensen model is caught inside a polytopic region and the model is built up by a linear combination of the linearized models derived in each polytopic point (covering the physiologic boundaries of the glucose-insulin interaction of the Sorensen-model).
Finally, using induced L_2-norm minimization technique, a robust controller is developed for insulin delivery in Type I diabetic patients. The robust control was developed taking input and output multiplicative uncertainties with two additional uncertainties from those used by (Parker et al., 2000). Comparative results are given and closed-loop simulation scenarios illustrate the applicability of the robust LPV control techniques.

1.5 Brief review of the article published by (Parker et al., 2000)

As in the current chapter a continuous comparison of the obtained results will be done with those obtained by (Parker et al., 2000), we considered useful to briefly summarize the mentioned article.
Although the first application of the H_∞ theory on the field of diabetic control was that of (Kienitz & Yoneyama, 1993), the publication of (Parker et al., 2000) can be considered a pioneer work in applying the H_∞ method for glucose-insulin control of Type I diabetic patients using the fundamental nonlinear Sorensen-model.
In (Parker et al., 2000) uncertainty in the nonlinear model was characterized by up to ±40% variation in eight physiological parameters and by sensitivity analysis it was identified that three-parameter set have the most significant effect on glucose and insulin dynamics. Controller performance was designed to track the normoglycemic set point (81.1 mg/dL) of the Sorensen-model in response to a 50 g meal disturbance (using the six hour meal disturbance function of (Lehmann & Deutsch, 1992)). By this way, glucose concentration was maintained within ±3.3 mg/dL of set point.

The results were compared to the results of (Kienitz & Yoneyama, 1993), who developed an H_∞ controller based on a third order linear diabetic patient model. Performance of (Kienitz & Yoneyama, 1993)'s controller in response to a meal disturbance was quantitatively similar to the nominal controller obtained by (Parker et al., 2000). However, the uncertainty-derived controller of (Parker et al., 2000) was tuned to handle significantly more uncertainty than that of (Kienitz & Yoneyama, 1993).

On the other hand, (Parker et al., 2000) underlined that a significant loss in performance appeared applying the potential uncertainty in the model in comparison to the nominal case. This could be mostly exemplified by the near physiologically dangerous hypoglycaemic episode, typically characterized as blood glucose values below 60 mg/dL (see Fig. 9 and Fig. 10 of (Parker et al., 2000) also captured by Fig. 2 of the current work).

Therefore, our goal was dual: applying nonlinear model-based LPV control methodology to design robust controller for Type I diabetic patients and to design a robust controller by taking into account two additional uncertainties from those used in (Parker et al., 2000), namely sensor noise and worst case design for meal disturbance presented in (Lehmann & Deutsch, 1992) (60 g carbohydrate).

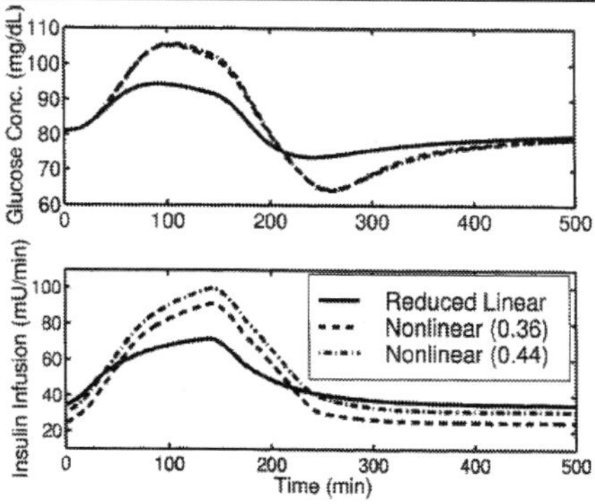

Fig. 2. Results obtained by (Parker et al., 2000) (taking from their work).

2. LPV modelling using polytopic description

The chapter suggests using Linear Parameter concepts with optimal and robust control scheme in order to show a candidate for diabetes Type I closed-loop control. First, the most important control related definition of such a system class is given. Solution of the robust control synthesis by Linear Matrix Inequalities (LMI) is briefly summarized.

2.1 LPV system definition

Linear Parameter Varying (LPV) system is a class of nonlinear systems, where the parameter could be an arbitrary time varying, piecewise-continuous and vector valued function denoted by $\rho(t)$, defined on a compact set $\mathcal{P}$. In order to evaluate the system, the parameter trajectory is requested to be known either by measurement or by computation. A formal definition of the parameter varying systems is given below.

Definition 1. For a compact $\mathcal{P} \subset \mathbf{R}^{s}$, the parameter variation set $F_{\mathcal{P}}$ denotes the set of all piecewise continuous functions mapping $\mathbf{R}^{+}$ (time) into $\mathcal{P}$ with a finite number of discontinuities in any interval. The compact set $\mathcal{P} \subset \mathbf{R}^{s}$ along with the continuous functions A: $\mathbf{R}^{s} \to \mathbf{R}^{n \times n}$, B: $\mathbf{R}^{s} \to \mathbf{R}^{n \times n_u}$, C: $\mathbf{R}^{s} \to \mathbf{R}^{n_y \times n}$, D: $\mathbf{R}^{s} \to \mathbf{R}^{n_y \times n_u}$ represent an nth order LPV system whose dynamics evolve as:

$$\begin{aligned} \dot{x}(t) &= A(\rho)x(t) + B(\rho)u(t) \\ y(t) &= C(\rho)x(t) + D(\rho)u(t) \end{aligned} \tag{1}$$

with $\rho(t) \in F_{\mathcal{P}}$ (Wu et al., 2000).
As a result, it can be seen that in the LPV model, by choosing parameter variables, the system's nonlinearity can be hidden. This methodology is used on different control solutions, like (Balas, 2002), which gave also a solution of the problem.
There are different descriptions of the LPV systems (Kulcsar, 2005). In the affine description possibility, a part of the x(t) states are equal with the ρ(t) parameters. However, due to the complexity of the Sorensen model, this representation is impossible to be developed.
Polytopic representation could be another description of the LPV systems. In this case, the validity of the model is caught inside a polytopic region and the model is built up by a linear combination of the linearized models derived in each polytopic point ($\Sigma_i = \begin{bmatrix} A_i & B_i \\ C_i & D_i \end{bmatrix}$) (Kulcsar, 2005):

$$\Sigma(t) \subset \{\Sigma_1, \ldots, \Sigma_2\} = \left\{ \sum_{i=1}^{j} \alpha_i \Sigma_i : \alpha_i \geq 0, \sum_{i=1}^{j} \alpha_i = 1 \right\} \tag{2}$$

Hence, the LPV system is given by the complex combination of the positive coefficients and the system Σ-s. The polytopic LPV model can be thought as a set of linear models on a vertex (a convex envelope of LTI systems), where the grid points of the description are LTI systems. The generation of a polytopic model is the derivation around an operating point of the general nonlinear state-space representation. The LPV polytopic model is valid only in a restricted domain, characterized by the range of the polytope (Kulcsar, 2005).
Therefore, the correct definition of the polytopic region (which is capable to describe the whole working area of the system) is a key point in this methodology.

2.2 Induced L_2 performance objective of LPV systems region

For a given compact set $\mathcal{P} \subset \mathbf{R}^{s}$ and a continuous bounded matrix function A: $\mathbf{R}^{s} \to \mathbf{R}^{n \times n}$ which describes the $\dot{x}(t) = A(\rho(t))x(t)$ LPV system ($\rho(t) \in \mathcal{P}$) and for a V Lyapunov function candidate, it can be written that the time derivative of V(x) (for $\forall \rho \in \mathcal{P}$ along the LPV system trajectories) is (Tan, 1997):

$$\frac{d}{dt} V(x(t)) = x^T(t)\left[A^T(\rho(t))P + PA(\rho(t))\right]x(t) \tag{3}$$

Defintion 2. Function A is quadratically stable over $\mathcal{P}$ if there exists a $P \in \mathbf{R}^{n \times n}$, $P = P^T > 0$ positive definite matrix, such that for $\forall \rho \in \mathcal{P}$ (Wu et al., 2000):

$$A^T(\rho(t))P + PA(\rho(t)) < 0 \tag{4}$$

It can be seen that the quadratic stability is a strong form of the robust stability with respect to time varying parameters as it is true for quick changes of the $\rho(t)$ parameter trajectory and for its definition it is enough a single quadratic Lyapunov-function.

Defintion 3. For a quadratically stable LPV system $\Sigma_{\mathcal{P}}$ and for zero initial conditions, the induced L_2-norm of an LPV system is defined as follows (Tan, 1997):

$$\|G_P\|_2 = \sup_{\rho \in P} \sup_{\substack{\|d\|_2 \neq 0 \\ d \in L_2}} \frac{\|e\|_2}{\|d\|_2} \tag{5}$$

As a result, $\|G_P\|_2$ represents the largest disturbance to error over the set of all causal linear operators described by $\Sigma_{\mathcal{P}}$.

Corollary 1. (Tan, 1997) Given the LPV system $\Sigma_{\mathcal{P}}$ and $\gamma > 0$ a positive scalar, if there exists an $X \in R^{n\times n}$, $X = X^T > 0$ such that for all $\rho \in \mathcal{P}$.

$$L = \begin{pmatrix} A^T(\rho)X + XA(\rho) & XB(\rho) & \gamma^{-1}C^T(\rho) \\ B^T(\rho)X & -I & \gamma^{-1}D^T(\rho) \\ \gamma^{-1}C(\rho) & \gamma^{-1}D(\rho) & -I \end{pmatrix} < 0 \tag{6}$$

then:

1. The function A is quadratically stable over $\mathcal{P}$.
2. There exists a $\beta < \gamma$ such that $\|G_P\|_2 \le \beta$.

The matrix inequality (6) can be rewritten in the more familiar Riccati inequality by taking Schur components (Tan, 1997):

$$\begin{aligned} &A^T(\rho)X + XA(\rho) + \gamma^{-2}C^T(\rho)C(\rho) + \left(XB(\rho) + \gamma^{-2}C^T(\rho)D(\rho)\right)\cdot \\ &\cdot\left(I - \gamma^{-2}D^T(\rho)D(\rho)\right)^{-1}\left(B^T(\rho)X + \gamma^{-2}D^T(\rho)C(\rho)\right) < 0 \end{aligned} \tag{7}$$

As a result, the aim of the induced L_2 performance minimization is to find $\min_X \gamma$, with $L_{\gamma^2} < 0$, $X > 0$ and $\gamma > 0$ constraints, where L_{γ^2} can be derived from (6):

$$L_{\gamma^2} = \begin{pmatrix} A^T(\rho)X + XA(\rho) & XB(\rho) & C^T(\rho) \\ B^T(\rho)X & -I & 0 \\ C(\rho) & 0 & -\gamma^2 I \end{pmatrix} < 0 \tag{8}$$

3. Results

Open- and closed-loop LPV results are shown to describe the Sorensen-model. First, a polytopic gridding method is provided, second a robust control design is performed subjected to the uncertain open-loop LPV system and additional frequency weightings.

3.1 Covering the Sorensen-model with a polytopic region

In case of the 19th order Sorensen model (Fig. 1) two inputs: Γ_{meal} (meal disturbance), Γ_{IVI} (injected insulin amount), and one output, the capillary heart-lungs glucose concentration, G_H^C can be delimited. However, we have considered also the peripheral insulin concentration in the capillaries, I_P^C as an additionally output.

Due to the high complexity of the Sorensen-model it was hard to investigate the global stability of the system (the Lyapunov function is a real function with 19 variables). Therefore, a solution could be to cover the working region with a set of linear systems and in this way to investigate the local stability of them.

Choosing the polytopic points we have restricted to the physiological meanings of the variables. The first point was the normoglycaemic point (glucose concentration $y = G_H^C$ = 81.1 mg/dL and calculated insulin concentration $I_{P\ init}^C$ = 26.6554 mU/L), while the others were deflections from this point (given below in %):

- glucose concentrations: 25%, 50%, 75%, 100%, 150%, 200%;
- insulin concentrations: 0%, 25%, 50%, 100%, 150%, 200%.

The glucagon and the additional values were kept at their normoglycaemic value.

In the points of the so generated polytopic region (36 points) we have determined one by one a linearized model and we have analyzed the stability, observability and controllability properties of them. Each system proved to be stable, and partially observable and controllable (the rank of the respective matrices were all 15 and 14 respectively) (Kovacs, 2008). Finally, we have simulated the so developed polytopic LPV system of the Sorensen model, and we have compared the results with those obtained by (Parker et al., 2000). After comparing the results it can be seen (Fig. 3) that the LPV model is approximating with an acceptable error the nonlinear system. However, it can be also observed that without an insulin injection the glucose concentration reaches an unacceptable value for a diabetic patient. Moreover, for the considered polytope the LPV system is stepping out from the defined region being unable to handle the uncovered region.

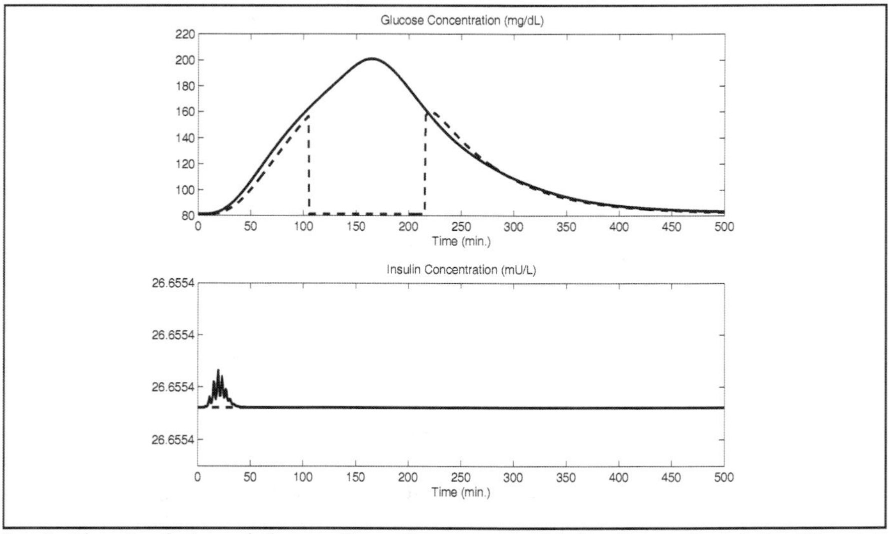

Fig. 3. The simulation of the nonlinear Sorensen model (continuous) and the 36 points polytope region (dashed).

Therefore, we had to extend the glucose concentration region of the considered polytope considering other grid points too, while the insulin concentration grid remained the same:

- glucose concentrations: 25%, 50%, 75%, 100%, 150%, 200%, 300%, 400%;
- insulin concentrations: 0%, 25%, 50%, 100%, 150%, 200%.

Using the newly generated polytopic region (48 points) and after the same investigation of each linear model (obtaining the same results: each system proved to be stable and partially observable and controllable) it can be seen that the LPV model remains inside the considered polytopic region (Fig. 4) and approximates with an acceptable error the nonlinear system (Kovacs, 2008).

For meal disturbance we have used the same six hour meal disturbance function of (Lehmann & Deutsch, 1992) (Fig. 5), filtered with a $\frac{1/60}{s+1/60}$ first order lag used by (Parker et al., 2000), while the insulin input was considered zero.

It can be seen, that in absence of control the open-loop simulation is going up to a very high glucose concentration value, unacceptable for a Type I diabetic patient.

3.2 LPV based robust control of the Sorensen-model

In case of robust control design, the results presented in (Parker et al., 2000) showed that a near hypoglycaemic situation appears for the considered uncertainties (Fig. 2). In case of a diabetic patient this could be also a dangerous situation (not only hyperglycaemia).

The aim of the control design is to minimize the meal disturbance level over the performance output for all possible variation of the parameter within the polytope $F_{\mathcal{P}}$.

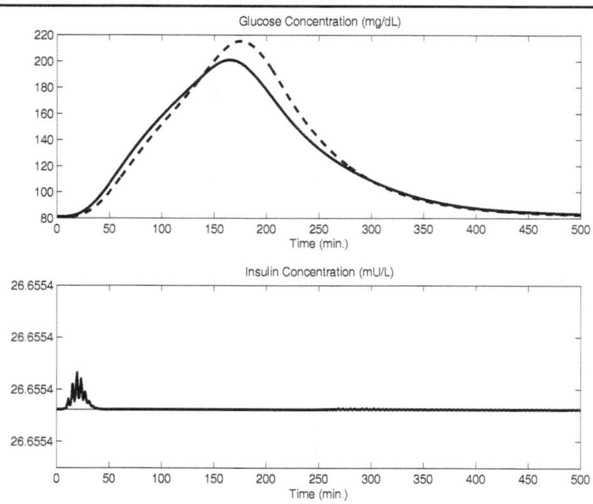

Fig. 4. The simulation of the nonlinear Sorensen model (solid) and the considered polytopic region (dashed).

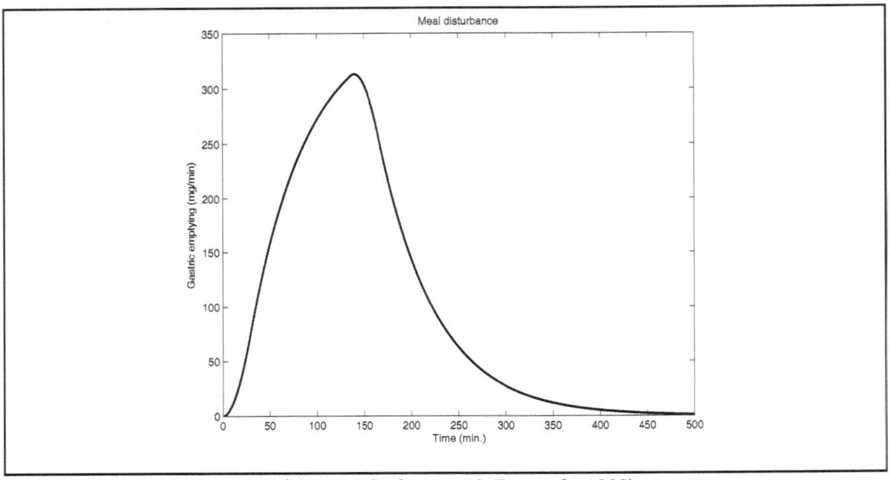

Fig. 5. The glucose emptying function (Lehmann & Deutsch, 1992).

$$\min_{K}\|G\| = \min_{K} \sup_{\rho \in F_p} \sup_{\|d\| \neq 0} \frac{\|z_{y1}\|}{\|d\|} \tag{9}$$

where d denotes the meal disturbance input and z describes the glucose variation. Priory information is injected to the controller throughout the augmentation of the nominal plant with extra dynamics, called weighting functions.

Therefore, the starting point of the control design was the appropriate choice of the weighting functions. Firstly, we have reproduced the results obtained by (Parker et al., 2000) with the dangerous near hypoglycemic episode, but using the LPV methodology (on the polytopic region presented in the previous section). Consequently, the weighting functions used were the followings:

- The multiplicative uncertainty of the insulin input, $W_i = \dfrac{s^2 + 0.47s + 0.015}{s^2 + 0.29s + 0.022}$;
- The multiplicative uncertainty of the glucose input, $W_{im} = \dfrac{1.63s^2 + 0.21s + 0.007}{s^2 + 0.52s + 0.010}$;
- The performance weighting function, $W_{perf} = \dfrac{\frac{1}{1.2}s + 0.25}{s + 0.01 * 0.25}$;
- The disturbance (glucose) input weighting function, $W_m = \dfrac{1}{6s+1}$.

However, as we mentioned above, we have additionally taken into account sensor noise too (neglected in (Parker et al., 2000), by considering it a 1/10000 value). We have considered that for insulin measurements a 5% error, while for glucose measurements a 2% error is tolerable (values taken from clinical experience).

As a result, the considered closed-loop interconnection of system can be illustrated by Fig. 6, while the obtained results obtained on the original nonlinear Sorensen-model can be seen in

Fig. 7. By the reproduced results of (Parker et al., 2000) we have proved that the obtained controller (designed for the created LPV model) works correctly.
Now, we have redesigned the control problem, to minimize the negative effects obtained by (Parker et al., 2000). Moreover, for meal disturbances we focused on the worst case of the (Lehmann & Deutsch, 1992) absorption taking into account a 60 g carbohydrate intake (in comparison with the 50 g carbohydrate considered by (Parker et al., 2000)).
To avoid the hypoglycaemic situation and take into account the two additional uncertainties mentioned above, we have extended the control loop with a weighting function for the control signal and an output uncertainty block (Fig. 8).

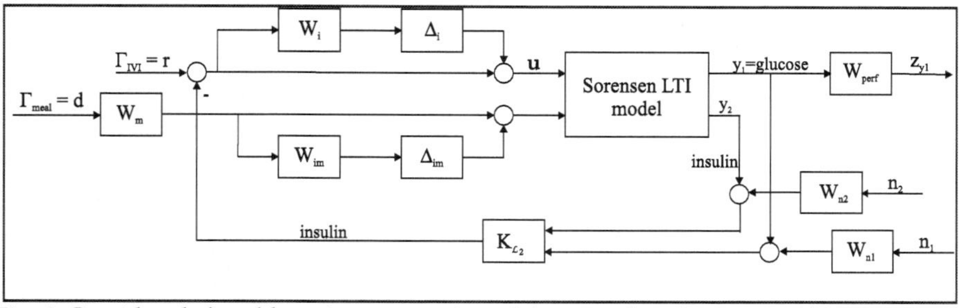

Fig. 6. Considered closed-loop interconnection of the reproduced situation of (Parker et al., 2000) extended with additionally considered sensor noise weighting functions.

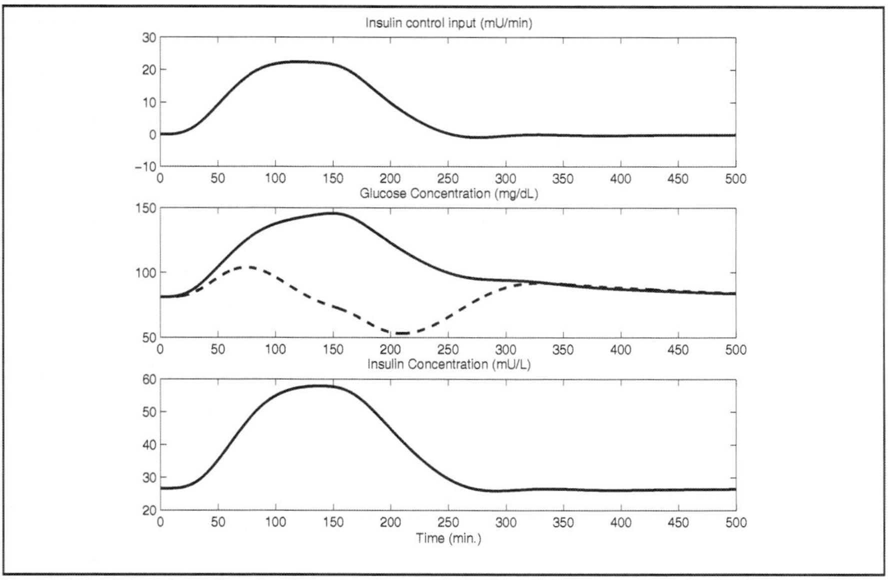

Fig. 7. The LPV based robust controller with induced L_2-norm minimization guarantee, using the same weighting functions as in (Parker et al., 2000): in case of the original nonlinear Sorensen model (solid) and the considered polytopic region (dashed) controller.

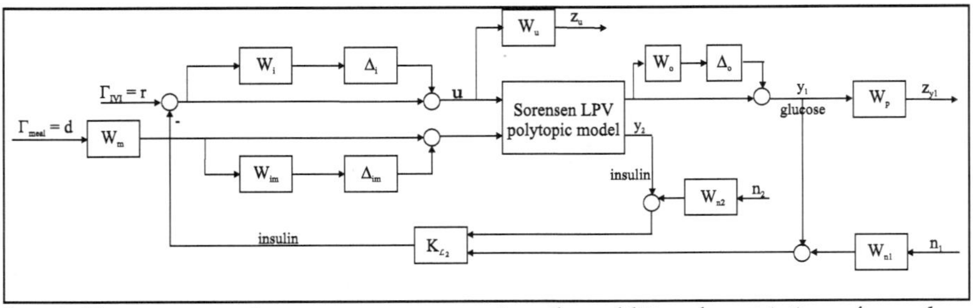

Fig. 8. The augmented system structure using the additional restrictions from those published in (Parker et al., 2000).

As a result, regarding the weighting functions used in (Parker et al., 2000), we have modified only the multiplicative uncertainty weighting functions (W_{im}, W_i) and the performance weighting function W_{perf}, while these were chosen only from engineering point of view. Now physiological aspects were taken also into account. The frequency response of the weighting functions can be seen in Fig. 9.

During the robust control design, a $\gamma = 1.0096$ solution was obtained. It can be seen (Fig. 10) that the hypoglycaemic situation is avoided and the glucose level is kept inside the normal 80-120 mg/dL range. Testing the controller on the original nonlinear Sorensen-model results are good too. Although in this case the glucose results are stepping out the normal range (160 mg/dL) this is acceptable (and similar to the healthy subjects).

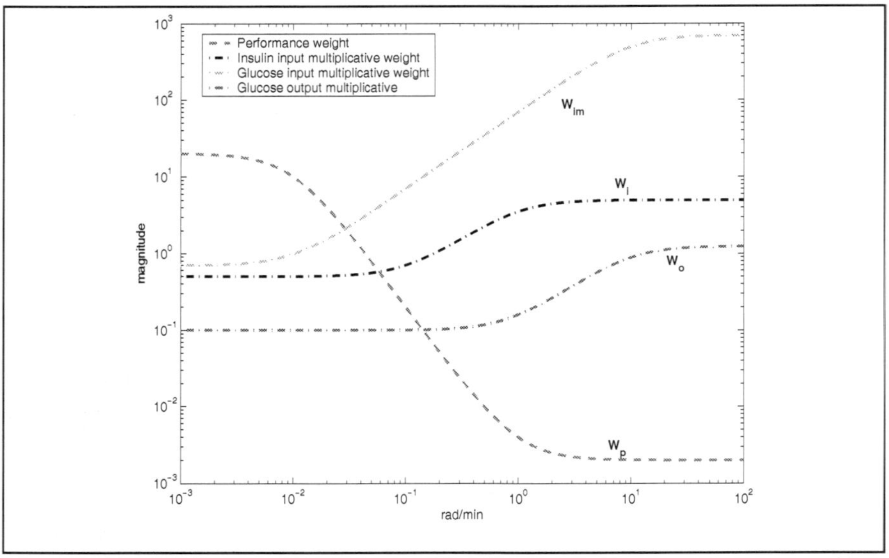

Fig. 9. Weighting functions used for the LPV-based induced L_2-norm minimization (those which have been modified from (Parker et al., 2000)).

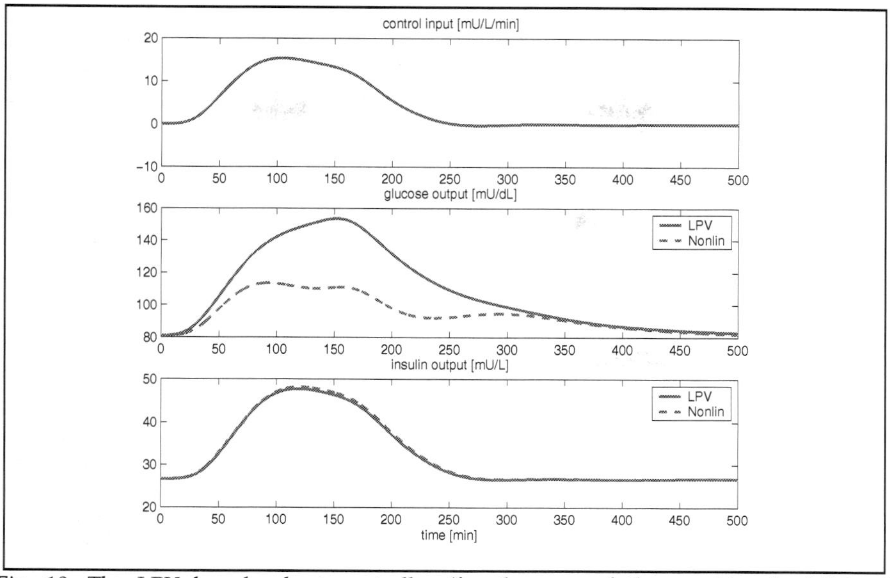

Fig. 10. The LPV based robust controller (for the case of the considered additional uncertainties) with induced L_2-norm minimization guarantee in case of the original nonlinear Sorensen model (solid) and the considered polytopic region (dashed).

4. Conclusions

In the current work a nonlinear model-based LPV control method was applied to design a robust controller for the high complexity Sorensen-model. The used methodology is more general than the classical linear H_∞ method as it deals directly with the nonlinear model itself. From the different descriptions of the LPV systems, polytopic representation was used, where the validity of the model was captured inside a polytopic region. In this way the model was built up by a linear combination of the linearized models derived in each considered polytopic point.

Using induced L_2-norm minimization technique, a robust controller was developed for insulin delivery in Type I diabetic patients. Considering the normoglycaemic set point (81.1 mg/dL), a polytopic set was created over the physiologic boundaries of the glucose-insulin interaction of the Sorensen-model.

The robust control was developed taking into account input and output multiplicative uncertainties, sensor noise and worst case meal disturbance (as additional restrictions from those applied in (Parker et al., 2000)). The obtained results showed that glucose level can be kept inside a normal range, avoiding hypoglycaemic episode (which was not possible with the control formalism applied in (Parker et al., 2000)). By the given comparative results and closed-loop simulation scenarios it was illustrated the applicability of the robust LPV control techniques.

Parameter dependency of the considered weighting functions could be considered in the future, which gives additional design freedom.

5. Acknowledgment

This research has been supported by Hungarian National Scientific Research Foundation, Grants No. OTKA T69055.

6. References

Balas, G.J. (2002). Linear, Parameter-Varying Control and Its Application to a Turbofan Engine. *International Journal of Robust and Nonlinear Control*, vol. 12, no. 9, pp. 763-796.

Benett, D.L. and Gourley, S.A. (2003). Asymptotic properties of a delay differential equation model for the interaction of glucose with plasma and interstitial insulin. *Applied Mathematics and Computation*, vol. 151, no. 1, pp. 189-207.

Bergman, B.N., Ider, Y.Z., Bowden, C.R. and Cobelli, C. (1979). Quantitive estimation of insulin sensitivity. *American Journal of Physiology*, vol. 236, pp. 667-677.

Bergman, R.N., Philips, L.S. and Cobelli, C. (1981). Physiologic evaluation of factors controlling glucose tolerance in man. *Journal of Clinical Investigation*, vol. 68, pp. 1456-1467.

Chbat, N.W. and Roy, T.K. (2005). Glycemic Control in Critically Ill Patients - Effect of Delay in Insulin Administration. in *Proc. of 27th IEEE EMBS Annual International Conference*, Shanghai, China, pp. 2506-2510.

Chee, F., Fernando, T.L., Savkin, A.V. and van Heeden, V. (2003). Expert PID control system for blood glucose control in critically ill patients. *IEEE Transactions on Information Technology in Biomedicine*, vol. 7, no. 4, pp. 419-425.

Chee, F. and Tyrone, F. (2007). *Closed-loop control of blood glucose*. Lecture Notes of Computer Sciences 368, Springer-Verlag, Berlin.

Cobelli, C., Federspil, G., Pacini, G., Salvan, A. and Scandellari, C. (1982). An integrated mathematical model of the dynamics of blood glucose and its hormonal control. *Mathematical Biosciences*, vol. 58, pp. 27-60.

Dazzi, D., Taddei, F., Gavarini, A., Uggeri, E., Negro, R. and Pezzarossa, A. (2001). The control of blood glucose in the critical diabetic patient: A neuro-fuzzy method. *Journal of Diabetes and Its Complications*, vol. 15, pp. 80-87.

Dalla Man, Ch., Caumo, A. and Cobelli, C. (2002). The Oral Glucose Minimal Model: Estimation of Insulin Sensitivity From a Meal Test. *IEEE Transactions on Biomedical Engineering*, vol. 49, no. 5, pp. 419-429.

Dalla Man, Ch., Toffolo, G., Basu, R., Rizza, R.A. and Cobelli, C. (2006a). A Model of Glucose Production During a Meal. in *Proc. of 28th IEEE EMBS Annual International Conference*, New York City, USA, pp. 5647-5650, 2006.

Dalla Man, Ch., Rizza, R.A. and Cobelli, C. (2006b). Mixed Meal Simulation Model of Glucose-Insulin System. in *Proc. of 28th IEEE EMBS Annual International Conference*, New York City, USA, pp. 307-310.

Fabietti, P.G., Canonico, V., Orsini Federici, M., Massi Benedetti, M. and Sarti, E. (2006). Control oriented model of insulin and glucose dynamics in type 1 diabetics. *Medical and Biological Engineering and Computing*, vol. 44, pp. 69–78.

Fernandez, M., Acosta D., Villasana M. and Streja, D. (2004). Enhancing Parameter Precision and the Minimal Modeling Approach in Type I Diabetes", in *Proc. of 26th IEEE EMBS Annual International Conference*, San Francisco, USA, pp. 797–800.

Fonyo, A. and Ligeti, E. (2008). *Physiology* (in Hungarian). 3rd ed., Ed. Medicina, Budapest.

de Gaetano, A. and Arino, O. (2000). Some considerations on the mathematical modeling of the Intra-Venous Glucose Tolerance Test. *Journal of Mathematical Biology*, vol. 40, pp. 136-168.

Guyton, J.R., Foster, R.O., Soeldner, J.S., Tan, M.H., Kahn, C.B., Koncz, L. and Gleason, R.E. (1978). A model of glucose-insulin homeostasis in man that incorporates the heterogeneous fast pool theory of pancreatic insulin release. *Diabetes*, vol. 27, pp. 1027.

Hernjak, N. and Doyle III, F.J. (2005). Glucose control design using nonlinearity assessment techniques. *AIChE Journal*, vol. 51, no. 2, pp. 544-554.

Hipszer, B.R. (2001). *A Type 1 Diabetic Model*. Master Thesis, Drexel University, USA, 2001.

Hovorka, R., Shojaee-Moradie, F., Carroll, P.V., Chassin, L.J., Gowrie, I.J., Jackson, N.C., Tudor, R.S., Umpleby, A.M. and Jones, R.H. (2002). Partitioning glucose distribution/transport, disposal, and endogenous production during IVGTT. *American Journal Physiology Endocrinology Metabolism*, vol. 282, pp. 992-1007.

Hovorka, R., Canonico, V., Chassin, L.J., Haueter, U., Massi-Benedetti, M., Orsini Federici, M., Pieber, T.R., Schaller, H.C., Schaupp, L., Vering, T. and Wilinska, M.E. (2004). Nonlinear model predictive control of glucose concentration in subjects with type 1 diabetes. *Physiological measurement*, vol. 25, pp. 905-920.

Ibbini, M. (2006). A PI-fuzzy logic controller for the regulation of blood glucose level in diabetic patients. *Journal of Medical Engineering and Technology*, vol. 30, no. 2, pp. 83-92.

Kienitz, K.H. and Yoneyama, T. (1993). A Robust Controller for Insulin Pumps Based on H-Infinity Theory. *IEEE Transactions on Biomedical Engineering*, vol. 40, no. 11, pp. 1133-1137.

Kovacs, L., Palancz, B., Benyo, B, Torok, L. and Benyo, Z. (2006). Robust blood-glucose control using Mathematica. in *Proc. of 28th EMBS Annual International Conference*, New York, USA, pp. 451-454.

Kovacs, L. and Palancz, B. (2007). Glucose-insulin control of Type1 diabetic patients in H_2/H_∞ space via Computer Algebra. *Lecture Notes in Computer Science*, vol. 4545, pp. 95–109.

Kovacs L., Kulcsar B., Bokor, J. and Benyo, Z. (2008). Model-based Nonlinear Optimal Blood Glucose Control of Type 1 Diabetes Patients. in *Proc. 30th IEEE EMBS Annual International Conference*, Vancouver, Canada, pp 1607-1610.

Kovacs, L. (2008). *New principles and adequate control methods for insulin dosage in case of diabetes*. PhD dissertation (in Hungarian). Budapest University of Technology and Economics, Budapest, Hungary.

Kulcsar, B. (2005). *Design of Robust Detection Filter and Fault Correction Controller*. PhD dissertation, Budapest University of Technology and Economics, Budapest, Hungary.

Lee, L.H. (1997). *Identification and Robust Control of Linear Parameter-Varying Systems*. PhD dissertation, University of California at Berkeley, USA.

Lehmann, E.D. and Deutsch, T.A. (1992). A physiological model of glucose-insulin interaction in Type1 diabetes mellitus. *Journal of Biomedical Engineering*, vol. 14, pp. 235-242.

Lin, J., Chase, J.G., Shaw, G.M., Doran, C.V., Hann, C.E., Robertson, M.B., Browne, P.M., Lotz, T., Wake, G.C. and Broughton, B. (2004). Adaptive bolus-based set-point regulation of hyperglycemia in critical care. in *Proc. of 26th IEEE EMBS Annual International Conference*, San Francisco, USA, pp. 3463-3466.

Morris, H.C., O'Reilly, B. and Streja, D. (2004). A New Biphasic Minimal Model. in *Proc. of 26th IEEE EMBS Annual International Conference*, San Francisco, USA, pp. 782–785.

Mougiakakou, S.G., Prountzou, A., Iliopoulou, D., Nikita K.S., Vazeou, A. and Bartsocas, Ch.S. (2006). Neural network based glucose - insulin metabolism models for children with type 1 diabetes. in *Proc. of 28th IEEE EMBS Annual International Conference*, New York, USA, pp. 3545-3548.

Ortiz-Vargas, M. and Puebla, H. (2006). A cascade control approach for a class of biomedical systems. in *Proc. of 28th IEEE EMBS Annual International Conference*, New York, USA, pp. 4420-4423.

Parker, R.S., Doyle III, F.J. and Peppas, N.A. (1999). A Model-Based Algorithm for Blood Glucose Control in Type I Diabetic Patients. *IEEE Transactions on Biomedical Engineering*, vol. 46, no. 2, pp. 148-157.

Parker, R.S., Doyle III, F.J., Ward, J.H. and Peppas, N.A. (2000). Robust H_∞ Glucose Control in Diabetes Using a Physiological Model. *AIChE Journal*, vol. 46, no. 12, pp. 2537-2549.

Parker, R.S., Doyle III, F.J. and Peppas, N.A. (2001). The intravenous route to blood glucose control. A review of control algorithms for noninvasive monitoring and regulation in type I diabetic patients. *IEEE Engineering in Medicine and Biology*, vol. 20, no.1, pp. 65-73.

Roy, A. and Parker, R.S. (2006a). Dynamic Modeling of Free Fatty Acid, Glucose, and Insulin: An Extended "Minimal Model". *Diabetes Technology & Therapeutics*, vol. 8, pp. 617-626.

Roy, A. and Parker, R.S. (2006b). Mixed Meal Modeling and Disturbance Rejection in Type I Diabetic Patients. in *Proc. of 28th IEEE EMBS Annual International Conference*, New York City, USA, pp. 323-326.

Ruiz-Velazquez, E., Femat, R. and Campos-Delgado, D.U. (2004). Blood glucose control for type I diabetes mellitus: A robust tracking H_∞ problem. *Elsevier Control Engineering Practice*, vol. 12, pp. 1179-1195.

Shamma, J. and Athans, M. (1991). Guaranteed properties of gain scheduled control for linear parameter varying plants. *Automatica*, vol. 27, no. 3. pp. 559-564.

Sorensen, J.T. (1985). *A physiologic model of glucose metabolism in man and its use to design and assess improved insulin therapies for diabetes*. PhD Thesis, Dept. of Chemical Eng. Massachusetts Institute of Technology, Cambridge, USA.

Tan, W. (1997). *Applications of Linear Parameter-Varying Control Theory*. MsC. thesis, University of California at Berekley, USA.

Thomaseth, K., Kautzky-Willer, A., Ludvik, B., Prager, R. and Pacini, G. (1996). Integrated mathematical model to assess β -cell activity during the oral glucose test. *Modeling in Physiology*, pp. 522-531.

Van Herpe, T., Pluymers, B., Espinoza, M., Van den Berghe, G. and de Moor, B. (2006). A minimal model for glycemia control in critically ill patients. in *Proc. 28th of IEEE EMBS Annual International Conference*, New York, USA, pp. 5432-5435.

Wild, S., Roglic, G., Green, A., Sicree, R. and King, H. (2004). Global prevalence of diabetes - Estimates for the year 2000 and projections for 2030. *Diabetes Care*, vol. 27, no. 5, pp. 1047-1053.

Wu, F., Grigoriadis, K.M. and Packard, A. (2000). Anti-windup controller design using linear parameter varying control methods. *International Journal of Control*, vol. 73, no. 12, pp. 1104-1114.

7. Appendix

7.1 Nomenclature and constants used in the Sorensen-model

In the current work the same nomenclature was used as it can be found in (Parker et al., 2000). The notations of the indexes used in the equations given below are:

- A - hepatic artery
- B - brain
- BU - brain uptake
- C - capillary space
- G - glucose
- H - heart and lungs
- HGP - hepatic glucose production
- HGU - hepatic glucose uptake
- I - insulin
- IHGP - insulin effect on HGP
- IHGU - insulin effect on HGU
- IVI - intravenous insulin infusion
- K - kidney
- KC - kidney clearance
- KE - kidney excretion
- L - liver
- LC - liver clearance
- N - glucagon
- NHGP - glucagon effect on HGP
- P – periphery (muscle / adipose tissue).
- PC - peripheral clearance
- PGU - peripheral glucose uptake
- PIR - pancreatic insulin release
- PNC - pancreatic glucagon clearance
- PNR - pancreatic glucagon release (normalized).
- RBCU - red blood cell uptake
- S – gut (stomach / intestine).
- SIA - insulin absorption into blood stream from subcutaneous depot
- SU - gut uptake
- T - tissue space

while the model variables notations are:

- A - auxiliary equation state (dimensionless).
- B - fractional clearance (I, dimensionless; N, L/min).
- G - glucose concentration (mg/dL).
- I - insulin concentration (mU/L).
- N - glucagon concentration (normalized, dimensionless).
- Q - vascular plasma flow rate (L/min).
- q - vascular blood flow rate (dL/min).
- T - transcapillary diffusion time constant (min).
- V - volume (L).
- v – volume (dL).
- Γ - metabolic source or sink rate (mg/min or mU/min).

The values of the used constants can be seen in Table 1.

[dL]	[L]	[dL/min]	[L/min]	[L/min]	[min]
$v_B^C = 3.5$	$V_B^C = 0.265$	$q_B = 5.9$	$Q_B = 0.45$	$F_{PNC} = 0.91$	$T_B = 2.1$
$v_B^T = 4.5$	$V_H^C = 0.985$	$q_H = 43.7$	$Q_H = 3.12$	$F_{LC} = 0.4$	$T_P^G = 5.0$
$v_H^C = 13.8$	$V_S^C = 0.945$	$q_S = 10.1$	$Q_S = 0.72$	$F_{KC} = 0.3$	$T_P^I = 20$
$v_S^C = 11.2$	$V_L^C = 1.14$	$q_L = 12.6$	$Q_L = 0.9$	$F_{PC} = 0.15$	
$v_L^C = 25.1$	$V_K^C = 0.505$	$q_A = 2.5$	$Q_A = 0.18$		
$v_K^C = 6.6$	$V_P^C = 0.735$	$q_K = 10.1$	$Q_K = 0.72$		
$v_P^C = 10.4$	$V_P^T = 6.3$	$q_P = 15.1$	$Q_P = 1.05$		
$v_P^T = 67.4$	$V_N = 9.93\ 1$				

Table 1. Parameter values for the Sorensen-model (Parker et al., 2000).

7.2 Equations of the Sorensen-model

The equations of the Sorensen-model can be structured in three parts:

- Glucose equations;
- Insulin equations;
- Glucagons production;

The eight equations of the glucose part are given below:

$$\dot{G}_B^C = \left(G_H^C - G_B^C\right)\frac{q_B}{v_B^C} - \left(G_B^C - G_B^T\right)\frac{v_B^T}{T_B v_B^C} \tag{A-1}$$

$$\dot{G}_B^T = \left(G_B^C - G_B^T\right)\frac{1}{T_B} - \frac{\Gamma_{BU}}{v_B^T} \tag{A-2}$$

$$\dot{G}_H^C = \left(G_B^C q_B + G_L^C q_L + G_K^C q_K + G_P^C q_P - G_H^C q_H - \Gamma_{RBCU}\right)\frac{1}{v_H^C} \tag{A-3}$$

$$\dot{G}_S^C = \left(G_H^C - G_S^C\right)\frac{q_S}{v_S^C} + \frac{\Gamma_{meal}}{v_S^C} - \frac{\Gamma_{SU}}{v_S^C} \tag{A-4}$$

$$\dot{G}_L^C = \left(G_H^C q_A + G_S^C q_S - G_L^C q_L\right)\frac{1}{v_L^C} + \frac{\Gamma_{HGP}}{v_L^C} - \frac{\Gamma_{HGU}}{v_L^C} \tag{A-5}$$

$$\dot{G}_K^C = \left(G_H^C - G_K^C\right)\frac{q_K}{v_K^C} - \frac{\Gamma_{KE}}{v_K^C} \tag{A-6}$$

$$\dot{G}_P^C = \left(G_H^C - G_P^C\right)\frac{q_P}{v_P^C} + \left(G_P^T - G_P^C\right)\frac{v_P^T}{T_P^G v_P^C} \tag{A-7}$$

$$\dot{G}_P^T = \left(G_P^C - G_P^T\right)\frac{1}{T_P^G} - \frac{\Gamma_{PGU}}{v_P^T} \tag{A-8}$$

where for simplification $k_B^C = G_B^C \frac{v_B^T}{T_B}$ and $k_B^T = G_B^T \frac{v_B^T}{T_B}$ notations can be introduced.

The seven insulin equations are:

$$\dot{I}_B^C = \left(I_H^C - I_B^C\right)\frac{Q_B}{V_B^C} \tag{A-9}$$

$$\dot{I}_H^C = \left(I_B^C Q_B + I_L^C Q_L + I_K^C Q_K + I_P^C Q_P - I_H^C Q_H + \Gamma_{IVI}\right)\frac{1}{V_H^C} \tag{A-10}$$

$$\dot{I}_S^C = \left(I_H^C - I_S^C\right)\frac{Q_S}{V_S^C} \tag{A-11}$$

$$\dot{I}_L^C = \left(I_H^C Q_A + I_S^C Q_S - I_L^C Q_L\right)\frac{1}{V_L^C} + \frac{\Gamma_{PIR}}{V_L^C} - \frac{\Gamma_{LC}}{V_L^C} \tag{A-12}$$

$$\dot{I}_K^C = \left(I_H^C - I_K^C\right)\frac{Q_K}{V_K^C} - \frac{\Gamma_{KC}}{V_K^C} \tag{A-13}$$

$$\dot{I}_P^C = \left(I_H^C - I_P^C\right)\frac{Q_P}{V_P^C} - \left(I_P^C - I_P^T\right)\frac{V_P^T}{T_P^I V_P^C} \tag{A-14}$$

$$\dot{I}_P^T = \left(I_P^C - I_P^T\right)\frac{1}{T_P^I} + \frac{\Gamma_{SIA}}{V_P^T} - \frac{\Gamma_{PC}}{V_P^T} \tag{A-15}$$

The remaining four equations compose the remaining states of the Sorensen model: the glucagon and three additional (dimensionless) variables. The use of the latter three variables is to highlight the glucagons dependent dynamics of the glycogen (synthesis or glycogenolyzes) which is also dependent by the actual blood glucose and insulin level:

$$\dot{N} = \left(\Gamma_{PNR} - N\right)\frac{F_{PNC}}{V_N} \tag{A-16}$$

$$\dot{A}_{IHGP} = \frac{1}{25}\left[1.2088 - 1.138\tanh\left(1.669\frac{I_L^C}{21.43} - 0.8885\right) - A_{IHGP}\right] \tag{A-17}$$

$$\dot{A}_{NHGP} = \frac{1}{65}\left[\frac{2.7\tanh(0.388N) - 1}{2} - A_{NHGP}\right] \tag{A-18}$$

$$\dot{A}_{IHGU} = \frac{1}{25}\left[2\tanh\left(0.549\frac{I_L^C}{21.43}\right) - A_{IHGU}\right] \tag{A-19}$$

It can be observed, that in the different equations different Γ_i parameters appear. These correspond for the different metabolic source and sinks:

$$\Gamma_{BU} = 70 \tag{A-20}$$

$$\Gamma_{RBCU} = 10 \tag{A-21}$$

$$\Gamma_{SU} = 20 \tag{A-22}$$

$$\Gamma_{HGP} = 155A_{IHGP}\left[2.7\tanh(0.388N) - A_{NHGP}\right]\cdot\left[1.425 - 1.406\tanh\left\{0.6199\left(\frac{G_L^C}{101} - 0.4969\right)\right\}\right] \tag{A-23}$$

$$\Gamma_{HGU} = 20A_{IHGP}\left[5.6648 + 5.6589\tanh\left\{2.4375\left(\frac{G_L^C}{101} - 1.48\right)\right\}\right] \tag{A-24}$$

$$\Gamma_{KE} = \begin{cases} 71 + 71\tanh\left[0.011\left(G_K^C - 460\right)\right] & ,\text{if } G_K^C < 460\dfrac{mg}{dl} \\ 0.872G_K^C - 300 & ,\text{if } G_K^C \geq 460\dfrac{mg}{dl} \end{cases} \tag{A-25}$$

$$\Gamma_{PGU} = \frac{35G_P^T}{86.81}\left[7.035 + 6.51623\tanh\left\{0.33827\left(\frac{I_P^T}{5.304} - 5.82113\right)\right\}\right] \tag{A-26}$$

$$\Gamma_{LC} = F_{LC}\left(I_H^C Q_A + I_S^C Q_S + \Gamma_{PIR}\right) \tag{A-27}$$

$$\Gamma_{PIR} = 0 \tag{A-28}$$

$$\Gamma_{KC} = F_{KC} I_K^C Q_K \tag{A-29}$$

$$\Gamma_{PC} = \frac{I_P^T}{\dfrac{1 - F_{PC}}{F_{PC}}\dfrac{1}{Q_P} - \dfrac{1}{T_P^I V_P^T}} \tag{A-30}$$

$$\Gamma_{PNR} = \left[1.3102 - 0.61016\tanh\left\{1.0571\left(\frac{I_H^C}{15.15} - 0.46981\right)\right\}\right]\cdot \\ \cdot\left[2.9285 - 2.095\tanh\left\{4.18\left(\frac{G_H^C}{91.89} - 0.6191\right)\right\}\right] \tag{A-31}$$

12

Towards Diagnostically Robust Medical Ultrasound Video Streaming using H.264

A. Panayides[1], M.S. Pattichis[2], C. S. Pattichis[1], C. P. Loizou[3], M. Pantziaris[4], and A. Pitsillides[1]
[1]*Department of Computer Science, University of Cyprus, Nicosia, Cyprus*
[2]*Department of Electrical and Computer Engineering, University of New Mexico, Albuquerque, New Mexico, USA*
[3]*Department of Computer Science, Intercollege, Limassol, Cyprus*
[4]*The Cyprus Institute of Neurology and Genetics, Nicosia, Cyprus*

1. Introduction

M-Health systems and services have seen significant growth over the past decade. Increasingly available bitrate through new wireless technologies linked with compression advances provided by current state-of-the-art H.264 advanced video coding standard, have brought rapid growth to the development of mobile health (m-Health) healthcare systems and services. Advances in nanotechnologies, compact biosensors, wearable devices and clothing, pervasive and ubiquitous computing systems have broadened the applicability areas of such systems and services. A recent overview of the current status, highlighting future directions, while also covering incorporated wireless transmission technologies, can be found in (Kyriacou et al., 2007; Istepanian et al., 2006).

Despite this momentum towards m-Health systems and especially e-Emergency systems, wireless channels remain error prone, while the absence of objective quality metrics (Wang & Bovik, 2009) limits the ability of providing medical video of adequate diagnostic quality at a required bitrate. Recently, new image and video quality metrics have been proposed, for evaluating the original and transmitted (or despeckled) (Loizou & Pattichis, 2008) video over a communication path, but these have not yet been applied to wireless transmission. The development of effective medical video streaming systems requires the implementation of error-resilient methods that are also diagnostically relevant. Although a plethora of studies has been published in video transmission, very few have focused on the difficulties associated with the wireless transmission of medical ultrasound video. In (Doukas & Maglogiannis, 2008), scalable coding is used for adaptive transmission of medical images and video snapshots over simulated wireless networks, while in (Tsapatsoulis et al., 2007), a saliency-based visual attention ROI for low bit-rate medical video transmission is proposed. Mathematically lossless (M-lossless) coding of the ROI after video denoising using motion compensated temporal filtering (MCTF) is practiced in (Rao & Jayant, 2005). A new rate control algorithm which takes into account a new motion complexity measure together with perceptual bit allocation is proposed in (Hongtao et al., 2005).

Here, we investigate different encoding schemes and packet loss rates in video transmission and provide recommendations regarding efficiency and the trade-off between bitrate and diagnostic quality. We propose the use of different frame type ordering schemes and provide methods for quantifying video quality for different packet loss rates. We also provide lower bounds for acceptable video quality and discuss how these bounds can be achieved by different frame type encoding schemes. A preliminary study appears in (Panayides et al., 2008).

Then, we are interested in exploiting new error resilience techniques and how they relate to diagnostic error resilient encoding. Loss tolerance is subject to the amount of clinical data recovered and whether this amount is suitable for providing acceptable diagnosis. Failure to do so may result in imprecise diagnosis. Consequently, the effort is directed towards maximizing error protection and recovery while at the same time conforming to channel limitations (bandwidth) and (varying) conditions (introducing delay, jitter, packet loss, and data corruption). We propose the development of effective wireless video transmission systems by extending the current state-of-the-art H.264/AVC standard to provide for video encoding that is driven by its intended diagnostic use.

Medical experts evaluating carotid ultrasound video are mainly interested in identifying possible stenosis of the carotid artery. Having diagnosed a stenosis, they aim at extracting atherosclerotic plaque (causing the stenosis) features, tracking of which in time can aid in the prediction of the severity of this abnormality. Intima media thickness (IMT) of the near and far wall also aid in this direction. The remaining regions of the video carry little, yet some diagnostic significance.

Bearing in mind the aforementioned, segmentation algorithms identifying these region(s) of diagnostic interest (ROIs) were developed by our group. The key concept is that once diagnostic ROIs have been defined, the remaining part of the video can be effectively compressed without significantly altering diagnosis. We investigate the use of a spatially-varying encoding scheme, where quantization levels are spatially varying as a function of the diagnostic significance of the video. To implement this approach, we use flexible macroblock ordering (FMO). Having derived the diagnostic ROIs of carotid ultrasound medical video, we use them as input for FMO type 2 slice encoding. We extend the FMO concept by enabling variable quality slice encoding (i.e. different quantization parameter for each ROI), tightly coupled by each region's diagnostic importance, targeting high diagnostic quality at a reduced bitrate. Subjective (clinical evaluation) as well as objective (PSNR) quality assessment shows considerable bitrate reductions while at the same not compromising diagnostic quality.

The rest of the chapter is organized as follows. Section 2 introduces the fundamental concepts of video streaming architecture and protocols. Section 3 briefly highlights H.264, describes frame types and encoding modes, as well as Flexible Macrblock Ordering. Section 4 illustrates the methodology while section 5 presents an analysis of the conducted experiments. Finally Section 6 provides some concluding remarks.

2. Video Streaming Architecture and Protocols

2.1 Architecture

Video streaming is the delivery of a video sequence over a network in real time, where video decoding starts before the entire video has been transmitted. That is, the client plays the incoming video stream in real time as the data is received. However, we should distinguish between live and on demand video streaming. Essentially, we have two different delivery methods: live video streaming where the live source (video) capture and encoding is done in real time, and on-demand video streaming, which tackles archived pre-encoded video.

A typical video streaming architecture is illustrated in Figure 1. The raw video is captured by a camera or ultrasound device, before it is fed to a source encoding software (i.e. H.264/AVC encoder). The resulting stream is then forwarded to the storage device of a server (encoding software and server can reside on the same computer, for example a laptop in an ambulance). The server is responsible for channel encoding and delivery of the stream to the client(s) through the network. The reverse procedure is followed at the client's side. After channel decoding the stream enters a playout buffer before it's forwarded to the decoder for source decoding and rendering of the transmitted video.

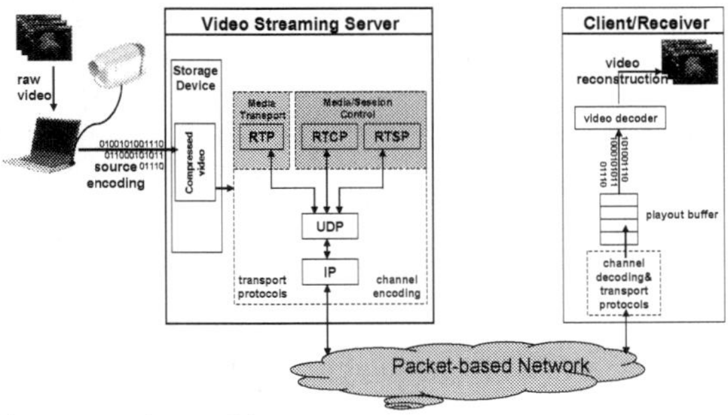

Fig. 1. A typical video streaming architecture.

2.2 Protocols

Unique requirements associated with video streaming impose strict time-delay constraints on video transmission. Video streaming protocols can be classified as follows: *session control* protocols, *transport* protocols and *network* protocols.

Session control protocols such as the Real Time Streaming Protocol (RTSP) (Schulzrinne et al., 1998), or alternative Session Initiation Protocol (SIP) (Hanfley et al., 1999) are responsible for session initialization between client and server.

Transport protocols are further distinguished in upper and lower layer, Real-Time Transport Protocol (RTP), and UDP/TCP respectively. Transmission control protocol (TCP) (Postel, 1981) uses retransmission and traffic monitoring to secure packet delivery to destination. This property constituted TCP highly efficient for HTTP (Fielding, 1999) applications. However, when streaming video, retransmission time may result in alternations of temporal relations between audio and video and is in most cases unacceptable. Given the fact that a limited number of packet losses are tolerable in video streaming and error resilience techniques are employed both at encoder and decoder, TCP's no loss tolerance simply introduces additional jitter and skew. The user datagram protocol (UDP) (Postel, 1980) on the other hand, does not provide any error handling or congestion control mechanisms, allowing therefore packets to drop out. Given the aforementioned, UDP is primarily established as the lower layer transport protocol.

The design of a new internet protocol that would enhance the existing protocols while being suitable for real time data delivery was more than essential. RTP (Schulzrinne, 1996) provides end-to-end delivery services for data with real time characteristics such as interactive video and audio. Despite being able to provide real time data delivery, RTP itself does not contain any mechanisms to ensure on time delivery. In the contrary it relies on UDP, TCP for doing so. It does provide however the appropriate functionality for carrying real time content such as time-stamping and control mechanisms that enable synchronization of different streams with timing properties. RTP payload contains the real time data being transferred while the RTP header contains information characterizing the payload such as timestamp, sequence number, source, size and encoding scheme. RTP distinguishes data delivery and control mechanisms and consists of basically two parts: the RTP part which carries the real time data and the Real Time Control Protocol (RTCP) part which is responsible for Quality of Service (QoS) monitoring and extracting information regarding the participants in an RTP session. This information can be later used to improve QoS as it can be supplied as feedback for the encoder to adapt to varying network conditions. As we have already mentioned, RTP packets are usually transferred over UDP.

The resulting packets are encapsulated using the internet protocol (IP), responsible for delivering a packet from source to destination through the network, hence RTP/UDP/IP headers.

3. H.264/AVC and related Error Resilience techniques

H.264/AVC is the current state of the art video coding standard (ITU-T Rec. H.264 | ISO/IEC 14496-10 AVC), and was jointly developed by the ISO/IEC MPEG and ITU-T VCEG experts, who formed the Joint Video Team (JVT). H.264 met the growing demand of multimedia and video services by providing enhanced compression efficiency significantly outperforming all prior standards (MPEG-1, 2 and 4, and H.262x). All features used together in a fashionably manner can provide for bitrate reductions of up to 50% for equivalent perceptual quality compared to its predecessors (Wiegand et al., 2003). Its design enables transportation over heterogeneous networks to be carried out in a friendly-manner. To attain the abovementioned, H.264 defines a video coding layer (VCL) and a network adaptation layer (NAL). VCL, as its name suggests, is responsible for video coding and is a unit already known from prior standards, maintaining its block-oriented coding functionality. Its enrichment and refinement resulted in the provided compression efficiency. On the other hand, NAL is novel concept aiming at a network-friendly adaptation of VCL content to candidate heterogeneous networks (or storage devices). NAL functionality is a substantial improvement constituting H.264 coding and transmission network-independent. As always, the scope of the standard is centered on the decoder. That is, only the decoder is standardized, allowing great flexibility to the encoder. H.264 offers a plethora of error resilience techniques with a wide range of applications. A thorough overview of the standard, error resilience features and discussion exploiting H.264 in the context of IP based networks can be found in (Wiegand et al., 2003; Wenger, 2003).

3.1 Encoding Modes and Frame types

Frame encoding modes can have a significant impact on both error propagation and video compression performance. We provide a summary of the different modes:

- Intra-mode: Intra-mode is the procedure where intra-prediction is used for coding a video frame (I-frame). That is, all the information used for coding, originates from the picture itself where block samples are predicted using spatially neighboring samples of previously coded blocks.
- Inter-mode: Inter-mode is the procedure where inter-prediction is used for coding a video frame.
  - P-mode: P-mode uses prediction from previously decoded frames. In inter-mode, the encoder's side provides all the necessary information for accurate motion estimation of the spatial displacement between the decoder's reference picture and the current picture in the sequence at the encoder. This procedure is described as motion compensation.
  - B-mode: Whereas in P-mode at most one motion compensated signal is employed, B-mode provides the ability to make use of two motion compensated signals for the prediction of a picture. B-mode is also referred to as bi-prediction as not only it allows the utilization of previously decoded pictures but also the utilization of forthcoming ones.

The extensive use of predictive coding (P-frames, B-frames) or not (I-frames), is application specific. Depending on time and quality constraints imposed, one mode may be preferred over the other and the other way round. Recent video coding standards have largely adopted predictive coding and it is considered one of the key components in the video streaming success. Intra coding on the other hand is mostly employed as en error resilience feature for periodic updates (i.e. inserting an I-frame every Group of Picture-GOP). The predictive coding question which arises next is the relationship (ratio) between P-frames and B-frames used, and is a matter of investigation in this particular study. P-frames employ unidirectional prediction as mentioned above whereas B-frames use bidirectional. For P-frames this is translated into less motion estimation time with more bits per picture. The opposite stands for B-frames where the prediction from both previous and forward frames results in greater motion estimation time during encoding but less bits per picture for transmission.

3.2 Flexible Macroblock Ordering

An innovative error resilient feature introduced by H.264/AVC is flexible macroblock ordering (Wenger, 2002; Wenger & Horowitz, 2002). FMO is essentially a slice structuring approach, where a frame is partitioned into independently transmitted and decoded slices. Each frame may be partitioned in up to eight different slices and a frame may still be decoded even if not all slices are present at the decoder. In this manner and in conjunction with proper utilization of the spatial relationships between error free slices and macroblocks (MBs) therein, concealment of errors becomes much more efficient. Seven different types of FMO are defined (i.e. patterns for MB to slice allocation). A macroblock allocation map (MBAmap) is used to keep track of macroblocks assigned to slices.

Figure 2 depicts FMO utilization of FMO type 1 (Figure 2a)) and FMO type 2 (Figure 2b)). FMO type 1 aims to evenly distribute errors throughout a frame in such a way that for every lost slice, the neighboring MBs of the lost slice's MBs residing in a different slice may be used for concealment, providing for a very efficient error recovery design. FMO type 2 is designed for defining rectangular slices as foreground(s) and leftover. A well suited scheme for region of interest coding and transmission. Slices may overlap but a MB may only belong to one slice, the first it was assigned. In the event that a packet carrying a whole slice is dropped, H.264/AVC allows the transmission of redundant slices (RS) (a redundant slice being a slice describing the same MBs in a bitstream). RS can be coded in a different manner with respect to the primary slices (i.e. different coding parameters) and are utilized in the absence of a clear primary slice. A thorough overview of FMO, performance evaluation and overhead analysis, can be found in (Wenger, 2003; Lambert et al., 2006).

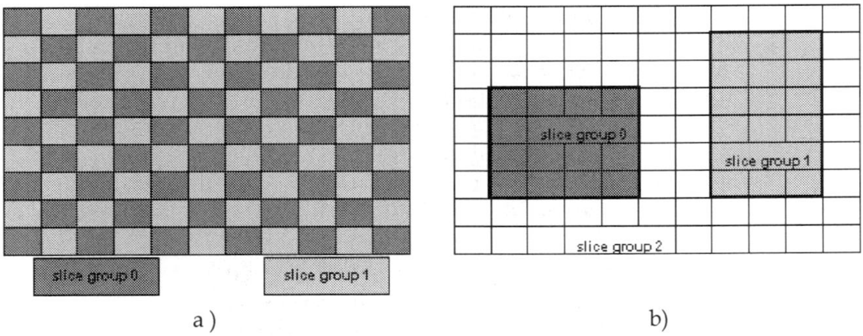

Fig. 2. Flexible Macroblock Ordering. a) Scattered Slices and b) Foreground(s) (ROIs) and leftover.

4. Methodology

4.1 Material and Video Acquisition

Cardiovascular disease accounts for about half of the deaths in the western world, with stroke being the third leading cause of death and disability worldwide. The predictive ability to identify which patients will have a stroke is poor, where the current practice of assessing the risk of stroke relies on measuring the thickness of the intima media (Intima-Media-Thickness, IMT) of the carotid artery wall or the artery lumen stenosis by identifying the plaque borders in the carotid artery. However, the IMT and the degree of stenosis do not provide adequate information of an individual stroke risk, and treatment of asymptomatic patients remains controversial. Thus the need exists for the development of new tools and techniques for the assessment of the risk of stroke.

Video analysis of the common carotid artery (CCA) can be used to analyze plaque motion patterns. Plaque motion analysis patterns can then be used to differentiate between asymptomatic and symptomatic atherosclerotic plaques. Diagnostically, the clinicians rely on visual evaluation of the CCA video motion to differentiate between asymptomatic and symptomatic plaques.

Ultrasound is widely used in vascular imaging because of its ability to visualize body tissue and vessels in a non invasive and harmless way and to visualize in real time the arterial lumen and wall, something that is not possible with any other imaging technique. B-mode ultrasound imaging can be used in order to visualize arteries longitudinally from the same subject in order to monitor the development of atherosclerosis.

CCA videos from B-mode longitudinal ultrasound segments were digitally recorded by the Philips ATL HDI-5000 ultrasound scanner (Advanced Technology Laboratories, Seattle, USA) with 256 gray levels, 768x576 resolution, having frame rate of 100 frames per second. For detailed technical characteristics of the ultrasound scanner (multi element ultrasound scan head, operating frequency, acoustic aperture, and transmission focal range), we refer to (Loizou et al., 2007).

4.2 Segmentation Procedure

For the purposes of this study, we use snake segmentation of the plaque region and use it to define a region of interest over the video (see section 4.3.2, Fig. 4). We begin with the basic definitions.

We delineate a segmentation region using a snake contour. A snake contour is represented parametrically by $v(s)=[x(s),y(s)]$, where $(x,y)\in\Re^2$ denotes the spatial coordinates of an image, and $s\in[0,1]$. The snake adapts itself by a dynamic process that minimizes an energy function defined as in (Williams & Shah, 1992):

$$E_{snake}(v(s))=E_{\text{int}}(v(s))+E_{image}(v(s))+E_{external}(v(s))=\int_s(\alpha(s)E_{cont}+\beta(s)E_{curv}+\gamma(s)E_{image}+E_{external})ds. \quad (1)$$

At each iteration step, the energy function in (1), is evaluated for the current point in $v(s)$, and for the points in an mxn neighborhood along the *arc* length s, of the contour. Subsequently the point on $v(s)$ is moved to the new position in the neighborhood that gives the minimum energy. The term $E_{\text{int}}(v)$ in (1) denotes the internal energy derived from the physical characteristics of the snake and is given by the continuity $E_{cont}(v)$, and the curvature term $E_{curv}(v)$. This term controls the natural behaviour of the snake. The internal energy contains a first-order derivative controlled by $\alpha(s)$, which discourages stretching and makes the model behave like an elastic string by introducing tension and a second order term controlled by $\beta(s)$, which discourages bending and makes the model behave like a rigid rod by producing stiffness. The weighting parameters $\alpha(s)$ and $\beta(s)$ can be used to control the strength of the model's tension and stiffness, respectively. Altering the parameters α, β, and γ, affect the convergence of the snake. The second term in (1) E_{image}, represents the image energy due to some relevant features such as the gradient of edges, lines, regions and texture (Williams & Shah, 1992). It attracts the snake to low-level features such as brightness and edge data. Finally the term $E_{external}$, is the external energy of the snake, which is defined by the user and is optional. In our study we used a modification of the greedy algorithm as presented in (Williams & Shah, 1992).

Figure 3 a) shows the first frame from an ultrasound video of the CCA, whereas Fig. 3b) shows the first frame of the blood flow video. After cross-correlating the first frame of the video with the first frame of the blood flow, the initial blood flow contour for the first video frame is extracted (see Fig, 3c)). The user then selects an area of interest defining a contour segment, which will be used as an initial contour for the snake. The snake then deforms and converges as shown in Fig. 3d). Figure 3e) shows the manual segmentation results made by an expert radiologist. Additionally, in order to help the snake to converge better the lsmv (local statistics filter based on mean and variance of the local neighborhood) despeckle filter (Loizou et al., 2005) was applied on the original video frame in Fig. 3a.

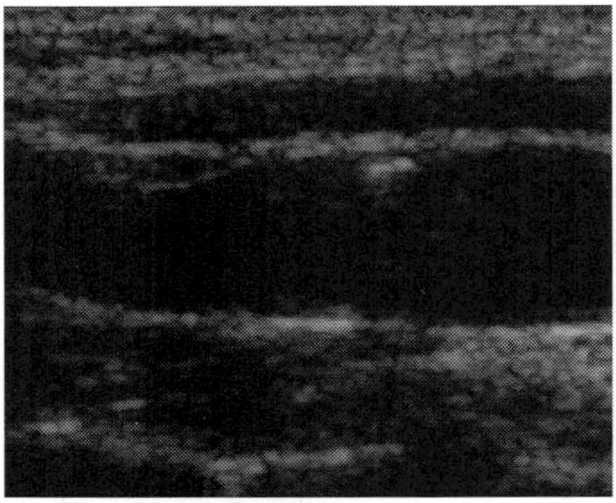

(a) Original B-mode image.

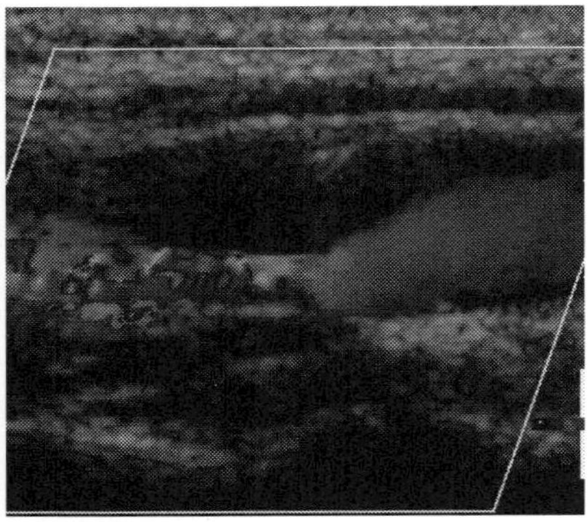

(b) Blood flow image.

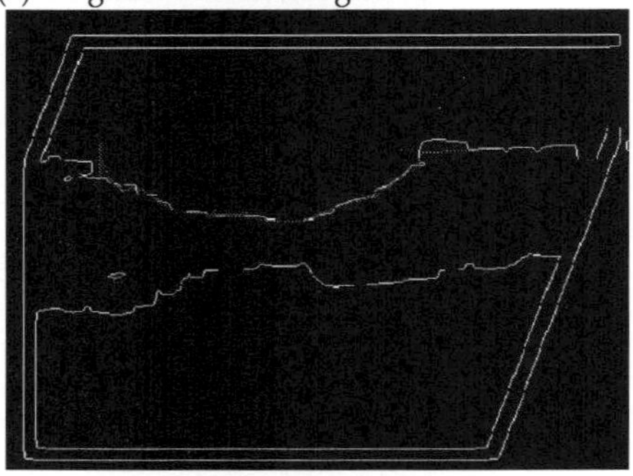

(c) Initial blood flow edge contour.

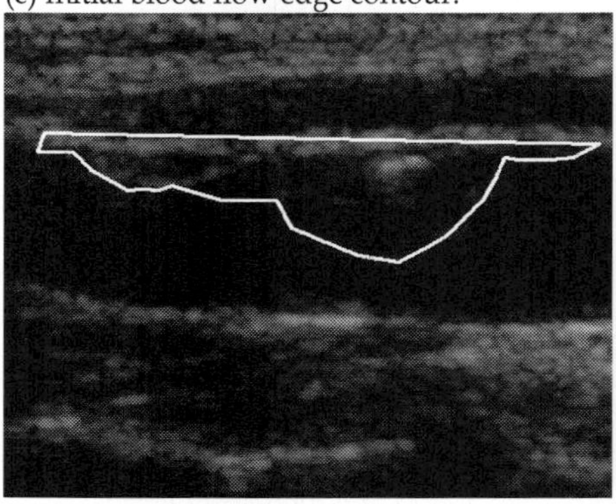

(d) Williams & Shah snakes segmentation results.

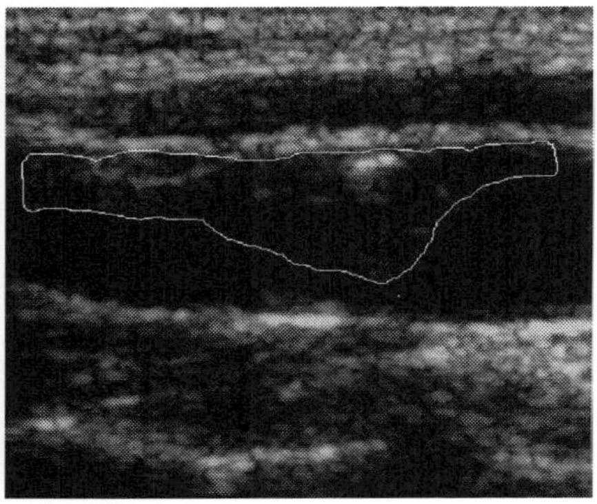

(e) Manual segmentation results.

Fig. 3. Plaque initialization using the blood flow image: (a) Original ultrasound B-mode image (first video frame) of a carotid artery with plaque at the far wall, (b) first frame of the blood flow video in a), (c) initial blood flow edge contour with the area for the initial contour selected by the user, (d) Williams & Shah snakes segmentation of plaque, and (e) manual segmentation of plaque.

The automated snakes segmentation system used for the segmentation of the CCA plaque in each video frame, was proposed and evaluated on ultrasound images of the CCA in (Loizou et al., 2007), and is based on the Williams & Shah snake as described above. Initially the plaque on the first video frame was segmented and then the segmentation of the first frame was used as an initialization for the next frame. This procedure was repeated until all video frames were segmented. The snake contour iterations in each frame varied from 10 to 22.

4.3 Encoding/ Decoding Procedure

4.3.1 Frame Encoding

Using the JM 15.1 Reference Software (http://iphome.hhi.de/suehring/tml/), we evaluated three different encoding schemes, namely IPPP, IBPBP and IBBPBBP. A series of four videos encoded at QCIF and CIF resolutions were used. The default JM rate control algorithm was applied to explore the trade-off between video quality and bitrate, performing frame level adaptation. Besides the target bitrate, initial quantization parameter (QP) is another fundamental parameter which impacts on rate control algorithms performance. The first frame is encoded using the provided QP and given the remaining frames and available bitrate, QPs of following frames are adjusted accordingly to try to match the target bitrate. The initial QP was selected according to the following formula (Li et al., 2003):

$$QP = \begin{cases} 40 & bpp \le 0.15 \\ 30 & 0.15 < bpp \le 0.45 \\ 20 & 0.45 < bpp \le 0.9 \\ 10 & bpp > 0.9 \end{cases} \tag{2}$$

where

$$bpp = \frac{R}{f \times N_{pixels}}. \tag{3}$$

Here, *bpp* denotes the target bits per pixel, *Npixels* is the number of pixels in the N-th frame, *R* is the target bitrate and *f* the frame rate of the encoded video sequence. Initial quantization parameters for QCIF and CIF resolutions are summarized in Table 1.

To evaluate the performance of the aforementioned encoding schemes in error prone wireless environments, the pseudo-random RTP packet loss simulator included in JM was modified to provide better random simulation performance by adding an implementation of the random number generator described in (Park & Miller, 1998). The simulator was also enhanced with a number of loss distributions. The uniform distribution was used throughout the experiments and all results were obtained by averaging 10 consecutive runs. The main encoding parameters are summarized in Table 2. Intra MB line update allows a fully intra coded frame every 11 and 18 frames for QCIF and CIF resolutions respectively. Simple frame copy error concealment method is applied at the decoder to reconstruct corrupted packets. Here, the use of this simple error-concealment scheme is allowed due to the fact that stenosis characteristics are only slightly affected by frame copying.

QCIF	Initial QP	CIF	Initial QP
32000	40	96000	40
64000	40	256000	40
128000	30	512000	30
256000	30	800000	30
400000	20	1200000	20
512000	20	1500000	20

Table 1. Target BitRate and Initial Quantization Parameters.

Parameters	Value	Parameters	Value
Profile	Main	MbLineIntraUpdate	1
FramesToBeEncoded	100	NumberBFrames	0/1/2
FrameRate	25	SymbolMode	CABAC
IntraPeriod	0	OutFileMode	RTP
SearchRange	32	RateControlEnable	1
NumberOfReferenceFrames	5	BasicUnit	99/396

Table 2. Encoding Parameters.

4.3.2 Variable QP Encoding

A modified version of the JM 15.1 Reference Software was used to support FMO type 2 variable quality slice encoding. FMO type 2 was selected amongst other FMO types since it's specifically designed for defining foreground(s) (ROIs) with leftover. By defining upper left and lower right corner points (on a MacroBlock basis) we select the rectangular diagnostic ROIs as illustrated in Figure 4. These bounds are defined at the beginning of each encoded sequence and are directly derived from the segmentation procedure. Taking plaque movement into account we select a slightly broader area as ROI, thus avoiding redefinition of the rectangular area further in the sequence (incorporating additional bits for picture parameter sets). Following a similar concept with MB Allocation Map (MBAmap), where each macroblock is allocated a slice id according to the slice group it belongs to, we define a QP Allocation Map (QPAmap), which stores the QP of each macroblock (see Figure 4). The QP of each ROI slice is parsed via the same configuration file used to define the boundaries of the rectangular ROIs. Each slice's QP is carried within its slice header during transmission, hence no additional bits are transmitted through picture or sequence parameter sets and the resulting bitstream is H.264/AVC compliant. Employing these minor adjustments achieves variable quality FMO slice encoding.

A series of four videos encoded at QCIF and CIF resolutions for QPs listed in Table 3 were used to evaluate our proposed approach. The videos were encoded using:

1) Constant QP throughout the sequence, which is the default encoding scheme. Here, we are interested in showing that despite achieving the best overall quality video, the required bitrate is a preventing factor, while at the same time not achieving the best diagnostic performance in the presence of errors.

2) FMO type 2 with variable QP according to the ROIs diagnostic importance (following a low to medium, medium and medium to high QP allocation pattern for non-important regions, IMT (and ECG when available) and atherosclerotic plaque slices respectively, see Table 3). The QP of the constant QP encoding and slice 0 (describing the plaque) are equal so as to be able to deduct conclusions regarding diagnostic quality. Our aim is to depict that the best diagnostic performance is attained at a significantly reduced bitrate.
3) Rate control encoding with target bit rate being the output bitrate of 2). In this manner we are able to compare the diagnostic performance of the latter two schemes for the same bitrate.

Packet loss simulation and decoding procedure are similar to the ones described in section 4.3.1. Encoding parameters are summarized in Table 4.

Constant QP Encoding	Variable QP FMO slice 3/ 2(1)/ 0	Rate Control
32	48/40/32	Target Bit Rate is the output Bit Rate of Variable QP FMO
28	44/36/28	
24	40/32/24	
20	36/28/20	
16	32/24/16	

Table 3. Quantization Parameters and Target BitRate.

Parameters	Value	Parameters	Value
Profile	Baseline	MbLineIntraUpdate	0/1*
FramesToBeEncoded	100	NumberBFrames	0
FrameRate	25	SymbolMode	UVLC
IntraPeriod	16/0*	OutFileMode	RTP
SearchRange	32	RateControlEnable	0/1*
NumberOfReferenceFrames	1	BasicUnit	99/396

Table 4. Encoding Parameters.

*IntraPeriod is enabled for Constant QP and Variable QP FMO encodings and disabled for RateControl encoding. The opposite stands for MbLineIntraUpdate and RateControlEnable.

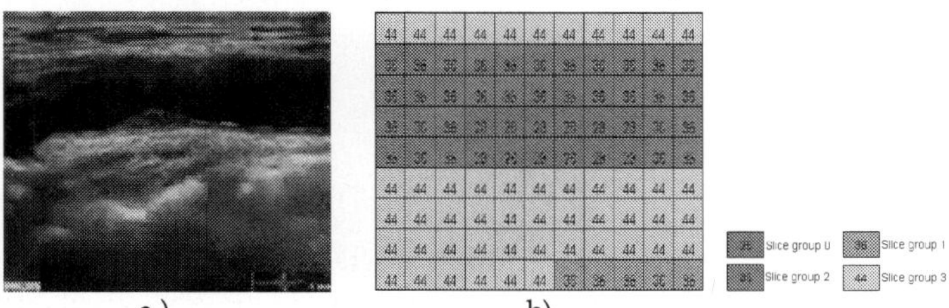

a) b)

Fig. 4. a) Frame 1 of compressed QCIF carotid ultrasound video using variable QP FMO. b) The corresponding Quantization Parameter Allocation map (QPAmap). Slice groups: 0: atherosclerotic plaque, 1: ECG, 2: Upper and lower intima media complex, including the lumen diameter, 3: other components.

5. Experimental Results

5.1 Frame Encoding

5.1.1 Technical Evaluation

Figure 5 depicts the trade-off between quality and bit rate for one of the investigated videos in QCIF and CIF resolutions. Naturally, the more bits that are allocated for source encoding using rate control, the higher PSNR quality is attained. IBPBP and IBBPBBP coding structures behave similarly, while IPPP coding structure achieves slightly lower PSNR values. Typically, bidirectional prediction requires fewer bits during encoding than single-directional prediction for the same quantization parameters, however, since we are using rate control, this is translated into increased quality. On the other hand, single-directional prediction is marginally quicker in terms of encoding time due to the increased motion estimation time required for bidirectional encoding.

Figures 6 and 7 demonstrate the performance of the three tested encoding schemes under losses of 2%, 5%, 8% and 10% of transmitted RTP packets for the same video, for QCIF and CIF resolutions respectively. For QCIF resolution, IBBPBBP achieves better PSNR output than IBPBP and IPPP, especially up to 5% loss rate. For 8% and 10%, IPPP coding structure attains higher PSNR ratings in some cases. For CIF resolution, bidirectional prediction (IBPBP and IBBPBBP) achieves slightly better results up to 5% loss rates, but then it is outperformed by single-directional (although for 8% loss rate, ratings are comparable with IBBPBBP). In general, in low-noise environments bidirectional prediction gives the best performance. However, as the noise level increases, the use of single-directional prediction provides for better error recovery and better results.

Another important aspect which was observed by examining the results obtained by averaging 10 consecutive runs for each scheme is that quality is directly affected by the loss ratio of P to B frames. High ratio (more P-frames dropped) is translated into poor quality, whereas low ratio (more B-frames dropped) results into better quality.

5.1.2 Clinical Evaluation

The tested coding structures' performance was also evaluated by a medical expert so as to provide the level of diagnostic quality. The videos were played back on a Laptop at their original pixel size dimensions.

The evaluation recorded that videos achieving PSNR ratings higher than 30.5 db may be suitable for providing diagnosis. That is, there is sufficient information in the ultrasound video that enables the medical expert to make a confident diagnosis regarding the presence of an atherosclerotic plaque and the degree of stenosis. This information was also available to videos attaining lower PSNR ratings in some cases. This was made possible when the medical expert freezed a relatively clean frame to use for diagnosis. Moreover, for bitrates of 128kbps for QCIF resolution and 512kbps for CIF resolution, the medical expert could almost identify as much diagnostic information in the compressed video as in the original video sequence. It is worth noting here that for the abovementioned bitrates, the initial QP switches from 40 to 30 (according to (2) and (3)) for the target bitrates chosen for this series of experiments.

We also observed motion delays when using bidirectional prediction (more obvious on IBBPBBP, in the presence of heavy loss rates). However, diagnostic quality is not affected by this observation. The medical expert was emphatic that the carotid ultrasound videos used in this particular study were very clear cases.

5.2 Variable QP Encoding

5.2.1 Technical Evaluation

Diagnostic quality for carotid ultrasound video evaluation can be defined as the PSNR over the (atherosclerotic) plaque, being the primary focus point of the clinical evaluation. In Figures 8 and 9 we provide rate-distortion curves of both entire video (Figures 8a) and 9a)) and atherosclerotic plaque (region of diagnostic importance, Figures 8b) and 9b)) and the impact that can have on bitrate.

As expected, the incorporated R-D curves differentiate only with respect to variable QP FMO encoding, as the latter is the only scheme to employ variable QP encoding. In Figures 8a) and 9a) constant QP encoding achieves the best overall performance with rate control encoding following, since both schemes employ equal QP throughout a frame. When it comes to diagnostic performance however (Figures 8b) and 9b)), variable QP FMO attains similar PSNR ratings with constant QP, the key observation being the drastically lower sequence bitrate it involves. Compared to rate control incorporating the same bitrate, variable QP FMO achieves higher PSNR ratings.

Figure 10 demonstrates the performance of the three tested encoding schemes when extracting the atherosclerotic plaque (diagnostic ROI) of the decoded video under losses of 5% of transmitted RTP packets. We have significant bandwidth requirement reductions without sacrificing diagnostic quality. Furthermore, FMO provides increased error resilience by coding diagnostically relevant regions independent of the rest. Figures 8-10 show the results of QCIF and CIF resolution video with ECG lead while Table 5 records indicative db gain and bitrate reductions for a video with no ECG lead. Results are video specific but the trend is the same for all investigated videos.

5.2.2 Clinical Evaluation

The evaluation recorded that all CIF resolution variable QP FMO encoding videos were well within the desired diagnostic range. The medical expert could identify the presence of a plaque (stenosis), come to conclusions regarding the degree of stenosis and quality of the plaque, and classify the plaque as echogenic or echolucent. Naturally, as the quality rose, diagnosis became easier and more precise. As the medical expert designated, all video qualities qualified for urgent clinical practice. Some distortion in ECG for 48/40/32 QPs (40 being the QP of the ECG) was observed, not present for lower QPs or affecting diagnostic quality.

Similar conclusions were drawn for constant QP encoding. Rate control encoding also performed quite well, however, for videos attaining PSNR ratings higher than 30.5db, corresponding to output bitrate of quantization parameters 40/32/24 of variable QP FMO and lower.

For QCIF resolution, the medical expert underlined that plaque classification could not be derived for all videos, irrespective of video quality, rather its dimensions. This of course is video specific but for the same video in CIF resolution classification could be obtained. Furthermore, in some cases, and under loss rates of 5%, 48/40/32 variable QP FMO corresponding to PSNR slightly lower than 31db, required extra attention to reach diagnosis. Again, all video qualities qualified for urgent clinical practice, however QPs of 44/36/28 is recommended. The same allegations stand for constant QP encoding, whereas for rate control, similar to CIF resolution, videos attaining PSNR higher than 30.5 db.

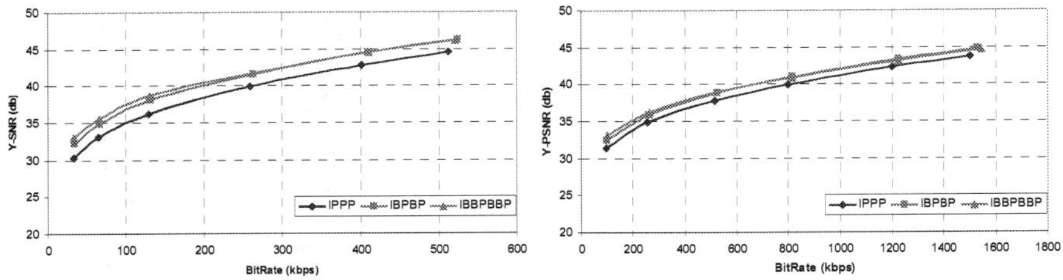

a) b)

Fig. 5. Rate-distortion curves for tested frame encoding schemes. a) QCIF and b) CIF.

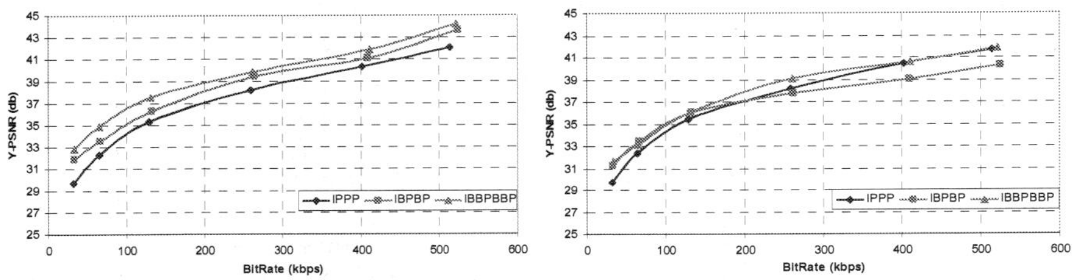

a) b)

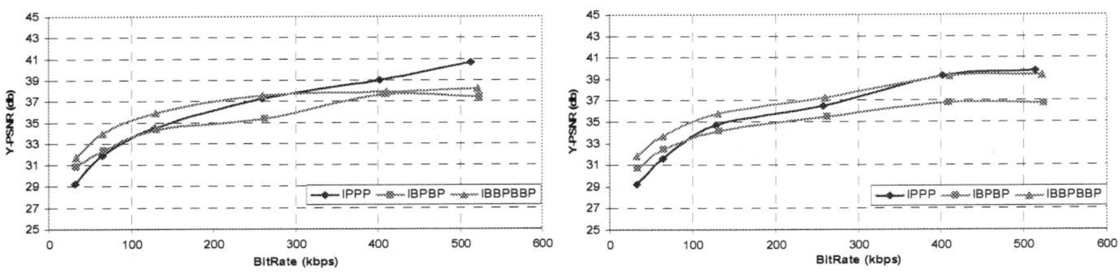

c) d)

Fig. 6. Rate-distortion curves for tested frame encoding schemes, QCIF resolution. a) 2%, b) 5%, c) 8% and d) 10% loss rates. IBBPBBP encoding scheme attains higher PSNR ratings in most cases, especially in low-noise (up to 5%) scenarios.

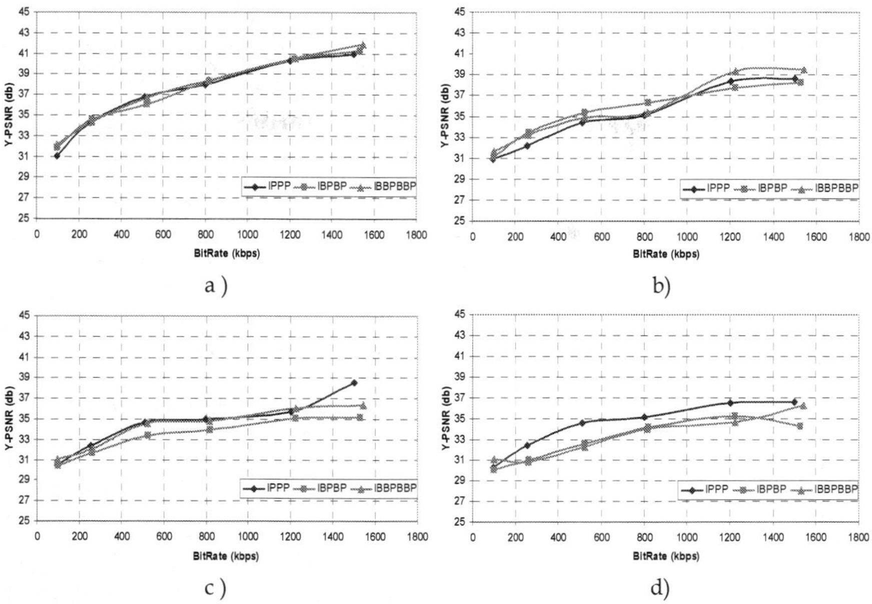

Fig. 7. Rate-distortion curves for tested frame encoding schemes, CIF resolution. a) 2%, b) 5%, c) 8% and d) 10% loss rates. Bi-directional prediction (IBPBP and IBBPBBP) achieves better results up to 5% loss rates (low-noise), whereas as the noise level increases, single - directional (IPPP) provides for better error recovery.

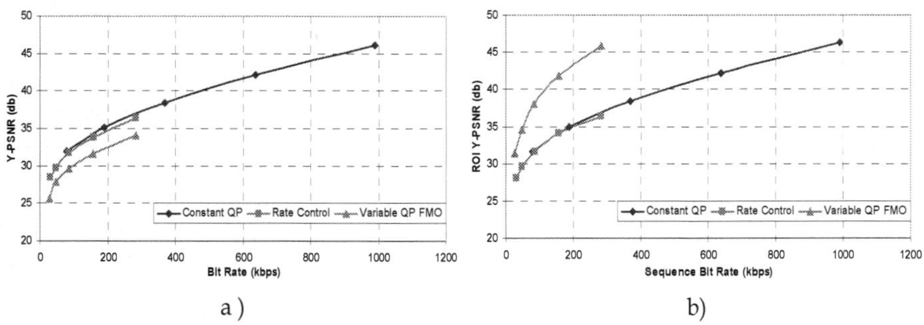

Fig. 8. Rate-distortion curves for a) entire video, QCIF resolution with ECG lead and b) atherosclerotic plaque extracted from QCIF resolution video with ECG lead (diagnostic ROI). Observe that Variable QP FMO encoding attains inferior quality for the whole video, when it comes to diagnostic quality however it outperforms rate control encoding, while it achieves similar PSNR ratings with constant QP encoding, the key observation being the drastically lower bitrate it involves.

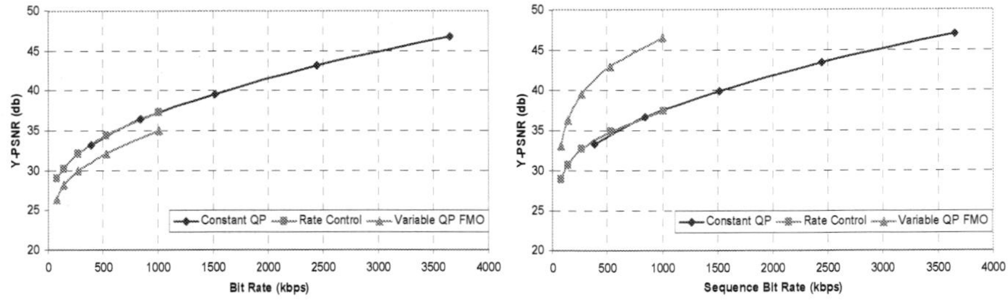

a) b)

Fig. 9. Rate-distortion curves for a) entire video, CIF resolution video with ECG lead and b) atherosclerotic plaque extracted from CIF resolution video with ECG lead (diagnostic ROI). Observe that Variable QP FMO encoding attains inferior quality for the whole video, when it comes to diagnostic quality however it outperforms rate control encoding, while it achieves similar PSNR ratings with constant QP encoding, the key observation being the drastically lower bitrate it involves.

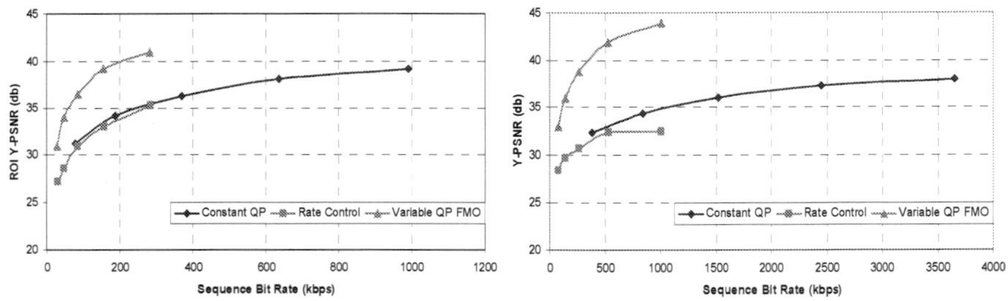

a) b)

Fig. 10. Rate-distortion curves for a) atherosclerotic plaque extracted from QCIF resolution video with ECG lead, 5% loss rate and b) atherosclerotic plaque extracted from CIF resolution video with ECG lead, 5% loss rate. Variable QP FMO encoding attains the best diagnostic performance. Better error recovery compared to constant QP encoding is due to the fact that FMO employs slice encoding. Bandwidth requirements reductions as to Figures 8-9.

Constant QP		Rate Control		Variable QP FMO		Constant QP vs Variable QP FMO		Rate Control vs Variable QP FMO	
PSNR	Seq. BitRate	PSNR	Seq. BitRate	PSNR	Seq. BitRate	Db Gain	BitRate Reduction	Db Gain	BitRate Reduction
33.08	235	29.19	82	33.19	82	0.11	153	4	Negligible
34.88	508	30.69	157	36.06	156	1.18	352	5.37	
36.51	960	33.01	302	38.65	301	2.14	659	5.64	
37.47	1642	33.67	562	40.77	561	3.30	1081	7.10	
38.04	2554	35.6	960	42.56	959	4.52	1595	6.96	

Table 5. Atherosclerotic plaque extracted from CIF resolution video, no ECG lead - 5% Loss Rate.

6. Conclusion and Future Work

M-Health systems and services facilitated a revolution in remote diagnosis and care. Driven by advances in networking, video compression and computer technologies, wide deployment of such systems and services is expected in the near future. Before such a scenario becomes a reality however, there are a number of issues that have to be addressed. Video streaming of medical video over error prone wireless channels is one critical issue that needs to be addressed. Remote diagnosis is very sensitive to the amount of clinical data recovered, hence the effort should be directed towards the provision of robust medical video at a required bitrate for the medical expert to provide a confident and accurate diagnosis.

H.264/AVC encompasses powerful video coding and error resilience tools, exploitation of which can significantly improve video quality. We present an evaluation of different frame types and encoding modes of H.264/AVC and how they relate to diagnostic performance. In addition, an efficient, diagnostically relevant approach is proposed for encoding and transmission of medical ultrasound video of the carotid artery. Driven by its diagnostic use, ultrasound video is segmented and encoded using flexible macroblock ordering (FMO). FMO type 2 concept is extended to support variable quality slice encoding. Diagnostic region(s) of interest are encoded in high quality whereas the remaining, non-diagnostic region, is heavily compressed. Both technical and clinical evaluation show that enhanced diagnostic performance is attained in the presence of errors while at the same time achieving significant bandwidth requirements reductions.

Future work includes the insertion of redundant slices (RS) describing diagnostically important region(s) in the resulting bitstream, maximizing medical video's error resilience under severe packet losses (Panayides et al., 2009). We will also explore the application of these technologies to other medical video modalities.

7. Acknowledgement

This work was funded via the project *Real-Time Wireless Transmission of Medical Ultrasound Video* of the Research and Technological Development 2008-2010, of the Research Promotion Foundation of Cyprus.

8. References

Doukas, C. & Maglogiannis, I. (2008). Adaptive Transmission of Medical Image and Video Using Scalable Coding and Context-Aware Wireless Medical Networks, *EURASIP Journal on Wireless Communications and Networking*, Vol. 2008, Article ID 428397, 12 pages. doi:10.1155/2008/428397.

Fielding, R.; Gettys, J.; Mogul, J.; Frystyk, H.; Masinter, L.; Leach, P. & Berners-Lee, T. (1999). Hypertext Transfer Protocol-HTTP/1.1., Internet Engineering Task Force, RFC 2616, 1999.

H.264/AVC JM 15.1 Reference Software, Available: http://iphome.hhi.de/suehring/tml/.

Handley, M.; Schulzrinne, H.; Schooler, E. & Rosenberg, J. (1999). SIP: Session Initiation Protocol, Internet Engineering Task Force, RFC 2543, Mar. 1999.

Hennerici, M. & Neuerburg-Heusler, D. (1998). *Vascular Diagnosis With Ultrasound*, Thieme, 0865776032, 9780865776036, Stutgart - New York.

Istepanian, R.H.; Laxminarayan, S. & Pattichis, C.S. (2006). *M-Health: Emerging Mobile Health Systems*, Springer, 0387265589, 9780387265582, New York.

Joint Video Team of ITU-T and ISO/IEC JTC 1. (2003). Draft ITU-T Recommendation and Final Draft International Standard of Joint Video Specification (ITU-T Rec. H.264 | ISO/IEC 14496-10 AVC), Joint Video Team (JVT) of ISO/IEC MPEG and ITU-T VCEG, JVTG050, Mar. 2003.

Kyriacou, E.; Pattichis, M.S.; Pattichis, C.S.; Panayides, A. & Pitsillides, A. (2007). M-Health e-Emergency Systems: Current Status and Future Directions [Wireless corner], *Antennas and Propagation Magazine, IEEE* , Vol. 49, No. 1, Feb. 2007, pp. 216-231, 1045-9243.

Lambert, P.; De Neve, W.; Dhondt, Y. & Van De Walle, R. (2006). Flexible macroblock ordering in H.264/AVC, *Journal of Visual Communication and Image Representation*, Vol. 17, No. 2, Apr. 2006, pp. 358-375, 10473203.

Li, Z.G.; Pan, F.; Lim, K.P.; Feng, G.N.; Lin X. & Rahardaj, S. (2003). Adaptive basic unit layer rate control for JVT, JVT-G012, 7th meeting, *Pattaya II, Thailand*, 7-14, Mar. 2003.

Loizou, C.P.; Pattichis, C.S.; Christodoulou, C.I.; Istepanian, R.S.H.; Pantziaris, M. & Nicolaides, A. (2005). Comparative evaluation of despeckle filtering in ultrasound imaging of the carotid artery, *IEEE Transactions on Ultrasonics Ferroelectrics and Frequency Control*, Vol. 52, No. 10, Oct. 2005, pp. 1653-1669, 0885-3010.

Loizou, C.P.; Pattichis, C.S.; Pantziaris, M. & Nicolaides, A. (2007). An integrated system for the segmentation of atherosclerotic carotid plaque, *IEEE Transactions on Information Technology in Biomedicine*, Vol. 11, No. 5, Nov. 2007, pp. 661-667, 1089-7771.

Loizou, C.P. & Pattichis C.S. (2008). Despeckle filtering algorithms and Software for Ultrasound Imaging, *Synthesis Lectures on Algorithms and Software for Engineering*, Ed. Morgan & Claypool Publishers, 13: 9781598296204, USA.

Panayides, A.; Pattichis, M. S. & Pattichis, C. S. (2008). Wireless Medical Ultrasound Video Transmission Through Noisy Channels, *Proceedings of the 30th Annual International Conference of the IEEE Engineering in Medicine and Biology Society (EMBC'08)*, pp. 5326-5329, 1557-170X, Aug. 2008, Vancouver, Canada.

Panayides, A.; Pattichis, M. S.; Pattichis, C. S.; Loizou, C. P.; Pantziaris, M. and Pitsillides, A. (2009). Robust and Efficient Ultrasound Video Coding in Noisy Channels Using H.264, to be published in *Proceedings of the 31st Annual International Conference of the IEEE Engineering in Medicine and Biology Society (EMBC'09)*, Sep. 2009, Minnesota, U.S.A.

Park S. & Miller, K. (1998). Random Number Generators: Good Ones Are Hard To Find, *Communications of the ACM*, Vol. 31, No. 10, Oct. 1988, pp. 1192 - 1201,0001-0782.

Postel, J. (1980). User Datagram Protocol, Internet Engineering Task Force, RFC 768, 1980.

Postel, J. (1981). Transmission Control Protocol, Internet Engineering Task Force, RFC 793, 1981.

Rao, S. & Jayant, N. (2005). Towards high quality region-of-interest medical video over wireless networks using lossless coding and motion compensated temporal filtering, *Proceedings of the fifth IEEE International Symposium on Signal Processing and Information Technology (ISSPIT'05)*, pp. 618-623, 0-7803-9313-9, Dec. 2005, Athens, Greece.

Schulzrinne, H.; Casner, S.; Frederick, R. & Jacobson, V. (1996). RTP: A Transport Protocol for Real-Time Applications, Internet Engineering Task Force, RFC 1889, Jan. 1996.

Schulzrinne, H.; Rao, A. & Lanphier, R. (1998). Real-Time Session Protocol (RTSP), Internet Engineering Task Force, RFC 2326, Apr. 1998.

Tsapatsoulis N.; Loizou, C. & Pattichis, C. (2007). Region of Interest Video Coding for Low bit-rate Transmission of Carotid Ultrasound Videos over 3G Wireless Networks, *Proceedings of the 29th Annual International Conference of the IEEE Engineering in Medicine and Biology Society (EMBC'07)*, pp. 3717-3720, 978-1-4244-0787-3, Aug. 2007, Lyon, France.

Wang Z. & C. Bovik, A. (2009) Mean squared error: love it or leave it? - A new look at signal fidelity measures, *IEEE Signal Processing Magazine*, Vol. 26, No. 1, Jan. 2009, pp. 98-117.

Wenger S. (2002). FMO: Flexible Macroblock Ordering, *ITU-T JVT-C089*, May 2002.

Wenger, S. & Horowitz, M. (2002). Flexible MB Ordering - A New Error Resilience Tool for IP-Based Video, *Proceedings of International Workshop on Digital Communications (IWDC'02)*, Sept. 2002, Capri, Italy.

Wenger, S. (2003). H.264/AVC over IP, *IEEE Transactions on Circuits and Systems for Video Technolology*, Vol. 13, No. 7, Jul. 2003, pp. 645–656, 1051-8215.

Wiegand, T.; Sullivan, G. J.; Bjøntegaard, G. & Luthra, A. (2003). Overview of the H.264/AVC video coding standard, *IEEE Transactions on Circuits and Systems for Video Technolology*, Vol. 13, No. 7, Jul. 2003, pp. 560–576, 1051-8215.

Williams, D. & Shah, M. (1992). A Fast Algorithm for Active Contour and Curvature Estimation, *GVCIP: Imag. Und.*, Vol. 55, No. 1, 1992, pp. 14-26.

Yu, H.; Lin, Z. & Pan, F. (2005). Applications and improvement of H.264 in medical video compression, *IEEE Transactions on Circuits and Systems I, Special issue on Biomedical Circuits and Systems: A New Wave of Technology*, Vol. 52, No. 12, Dec. 2005, pp. 2707-2716, 1549-8328.

Contact-less Assessment of In-vivo Body Signals Using Microwave Doppler Radar

Shahrzad Jalali Mazlouman, Kouhyar Tavakolian, Alireza Mahanfar and Bozena Kaminska
Simon Fraser University, School of Engineering Science
8888 University Drive, V5A 1S6
Burnaby, BC, Canada

1. Introduction

Every seven minutes in Canada, someone dies from heart disease or stroke. Cardiovascular disease (heart disease, diseases of the blood vessels and stroke) accounts for the death of more Canadians than any other disease (Heartandstroke, 2004). Early detection and treatment of symptoms and abnormalities can significantly decrease this rate. Therefore, the heart-related signals are the most important vital signals to monitor. For many years, extensive work has been devoted to finding low-cost, convenient, ubiquitous solutions to monitor heart signals in the everyday life. While these devices are beneficial, they have the disadvantage of requiring physical contact with the patient. Examples include chest straps to monitor the electrocardiogram (ECG) signal, gel for ultrasounds (echocardiography), heavy accelerometer sensor for seismocardiogram and electrodes for impedance cardiography (ICG) and oximetery. In addition, most of the existing methods require special expertise to use. The ideal solution would include a non-obtrusive method that can be used continuously and in everyday life without touching the patient and without requiring special expertise.

From another point of view, seniors are becoming the fastest growing segment of the population in North America (Michahelles et al., 2004). This trend creates a new demand for health care. Availability of cost-efficient, wearable, non-invasive, real-time methods of monitoring body signals that can be used at home can save a significant fraction of costs for the health care system while providing efficient care to the elderly. Consequently, there is a growing demand for devices that allow remote monitoring of health related parameters and transferring the recorded data to a physician via telephone, internet, or cellular phone networks, in case of sensing any abnormalities or symptoms.

Such non-invasive methods can also be beneficial for monitoring the effectiveness of treatment procedures for patients in the hospital or at home without requiring physical contact, thereby allowing long-term health care monitoring at almost no compromise in the patient's mobility or ordinary lifestyle. As an example, in this chapter, a new method for monitoring of congestive heart failure patients using the radar technology is proposed. In addition, in-vivo body signals monitoring, in particular heart and breathing rate monitoring, can provide safety in critical situations such as car driving, by initiating actions such as automatic control, stop and urgent call upon reading of an emergency call by the developed sensor (Michahelles et al., 2004).

In this chapter, the basics of Microwave Doppler radar systems are investigated as a cost-efficient, non-invasive, and ubiquitous solution for continuous monitoring of in-vivo body signals; in particular, non-invasive sensing of cardiac, respiratory, and arterial movements. Microwave Doppler radar can detect motions and velocity based on Doppler effect; therefore, a variety of body signals including the mechanical motions of the chest because of heart beat (the radar seismocardiogram, R-SCG) as well as the blood flow velocity in major blood vessels can be monitored. Parameters such as heart-rate, hemodynamic parameters, blood flow velocity and respiration rate can be measured using these devices. Microwave Doppler radar systems do not require direct contact with the body and can function through blankets or clothing.

Although laboratory demonstrations of the use of Doppler radar for cardiovascular and respiratory measurements date back to the late 1970's and early 1980's (Lin, 1975; Lin, 1979), cost-efficient, wearable body signal monitoring devices have not been reported until very recently; when implementation of low-cost, low-power, battery-operated devices is more feasible than ever by virtue of the availability and advances in high-integration technologies, signal processing techniques, and high-speed communication networks.

Depending on the application, Microwave Doppler radar systems may use a continuous-wave or a time-gated radar signal. Continuous-wave Doppler radar have been shown to be comparable and even exceeding the conventional impedance cardiography methods for measuring the mechanical activity of the heart, as well as for measuring the heart-rate variability (HRV) (Staderini, 2002a). In fact, the derivative of the radar signal shows better correlations with the impedance cardiogram signal (ICG) (Thijs et al., 2005). Some signals have been confirmed to be more clear on the captured radar signal than on the ICG, for example, the opening of the atrium and the mitral valve (Thijs et al., 2005).

A continuous Microwave Doppler radar based system was developed in the centre for integrative bio-engineering research (CiBER lab) of Simon Fraser University (Tavakolian et al, 2008a). The developed device is completely implemented on board and is the first reported device that can be used independently as a stand-alone system or can be connected to a PC. This device was tested to measure the heart and respiration rate of human subjects and demonstrated a noticeable accuracy of 91.35% for respiration rate, and 92.9% for heart rate. More importantly, this system was used to extract R-SCG signal as is discussed in the next sections.

The structure of this book chapter is as follows. In Section 2, body signals that can potentially be measured using the Doppler radar system are introduced. Special emphasize has been given to a class of infrasonic cardiac signals, that radar extracted R-SCG signal belongs to it. In this section technical background such as the Doppler Effect, the radar system, and the ultra-wideband radar are discussed. In Section 3, details of the Microwave Doppler radar systems are discussed and analyzed and the related equations are derived. The building blocks are introduced and design specifications and requirements are calculated. Section 4 is devoted to practical implementation of the Microwave Doppler radar based system that was designed and implemented in the CiBER lab.

2. Background

2.1 Infrasonic Cardiac Signals

Radar seismocardiogram (R-SCG) belongs to a category of cardiac signals that have their main components in the infrasonic range (less than 20 Hz) and reflect the mechanical function of the heart as a pump. During the past century, extensive research has been conducted on interpretation of these signals in terms of their relationship to cardiovascular dynamics and their possible application in cardiac abnormality diagnostics. Signals such as ballistocardiogram (BCG), seismocardiogram (SCG), apexcardiogram (ACG) and radar seismocardiogram reflect the displacement, velocity, or acceleration of the body in response to the heart beating.

Different methods that were used to acquire these signals are shown in Fig. 1. R-SCG is recorded by contactless radar method, SCG and ACG are recorded by attaching sensors to the chest and BCG is recorded by measuring the changes of the center of mass of the whole body. The ACG acquisition is very similar to SCG, except for the recording site on the chest, which is the point of maximum impulse for ACG and the sternum for most SCG definitions, as is explained in the next section. A contactless method of recording ACG has also been proposed using microwave radar (Lin, 1979).

The recorded signal morphology will vary with the method employed, but all the techniques appear to signal basically the same events in the cardiac cycle. The basic physiology behind all these signals are as follows: with each heart beat, blood rushes upward and strikes the aortic arch. The impact is great enough to give the whole body an upthrust. When the descending blood slows down, there is a rebound effect which gives the body a downthrust, not as intense as the earlier upthrust.

These signals are normally recorded together with ECG thus, an understanding of the electromechanical performance of the heart can be achieved. In order to better understand the genesis of waves in R-SCG signal, for the first time in this writing, we study these signals in the same context and briefly investigate their simillarities and differences.

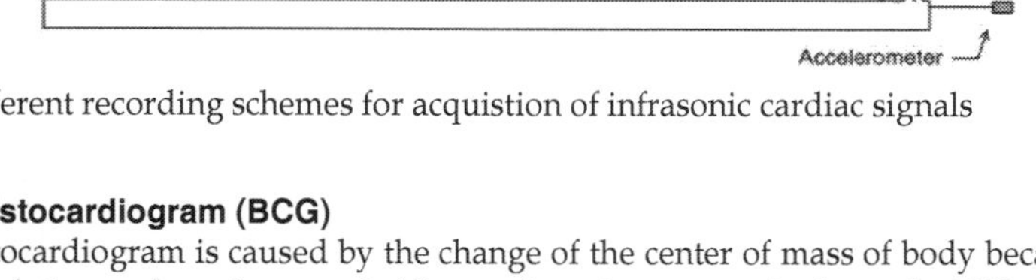

Fig. 1. Different recording schemes for acquistion of infrasonic cardiac signals

2.1.1 Ballistocardiogram (BCG)

The ballistocardiogram is caused by the change of the center of mass of body because of the blood circulation and can be recorded by noninvasive means. In the early 1930s Isaac Starr recognized that the BCG signals closely reflect the strength of myocardial contraction and function of the heart as a pump. As a result of his valuable research, clinicians and medical experts for almost three decades studied the effects of different heart malfunctions using BCG and proved that these malfunctions can be related to typical patterns on the BCG signal morphology (Starr & Noordergraaf, 1967).

Most types of BCG involve a platform upon which a subject lies supinely. BCG systems were categorized by their natural frequency with respect to the heart's own natural frequency of about 1 Hz. Those BCG apparatuses with higher natural frequencies of 10 Hz to 15 Hz are high frequency BCG (HF-BCG). Those with natural frequencies of approximately 1 Hz are low frequency (LF-BCG) and those lower than 1 Hz are ultra-low frequency (ULF-BCG). Binding and dampening of the BCG apparatus can be thought of as filtering its resultant signal such that frequencies below its natural frequency are removed. Thus, HF-BCG removes more of the low frequency spectrum, and so it reflects forces, whereas ULF-BCG measures displacement better. The physical basis of these BCG apparatuses is examined in elegant detail by Noordergraaf (Starr & Noordergraaf, 1967).

The ideal BCG waveform consists of seven waveforms peaks labeled G through N as defined by the American Heart Association. H is the first upward deflection after electrocardiograph (ECG) R-wave on the acceleration BCG when recorded simultaneously. The letter I is the downward wave immediately after H, and lastly the letter J is the upward wave after I. The L, M and N waves correspond to the diastolic phase of the cardiac cycle, all the waves can be seen in Fig. 2. (Scarborough & Talbot 1956).

In addition to a number of clinical studies that have been performed with BCG, specialized BCG instruments, including beds (Jensen et al., 1991), chairs (Junnila et al., 2008) and weight scale (Inan et al., 2008), have been developed by different research groups. However, due to the unrefined nature of the previous BCG signal acquisition technologies, the lack of interpretation algorithms, and the lack of practical devices, the current health care systems do not use BCG for clinical purposes.

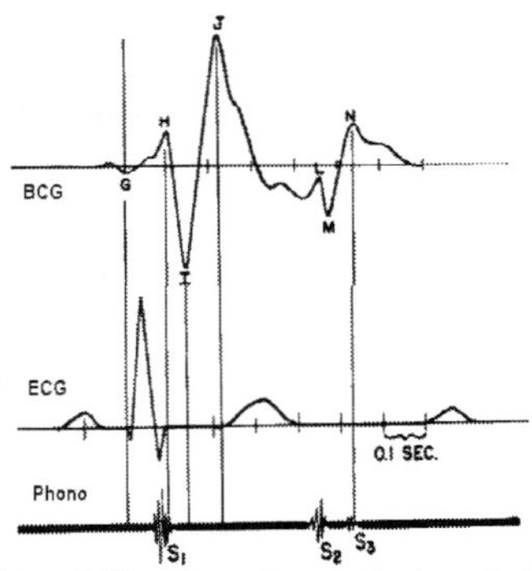

Fig. 2. Simulaneous BCG, ECG and Phonocardiograph signals (Scarborough & Talbot 1956)

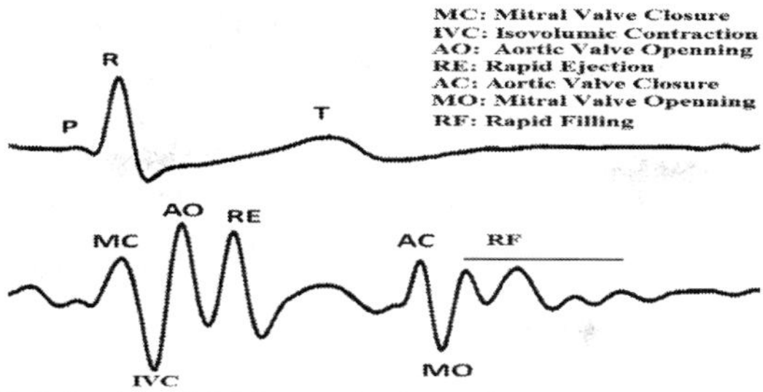

Fig. 3. A cycle of ECG (top) and SCG signals, from the second author, and the sequence of cardiac events assigned to it based on Salerno's research (Crow et al. 1994)

2.1.2 Seismocardiogram (SCG)

Seismocardiography is a technique used for analyzing the vibrations generated by the heart and it is recorded from the surface of the body using accelerometers. The seismocardiography was first introduced to clinical medicine by J. Zanetti (earthquake seismologist) and D. Salerno (cardiologist) in 1987. They borrowed the technology used in seismology to record the cardiac induced vibration from the surface of the body (Salerno & Zanetti, 1990a). This signal was also given the name Sternal Ballistocardiography as it was recorded from the sternum and had similarities to the ballistocardiogram (Mckay et al., 1999) (Tavakolian et al., 2008b). A cycle of synchronous SCG and ECG is shown in Fig. 3.

It was shown later on that changes in SCG after exercise was more sensitive for detection of moderate coronary artery stenosis than ECG. Later, the same claim was proven on more number of patients, 505, that the qualitative seismocardiography was more accurate, both in sensitivity and specificity, than electrocardiography for detection of coronary artery stenosis. This was true for severe, multivessle disease as well as for moderate disease and also for presence or absence of myocardial infarction (Salerno et al., 1990b).

There are two different subgroups of signals that have been introduced so far as seismocardiogram. In the first group, which consists the majority of the papers, the signal is recorded by positioning of an accelerometer on the sternum while in the second group other places on the torso such as left clavicle (Castiglioni et al. 2007) or hip (Trefny, 2005) were used. Thus, in a wider sense seismocardiogram is recording of cardiac induced vibrations on the upper part of the body while in a particular definition given by Salerno and his group seismocardiogram, is just limited to the vibration signals recorded from the sternum.

The first commercial SCG instrument was a failure as it required a heavy and bulky seismology sensor on the sternum which was cumbersome to tolerate for a long time. New sensor technologies have provided new possibilities for portable and wireless sensors that can be worn under clothing to record the SCG signal during daily activities. A new line of research has emerged aiming to re-introduce SCG as a clinical instrument that can be used to noninvasively and inexpensively diagnose cardiac abnormalities (Akhbardeh et al., 2007) (Castiglioni et al. 2007) (Tavakolian et al. 2008b).

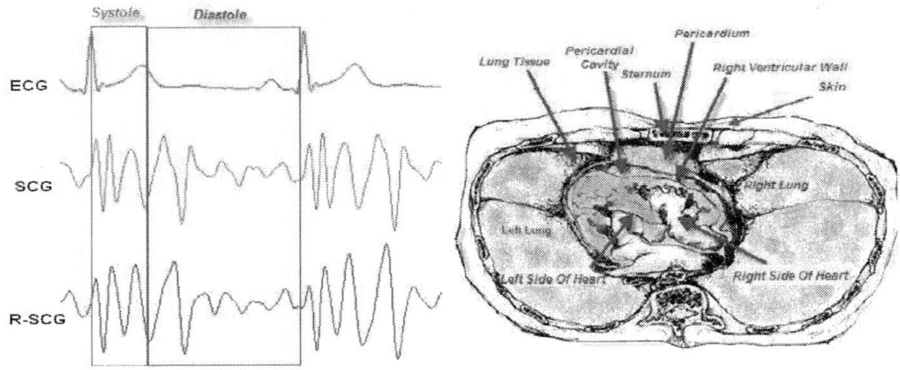

Fig. 4. Right: Positioning of different layers of tissues that the radar signal will go through. Left: two cycles of the R-SCG, SCG and ECG signals (Tavakolian et al., 2008a).

2.1.3 Radar seismocardiogram (R-SCG) and its Medical Relevance

Radar seismocardiogram also known as radarcardiogram (Geisheimer & Greneker, 1999) and mechanocardiogram (Tavakolian et al., 2008a) reflects the mechanical dynamics of the heart recorded by contactless methods. While monitoring the heart away from the chest the signal passes through only a few layers of different tissues between the sternum and the heart which can be seen in Fig.4. The tissue layers between the sensor and heart muscle include: skin, sternum, lung and pleural tissue, pericardium and pericardial space. From the sternum position these tissue layers are thinner compared to the other positions. Therefore, the best position to record the heart's R-SCG signal is from the sternum. R-SCG signal has close relationship to SCG signal as can be seen in Fig 4. In other words, proper processing of the radar signal reflected from the chest will enable us to extract a signal (R-SCG) which is very similar in morphology to SCG thus, a better understanding of SCG mechanism helps us understand R-SCG signal as well.

Some hemodynamic parameters can be extracted from either the amplitute or timings of R-SCG signal as can be seen in Fig. 5. The amplitute of R-SCG is an indication of the cardiac contractility thus, it is correlated with stroke volume and cardiac output (Mckay et al. 1999). The time intervals between the R-SCG peaks is correlated with cardiac intervals such as isovolumic contraction and relaxation times and ventricular ejection time. Calculation of these three cardiac intervals from R-SCG will provide us with the possibility of noninvasive calculation of a combined myocardial performance index called Tei-index.

Tei index equals isovolumic contraction time plus isovolumic relaxation time divided by ejection time. Congestive heart failure is related to contraction and relaxation abnormalities of the ventricle. Isolated analysis of either mechanism may not be reflective of overall cadiac dysfunction. Tei-index has been described to be more effective for analysis of global cardiac dysfunction than systolic and diastolic measures alone. Tei-Index is evaluated against invasive examinations and proved to be a sensitive indicator of overall cardiac dysfunction in patients with mild-to-moderate congestive heart failure (Brush et al., 2000).

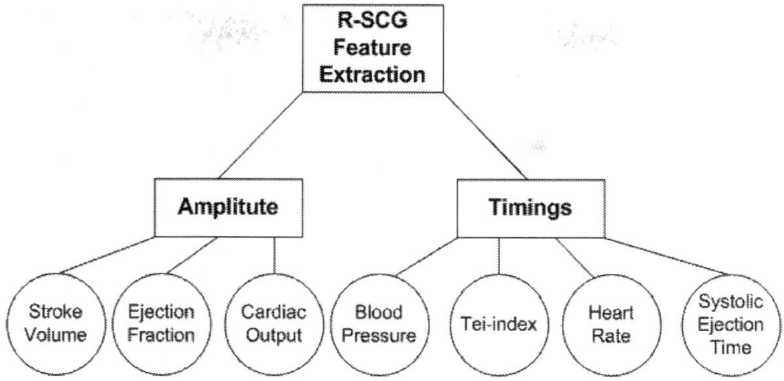

Fig. 5. Possible extraction of clinical parameters from R-SCG.

Vital signs are measures of various physiological statistics in order to monitors the most basic body functions. There are four standard vital signs: heart rate, respiratory rate, blood pressure and body temprature. Blood pressure is the pressure of the blood in the arteris and is created by the contraction of the heart. In clincs the blood presure is normally reported by two numbers. The higher number correponds to the systolic blood presure and is measured after the heart contracts and the other one is diastolic blood pressure and is measured befor the heart contraction.

Using R-SCG heart and breathing rates, can be reliably estimated. Further improvement of the current technolgy can enable us to estimate blood pressure from the R-SCG signal in future. The interval between the openning of aorta to the point of maximum systolic ejection is inversely proportional to the blood presure and can be used for the estimation of systolic blood pressure. In a novel study, from BCG signals acquired from bathroom scale, the interval between the R wave of ECG signal to the rapid ejection point of BCG was used for this estimation (Kim et al. 2006). Thus, except for temprature R-SCG can enable us to monitor three of the four vital signs as mentioned above.

2.1.4. Comparison Study of Infrasonic Cardiac Signals

As mentioned before, BCG signal is the most studied signal in the field of infrasonic cardiac signals and has been around for about a century. BCG is different compared to R-SCG and SCG as it reflects the movement of the center of gravity of the whole body and its support while the SCG and R-SCG signals reflect the mechanical vibration of the upper part of the body as recorded from its surface. Fig. 1. shows the differnt setups that were used for the acquistion of these signals.

The SCG and R-SCG signals are recorded from positions closer to the heart thus, there are less mechanical damping of the cardiac vibration compared to classical BCG in which, the heart moves the whole body and the recording system (Bed, chair and weight scale). This finds more importance in the sense that, being close to the heart, SCG and R-SCG are able to trace valvular activities while these tiny movements gets dampen out by the classical BCG beds. Thus, in terms of evaluation of timings of valvular events SCG and R-SCG are a better reference compared to BCG.

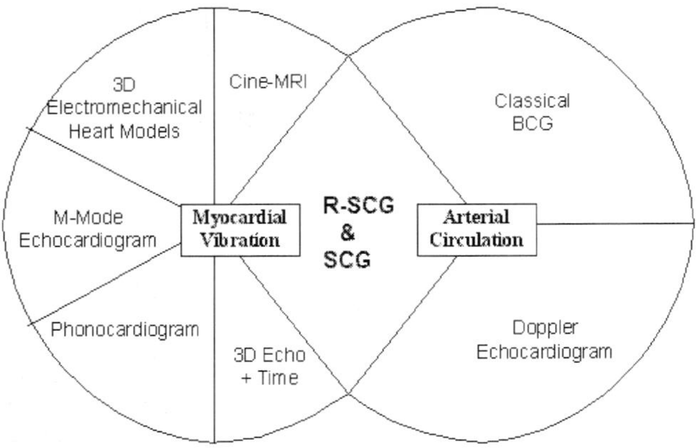

Fig. 6. The two main factors determining the R-SCG and SCG morphology and the possible tools for investigating them.

On the other hand, as BCG is a record of the sum of all the cardiovascular forces exerted on the body thus, its amplitude is a more faithful representation of the force of cardiac system compared to SCG and R-SCG which reflect a portion of this force that affects the upper body thus, BCG is a better candidate to estimate stroke volume and cardiac output compared to SCG. The old BCG instruments were quite bulky and required the patients to lie down on beds suspended from the ceiling while SCG and R-SCG facilitate signal recording and thus, provide alternative possibilities that BCG was inherently unable to.

Using R-SCG, on the other hand, provides a unique advantage, over other infrasoinc cardiac signals, that it does not require any mechanical contact to the body. Thus, in applications such as monitoring new born babies, to avoid sudden infant death syndrome (SIDS), R-SCG contactless recording is an advantage.

2.2. The Genesis of R-SCG waves

As mentioned previously the R-SCG morphology has close resemblance to SCG and it basically signals the same events in the cardiac cycle as SCG does. Thus, in this section, we briefly introduce different methods used for understanding of the genesis of SCG waves, assuming that this knowledge can be transferred to the R-SCG field as well.

The waves observed on R-SCG and SCG signals originate from two main cardiovascular phenomenons of myocardial contraction and arterial circulation. In other words, some components of the R-SCG are due to vibration waves directly created by the heart contractions and transferred to the surface of the body, and some other components are because of the recoil created by the circulation of blood in the arteries.

In a study conducted by Salerno the SCG signal was simultaneously recorded together with echocardiograph images for 39 subjects and it was shown that aortic and mitral valve opening and closures could be corresponded to peaks and valleys on the SCG signal (Crow et al. 1994). An example of SCG traces recorded in CiBER and annotated based on Salerno's work can be seen in Fig. 3. After the P wave on ECG and during the QRS complex there is a local maximum correponding to the Mitral valve closure (MC) the interval between this point and the next maximum (The aortic valve opening) is the iso-volumic contraction interval. Rapid systolic ejection point (RE) is the next maximum after that, as it can also be identified in the Doppler echocardiogram on the left side of Fig.7 At the end of the sytole the aorta closes (AC) followed by the opening of the Miral valve (MO). The interval between AC and MO is defined as iso-volumic relaxation time.

The simultaneous echocardiogram and SCG and ECG signal used for investigation of cardiac events as recorded on the SCG signal can be seen in Fig. 7. On the left side of the figure by using Doppler echocardiogram and SCG; point of rapid systolic ejection is shown by a vertical red line in two consecutive cycles. On the right side of Fig. 7 the M-mode echocardiogram is shown and the aortic valve opening time is shown by a vertical green line and the aortic valve closure with a dotted blue line. The Echocardiograms were recorded in Burnaby General Hospital, Canada, using a GE vivid 7 system.

Echocardiograph is still the gold standard for investigation of the origin of the waves observed on R-SCG and SCG signals but there are two reasons to investigate for alternative solutions besides echocardiography. Firstly, echocardiography has limitations: being operator dependant, being dependant on the position of the transducer, and being limited to a few numbers of beats. Secondly, by using the Echo images alone we still do not clearly know how the underlying cardiac events create the waves observed on the signal recorded from the chest. The reason is the fact that these cardiac events superimpose on each other and sometimes amplify or decrease each other's effects. Thus, as can be seen in Fig. 6, other methodologies such as Cine-MRI and 3D, finite element, electromechanical model of the heart have been proposed to study the effect of cardiac contraction (Akhbardeh et al. 2009) and, on the other hand, classical BCG and Doppler echocardiogram have been proposed to study the effects of blood circulation on the SCG morphology (Ngai et al. 2009).

Phonocardiogram can also be used to study the effects of cardiac vibrations on the R-SCG morphology as can be seen in Fig. 10. The heart sounds as observed on phonocardiogram can be used to study the effects of valvular events on the morphology of the signal. Two cycles of synchronous radar R-SCG, Phonocardiograph and ECG signal showing the correlation of cardiac cycle events to R-SCG signal. Systolic and diastolic complexes can be identified in the radar R-SCG signal corresponding to S1 and S2 of heart sounds.

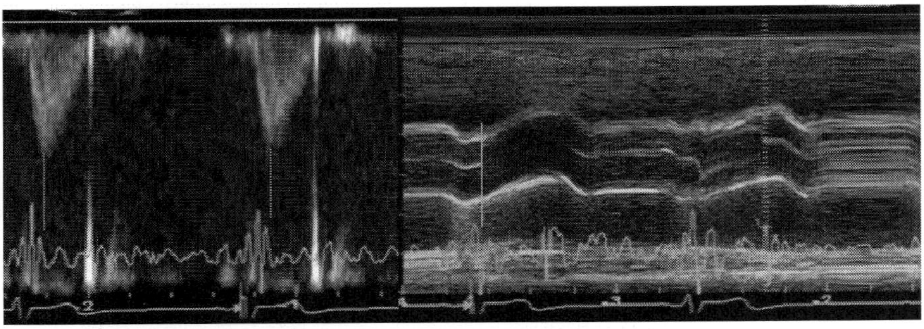

Fig. 7. left: Doppler echocardiogram and SCG; right: M-mode echocardiogram

2.3 Doppler Based Radar System

Radio detection and ranging (Radar) systems are used to identify the range, direction, or speed of both moving and fixed objects such as aircrafts, vehicles and terrains. These systems are usually comprised of an RF/Microwave transceiver to transmit the Electromagnetic signal to the object under test and receive the reflected wave carrying the required data. Depending on the application, this data is further processed using basic or advanced signal processing techniques. Microwave Doppler radar-based systems are one of the most common applications of radar in everyday life. These systems will be discussed in detail in Section 3.

A class of radars utilize Doppler Effect to measure the velocity of moving objects. This kind of approach has long been used to estimate the velocity of moving vehicles for speed control and other purposes. The Doppler principle has been used in different modalities including microwave, laser and ultrasound. Doppler radars are commercially used in air defence, air traffic control, sounding satellites, and even police speed guns.

Microwave electromagnetic waves can propagate through the body and are reflected at the interfaces between different tissue layers. By the Doppler Effect for Microwave radar, if a radio frequency wave is transmitted to a moving surface, the reflected wave undergoes a frequency shift proportional to the surface velocity. If the surface has periodic motion, like that of the heart and chest, this can also be seen as a phase shift proportional to the surface displacement. If this displacement is small compared to the wavelength, a low-frequency component can be extracted from downconversion and filtering (removing the high-frequency component) the reflected wave that is directly proportional to the object displacement.

The Doppler Effect can be written as (Skolnik, 1990):

$$\omega_r = \omega_0(1 + \frac{v}{c} Cos\alpha) \tag{1}$$

where ω_r corresponds to the reflected wave frequency, ω_0 corresponds to the transmitted wave frequency, v corresponds to the relative speed, c corresponds to the prorogation speed of the wave (in this case, the Electromagnetic wave speed which is 3×10^8 m/s in free space) and finally, *a* corresponds to the angle of the reflected wave versus the moving object. If the transmitter and the moving object are approaching each other, then the reflected wave frequency is higher than the transmitted wave frequency ($\omega_r > \omega_0$) and if they are departing from each other, then the reflected wave is lower than the transmitted wave frequency ($\omega_r < \omega_0$). Assuming the transmitted wave direction to be along the movement direction of the object under test ($a=0$), the Doppler Effect for a return way can be re-written as:

$$\omega_r = \omega_0 + \omega_D = \omega_0 (1 + \frac{2v}{c}) \tag{2}$$

Therefore, the speed of the moving object can be calculated. The operation of the Microwave radar based systems will be further analysed in Section 3.3.

2.4 The Ultra-wideband (UWB) Radar for Biomedical Applications

In 2002, the Federal Communications Commission (FCC) allocated the 3.1 to 10.6GHz band to ultra-wideband (UWB) communication systems in which the systems have a bandwidth greater than 500MHz and a maximum equivalent isotropic radiated power (EIRP) spectral density of −41.3dBm/MHz (FCC, 2002). This broad definition has encouraged a variety of UWB variants for different applications including UWB Doppler radar for vital signal sensing (Staderini, 2002a). UWB power levels are very low and therefore reduce the risk of molecular ionization (Jauchem et al., 1998). In addition, advances in modern silicon integration technologies with high cutoff frequencies allow for small, low-power implementation of UWB sensors. Time-gating of short radar UWB pulses allows for additional power efficiency; however, as explained in section 3.2., new design challenges on the control of sampling at the receiver is introduced.

Doppler radar-based systems for cardiovascular and respiratory measurements date back to the late 1970's and early 1980's for the X-band (around 10GHz) (Lin, 1975; Lin, 1979; Chen et al., 1986). In mid-1980s, a frequency-modulated-continuous wave (FM-CW) system was developed to detect the vital signs of a wounded soldier in live fire situations at distances of up to 100 meters (Greneker, 1997). Despite its severe limitations such as sensitivity to surrounding objects, this device was the first of the many later developed radar vital signs monitor (RVSM) devices (Thansandote et al., 1983).

RVSM devices are capable of detecting human heart beat and respiration rate in a contact-less manner, by transmitting a radio frequency signal to the subject and measuring the phase shift in the reflected signal based on the Doppler Effect. During the 1996 Olympics, a variant of the RVSM, developed by Georgia Tech Research Institute (GTRI), (Greneker, 1997), was developed for assessment of the performance of the athletes in the archery and rifle competitions. Human heartbeat and respiration signals were measured at ranges exceeding 10 meters using this RVSM that was mounted onto a 0.6m parabolic dish antenna and transmitted an output power of 30mW at 24.1 GHz. Other suggested applications for these devices include home telemedicine monitoring systems and security applications. Major problems with these devices include sensitivity to surroundings due to weak signal processing and their high cost due to bulkiness.

In (Thansandote et al., 1983), a microwave Doppler radar system was reported for continuously monitoring time-varying biological impedances. The radar compares the phase of the signal scattered from the biological tissue with that of the transmitted signal.

The phase variations of the scattered signal are indicate the net impedance changes in the test region due to physiological processes, e.g. movements of blood vessels during the cardiac cycle. The system operation at both frequencies of 3GHz and 10.5GHz was tested with healthy human subjects. The 3GHz operation frequency for the Doppler radar system was shown to have significantly greater penetration in tissues but was less sensitive to changes of the biological impedance than the 10.5GHz system.

A simple add-on module was reported in (Lubecke et al., 2002) that allows the Doppler radar based detection of human respiration and heart activity using the 2.4 GHz cordless telephone system without requiring modifications in the existing telephone infrastructure. This module includes an inverted F-type antenna combined with a Schottky diode as the mixing element. The implemented module is very small in size but does not implement the complete system and the receiver baseband section is implemented on a digitizing oscilloscope.

A digital signal processor was described in (Lohman et al., 2002) for the determination of respiration and heart rates in Doppler radar measurements for remote monitoring. The processor can reliably calculate both rates for a subject at distances of 2m. Several enhancement techniques such as autocorrelation and center clipping are used. The calculated heart rates agree for over 88% of the cases, within a 2% margin, for all datasets.

The first single-chip radios for the remote sensing of vital signs using direct-conversion radars integrated in low-cost silicon technologies were implemented in (Droitcour et al., 2001). Two Doppler radar systems operating at 1.6GHz were fabricated using CMOS/BiCMOS technologies with more than 83% agreement with references. Despite the high phase noise of the integrated oscillators, heart and respiration rates were detected remotely, using phase noise reduction through range correlation (Droitcour et al., 2001).

In (Thijs et al., 2005), the data obtained from a commercially available continuous-wave Doppler radar sensor (KMY24) was compared to an ICG device using a Cardiac Output Monitor (Medis Niccomo). The obtained data was shown to be clearer on the captured radar signal than on the ICG, for example, the opening of the atrium and the mitral valve (Thijs et al., 2005).

An infant vital sign monitor device is reported in (Li et al., 2009). This device operates at 5.8 GHz and monitors the existence of the infant's heart and respiration rate. Therefore, the signal processing required for this device is simplified.

Several UWB Microwave Doppler radar based implementations have also been reported in the literature based on (McEwan, 1994). A bread-board UWB prototype is implemented in (Michahelles et al., 2004) that can determine the heart-rate at a distance of up to 15cm with a relative error of 5% compared to oximeter measurements.

Another UWB prototype was developed in (Staderini, 2002b) using a dipole antenna that emits 2ns pulses with a mean pulse repetition frequency (PRF) of 2MHz. This prototype is used to measure the HRV signal. Using fast Fourier transform (FFT), the spectral content of the radar captured signal is compared to an ECG-derived HRV signal and good correlations are confirmed.

UWB radar systems have also been reported to detect human beings behind walls Meyerhoff, 2007), or as lie detectors (Staderini, 2002b), or as human activity monitoring, e.g., detection of walking, running, sleeping, etc., (Dutta et al., 2006; Such et al., 2006; Chia et al., 2005) using the body signals.

A system-on-chip (SoC) implementation of a UWB vital signal sensor is in progress funded by the European Union (Zito et al., 2007; Zito et al., 2008). In this project, a wearable UWB radar wireless sensor for detection of heart and breath rates is to be implemented using CMOS 90nm technology. Short pulses of 200-300ps duration with a PRF of 1-10 MHz are used (Zito et al., 2008). An IEEE 802.15.4 ZigBee (ZigBee Alliance, 2004) low-power radio interface is used for wireless data communication.

3. The Microwave Doppler-Based Radar System Blocks and Specifications

A block diagram depicting the main blocks of the Microwave Doppler-based radar system is shown in Fig. 8. As shown in this figure, these devices are generally composed of two main stages: The RF stage and the baseband signal processing stage. The RF stage includes an RF/UWB transceiver block to transmit the radar wave and receive the reflected wave. The received wave includes the frequency shift due to the motion/velocity of the target (e.g. thorax, blood flow). The received signal is down-converted and low-pass filtered to extract the baseband shifting data. This baseband signal is further amplified, digitized, and processed in the baseband stage. The digital signal processing techniques can be implemented in hardware or software.

In this section, the Doppler based Radar system is analyzed, the main stages as shown in Fig. 8 are reviewed, and some major reported ideas for on-board and CMOS integrated implementation of these blocks are discussed.

3.1 The RF Stage

As shown in Fig. 1, on the transmit side, the RF stage includes a pulse generator (Gaussian pulse, in case of UWB system), a mixer (LO) to modulate the pulse, a power amplifier (PA) to radiate the modulated pulse, and finally a transmitting antenna. The transmitted signal can be a continuous wave monochrome (single frequency) non-modulated sinusoidal radar signal. In this case the system is simplified to the non-dashed blocks and only the signal generated at the LO is transmitted (no pulse generator or mixer stage required).

On the receive side, the reflected beams are captured by the receiving antenna, followed by a low-noise amplifier (LNA), a downconversion mixer, and a low-pass filter. The downconversion mixer multiplies the received signal by a replica (a delayed replica if time-gating is used) of the same signal as the one at the transmit side to demodulate it. The signal is then filtered to extract the low frequency component that includes the shift depending on the object motion data. Similar to the transmit side, if monochrome radar is used, no downconversion mixer stage is required.

The choice of a proper frequency is a compromise and depends on the test objectives, as a higher frequency enables a larger Doppler shift and therefore a higher resolution, but also results in a lower tissue penetration depth. In many reported works, the 2.45GHz frequency is chosen to exploit the commercially available components, e.g. (Lubecke et al., 2002). The frequency of the transmitted beam is adjusted by the mixer signal provided by the local oscillator (LO) block. The LO signal can be a voltage controlled oscillator (VCO) or simply a crystal oscillator. In the case of UWB radar systems, a short Gaussian monopulse is generated with a pulse-width in the order of magnitude of a few nanoseconds. Several short pulse generators have been reported in the literature. For example, digital pulse generators have been suggested in (Wentzeloff & Chandrakasan, 2006), for on-chip or on-board implementation based on a short delay between two NAND gates.

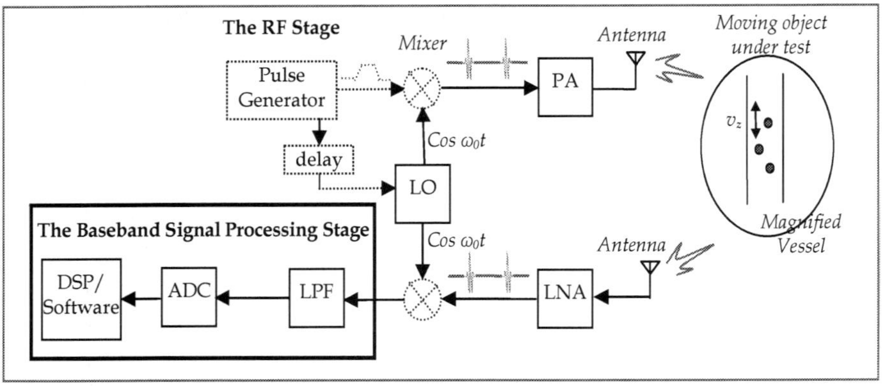

Fig. 8. The Microwave Doppler Radar-based system block diagram

The modulated signal is amplified by the PA and propagated by the transmitting antenna. In (Zito et al., 2008), a system-on-chip UWB sensor is implemented using a shaper block for the mixer and an integrator to sample and low-pass filter the received signal. In (Prak et al, 2007), quadrature mixers are used for the modulation/demodulation stages to increase accuracy and arctangent demodulation and dc-cancellation methods are used.

3.2 Time-Gating

To reduce power, in particular where battery-operated wireless handheld devices are implemented, the same antenna and mixing stage can be time-gated between the transmitting and the receiving stage. For example, by assigning a 50% duty cycle to a generated square pulse, the system can transmit the illuminating monochrome signal for the first half of the pulse width and receive the reflected signal for the second half of the pulse width. Note that in this case the dashed blocks are used in Fig. 1. A switch or a circulator can be used to implement the time-gating with the desired time-span.
UWB short-pulse systems are usually implemented using this structure and pulses as short as a few nanoseconds are used. As shown in Fig. 1, the pulse generator also activates a delay line block. This block controls proper sampling of the received signals from the object. The receiver only samples at short time intervals triggered by the delay line block. Proper timing of this triggering is essential to ensure sampling only when the received signals from a certain distance are received, for example, only when echoes of the heart-wall are expected (Michahelles et al., 2004). Intuitively, this delay should be equal to the flight time of the pulse from the radar to the heart and then from the heart to the radar. Note that time gating and adjusting the sampling time increases the signal-to-noise-ratio at the receiver as less interference signals due to body movements and other moving objects are sampled. Therefore, the effect of the interferences is less pronounced.
Time-gating is specified by the pulse repetition frequency (PRF). The PRF is defined as the number of pulses transmitted per second. It should be noted that depending on the velocity

of the object under test and the application, a minimum PRF should be met that depends on the radar range and the speed of the radar waves (in this case, c, for electromagnetic waves). To avoid ambiguity and increase the velocity measurement accuracy, sufficient observation time is required, which is possible by choosing proper PRF (Skolnik, 1990).

3.3 Analysis

For simplicity and without loss of generalization, assume a monochrome continuous RF-modulated signal, $x(t)$, is chosen as the radar transmitting signal:

$$x(t)=A \cdot Cos(\omega_0 t) \tag{3}$$

The reflected signal captured at the receive side will include the transmitted signal provided by the signal generator, with a frequency shift, ω_d, that is proportional to the velocity of the blood flow. The received signal will therefore include a term:

$$y(t)=A \cdot Cos[(\omega_0+ \omega_d)t] \tag{4}$$

plus some noise terms, where,

$$\omega_d = \frac{2v\omega_0}{c} \tag{5}$$

where ω_0 is the mixer frequency, c is the speed of light, and v is the velocity of the moving object under test; for example blood-flow velocity in arteries and veins, or the heart wall.
The frequency displacement resulting from the motion of the object under test can also be modelled as a phase shift, $\Phi(t)$, that depends on the velocity: (Thijs et al., 2005; Thansandote et al., 1983; Lohman et al., 2002)

$$\Phi(t) = \frac{2\pi}{\lambda}\int_0^t v(\tau)d\tau = \frac{4\pi}{\lambda}s(t) \tag{6}$$

where λ is the wavelength and $s(t)$ is the movement amplitude. Therefore, the vital signals such as the movement of the Thorax can be sensed.
In the case of UWB radar, the transmitted signal would be the product of a narrow Gaussian pulse by the mixer signal:

$$x(t) = Cos(\omega_0 t).\sum_{n=0}^{\infty}\exp\left[-\frac{(t-\mu-nT_p)^2}{2\sigma^2}\right] \tag{7}$$

and the reflected, received signal will include the Doppler shifted component,

$$y(t) = Cos(\omega_0+\omega_d)t\cdot\sum_{n=0}^{\infty}\exp\left[-\frac{(t-\mu-nT_p)^2}{2\sigma^2}\right] \tag{8}$$

where ω_0 is angular frequency of UWB modulation signal, ω_d is the Doppler shift frequency, μ represents Gaussian envelope phase, σ represents the pulse width and T_p is the pulse repetition period (corresponding to the PRF). Here, the added noise components not taken into account.

To extract the velocity of the object under test from the received signal, $y(t)$ is downconverted by $Cos(\omega_0 t)$, as (ignoring the mismatch errors)

$$y(t) = Cos((\omega_0 + \omega_d)t) \cdot Cos(\omega_0 t) \sum_{n=0}^{\infty} \exp\left[-\frac{(t-\mu-nT_p)^2}{2\sigma^2} \right] \quad (9)$$

That can be rewritten as:

$$y(t) = \left[Cos((2\omega_0 + \omega_d)t) + Cos(\omega_d t) \right] \cdot \sum_{n=0}^{\infty} \exp\left[-\frac{(t-\mu-nT_p)^2}{2\sigma^2} \right] \quad (10)$$

Therefore, the high frequency component can be filtered and the remaining baseband term that includes the shift data, i.e.,

$$y(t) = Cos(\omega_d t) \cdot \sum_{n=0}^{\infty} \exp\left[-\frac{(t-\mu-nT_p)^2}{2\sigma^2} \right] \quad (11)$$

is transferred to the following baseband signal processing stage.

3.4 The Baseband Stage

The baseband signal processing stage is the last stage in the Microwave Doppler radar-based system. In this stage, the frequency shift data and therefore the velocity/motion rate of the object under test is extracted from the signal received at the output of the lowpass filtering stage. Depending on the application, the received signal is processed through various digital signal processing (DSP) techniques. Usually, the received signal at the baseband stage is first amplified and converted into digital by an analog-to-digital converter stage (ADC) and then processed by further DSP techniques in the digital domain, where more flexible, simpler, and potentially lower cost implementations are possible. DSP techniques in the time-domain or frequency-domain such as fast Fourier transform (FFT), autocorrelation and noise cancellation methods, as well as several digital filtering stages can be used to increase coherency, attenuate the noise terms (such as echo), cancel motion artefacts due to other movements in the body and surrounding objects, and extract the target data.

The DSP techniques can be implemented in hardware (board-level or integrated), or in software, using a PC (e.g. MatLab™ DSP toolbox), or both, depending on the application. The DSP blocks can be implemented in hardware, on an FPGA, or on a DSP module, depending on their complexity. Also, several DSP prototype development boards are available by Texas Instruments Inc., and Altera Co. that can accommodate various applications.

In order to select proper hardware for a specific application, requirements on the maximum measurement frequency and resolution should be decided. Body signal such as blood flow rate or heart rate are usually not high frequency and therefore the requirements are not tight. However, some applications may require better resolutions. The Nyquist-rate requirement for proper sampling by the ADC is specified as:

$$f_s \geq 2 f_{\max} \quad (12)$$

where f_{max} is the maximum measurement frequency and f_s is the sampling frequency of the ADC. Oversampling can help increase the signal-to-noise-ratio (SNR) and therefore the resolution of the digitized signal (Northworthy et al., 1996). Note that these two parameters are related as (Northworthy et al., 1996):

$$SNDR = 6.02n + 1.76\, dB \quad (13)$$

where n is the effective number of bits (ENOB) of an ADC, known as the resolution of the ADC. As an example, in case of the heart signals measurements, a baseband signal of less than 30 Hz is expected at the output of the RF stage, therefore a sample rate of 80-100Hz for the ADC would be required.

4. The Developed R-SCG System and Measurement Results

The principal design of the radar-based R-SCG device is shown in the block diagram of Fig 9. The antenna mounted on the device is HFMD24 by Siemens and contains a transmitter and a receiver in the same housing. The operating frequency is 2.45GHz. The transmitter transmits continuous wave radio frequency energy towards subject body. The output signal from the receiver is filtered and amplified, signal conditioning block. The cut-off frequencies for the band-pass filter are 1Hz and 100Hz and the gain of the amplifier is around 800. After filtering and amplifying, the R-SCG signal is sent to the A/D unit and then to the ATMEL CPU for further processing. The CPU is connected to a thin-film transistor (TFT) display via its SPI (Serial Peripheral Interface) port. The R-SCG device operates with two AA batteries (2.45V) (Tavakolian et al, 2008a).

Considering that the R-SCG device has its own CPU and monitor, it can be used stand alone to acquire and process the R-SCG signal. There is also another option of sending the data to a personal computer for more advanced processing of the data using Matlab. To have this option on our device, the digitized R-SCG signal is transformed to packets and sent through UART to the USB and finally to the host personal computer for possible further processing.

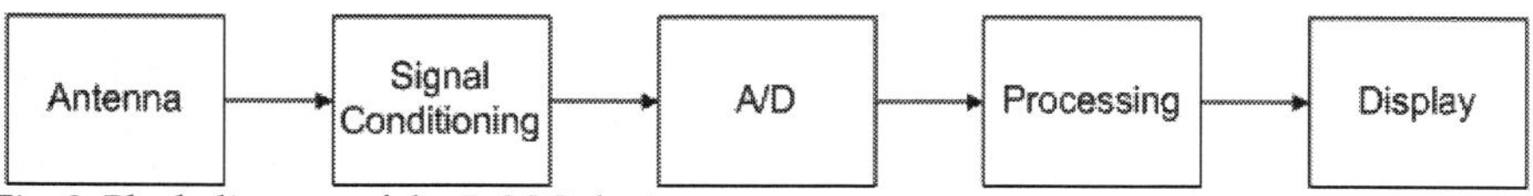

Fig. 9. Block diagram of the R-SCG device

The R-SCG signal was acquired by the sensor, 10cm away from the subject chest. The data acquisition involved the measurement of ECG and respiration signals too. RF signal with the carrier frequency of 2.45 GHz was transmitted toward the subject's chest and the reflected signal was band-passed filtered between 0.5 to 25 Hz. The filtered signal was differentiated and then band-pass filtered again between 4 Hz to 20 Hz. The comparison of the processed R-SCG signal to the SCG signal recorded simultaneously from the sternum can be seen in Fig. 4 together with the synchronized ECG signal.

It can be observed that there is a close correlation between the signal acquired from the radar-based R-SCG device and the simultaneous signal recorded from the SCG sensor attached to the sternum. The systolic and diastolic phases of cardiac cycle are shown to identify the correlations of these mechanical signals to the heart functioning. As explained before in section two, due to this close resemblance of the signal to SCG we are able to transfer the knowledge in the SCG field, about the genesis of waves, to R-SCG analysis.

Phonocardiograph signal reflects the heart sounds that can be hared using stethoscope. Heart sound S1 corresponds to systolic phase of the heart cycle and S2 corresponds to the diastolic phase of it. For the comparison purpose, the R-SCG signal was acquired synchronously with phonocardiogram signal and it was observed that S1 and S2 sounds of the phonocardiograph signal corresponded to the similar complexes on the R-SCG displacement signal as can be seen in Fig.10.

The data from subjects were recorded at Burnaby General Hospital. For the heart rate measurement the experimental setup included the acquisition of the R-SCG signal and two leads of ECG as a reference. For respiration rate measurement the setup included the acquisition of R-SCG signal together with the respiration signal as the reference. Eight subjects took part in the respiration measurement tests and six of these subjects took part in the heart rate measurement tests too. Breathing rate measurement experiments were 60 seconds long while heart rate measurement experiments were 15 seconds long.

For detection of breathing rate the radar signal was low pass filtered under 0.4Hz and the peaks were counted and compared to the results acquired from a strain gauge transducer that measures the changes in thoracic circumference, using a belt which is fastened to the subject's thorax. The accuracy of respiration rate measurement was 91.35 percent over all eight subjects. The heart rate was measured using radar-based R-SCG device and was compared to the heart rate calculated from the simultaneous ECG signal for six subjects. The average of the heart rate accuracy on these subjects was calculated to be 92.9 percent.

4.1 Safety Issues

In order to standardize and commercialize the developed device, the radar sensor's SAR (specific absorption rate) should be determined. SAR measurements are usually used for cellphone handsets to assess the thermal effect on the human body tissue due to cellphone radiation. It is also a measure of the amount of energy absorbed by the human body. The SAR value for similar sensors have been measured to be lower than a standard cellphone handset (Thijs et al., 2005).

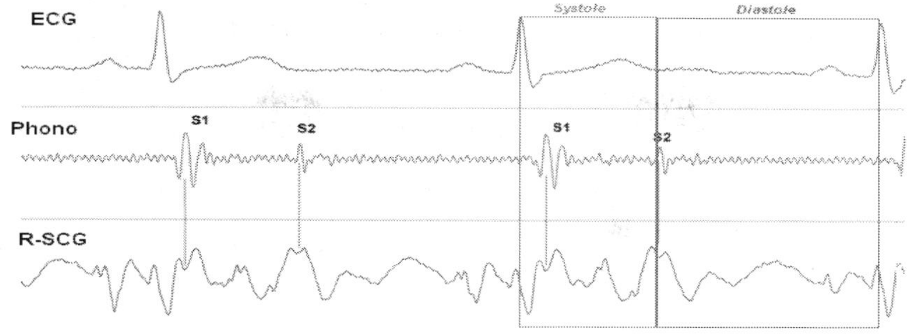

Fig. 10. Synchronous radar displacement R-SCG, Phonocardiograph and ECG signals (Tavakolian et al, 2008a)

5. Concluding Remarks and Future Work

Microwave Doppler radar-based systems can be used to monitor vital signs such as heart and breathing rate and to extract Radar seismocardiogram, by which, several other cardiac dynamic parameters can be estimated. Thus, in this chapter, a brief review of reported devices using continuous-time, and Ultra-wideband Microwave Doppler radar is presented as the technical basis of R-SCG device. Basic system design and implementation criteria are discussed and measurement results are shown. As an example, a system developed in the Simon Fraser University is discussed. On the other hand, the category of infrasonic cardiac signals has been investigated to further clarify the possible application of the recorded R-SCG signal in estimation of hemodynamic parameters.

Preliminary studies and measurements confirm that these systems can also be used to monitor cerebral blood flow, arterial blood flow and blood flow in bones. Compared to the conventional ultrasound methods, Microwave Doppler radar offers the advantage of ability to detect blood flow under bony tissues. A feasibility analysis for measuring cerebral blood flow using Microwave Doppler radar based devices can be found in (Jalali Mazlouman et al., 2009).

Although there are a variety of applications for vital signals monitoring where movement is not an issue, such as avalanche victims, and wireless monitoring of patients in a hospital or the elderly overnight, future work should focus on methods to detect and classify body movements, as also recommended in (Michahelles et al., 2004). For this purpose, more elaborate signal processing methods can be used to decrease the effects of the motion artefacts due to other body motions or movements of objects in the surrounding (Morgan & zierdt, 2009). To name a few, multiple antenna methods are recommended in (Li et al., 2009), to eliminate the noise caused by random body movements and clutter. A more recently used parametric and cyclic optimization algorithm, referred to as RELAX algorithm is suggested in (Li & Stocia, 1996) for spectral analysis of the captured signals. Blind source separation techniques using direct conversion Doppler radar and multiple antennas are recommended in (Vergara et al., 2008) to suppress the effect of other body motions and to capture real-time

Cardiopulmonary signals. Random body movement cancellation methods using complex quadrature demodulation and arctangent demodulation techniques are presented in (Li & Lin, 2008).

6. Acknowledgement

We would like to thank Alireza Akhbardeh and Brandon Ngai for helping us in preparation of this chapter.

7. References

Akhbardeh, A.; Junnila, S.; Koivuluoma, M.; Koivistoinen, T.; Turjanmaa, V. Kööbi, T.; Värri, A. (2007) Towards a Heart Disease Diagnosing System based on Force Sensitive chair's measurement, Biorthogonal Wavelets and Neural Network classifiers. *Engineering Applications on Artificial Intelligence*, Vol. 20, Issue 4, pp. 493.

Akhbardeh, A.; Tavakolian, K.; Gurev, V.; Lee, T.; New. W.; Kaminska, B.; Trayanova, N. (2009). Comparative Analysis of Three Different Modalities for Characterization of the Seismocardiogram" submitted to *31st IEEE Engineering in Medicine and Biology conference 2009.*

Bruch, C.; Schmermund, A.; Marin, D.; Katz, M.; Bartel, T.; Schaar, J.; Erbel, R; (2000). Tei-Index in patients with mild-to-moderate congestive heart failure. *European Heart Journal* (2000) 21, 1888–1895.

Castiglioni, P.; Faini, A.; Parati, G.; Rienzo, M.D. (2007). Wearable Seismocardiography. 29th IEEE EMBS, Lyon, France, August 2007, pp 3954-3958.

Chen, K.; Misra, D.; Wang, H.; Chuang, H. & Postow, E. (1986). An X-Band Microwave Life-Detection System. *Biomedical Engineering, IEEE Trans.*, BME-33, no.7, pp.697-701, July 1986.

Chia, M. Y. W.; Leong, S. W.; Sim, C. K. & Chan, K. M. (2005). Through-wall UWB radar operating within FCC's mask for sensing heart beat and breathing rate. *Microwave Conf., European*, Vol.3, pp. 4-6, Oct. 2005.

Crow, R.S.; Hannan, P.; Jacobs, D.; Hadquist, L. Salerno D.M. (1994). Relationship between Seismocardiogram and Echocardiogram for Events in Cardiac Cycle., *American Journal of Noninvasive Cardiology*, Vol. 8, pp.39-46, 1994.

Droitcour, A.; Lubecke, V.; Jenshan Lin & Boric-Lubecke, O. (2001). A microwave radio for Doppler radar sensing of vital signs. *Microwave Symp. Digest, 2001 IEEE MTT-S Int.*, Vol.1, pp.175-178, 2001.

Dutta, P.K.; Arora, A.K.& Bibyk, S.B. (2006). Towards radar-enabled sensor networks. *5th Int. Conf. on Information Processing in Sensor Networks (IPSN)*, Nashville, Tennessee, USA, April 2006.

FCC (2002), Federal Communications Commission, *Revision of part 15 of the commission's rules regarding ultra wideband transmission systems*. April 2002, www.fcc.gov/Bureaus/Engineering _Technology/Orders/2002/fcc02048.pdf.

Greneker, E.F. (1997). Radar Sensing of Heartbeat and Respiration at a Distance with Applications of the Technology, *IEEE Conference on Radars*, UK, pp 150-154, 1997.

Geisheimer, J.; Greneker, G. (1999). Applications of neural networks to the radarcardiogram (RCG), SPIE Conference on Applications and Science of Computational Intelligence Orlando, Florida, April 1999, SPIE Vol. 3722.

Heart and Stroke (2004), http://www.heartandstroke.com/site/c.ikIQLcMWJtE/b.3483991/k.34A8/Statistics.htm#heartdisease

Inan, O.T.; Etemadi, M.; Wiard, R. M.; Kovacs, G. T. A. & Giovangrandi, L. (2008). Non-Invasive Monitoring of Valsalva-Induced Hemodynamic Changes Using a Bathroom ScaleBallistocardiograph," *30th Annual IEEE Engineering in Medicine and Biology Conference*, Vancouver, B.C., August, 2008.

Jalali Mazlouman, S.; Mahanfar, A. & Kaminska, B. (2009). Contact less Monitoring of the major blood vessels supplying head and brain (Carotid Arteries). *Nanotech09*, Houston, Texas, May 2009.

Jauchem, J.R.; Seaman, R.L.; Lehnert, H.M.; Mathur, S.P.; Ryan, K.L.; Frei, M.R. & Hurt, W.D. (1998). Ultra-wideband electromagnetic pulses: lack of effects on heart-rate and blood pressure during two-minute exposures of rats. *Bio-electromagnetics*, vol. 19, No. 5, pp. 330-333, 1998.

Jensen, B.H.; Larsen B.H. & Shankar,K. Monitoring of the Ballistocardiograph with the Static Charge Sensetive Bed (1991). *IEEE Transaction on Biomedical Engineering*, Vol. 38, No. 8, August 1991.

Junnila, S.; Akhbardeh, A. & Värri, A. (2008). An Electromechanical Film Sensor Based Wireless Ballistocardiographic Chair: Implementation and Performance, Journal of Signal Processing Systems, Springer New York, pp. November 11, 2008

Kim, J.S.; Chee, Y.J.; Park, J.W.; Choi, J.W.; Park, K.S. (2006). A new approach for non-intrusive monitoring of blood pressure on a toilet seat. *Journal of Physiological Measurement*, Institute of Physics 27 (2006) 203–211.

Li, C. & Lin, J. (2008). Random Body Movement Cancellation in Doppler Radar Vital Sign Detection, *Microwave Theory and Techniques, IEEE Trans.*, Vol.56, No.12, pp.3143-3152, Dec. 2008.

Li, C.; Cummings, J.; Lam, J.; Graves, E. & Wu, W. (2009). Radar Remote Monitoring of Vital Signs. *Microwave Magazine, IEEE* , Vol.10, No.1, pp.47-56, Feb. 2009.

Lin, J.C. (1975). Non-invasive Microwave Measurement of Respiration, *Proceedings of the IEEE*, vol. 63, pp. 1530, 1975.

Li J. & Stoica, P. (1996). Efficient mixed-spectrum estimation with applications to target feature extraction, *Signal Processing, IEEE Trans.*, Vol.44, No.2, pp.281-295, Feb 1996.

Lin, J.C.; Kiernicki, J.; Kiernicki, M. & Wollschlaeger, P.B. (1979). Microwave Apexcardiography, *Microwave Theory and Techniques, IEEE Trans.*, vol.27, no.6, pp. 618-620, Jun 1979.

Lohman, B.; Boric-Lubecke, O.; Lubecke, V.M.; Ong, P.W. & Sondhi, M.M. (2002). A Digital Signal Processor for Doppler Radar Sensing of Vital Signs. *IEEE Engineering in Medicine and Biology*, 2002.

Lubecke, V.; Boric-Lubecke, O. & Beck, E. (2002). A compact low-cost add-on module for Doppler radar sensing of vital signs using a wireless communications terminal. *Microwave Symp. Digest, IEEE MTT-S Int.*, Vol.3, pp.1767-1770, 2002.

McEwan, T. E. (1994). Ultra-wideband radar motion sensor.*US Patents* #5361070, 1994.

McKay, W.P.S.; Gregon, P.H.; McKay, B.; Militzer, J; (1999) Sternal Acceleration Ballistocardiography and Arterial Pressure Wave Analysis to Determine Stroke Volume. Clin Invest Med; 22(1), pages 4-14, 1999.

Meyerhoff, N.J. (2007). Intrusion Detection by Ultra-Wide Bandwidth Radar. *Technologies for Homeland Security, IEEE Conf.*, pp.81-84, 16-17 May 2007.

Michahelles, F.; Wicki, R. & Schiele, B. (2004). Less contact: Heart-rate Detection Without Even Touching the User, *Proceedings of Wearable Computers (ISWC 2004) 8th Int. Symp.*, vol.1, pp. 4-7, 31 Oct.-3 Nov. 2004.

Morgan, D.R. & Zierdt, M.G. (2009). Novel Signal Processing Techniques for Doppler Radar Cardiopulmonary Sensing, *Signal Processing J.*, Vol. 89, No.1, Jan. 2009, pp. 45-66, ISSN 0165-1684, DOI: 10.1016/j.sigpro.2008.07.008.

Norsworthy, S. R.; Schreier, R., & Temes G. C. (1996). *Delta-Sigma Data Conversions*, Wiley-IEEE Press, ISBN: 978-0780310452.

Ngai, B.; Tavakolian, K.; Akhbardeh, A.; Blaber, A.P.; and Kaminska, B. Comparative Analysis of Seismocardiogram Waves with the Ultra-Low Frequency Ballistocardiogram. Submitted to 31st *IEEE Engineering in Medicine and Biology conference 2009.*

Park, B.K.; Boric-Lubecke, O.; Lubecke, V.M. (2007). Arctangent Demodulation With DC Offset Compensation in Quadrature Doppler Radar Receiver Systems, *Microwave Theory and Techniques, IEEE Trans.*, Vol.55, No.5, pp.1073-1079, May 2007.

Salerno, D.; Zanetti, J. (1990a). Seismocardiography: A new technique for recording cardiac vibration. Concept, method and initial observation", *J Cardiovasc Technol*, Vol. 9, pp. 111–117, 1990.

Salerno, D.; Zanetti, J.; Green, L. (1990b). Qualitative exercise seismocardiography for detection of moderate and severe multivessel coronary artery disease. *J Am Coll Cardiol* 1990; 15:44A.

Scarborough, W.R.; Talbot, S.A. (1956) proposal for ballistocardiographic nomenclature and conventions: revised and extended. Circulation 1956;14:435-50.

Skolnik, M.I. (1990), *Radar Handbook*, 2nd Ed., R-SCGraw-Hill, New York, 1990.

Staderini, E.M. (2002a). UWB radars in medicine. *Aerospace and Electronic Systems Magazine, IEEE*, Vol. 17, No.1, pp. 13-18, Jan 2002.

Starr, I.; Noordergraaf, A. (1967) *Ballistocardiography in Cardiovascular Research.* Philadelphia: Lippincott, 1967.

Staderini, E.M. (2002b). An UWB radar based stealthy 'lie detector'. *Second Virtual Congress of HRV Scientific Material,* 2002.

Such, O., et al. (2006). On-body sensors for personal healthcare, in B. Spekowius and T. Wendler editors, *Advances in Health Care Technology: Shaping the Future of Medical Care*, Vol. 6, pp. 436–488, Springer, 2006.

Tavakolian, K.; Zadeh, F.M.; Chuo, Y.; Vaseghi, A. & Kaminska, B. (2008a). Development of a Novel Contactless Mechanocardiograph Device. *Int. J. Telemedicine Appl.*, 2008:436870.

Tavakolian, K.; Vaseghi, A.; Kaminska, B. (2008b). "Improvement of ballistocardiogram processing by inclusion of respiration information" *Journal of Physiological Measurement*, Institute of Physics, 29 (2008) 771-781.

Thansandote, A.; Stuchly, S.S.; Smith A.M. (1983). Monitoring variations of biological impedances using microwave Doppler radar. *Physics in Medicine & Biology*, 1983.

Thijs, J.A.J.; Muehlsteff, J.; Such, O.; Pinter, R.; Elfring, R. & Igney, C.H. (2005). A Comparison of Continuous Wave Doppler Radar to Impedance Cardiography for Analysis of Mechanical Heart Activity, *Engineering in Medicine and Biology Society (IEEE-EMBS), 27th Annual Int. Conf.*, Sep. 2005.

Subspace Techniques for Brain Signal Enhancement

Nidal S. Kamel and Mohd Zuki-Yusoff
Universiti Teknologi Petronas
Malaysia

1. Introduction

Human bodies can be considered as electrical generators that produce various biomedical signals. Examples of the biomedical signals that can be generated by the brain are evoked potentials, which include visual evoked potentials (VEPs), brainstem auditory evoked potentials (BAEPs), and somatosensory evoked potentials (SSEPs). In clinical environments, these potentials are used by clinicians as *signatures* to check the nerve signals (vision-, hearing-, or feel-triggered) that are transmitted to the brain and spinal cord.

Extracting the evoked potentials (EPs) from the brain is generally very difficult. The problem is caused by the presence of the spontaneous electroencephalograph (EEG) which contaminates heavily the desired signals. The ongoing EEG can be considered as colored noise since its frequency spectrum overlaps with that of the wanted signals. The EEG may degrade the overall signal-to-noise ratio (SNR) to as low as -10 dB (Regan, 1989; Henning, 1995).

The conventional method of "multi-trial" ensemble averaging (EA) does improve the SNR, but at the expense of longer recording time causing discomfort and fatigue to the subject under study. In fact, hundreds of response trials need to be gathered to obtain a satisfactorily clean estimate of EPs. Most importantly, EA introduces significant distortion and information loss since EPs are time varying (i.e., non-stationary) signals (Cui et al., 2004). In other words, since the waveform morphology (i.e., amplitude and shape) is not constant from one trial to another as experimented by (John et al., 1964), the averaging techniques tend to eliminate the trial-to-trial variations of the VEP signals which may prove useful to clinicians and other researchers.

For EP estimation, researchers have proposed various techniques utilizing different sorts of averaging and filtering which include Kalman filtering, Wiener filtering, wavelets, cumulants, etc. In this chapter, we discuss the subspace based EP extraction techniques and their potentials as single-trial estimators to replace the multi-trial based ones.

In subspace techniques for signal enhancement, the eigendecomposition of the covariance matrix of the noisy signal is used to decompose the matrix space into signal and noise subspaces. Retaining only the information in the signal subspace eigenvectors, that is, forming a lower-rank approximation of the covariance matrix effectively enhances the SNR because of the omission of the contribution of power in noise subspace. Many subspace techniques have been proposed over the last decade for EP extraction using the signal subspace, with different degrees of success. In this chapter, we outline the foundations of the proposed subspace techniques, through the aspects of bio-signal model development, creation and/or selection of the pertinent vector(s) and/or matrices, contaminated signal decorrelation and desired signal reconstruction processes. Three subspace techniques, especially designed for EP extraction, are discussed and compared in performance. The techniques are the generalized subspace approach (GSA) (Nidal-Kamel & Zuki-Yusoff, 2008), the subspace regularization method (SRM) (Karjalainen et al., 1999), and the subspace dynamical estimation method (SDEM) (Georgiadis et al., 2007). Furthermore, a criterion for defining the signal subspace dimension is suggested and analyzed.

The chapter is organized as follows. The fundamental concepts of subspace techniques are presented in section 2. The three subspace techniques namely GSA, SRM and SDEM are discussed in section 3. Section 4 describes the results in simulated and real environments and section 5 concludes the chapter.

For clarity, an attempt has been made to adhere to a standard notational convention. Lower case **boldface** characters will generally refer to vectors. Upper case **BOLDFACE** characters will generally refer to matrices. Vector or matrix transposition will be denoted using $(.)^T$ and $(.)^*$ denotes conjugation for complex valued signals. $\Re^{K \times K}$ denotes the real vector space of $K \times K$ dimensions.

2. Fundamental Concepts of Subspace Techniques

Consider $\boldsymbol{A} \in \Re^{MxM}$ as the autocorrelation matrix of the noisy EP signal. It has been found in many signal processing applications that the eigendecomposition of the matrix $\boldsymbol{A}$ can be used to decompose the matrix space into principal or signal subspace and noise subspace. This distinctive separation can be used to improve methods of signal enhancement and signal parameter estimation.

Principal component analysis, originating in work by Karl Pearson around the turn of the last century and further developed in 1930s by Harold Hoteling, consists of finding an orthogonal transformation of the original - stochastic- variables to a new set of uncorrelated variables, which are derived in non-increasing order of importance. These so-called principal components are linear combinations of the original variables such that their first few components will account for most of the variations in the original data, effectively reducing the dimensionality of the data (Deprettere, 1989). Since, the concept of oriented energy is closely related to principal components analysis, we start our work using this definition.

2.1 Oriented Energy

The column vectors of an $M \times M$ matrix $\boldsymbol{A}$ are considered to form an indexed set of M vectors, denoted by $\{\boldsymbol{a}_k\}$, $k = 1, 2, \ldots, M$. An M-dimensional vector $\boldsymbol{q}$ and the direction it represents in a vector space are used as synonyms.

Definition 1. Energy of a vector sequence.

Consider a sequence of M-vectors $\{\boldsymbol{a}_k\}$, $k = 1, 2, \ldots, M$ and associated real $M \times M$ matrix $\boldsymbol{A}$. Its total energy $E[\boldsymbol{A}]$ is defined via Frobenius norm of the $M \times M$ matrix $\boldsymbol{A}$:

$$E(\boldsymbol{A}) = \|\boldsymbol{A}\|_F^2 = \sum_{i=1}^{M} \sum_{j=1}^{M} \boldsymbol{a}_{ij}^2 \tag{1}$$

Definition 2. Oriented energy.

Let $\boldsymbol{A}$ be an $M \times M$ matrix and denote its M column vectors as $\boldsymbol{a}_k$, $k = 1, 2, \ldots, M$. For the indexed vector set $\{\boldsymbol{a}_k\}$ of M-vectors $\boldsymbol{a}_k \in \Re^M$ and for any unit vector $\boldsymbol{q} \in \Re^M$, the energy E_q measured in direction $\boldsymbol{q}$, is defined as:

$$E_q(\boldsymbol{A}) = \sum_{k=1}^{M} (q^T \bullet \boldsymbol{a}_k)^2 \tag{2}$$

More generally, the energy E_Q measured in a subspace $Q \subset \Re^M$, is defined as:

$$E_Q(\boldsymbol{A}) = \sum_{k=1}^{M} \|P_Q(\boldsymbol{a}_k)\|^2 \tag{3}$$

where $P_Q(\boldsymbol{a}_k)$ denotes the orthogonal projection of $\boldsymbol{a}_k$ into the subspace Q and $\|\cdot\|$ denotes the Euclidean norm. In other words, the oriented energy of a vector sequence $\{\boldsymbol{a}_k\}$, measured in the direction $\boldsymbol{q}$ (subspace Q) is the energy of the signal, projected orthogonally on to the vector $\boldsymbol{q}$ (subspace Q).

2.2 Oriented Energy and Eigendecomposition of $A \in \Re^{MxM}$

In section 2.1, attention was given to the basic concepts of the oriented energy distribution. In this section, the tools which allow numerical characterization of the oriented energy concept will be studied.

The eigenvalue decomposition (ED) of matrix $\boldsymbol{A} \in \Re^{MxM}$, is a factorization process where a diagonalizable matrix is represented in terms of its eigenvectors and eigenvalues. The eigenvectors are represented by a non-singular matrix whose columns represent individual eigenvectors that are orthonormal to each other. The eigenvectors' corresponding eigenvalues are held and represented diagonally by a singular matrix.

Theorem 1. Let the columns $v_1, v_2, \ldots, v_M$ be the eigenvectors corresponding to the set of eigenvalues $\lambda_1, \lambda_2, \ldots, \lambda_M$ of the square basis matrix $\boldsymbol{A} \in \Re^{MxM}$. Let $\boldsymbol{V} \in \Re^{MxM}$ be the matrix that holds the eigenvectors such that

$$\boldsymbol{V} = \begin{bmatrix} v_1 & v_2 & \cdots & v_M \end{bmatrix} \in \mathcal{R}^{M \times M} \tag{4}$$

and Λ be the diagonal that holds the eigenvalue entries such that

$$\Lambda = diag\begin{bmatrix} \lambda_1 & \lambda_2 & \cdots & \lambda_M \end{bmatrix} \tag{5}$$

in which, the eigenvalues have been ordered in decreasing values $\lambda_1 \geq \lambda_2 \geq \cdots \lambda_M$. Then the matrix $\boldsymbol{A}$ will have a linearly independent set of M eigenvectors if and only if $\boldsymbol{A}$ can be expressed as

$$\boldsymbol{A} = \boldsymbol{V}\Lambda\boldsymbol{V}^{-1} \tag{6}$$

If the nonsingular matrix $\boldsymbol{A}$ also has Hermitian symmetry, then $\boldsymbol{V}^{-1} = \boldsymbol{V}^H$ and $\Lambda = \Lambda^H$. This means that a Hermitian matrix has real eigenvalues and that, if all the eigenvalues are distinct, the eigenvectors form an orthogonal set, because $\boldsymbol{V}\boldsymbol{V}^H = \sum v_i v_i^H = \boldsymbol{I}$, that is, $\boldsymbol{V}$ is a unitary matrix. Thus the Hermitian matrix $\boldsymbol{A}$ which is diagonalized by a unitary transformation, will have the unique eigendecomposition (ED)

$$\boldsymbol{A} = \boldsymbol{V}\Lambda\boldsymbol{V}^H \tag{7}$$

Proof. A proof of the ED theorem is given in (Golub & Van Loan, 1989).

Lemma 1: The number of non-zero eigenvalues is equal to the algebraic rank of the matrix $\boldsymbol{A}$.

Lemma 2: Via the ED, the matrix $\boldsymbol{A}$ can be written as the sum of r = rank($\boldsymbol{A}$) rank-one matrices; that is

$$\boldsymbol{A} = \sum_{i=1}^{r} v_i \lambda_i v_i^{-1} \tag{8}$$

where $(v_i, \lambda_i, v_i^{-1})$ is the ith eigen triplet of $\boldsymbol{A}$.

Lemma 3: The Frobenius norm of $\boldsymbol{A} \in \Re^{MxM}$ of rank r is

$$\|\boldsymbol{A}\|_F^2 = \sum_{i=1}^{M}\sum_{j=1}^{M} a_{ij}^2 = \sum_{k=1}^{r} \lambda_k \tag{9}$$

where λ_k are the eigenvalues of $\boldsymbol{A}$.

The total energy in a vector sequence $\{\boldsymbol{a}_k\}$ associated with matrix $\boldsymbol{A}$, as stated in Definition 1, is equal to the energy in the eigenspectrum.

The smallest non-zero eigenvalue corresponds to the distance (in Frobenius norm) of the matrix to the closest matrix of lower rank. This property makes ED attractive tool in segregating the signal subspace from the noise subspace.

2.2.1 Conceptual relations between ED and oriented energy

We are now in the position to establish the link between the eigendecomposition and the concept of oriented energy distribution.

Define the unit ball UB in $\Re^M$ as $\text{UB} = \left\{ q \in \Re^M \middle| \, \|q\|_2 = 1 \right\}$.

Theorem 2. Consider a sequence of M-vectors $\{a_k\}$, $k = 1, 2, \ldots, M$ and the associated $M \times M$ matrix $\boldsymbol{A}$ with ED as defined in Eq. (6). Then,

$$E_{v_i}(\boldsymbol{A}) = \lambda_i \tag{10}$$

$\forall q \in \text{UB}$: if $q = \sum_{i=1}^{M} \gamma_i \cdot v_i$, then

$$E_q(\boldsymbol{A}) = \sum_{i=1}^{M} \gamma_i \cdot \lambda_i \tag{11}$$

Proof. Trivial from Theorem 1.

Based on Theorem 2, the following observations can be made:

- The oriented energy measured in the direction of the ith eigenvector of $\boldsymbol{A}$ is equal to the ith eigenvalue.
- The energy in an arbitrary direction q is the linear combination of the "orthogonal" oriented energies associated with the eigenvectors. If $\boldsymbol{A}$ is rank deficient, then there exists directions in $\Re^M$ that contains no energy at all.

Furthermore, Theorem 2 can be used to obtain the directions and spaces of extremal energies.

Corollary 1: Under the assumptions of Theorem 2, the following properties follow:

Property 1 $\quad \max_{q \in \text{UB}} E_q(\boldsymbol{A}) = E_{v_1}(\boldsymbol{A}) = \lambda_1$

Property 2 $\quad \min_{q \in \text{UB}} E_q(\boldsymbol{A}) = E_{v_M}(\boldsymbol{A}) = \lambda_M$

Property 3 $\quad \max_{Q^r \subset \Re^M} E_{Q^r}(\boldsymbol{A}) = E_{S_V^r}(\boldsymbol{A}) = \sum_{i=1}^{r} \lambda_i$

Property 4 $$\min_{Q^r \subset \Re^M} E_{Q^r}(\boldsymbol{A}) = E_{\left(S_V^{M-r}\right)^{\perp}}(\boldsymbol{A}) = \sum_{i=M-r+1}^{M} \lambda_i$$

where "max" and "min" denote operators, respectively maximizing or minimizing the overall r-dimensional subspace Q^r of $\Re^M$; S_V^r is the r-dimensional principal subspace of $\boldsymbol{A}$; and $\left(S_V^{M-r}\right)^{\perp}$ represents the R-dimensional orthogonal complement of S_V^{M-r}.

Proof. Properties 1 through 4 follow immediately from the ED Theorems 1 and 2.

In words, Properties 1and 2 relate the ED to the minima and maxima of the oriented energy distribution. The r-th principal subspace S_V^r is the one, among all r-dimensional subspaces of $\Re^M$, that senses a maximal oriented energy (Property 3). Properties 3 and 4 show that the orthogonal decomposition of the energy via the eigenvalue decomposition is canonical in the sense that it allows subspaces of dimension r to be found where the sequence has minimal and maximal energy. This decomposition of the ambient space, as the direct sum of a space of maximal and minimal energy for a given vector sequence, leads to very interesting rank consideration.

Now, if $\boldsymbol{A}$ ($M\times M$) represents the autocorrelation matrix of data corrupted by additive white noise, then it can be written as

$$\boldsymbol{A} = \boldsymbol{S} + \boldsymbol{N} \tag{12}$$

in which **S** is the signal correlation matrix and $\boldsymbol{N}$ is the noise autocorrelation matrix, given in the case of white noise as

$$\boldsymbol{N} = \sigma^2 \boldsymbol{I} \tag{13}$$

where σ^2 is the noise variance.

The signal matrix will have the eigendecomposition

$$\boldsymbol{S} = \sum_{i=1}^{r} \lambda_i \boldsymbol{v}_i \boldsymbol{v}_i^H \tag{14}$$

The eigenvectors $v_1, v_2, \ldots, v_r$, known as the principal subspace (as previously indicated), span the same signal subspace.

The noise matrix has the eigendecomposition

$$\boldsymbol{N} = \sum_{i=r+1}^{M} \lambda_i \boldsymbol{v}_i \boldsymbol{v}_i^H = \sigma^2 \sum_{i=r+1}^{M} \boldsymbol{v}_i \boldsymbol{v}_i^H \tag{15}$$

Substitution of Eqs. (14) and (15) into Eq. (12) yields the eigendecomposition of the autocorrelation matrix

$$\boldsymbol{A} = \sum_{i=1}^{r} \lambda_i v_i v_i^H + \sigma^2 \sum_{i=r+1}^{M} v_i v_i^H = \sum_{i=1}^{r} \left(\lambda_i + \sigma^2\right) v_i v_i^H + \sum_{i=r+1}^{M} \sigma^2 v_i v_i^H \tag{16}$$

Thus, the eigenvectors $v_{r+1}, v_{r+2}, \ldots, v_M$, span the noise subspace of $\boldsymbol{A}$, all with the identical eigenvalue σ^2. The principal eigenvectors $v_1, v_2, \ldots, v_r$ span the signal subspace of both $\boldsymbol{A}$ and **S**, with eigenvalues of $\lambda_1 + \sigma^2, \lambda_2 + \sigma^2, \cdots, \lambda_r + \sigma^2$.

The eigendecomposition of the autocorrelation matrix in Eq. (16) can be exploited in the following way to generate improved signal estimators. Retaining only the information in the signal subspace eigenvectors, that is, forming a lower-rank approximation of $\boldsymbol{A}$, effectively enhances the SNR because of the omission of the contribution of power in the noise subspace components. This is the basis of principal component (signal subspace) signal estimators.

Having established the link between the principal subspace (signal subspace) and the maximal energy of the signal, and between the noise subspace and the energy of the noise, we are in a position to show how this link is utilized by the different subspace techniques for EP enhancement.

3. The Subspace Techniques

3.1 The Generalized Subspace Approach

The generalized subspace approach (GSA) was proposed by (Nidal-Kamel & Zuki-Yusoff, 2008) as a subspace technique for EP signal enhancement in colored noise environment. This approach is an extension of (Ephraim & Van Trees, 1995) towards colored noise without the need for prewhitening. Other variations of subspace approaches to extract EPs can be found in (Zuki-Yusoff et al., 2009; Zuki-Yusoff et al., 2008; Zuki-Yusoff et al., 2007). The considered problem is to extract the clean EP signal $x(t)$ from the degraded EP signal by the brain background colored noise, $y(t)$. A K-dimensional vector of VEP samples $\boldsymbol{y}$ is defined as follows:

$$\boldsymbol{y}(k) = \left[y\left(\frac{0}{f_s}\right), y\left(\frac{1}{f_s}\right), \cdots, y\left(\frac{K-1}{f_s}\right) \right]^T \tag{17}$$

where f_s is the sampling frequency and $(.)^T$ denotes the transpose operation. Also, let $\boldsymbol{y}$ denote the corresponding K-dimensional vector of the noisy EP. Since noise is assumed to be additive, we have

$$\boldsymbol{y}(k) = \boldsymbol{x}(k) + \boldsymbol{n}(k) \tag{18}$$

where $\boldsymbol{x}$ is the K-dimensional vector of the original (clean) EP signal, and $\boldsymbol{n}$ is the K-dimensional noise vector. Now, let $\boldsymbol{H}$ be a $K \times K$ linear estimator of the clean EP vector as follows:

$$\hat{\boldsymbol{x}}(k) = \boldsymbol{H}(k) \bullet \boldsymbol{y}(k) \tag{19}$$

It is to be noted that the time index k shown in Eqs. (18) and (19) is for comprehensiveness and clarity. In the subsequent discussions, any vector or matrix that appears without a time index should be visualized as having k as its time index.

The error signal obtained in this estimation is given by

$$\begin{aligned}\varepsilon &= \hat{x} - x \\ &= Hy - x \\ &= (H - I)x + Hn \\ &= \varepsilon_x + \varepsilon_n \qquad \text{where } \varepsilon_x = (H - I)x \quad \text{and } \varepsilon_n = Hn\end{aligned} \tag{20}$$

where ε_x represents signal distortion and ε_n represents residual signal. Let

$$\begin{aligned}\bar{\varepsilon}_x^2 &= E\{\varepsilon_x^T \varepsilon_x\} = \mathrm{tr}\left(E\{\varepsilon_x \varepsilon_x^T\}\right) \\ &= \mathrm{tr}\left((H - I)R_x (H - I)^T\right)\end{aligned} \tag{21}$$

be the energy of the signal distortion vector. Similarly, let

$$\begin{aligned}\bar{\varepsilon}_n^2 &= E\{\varepsilon_n^T \varepsilon_n\} = \mathrm{tr}\left(E\{\varepsilon_n \varepsilon_n^T\}\right) \\ &= \mathrm{tr}\left(HR_n H^T\right)\end{aligned} \tag{22}$$

denote the energy of the residual noise, so that the total residual energies $\bar{\varepsilon}^2$ become

$$\bar{\varepsilon}^2 = \bar{\varepsilon}_x^2 + \bar{\varepsilon}_n^2 \tag{23}$$

The terms R_x and R_n in Eq. (21) and Eq. (22) refer to the covariance matrices of the clean signal and noise vectors, respectively. Since the EP and noise signals are independent as illustrated in Eq. (18), their covariance matrices also add linearly to produce the covariance matrix of the noisy EP R_y; that is,

$$R_y = R_x + R_n \tag{24}$$

In practice, the covariance matrix of the noisy signal R_y can be estimated directly from the observed (noisy) EP samples. Also, the noise covariance matrix R_n can be computed using the pre-stimulation EEG samples during which the EP signals are absent. Indirectly, R_x can be calculated by subtracting R_n from R_y. Now that R_x and R_n are known, the optimum linear estimator with time domain constraints on the residual noise is defined as follows (Ephraim & Van Trees, 1995):

$$H_{opt} = \min_{H} \ \bar{\varepsilon}_x^2 \qquad \text{subject to} : \bar{\varepsilon}_n^2 \le K\sigma^2 \tag{25}$$

where K is the dimension of the noisy vector space and σ^2 is a positive constant noise threshold level. The σ^2 in Eq. (25) dictates the amount of the residual noise allowed to remain in the linear estimator. Reducing noise in the given noisy EP signal causes some distortion in the extracted EP components. In the above optimization, by decreasing the noise threshold level σ^2, we can decrease the amount of the residual noise and therefore, increase the amount of distortion and vice versa. Therefore, an acceptable value of σ^2 needs to be chosen so that the EP signal distortion is minimal and the EEG colored noise residue is not excessive. The optimal distortion in the sense of Eq. (25) can be found using *Kuhn-Tucker* necessary conditions for constrained minimization. Specifically, H is a stationary feasible point and hence a minimizer, if it satisfies the gradient equation of the Lagrangian

$$L(\boldsymbol{H}, \mu) = \overline{\boldsymbol{\varepsilon}}_x^2 + \mu(\overline{\boldsymbol{\varepsilon}}_n^2 - K\sigma^2) \tag{26}$$

and

$$\mu(\overline{\boldsymbol{\varepsilon}}_n^2 - K\sigma^2) = 0 \quad \text{for } \mu \geq 0 \tag{27}$$

where μ is the Lagrangian multiplier. By setting the gradient equation $\nabla_{\boldsymbol{H}} L(\boldsymbol{H}, \mu) = 0$, we obtain

$$\begin{aligned} &\frac{\partial L(\boldsymbol{H}, \mu)}{\partial \boldsymbol{H}} = 0 \\ &\Rightarrow \frac{\partial}{\partial \boldsymbol{H}}[\text{tr}\left((\boldsymbol{H} - \boldsymbol{I})\boldsymbol{R}_x(\boldsymbol{H} - \boldsymbol{I})^T\right)] + \frac{\partial}{\partial \boldsymbol{H}}[\mu\text{tr}\left(\boldsymbol{H}\boldsymbol{R}_n\boldsymbol{H}^T\right)] = 0 \\ &\Rightarrow (\boldsymbol{H} - \boldsymbol{I})\boldsymbol{R}_x + \mu\boldsymbol{H}\boldsymbol{R}_n = 0 \\ &\Rightarrow \boldsymbol{H}(\boldsymbol{R}_x + \mu\boldsymbol{R}_n) - \boldsymbol{R}_x = 0 \end{aligned} \tag{28}$$

Subsequently, the gradient equation in Eq. (28) fulfilling Eq. (25) can be solved to yield the following estimator

$$\boldsymbol{H} = \boldsymbol{R}_x(\boldsymbol{R}_x + \mu\boldsymbol{R}_n)^{-1} \tag{29}$$

Next, the values for μ and σ^2 satisfying Eq. (27) need to be determined. Equation (27) can be simplified to yield

$$\overline{\boldsymbol{\varepsilon}}_n^2 = K\sigma^2 \tag{30}$$

The following expression for σ^2 is obtained by equating Eq. (30) with Eq. (22):

$$\begin{aligned} &\overline{\boldsymbol{\varepsilon}}_n^2 = K\sigma^2 = \text{tr}\left(\boldsymbol{H}\boldsymbol{R}_n\boldsymbol{H}^T\right) \\ &\Rightarrow \sigma^2 = \frac{1}{K}\text{tr}\left(\boldsymbol{H}\boldsymbol{R}_n\boldsymbol{H}^T\right) \end{aligned} \tag{31}$$

A meaningful relationship between σ^2 and μ is established by putting $\boldsymbol{H}$ computed in Eq. (29) into Eq. (31).

$$\sigma^2 = \frac{1}{K}\text{tr}\left(\boldsymbol{R}_x^2(\boldsymbol{R}_x + \mu\boldsymbol{R}_n)^{-2}\boldsymbol{R}_n\right) \tag{32}$$

One issue that arises from Eq. (32) is whether to first specify the permissible level of residual noise σ^2, or the Lagrange multiplier μ. The first approach is specify σ^2 in Eq. (32) and calculate μ from it. On the other hand, μ can be carefully chosen so that σ^2 can be calculated. Practically, the latter approach is normally used since μ can be computed without using Eq. (32) which is computationally expensive. Nonetheless, it is crucial to meet the necessary conditions stipulated in Eq. (32). From Eq. (32), we observe that $\sigma^2 \in [0, \sigma^2_{\max}]$ when $\mu \in [0, \infty]$, where $\sigma^2 = 0$ implies that $\mu = \infty$, and $\sigma^2 = \sigma^2_{max} = \frac{1}{K}\text{tr}(\boldsymbol{R}_n)$ yields $\mu = 0$. Therefore, μ which satisfies Eq. (32) also satisfies Eq. (27). Hence, μ must also be the Lagrange multiplier for the time-domain-constrained (TDC) optimization problem of

Eq. (25). Further, there is a sufficient condition to be satisfied in order for $\boldsymbol{H}$ to be a minimizer; that is, the following second derivative must be positive definite.

$$\begin{aligned} L''(\boldsymbol{H},\mu) &= \frac{\partial^2 L(\boldsymbol{H},\mu)}{\partial \boldsymbol{H}^2} \\ &= \boldsymbol{R}_x + \mu \boldsymbol{R}_n \end{aligned} \tag{33}$$

The noise covariance matrix $\boldsymbol{R}_n$ in Eq. (33) is always positive definite. However, it is not always the case for the signal covariance matrix $\boldsymbol{R}_x$, which is initially derived by subtracting $\boldsymbol{R}_n$ from $\boldsymbol{R}_y$. For a relatively high SNR, $\boldsymbol{R}_x$ is positive definite. As the SNR drops, $\boldsymbol{R}_x$ can be negative semidefinite. Nonetheless, μ is a positive number and $\boldsymbol{R}_n$ is still greater (for SNR < 0 dB) than $\boldsymbol{R}_x$ in any case, guaranteeing $\boldsymbol{L}''(\boldsymbol{H}, \mu)$ to be positive definite all the time and enabling $\boldsymbol{H}$ to be a minimizer.

It is clear that the filter matrix $\boldsymbol{H}$ derived in Eq. (29) is dependent on three parameters namely $\boldsymbol{R}_x$, $\boldsymbol{R}_n$ and μ. Without further manipulation, $\boldsymbol{H}$ stated in Eq. (29) will function as a fixed filter; it will perform well to estimate the desired signal for a relatively high SNR value. As the SNR value degrades, it is desirable if $\boldsymbol{H}$ can be adjusted accordingly to minimize the noise residues while keeping the signal distortion at a minimal level.

One possible way to achieve an adjustable $\boldsymbol{H}$ is by taking the eigendecomposition of the $\boldsymbol{R}_x$ and $\boldsymbol{R}_n$ terms in Eq. (29). When the $\boldsymbol{R}_x$ and $\boldsymbol{R}_n$ are represented by their respective eigenvectors and eigenvalues, the fixed filter matrix $\boldsymbol{H}$ then becomes adjustable. If the dimension of the $\boldsymbol{R}_x$ eigenvalues is not lowered, the filter $\boldsymbol{H}$ functions exactly as that denoted in Eq. (29) — keeping signal distortion to its very minimum and noise energy to its maximum. However, when the dimension of $\boldsymbol{R}_x$ is lowered to a certain rank, the filter $\boldsymbol{H}$ will eliminate certain noise portions. If the proper dimension L of the $\boldsymbol{R}_x$ eigenvalues is chosen such that L spans only the signal subspace, the component in the "noise only" subspace will get nulled. The component that remains available at the output of the filter $\boldsymbol{H}$ is the wanted signal from the "signal" subspace. Of course, the wanted signal may not be completely free from noise since the "signal" subspace is actually a "signal plus noise" subspace. Nevertheless, the wanted signal is now clearly visible as the SNR value gets improved due to the subspace filtering technique.

For colored noise, an explicit prewhitening stage is normally required to prewhiten the corrupted data. For example, the covariance matrix $\boldsymbol{R}_x$ can be explicitly whitened by multiplying it with the $\boldsymbol{R}_n^{-1/2}$ or $\boldsymbol{R}_n^{-1}$ term. Alternatively, the prewhitening process can be implicitly performed by means of the generalized eigendecomposition of $\boldsymbol{R}_x$ and $\boldsymbol{R}_n$ (Nidal-Kamel & Zuki-Yusoff, 2008). In other words, the eigendecomposition of a matrix can be generalized to a decomposition of the matrix pair $(\boldsymbol{R}_x,\boldsymbol{R}_n)$, as follows:

$$\boldsymbol{R}_x \boldsymbol{V} = \boldsymbol{R}_n \boldsymbol{V} \boldsymbol{\Lambda} \tag{34}$$

where $\boldsymbol{D}$ diagonal $K \times K$ matrix that contains the generalized eigenvalues $\boldsymbol{D}$ and $\boldsymbol{V}$ contains the generalized non-unitary eigenvectors. The following relationships are also established from the generalized ED:

$$R_x = V^{-T} D V^{-1} \tag{35}$$

$$R_n = V^{-T} I V^{-1} \tag{36}$$

An optimal estimator H_{GSA} based on the generalized subspace approach (GSA) can then be obtained by applying Eq. (35) and Eq. (36) to Eq. (29):

$$\begin{aligned} H_{GSA} &= V^{-T} D V^{-1} \left(V^{-T} D V^{-1} + \mu V^{-T} I V^{-1}\right)^{-1} \\ &= V^{-T} D (D + \mu I)^{-1} V^{+T} \\ &= V^{-T} G V^{T} \qquad \text{where } G = D(D + \mu I)^{-1} \end{aligned} \tag{37}$$

Based on Eq. (19) and Eq. (37), the EP is then estimated as

$$\begin{aligned} \hat{x} &= H_{GSA} \, . \, y \\ &= V^{-T} G V^{T} \cdot y \qquad \text{where } G = D(D + \mu I)^{-1} \end{aligned} \tag{38}$$

At a glance, the structure of Eq. (38) looks similar to the Karhunen Loeve transform (KLT) and inverse Karhunen Loeve transform (IKLT), with Eq. (38) having the extra signal subspace gain matrix G. However, the KLT and IKLT operation caters only for unitary eigenvectors. The eigenvectors V produced by the generalized ED process are not unitary; nevertheless, complete decorrelation is still achievable using these non-unitary eigenvectors. In brief, the corrupted VEP signal y in Eq. (38) is decorrelated by the non-KLT matrix V^T. Then, the transformed signal is modified by the matrix G. Next, the modified signal is retransformed back into the original form by the non-IKLT matrix V^{-T} to obtain the desired signal.

3.1.1 Configuration of critical parameters

In the GSA and other subspace techniques, there are several critical parameters that need to be configured properly to achieve optimized enhancement of the desired signal. Among the most important parameters requiring special attentions are frame length, correlation matrix dimension, and subspace dimension.

Frame length

The frame length is very important because it somehow dictates the dimension of the corresponding correlation matrix. In turn, the matrix size influences the statistical contents and the usefulness of the correlation matrix, which will be used later in the signal and noise separation. The frame length N must be larger than the order of the assumed signal model, or the dimension of the signal subspace. This is to ensure that a reasonable correlation matrix size bearing sufficient statistics can be generated from the given frame length. As a general rule, N should not be too small or too large. If N is too small, then the amount of statistical data in the correlation matrix will be affected; too large a value will be computationally expensive on the ED of the correlation matrix. In general, N is taken to be three to four times the order of the signal model.

Correlation matrix dimension

The correlation matrix dimension is carried out to $0.4m$ (rounded to the nearest integer) for each side of the autocorrelation curve shown in Fig. 1 below, where $-(N-1) \leq m \leq N-1$; N is the frame length and m is the distance or *lag* between data points. The region bounded by $-0.4m$ and $+0.4m$ contains majority of the statistical information about the signal under study. Beyond the shaded region the autocorrelation pairs at the positive and corresponding negative lags diminishes radically, making the calculation unreliable.

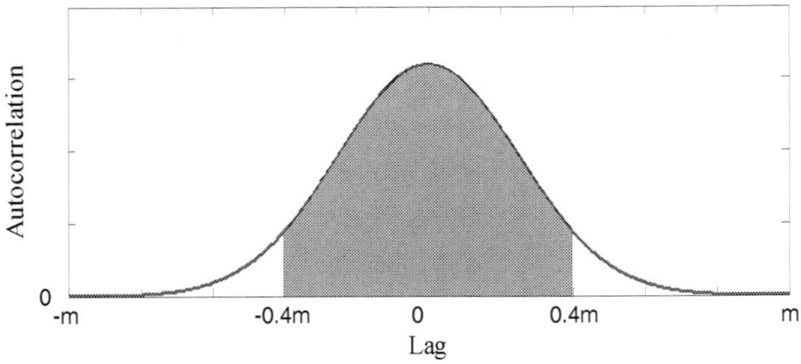

Fig. 1. The shaded area containing reliable statistical information for the correlation (covariance) matrix computation.

Dimension of signal subspace

In general, the dimension (i.e., rank) of the signal subspace is not known *a-priori*. The proper dimension of the signal subspace is critical since too low or too high an estimated dimension yield inaccurate VEP peaks. If the dimension chosen is too low, a highly smoothed spectral estimate of the VEP waveform is produced, affecting the accuracy of the desired peaks. On the other hand, too high a dimension introduces a spurious detail in the estimated VEP waveform, making the discrimination between the desired and unwanted peaks very difficult. It is crucial to note that as the SNR increases, the separation between the signal eigenvalues and the noise eigenvalues increases. In other words, for reasonably high SNRs (≥ 5dB), the signal subspace dimension can be readily obtained by observing the distinctive gap in the eigenvalue spectrum of the basis matrix covariance. As the SNR reduces, the gap gets less distinctive and the pertinent signal and noise eigenvalues may be significantly larger than zero.

As such, the choice of the dimension solely based on the non-zero eigenvalues as devised by some researchers tends to overestimate the actual dimension of the signal subspace. To overcome the dimension overestimation, some criteria need to be utilized so that the actual signal subspace dimension can be estimated more accurately, preventing information loss or suppressing unwanted details in the recovered signal. There exist many different approaches for information theoretic criteria for model identification purposes. Two well known approaches are Akaike information criteria (AIC) by (Akaike, 1973) and minimum description length (MDL) by (Schwartz, 1978) and (Rissanen, 1978). In this study, the criteria to be adapted is the AIC approach which has been extended by (Wax & Kailath, 1985) to handle the signal and noise subspace separation problem from the N snapshots of the corrupted signals. For our purpose, we consider only one snapshot (N = 1) of the contaminated signal at one particular time. Assuming that the eigenvalues of the observed signal (from one snapshot) are denoted as $\lambda_1 \geq \lambda_2 \geq \ldots \geq \lambda_p$, we obtain the following:

$$AIC(k) = 2\ln\left(\frac{\left[\frac{1}{P-k}\sum_{j=k+1}^{P}\lambda_j\right]^{P-k}}{\prod_{j=k+1}^{P}\lambda_j}\right) + 2k(2P-k) \tag{39}$$

The desired signal subspace dimension L is determined as the value of $k \in [0, P\text{–}1]$ for which the AIC is minimized.

3.1.2 The implementation of GSA technique

Step 1. Compute the covariance matrix of the brain background colored noise $\boldsymbol{R}_n$, using the pre-stimulation EEG sample.

Step 2. Compute the noisy VEP covariance matrix $\boldsymbol{R}_y$, using the post-stimulation EEG sample.

Step 3. Estimate the covariance matrix of the noiseless VEP sample as $\boldsymbol{R}_x = \boldsymbol{R}_y - \boldsymbol{R}_n$.

Step 4. Perform the generalized eigendecomposition on $\boldsymbol{R}_x$ and $\boldsymbol{R}_n$ to satisfy Eq. (34) and obtain the eigenvector matrix $\boldsymbol{V}$ and the eigenvalue matrix $\boldsymbol{D}$.

Step 5. Estimate the dimension L of the signal subspace using Eq. (39).

Step 6. Form a diagonal matrix $\boldsymbol{D}_L$, from the largest L diagonal values of $\boldsymbol{D}$.

Step 7. Form a matrix $\boldsymbol{V}_L$ by retaining only the eigenvectors of $\boldsymbol{V}$ that correspond to the largest L eigenvalues.

Step 8. Choose a proper value for μ as a compromise between signal distortion and noise residues. Experimentally, $\mu = 8$ is found to be ideal.

Step 9. Compute the optimal linear estimator as outlined in Eq. (37).

Step 10. Estimate the clean VEP signal using Eq. (38).

3.2 Subspace Regularization Method

The subspace regularization method (SRM) (Karjalainen et al., 1999) is combining regularization and Bayesian approaches for the extraction of EP signals from the measured data.

In SRM, a model for the EP utilizing a linear combination of some basis vectors as governed by Eq. (18), is used. Next, the linear observation model of Eq. (18) is further written as

$$y = H\theta + n \tag{40}$$

where, $\theta \in \Re^L$ represents an L-dimensional parameter vector that needs to be estimated; $H \in \Re^{K \times L}$ is defined as the K x L-dimensional basis matrix that does not contain parameters to be estimated. H is a predetermined pattern based on certain assumptions to be discussed below. As can be deduced from Eq. (40), the estimated EP signal x in Eq. (18) is related to H and θ in the following way:

$$x = H\theta \tag{41}$$

The clean EP signal x in Eq. (41) is modeled as a linear combination of basis vectors Ψ_i which make up the columns of the matrix $H = [\Psi_1, \Psi_2, \cdots, \Psi_p]$. In general, the generic basis matrix H may comprise equally spaced Gaussian-shaped functions (Karjalainen et al., 1999) derived from the individual Ψ_i, given by the following equation:

$$\Psi_i(t) = e^{\frac{-(t-\tau_i)^2}{2d^2}} \quad \text{for } t = 1, 2, \cdots, K \tag{42}$$

where d represents the variance (width) and τ_i represents the mean (position) of the function peak for the given i = 1, 2, ..., p. Once the parameter H is established and θ is estimated, the single-trial EP can then be determined as follows:

$$\hat{x} = H\hat{\theta} \tag{43}$$

where the hat (^) placed over the x and θ symbols indicates the "estimate" of the respective vector.

3.2.1 Regularized least squares solution

The parameter θ can be approximated by using a generalized Thikonov regularized least squares solution stated as:

$$\hat{\theta}_\alpha = \arg \min_{\theta} \left\{ \left\| L_1(y - H\theta) \right\|^2 + \alpha^2 \left\| L_2(\theta - \theta^*) \right\|^2 \right\} \tag{44}$$

where L_1 and L_2 are the regularization matrices; α is the value of the regularization parameter; θ^* is the initial (prior) guess for the solution. The solution in Eq. (44) is in fact the most commonly used method of regularization of ill-posed problems; Eq. (44) is a modification of the ordinary weighted least squares solution given as

$$\hat{\theta}_{LS} = \arg\min_{\theta} \left\{ \| L_1 (y - H\theta) \|^2 \right\} \tag{45}$$

Furthermore, the regularization parameter α in Eq. (44) controls the weight of the side constraint

$$\left\| L_2 (\theta - \theta^*) \right\|^2 \tag{46}$$

so that minimization is achieved. Subsequently, Eq. (44) can be simplified further (Karjalainen et al., 1999) to yield

$$\hat{\theta}_{\alpha} = (H^T W_1 H + \alpha^2 W_2)^{-1} (H^T W_1 y + \alpha^2 W_2 \theta^*) \tag{47}$$

where, $W_1 = L_1^T L_1$ and $W_2 = L_2^T L_2$ are positive definite weighting matrices.

3.2.2 Bayesian estimation

The regularization process has a close relationship with the Bayesian approach. In addition to the current information of the parameter (e.g. θ) under study, both methods also include the previous parameter information in their computation. In Bayesian estimation, both θ and n in Eq. (40) are treated as random and uncorrelated with each other. The estimator $\hat{\theta}$ that minimizes the mean square Bayes cost

$$B_{MS} = E\left\{ \left\| \theta - \hat{\theta} \right\|^2 \right\} \tag{48}$$

is given by the conditional mean

$$\hat{\theta} = E\{\theta \mid y\} \tag{49}$$

of the posterior distribution

$$p(\theta \mid y) \propto p(y \mid \theta) p(\theta) \tag{50}$$

Subsequently, a linear mean square estimator, known in Bayesian estimation as the maximum a posteriori estimator (MAP) is expressed as

$$\hat{\theta}_{MS} = (H^T R_n^{-1} H + R_{\theta}^{-1})^{-1} (H^T R_n^{-1} y + R_{\theta}^{-1} \eta_{\theta}) \tag{51}$$

where, R_n is the covariance matrix of the EEG noise n; R_{θ} and η_{θ} are the covariance matrix and the mean of the parameter θ, respectively—they represent the initial (prior) information for the parameters θ. Equation (51) minimizes Eq. (48) providing that

- the errors n are jointly Gaussian with zero mean.
- the parameters θ are jointly Gaussian random variables.

The covariance matrix R_{θ} can be assumed to be zero if it is not known. In this case, the estimator in Eq. (51) reduces to the ordinary minimum Gauss-Markov estimator given as

$$\hat{\theta}_{GM} = (H^T R_n^{-1} H)^{-1} H^T R_n^{-1} y \tag{52}$$

Next, the estimator in Eq. (52) is equal to the ordinary least squares estimator if the noise are independent with equal variances (i.e., $R_n = \sigma_n^2 I$); that is

$$\hat{\theta}_{LS} = (H^T H)^{-1} H^T y \tag{53}$$

As a matter of fact, Eq. (53) is the Bayesian interpretation of Eq. (47).

3.2.3 Computation of side constraint regularization matrix

As stated previously, the basis matrix H could be produced by using sampled Gaussian or sigmoid functions, mimicking EP peaks and valleys. A special case exists if the column vectors that constitute the basis matrix H are mutually orthonormal (i.e., $H^T H = I$). The least squares solution in Eq. (53) can be simplified as

$$\hat{\theta}_{LS} = H^T y \tag{54}$$

For clarity, let J be a new basis matrix that represents mutually orthonormal basis vectors. Now, the least squares solution in Eq. (54) is modified as

$$\hat{\theta}_{LS} = J^T y \tag{55}$$

The regularization matrix L_2 is to be derived from an optimal number of column vectors making up the basis matrix J. The reduced number of J columns, representing the optimal set of the J basis vectors, can be determined by computing the covariance of $\hat{\theta}_{LS}$ in Eq. (55); that is,

$$\begin{aligned} R_\theta &= E\{\hat{\theta}_{LS}\hat{\theta}_{LS}^T\} = E\{J^T y (J^T y)^T\} \\ &= E\{J^T y y^T J\} = J^T R_y J \\ &= \mathrm{diag}(\lambda_1, \lambda_2, \cdots, \lambda_q) = \Lambda_y \end{aligned} \tag{56}$$

where λ_1 through λ_q represent the diagonal eigenvalues of Λ_y. Equation (56) reveals that the correlation matrix R_θ is related to the observation vector correlation matrix R_y. Specifically, R_θ is equal to the the q x q-dimensional eigenvalue matrix Λ_y. In other words, R_θ is the eigenvalue matrix of R_y, which is the observation vector correlation matrix. Also, the q x q-dimensional matrix J is actually the eigenvector matrix of R_y. Even though there are q diagonal eigenvalues, the reduced basis matrix J, denoted as J_x, is the q x p dimensional eigenvectors that are associated with the p largest (i.e., non-zero) eigenvalues of Λ_y. It is further assumed that J_x contains an orthonormal basis of the subspace P. It is desirable that the EP $x = H\theta$ is closely within this subspace. The projection of x onto P is denoted as $(J_x J_x)H\theta$. The distance between x and P is

$$\| H\theta - (J_x J_x^T)H\theta \| = \| (I - J_x J_x^T)H\theta \| \tag{57}$$

The value of L_2 should be carefully chosen to minimize the side constraint in Eq. (46) which reduces to $\|L\theta\|$ for $\theta^* = 0$. From the inspection of Eq. (57), it can be stated that $L_2 = (I - J_x J_x^T)H$. It is now assumed that L_2 is *idempotent* and *symmetric* such that

$$\begin{aligned} W_2 = L_2^T L_2 &= \left((I - J_x J_x^T)H\right)^T (I - J_x J_x^T)H \\ &= H^T (I - J_x J_x^T)^T (I - J_x J_x^T)H \\ &= H^T (I - J_x J_x^T)H \end{aligned} \tag{58}$$

3.2.4 Combination of regularized solution and Bayesian estimation

A new equation is to be generated based on Eq. (47) and Eq. (51); comparisons between these two equations reveal the following relationships:

- $R_n^{-1} = W_1$, where $W_1 = L_1^T L_1$.
- $R_\theta^{-1} = \alpha^2 W_2$, where $W_2 = L_2^T L_2$.
- $\eta_\theta = \theta^*$.

The weight $W_1 = L_1^T L_1$ can be represented by R_n^{-1} since the covariance of the EEG noise R_n can be estimated from the pre-stimulation period, during which the EP signal is absent. On the contrary, the term R_θ^{-1} is represented by its equivalent $W_2 = L_2^T L_2$ term obtained from Eq. (58). The new solution based on Eq. (47) and Eq. (51) can now be written as

$$\hat{\theta} = \left(H^T R_n^{-1} H + \alpha^2 H^T (I - J_x J_x^T)H\right)^{-1} \left(H^T R_n^{-1} y + \alpha^2 H^T (I - J_x J_x^T) H \theta^*\right) \tag{59}$$

Equation (59) is simplified further by treating the prior value θ^* as zero:

$$\hat{\theta} = \left(H^T R_n^{-1} H + \alpha^2 H^T (I - H_x H_x^T)H\right)^{-1} H^T R_n^{-1} y \tag{60}$$

Therefore, the estimated VEP signal, $\hat{x}$, from Eq. (43) can be expressed as

$$\begin{aligned} \hat{x} &= H\hat{\theta} \\ &= H\left(H^T R_n^{-1} H + \alpha^2 H^T (I - J_x J_x^T)H\right)^{-1} H^T R_n^{-1} y \end{aligned} \tag{61}$$

3.2.5 Strength of the SRM algorithm

The structure of the algorithm in Eq. (61) resembles that of the Karhunen-Loeve transform, with H^T as the KLT matrix and H as the inverse KLT matrix. Equation (61) does have extra terms (besides H^T and H) which are used for fine tuning. The inclusion of the R_n^{-1} term indicates that a pre-whitening stage is incorporated, and the algorithm is able to deal with both white and colored noise.

3.2.6 Weaknesses of the SRM algorithm

The basis matrix, which serves as one of the algorithm parameters, needs to be carefully formed by selecting a generic function (e.g., Gaussian or sigmoid) and setting its amplitudes and widths to mimic EP characteristics. Simply, the improper selection of such a parameter with a predetermined shape (i.e., amplitudes and variance) somehow pre-meditates or influences the final outcome of the output waveform.

3.3 Subspace Dynamical Estimation Method

The subspace dynamical estimation method (SDEM) has been proposed by (Georgiadis et al., 2007) to extract EPs from the observed signals.

In SDEM, a model for the EP utilizes a linear combination of vectors comprising a brain activity induced by stimulation and other brain activities independent of the stimulus. Mathematically, the generic model for a single-trial EP follows Eq. (18) and Eq. (40), as this work is an extension of that proposed earlier by (Karjalainen et al., 1999).

3.3.1 Bayesian estimation

The SDEM scheme makes use of Eq. (48) through Eq. (53) that lead to Eq. (54). In SDEM, the regularized least squares solution is not included. Also, the basis matrix $\boldsymbol{H}$ is not produced by using sampled Gaussian or sigmoid functions; the basis matrix will solely be based on the observed signal under study. For clarity, let $\mathbf{Z}$ be a new basis matrix that represents mutually orthonormal basis vectors to be determined. Now, the least squares solution in Eq. (55) is modified as

$$\hat{\theta}_{LS} = \mathbf{Z}^T \boldsymbol{y} \tag{62}$$

Based on Eq. (56), it can be deduced that $\mathbf{Z}$ in Eq. (62) is actually the eigenvector matrix of $\mathbf{R}_y$. The $\mathbf{Z}$ term in Eq. (62) can now be represented by its reduced form $\mathbf{Z}_x$ which is associated with the p largest (i.e., non-zero) eigenvalues of Λ_y. It is also assumed that $\mathbf{Z}_x$ contains an orthonormal basis of the subspace P. Equation (62) is therefore written as

$$\hat{\theta} = \mathbf{Z}_x^T \boldsymbol{y} \tag{63}$$

Therefore, the estimated VEP signal, $\hat{x}$, from Eq. (43) can be expressed as

$$\hat{x} = \mathbf{Z}_x \cdot \mathbf{Z}_x^T \cdot \boldsymbol{y} \tag{64}$$

The structure in Eq. (64) is actually the Karhunen Loeve transform (KLT) and inverse Karhunen Loeve transform (IKLT), since the eigenvectors $\mathbf{Z}$ which is derived from the eigendecomposition of the symmetric matrix $\mathbf{R}_y$ is always unitary. What is achieved in Eq. (64) is that the corrupted EP signal $\boldsymbol{y}$ is decorrelated by the KLT matrix $\mathbf{Z}_x^T$. Then, the transformed signal (matrix) is truncated to a certain dimension to suppress the noise segments. Next, the modified signal is retransformed back into the original form by the IKLT matrix $\mathbf{Z}_x$ to obtain the desired signal.

3.3.2 Strength of the SDEM algorithm

The state space model is dependent on a basis matrix to be directly produced by performing eigendecomposition operation on the correlation matrix of the noisy observation. Contrary to SRM, SDEM makes no assumption about the nature of the EP.

3.3.3 Weaknesses of the SDEM algorithm

The SDEM algorithm will work well for any signal that is corrupted by white noise since the eigenvectors of the corrupted signal is assumed to be the eigenvectors of the clean signal and white noise. When the noise becomes colored, the assumption will no longer hold and the algorithm becomes less effective.

4. Results and Discussions

The three subspace techniques discussed above are tested and assessed using artificial and real human data.

The subspace methods under study are applied to estimate visual evoked potentials (VEPs) which are highly corrupted by spontaneous electroencephalogram (EEG) signals. Thorough simulations using realistically generated VEPs and EEGs at SNRs ranging from 0 to -10 dB are performed. Later, the algorithms are assessed in their abilities to detect the latencies of the P100, P200 and P300 components.

Next, the validity and the effectiveness of the algorithms to detect the P100's (used in objective assessment of visual pathways) are evaluated using real patient data collected from a hospital. The efficiencies of the studied techniques are then compared among one another.

4.1 Results from Simulated Data

In the first part of this section, the performances of the GSA, SRM, and SDEM in estimating the P100, P200, and P300 are tested using artificially generated VEP signals corrupted with colored noise at different SNR values.

Artificial VEP and EEG waveforms are generated and added to each other in order to create a noisy VEP. The clean VEP, $x(k) \in \Re^M$, is generated by superimposing J Gaussian functions, each of which having a different amplitude (A), variance (σ^2) and mean (μ) as given by the following equations (Andrews et al., 2005).

$$x(k) = \left[\sum_{n=1}^{J} g_n(k) \right]^T \tag{65}$$

where $g_n(k) = [g_{n1}, g_{n2}, \ldots, g_{nM}]$, for $k = 1, 2, \ldots, M$, with the individual g_{nk} given as

$$g_{nk} = \frac{A_n}{\sqrt{2\pi\sigma_n^2}} e^{\frac{-(k-\mu_n)^2}{2\sigma_n^2}} \tag{66}$$

The values for A, σ and μ are experimentally tweaked to create arbitrary amplitudes with precise peak latencies at 100 *ms*, 200 *ms*, and 300 *ms* simulating the real P100, P200 and P300, respectively.

The EEG colored noise $e(k)$ can be characterized by an autoregressive (AR) model (Yu et al., 1994) given by the following equation.

$$e(k) = 1.5084e(k-1) - 0.1587e(k-2) - 0.3109e(k-3) - 0.0510e(k-4) + w(k) \qquad (67)$$

where w(k) is the input driving noise of the AR filter and e(k) is the filter output. Since noise is assumed to be additive, Eq. (65) and Eq. (67) are combined to obtain

$$y(k) = x(k) + e(k) \qquad (68)$$

As a preliminary illustration, Fig. 2 below shows, respectively, a sample of artificially generated VEP, a noisy VEP at SNR = -2 dB, and the extracted VEPs using the GSA, SRM and SDEM techniques.

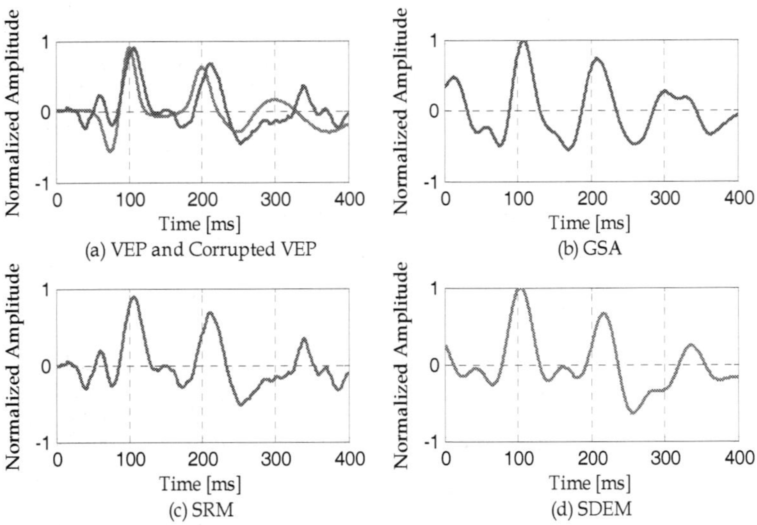

Fig. 2. (a) clean VEP (lighter line/color) and corrupted VEP (darker line/color) with SNR = -2 dB; and the estimated VEPs produced by (b) GSA; (c) SRM; (d) SDEM.

To compare the performances of the algorithms in statistical form, SNR is varied from 0 dB to -13 dB and the algorithms are run 500 times for each value. The average error in estimating the latencies of P100, P200, and P300 are calculated and tabulated along with the failure rate in Table 1 below. Any trial is noted as a failure with respect to a certain peak if the waveform fails to show clearly the pertinent peak.

SNR [dB]	Peak	Failure rate [%]			Peak	Average error		
		GSA	SRM	SDEM		GSA	SRM	SDEM
0	P100	0.6	0.5	1.6	P100	3.7	3.9	4.1
	P200	0.4	2.6	3.2	P200	3.9	4.2	4.3
	P300	17.8	53.2	40.2	P300	6.5	12.9	9.8
-2	P100	2.2	2.0	2.6	P100	4.1	4.1	4.5
	P200	1.4	7.2	9	P200	4.0	5.1	5.3
	P300	17.8	55.4	46	P300	6.3	13.3	10.8
-4	P100	3.2	2.8	6.6	P100	4.2	4.2	5.1
	P200	5.6	12.2	15.2	P200	4.8	5.8	6.3
	P300	21.4	61.4	48.4	P300	6.6	13.8	11.6
-6	P100	5.5	5.7	13.6	P100	4.2	4.5	6.9
	P200	4.8	22	22.8	P200	4.5	7.6	8
	P300	18.2	60	52.2	P300	6.1	14.0	12.7
-8	P100	8.2	9.8	22.2	P100	4.8	5.7	8.4
	P200	8.2	34.8	34.4	P200	4.7	10.0	10.4
	P300	17.4	59.6	52.4	P300	6.3	14.5	13
-10	P100	6	16.4	28.8	P100	4.4	7.1	9.6
	P200	12.8	37	39.4	P200	5.0	10.6	11.3
	P300	18.6	58.4	56.4	P300	6.1	15.2	13.3

Table 1. The failure rate and average errors produced by GSA, SRM and SDEM.

From Table 1, SRM outperforms GSA and SDEM in terms of failure rate for SNRs equal to 0 through -4 dB; however, in terms of average errors, GSA outperforms SRM and SDEM. From -6 dB and below, GSA is a better estimator compared to both SRM and SDEM.

Overall, it is clear that the proposed GSA algorithm outperforms SRM and SDEM in terms of accuracy and success rate. All the three algorithms display their best performance in estimating the latency of the P100 components in comparisons with the other two peaks.

Further, Fig. 3 below illustrates the estimation of VEPs at SNR equal to -10 dB.

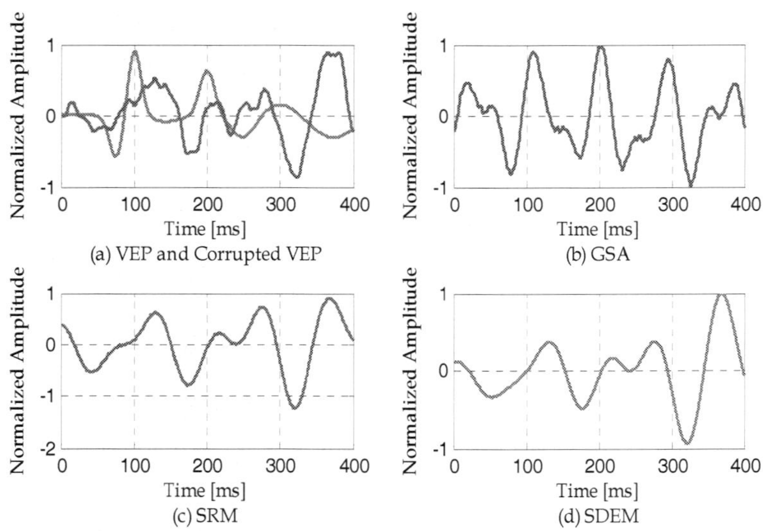

Fig. 3. (a) clean VEP (lighter line/color) and corrupted VEP (darker line/color) with SNR = -10dB; and the estimated VEPs produced by (b) GSA; (c) SRM; (d) SDEM.

4.2 Results of Real Patient Data

This section reveals the accuracy of the GSA, SRM and SDEM techniques in estimating human P100 peaks, which are used by doctors as objective evaluation of the visual pathway conduction. Experiments were conducted at Selayang Hospital, Kuala Lumpur using RETIport32 equipment, and carried out on twenty four subjects having **normal** (P100 < 115 ms) and **abnormal** (P100 > 115 ms) VEP readings. They were asked to watch a pattern reversal checkerboard pattern (1° full field), the stimulus being a checker reversal (N = 50 stimuli). Scalp recordings were made according to the International 10/20 System, with one eye closed at any given time. The active electrode was connected to the middle of the occipital (O1, O2) area while the reference electrode was attached to the middle of the forehead. Each trial was pre-filtered in the range 0.1 Hz to 70 Hz and sampled at 512 Hz.

In this study, we will show the results for artifact-free trials of these subjects taken from their right eyes only. Eighty trials for each subject's right eye were processed by the VEP machine using ensemble averaging (EA). The averaged values were readily available and directly obtained from the equipment. Since EA is a multi-trial scheme, it is expected to produce good estimation of the P100 that can be used as a baseline for comparing the performance of the GSA, SRM and SDEM estimators. Further, GSA and SRM require unprocessed data from the machine. Thus, the equipment was configured accordingly to generate the raw data. The recording for every trial involved capturing the brain activities for 333 ms before stimulation was applied; this enabled us to capture the colored EEG noise alone. The next 333 ms was used to record the post-stimulus EEG, comprising a mixture of the VEP and EEG. The same process was repeated for the consecutive trials.

For comparisons with EA, the eighty different waveforms per subject produced by SSM were also averaged. Again, the strategy here was to look for the highest peak from the averaged waveform. The purpose of averaging the outcome of the SSM was to establish the performance of GSA, SRM and SDEM as single-trial estimators; any mean peak produced by any algorithm will be compared with the EA value. The comparisons shall establish the degree of accuracy of the estimators' individual single-trial outcome.

Illustrated in Fig. 4 below is the estimators' extracted Pattern VEPs for S7 from trial #1.

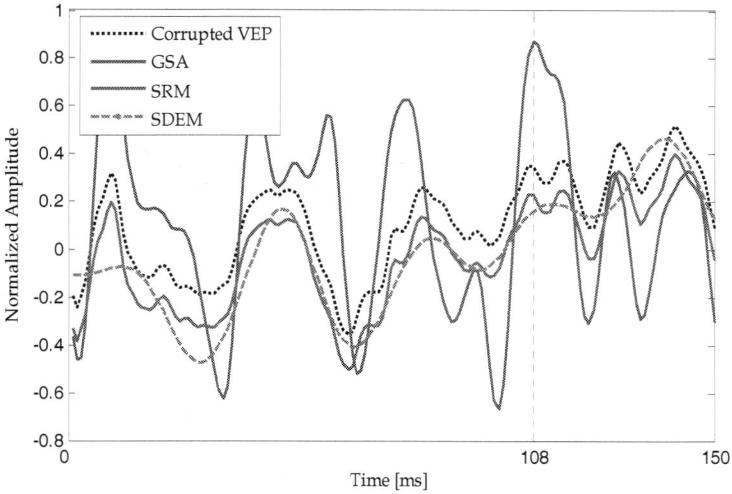

Fig. 4. The P100 of the seventh subject (S7) taken from trial # 1 (note: the P100 produced by the EA method is at 108 ms as indicated by the vertical dotted line).

It is to be noted that any peaks that occur below 90 ms are noise and are therefore ignored. Attention is given to any dominant (i.e., highest) peak(s) from 90 to 150 ms. From Fig. 4, the corrupted VEP (unprocessed raw signal) contains two dominant peaks at 107 and 115 ms, with the one at 115 ms being slightly higher. The highest peak produced by GSA is at 108 ms, which is the same as that obtained by EA. The SRM estimator produces two peaks at 107 and 115 ms, with the most dominant peak at 115 ms. The SDEM algorithm shows the dominant peak at 112 ms. In brief, our GSA technique frequently produces lower mean errors in detecting the P100 components from the real patient data.

Further, Table 2 below summarizes the mean values of the P100's by EA, GSA, SRM and SDEM for the twenty four subjects.

Subject	EA	Latency [ms]			Mean Error		
		GSA	SRM	SDEM	GSA	SRM	SDEM
S1	99	99	101	138	0	2	39
S2	100	100	101	101	0	1	1
S3	119	119	118	117	0	1	2
S4	128	130	125	96	2	3	32
S5	99	118	98	98	19	1	1
S6	107	104	103	103	3	4	4
S7	108	110	110	91	2	2	17
S8	107	103	105	105	4	2	2
S9	130	144	155	155	14	25	25
S10	117	107	106	105	10	11	12
S11	119	115	123	98	4	4	21
S12	114	113	114	116	1	0	2
S13	102	96	100	117	0	2	20
S14	123	118	118	90	5	5	33
S15	102	96	108	117	6	6	15
S16	108	108	107	106	0	1	2
S17	107	107	107	106	0	0	1
S18	107	108	110	111	1	3	4
S19	110	106	104	104	4	6	6
S20	130	130	121	128	0	9	2
S21	109	102	102	101	7	7	8
S22	130	135	148	138	5	13	8
S23	102	104	133	133	2	31	31
S24	102	102	102	102	0	0	0

Table 2. The mean values of the P100's produced by GSA, SRM and SDEM for twenty four subjects.

From Table 2, it is quite clear that GSA outperforms the SRM and SDM techniques in estimating the P100.

5. Conclusion

In this chapter the foundations of the subspace based signal enhancement techniques are outlined. The relationships between the principal subspace (signal subspace) and the maximum energy, and between the complementary subspace (noise subspace) and the minimum energy, are defined. Next, the eigendecomposition of the autocorrelation matrix of data corrupted by additive noise, and how it is used to enhance SNR by retaining only the information in the signal subspace eigenvectors, is explained. Since, finding the dimension of signal subspace is a critical issue to subspace teachings, the Akaike information criteria is suggested to be used. Three subspace based techniques, GSA, SRM and SDEM, exploiting the concept of signal and noise subspaces in different ways, in order to effectively enhance the SNR in EP environments, are explained. The performances of the techniques are compared using both artificially generated data and real patient data.

In the first experiment, the techniques are used to estimate the latencies of P100, P200, and P300, under SNR varying from 0 dB to -10 dB. The EPs are artificially generated and corrupted by colored noise. The results show better performance by the GSA in terms of both accuracy and failure rate. This is mainly due to the use of the generalized eigendecomposition for simultaneous diagonalization of signal and noise autocorrelation matrices.

In the second experiment the performances are compared using real patient data, and ensemble averaging is used as a baseline. The GSA is showing closer results to the EA, in comparisons with SRM and SDEM. This makes the single-trial GSA technique perform like the multi-trial ensemble averaging in VEP extraction, with the added advantages of recovering the desired peaks of the individual trial, reducing recording time, and relieving subjects from fatigue.

In summary, subspace techniques are powerful if used properly to extract biomedical signals such as EPs which are severely corrupted by additive colored or white noise. Finally, the signal subspace dimension and the Lagrange multiplier are two crucial parameters that influence the estimators' performances, and thus require further studies.

6. Acknowledgment

The authors would like to thank Universiti Teknologi PETRONAS for funding this research project. In addition, the authors would like to thank Dr. Tara Mary George and Mr. Mohd Zawawi Zakaria of the Ophthalmology Department, Selayang Hospital, Kuala Lumpur who acquired the Pattern Visual Evoked Potentials data at the hospital.

7. References

Akaike, H. (1973). Information Theory and an Extension of the Maximum Likelihood Principle, *Proceedings of the 2nd Int'l. Symp. Inform. Theory, Supp. to Problems of Control and Inform. Theory*, pp. 267-281, 1973.

Andrews, S.; Palaniappan R. & Kamel N. (2005). Extracting Single Trial Visual Evoked Potentials using Selective Eigen-Rate Principal Components. *World Enformatika Society Transactions on Engineering, Computing and Technology*, vol. 7, August 2005.

Cui, J.; Wong, W. & and Mann, S. (2004). Time-Frequency Analysis of Visual Evoked Potentials by Means of Matching Pursuit with Chirplet Atoms, *Proceedings of the 26th Annual International Conference of the IEEE EMBS*, San Francisco, CA, USA, pp. 267-270, September 1-5, 2004.

Deprettere, F. (ed.) (1989). *SVD and Signal Processing: Algorithms, Applications and Architectures*, North-Holland Publishing Co., 1989.

Ephraim, Y. & Van Trees, H. L (1995). A Signal Subspace Approach for Speech Enhancement. *IEEE Transaction on Speech and Audio Processing*, vol. 3, no. 4, pp. 251-266, July 1995.

Georgiadis, S.D.; Ranta-aho, P. O.; Tarvainen, M. P. & Karjalainen, P. A (2007). A Subspace Method for Dynamical Estimation of Evoked Potentials. *Computational Intelligence and Neuroscience*, vol. 2007, article ID 61916, pp. 1-11, September 18, 2007.

Gharieb, R. R. & Cichocki, A (2001). Noise Reduction in Brain Evoked Potentials Based on Third-Order Correlations. *IEEE Transactions on Biomedical Engineering*, vol. 48, no. 5, pp. 501-512, May 2001.

Golub, G. H. & Van Loan, C. F. (1989). *Matrix Computations*, The Johns Hopkins University Press, 2nd edition, 1989.

Henning, G. & Husar, P. (1995). Statistical Detection of Visually Evoked Potentials. *IEEE Engineering in Medicine and Biology*, July/August 1995.

John, E.; Ruchkin, D. & and Villegas, J. (1964). Experimental background: signal analysis and behavioral correlates of evoked potential configurations in cats. *Ann. NY Acad. Sci.*, vol. 112, pp. 362-420, 1964.

Karjalainen, P. A.; Kaipio, J. P.; Koistinen, A. S. & Vauhkonen, M. (1999). Subspace Regularization Method for the Single-Trial Estimation of Evoked Potentials. *IEEE Transactions on Biomedical Engineering*, vol. 46, no. 7, pp. 849-860, July 1999.

Nidal-Kamel & Zuki-Yusoff, M. (2008). A Generalized Subspace Approach for Estimating Visual Evoked Potentials, *Proceedings of the 30th Annual Conference of the IEEE Engineering in Medicine and Biology Society (IEEE EMBC'08)*, Vancouver, Canada, Aug. 20-24, 2008, pp. 5208-5211.

Regan, D. (1989). *Human brain electrophysiology: evoked potentials and evoked magnetic fields in science and medicine*, Elsevier, New York: Elsevier.

Rissanen, J. (1978). Modeling by shortest data description. *Automatica*, vol. 14, pp. 465-471, 1978.

Schwartz, G. (1978). Estimating the dimension of a model. *Ann. Stat.*, vol. 6, pp. 461-464, 1978.

Wax, M. & Kailath, T. (1985). Detection of Signals by Information Theoretic Criteria. *IEEE Transactions on Acoustics, Speech, and Signal Processing*, vol. ASSP-33, no. 2, pp. 387-392, April 1985.

Yu, X. H.; He, Z. Y. & and Zhang, Y. S (1994). Time-Varying Adaptive Filters for Evoked Potential Estimation. *IEEE Transactions on Biomedical Engineering*, vol. 41, no. 11, November 1994.

Zuki-Yusoff, M. & Nidal-Kamel (2009). Estimation of Visual Evoked Potentials for Measurement of Optical Pathway Conduction (accepted for publication), *the 17th European Signal Processing Conference (EUSIPCO 2009)*, Glasgow, Scotland, Aug. 24-28, 2009, to be published.

Zuki-Yusoff, M.; Nidal-Kamel & Fadzil-M.Hani, A. (2008). Single-Trial Extraction of Visual Evoked Potentials from the Brain, *Proceedings of the 16th European Signal Processing Conference (EUSIPCO 2008)*, Lausanne, Switzerland, Aug. 25-29, 2008.

Zuki-Yusoff, M.; Nidal-Kamel & Fadzil-M.Hani, A. (2007). Estimation of Visual Evoked Potentials using a Signal Subspace Approach, *Proceedings of the International Conference on Intelligent and Advanced Systems 2007 (ICIAS 2007)*, Kuala Lumpur, Malaysia, Nov. 25-28, 2007, pp. 1157-1162.

Classification of Mental Tasks using Different Spectral Estimation Methods

Pablo F. Diez[1], Eric Laciar[1], Vicente Mut[2], Enrique Avila[1], Abel Torres[3]
[1] *Gabinete de Tecnología Médica, Universidad Nacional de San Juan*
[2] *Instituto de Automática, Universidad Nacional de San Juan*
[3] *Departament ESAII, Universitat Politècnica de Catalunya*
[1,2]*Argentina*, [3]*Spain*

1. Introduction

The electroencephalogram (EEG) is the non-invasive recording of the neuronal electrical activity. The analysis of EEG signals has become, over the last 20 years, a broad field of research, including many areas such as brain diseases (Parkinson, Alzheimer, etc.), sleep disorders, anaesthesia monitoring and more recently, in new augmentatives ways of communication, such as Brain-Computer Interfaces (BCI).

BCI are devices that provide the brain with a new, non-muscular communication channel (Wolpaw *et al.*, 2002), which can be useful for persons with motor impairments. A wide variety of methods to extract features from the EEG signals can be used; these include spectral estimation techniques, wavelet transform, time-frequency representations, and others. At this moment, the spectral estimation techniques are the most used methods in the BCI field.

The processing of EEG signals is an important part in the design of a BCI (Wolpaw *et al.*, 2002). It is commonly divided in the features extraction and the feature translation (Mason & Birch, 2003). In this work, we will focus in the EEG features extraction using three different spectral estimation techniques.

In many studies, the researchers use different spectral estimation techniques like Fourier Transform (Krusienski *et al.*, 2007), Welch periodogram (Millán *et al.*, 2002); (Millán *et al.*, 2004) or Autoregressive (AR) modeling (Bufalari *et al.*, 2006); (Krusienski *et al.*, 2006); (Schlögl *et al.*, 1997) in EEG signals. A review of methods for features extraction and features translation from these signals can be found in a review from the Third BCI meeting (McFarland *et al.*, 2006). A comparison between the periodogram and the AR model applied to EEG signals aimed to clinical areas is presented in (Akin & Kiymik, 2000). Finally, an extended comparison of classification algorithms can be found in (Lotte *et al.*, 2007).

In this chapter, we compare the performance of three different spectral estimation techniques for the classification of different mental tasks over two EEG databases. These techniques are the standard periodogram, the Welch periodogram (both based on Fourier transform) and Burg method (for AR model-based spectral analysis). For each one of these methods we compute two parameters: the mean power and the root mean square (RMS) in different frequency bands. Both databases used in this work, are composed by a set of EEG signals acquired on healthy people. One database is related with motor-imagery tasks and the other one is related with math and imagery tasks.

The classification of the mental tasks was conducted with different classifiers, such as, linear discriminate analysis, learning vector quantization, neural networks and support vector machine.

This chapter is organized as follows. In the next section the databases utilized in this work are explained. The section 3 contains a description of the estimation spectral methods used. An explanation of the procedure applies to each database is arrived in section 4. The different classifiers are briefly described in section 5 and the obtained results are shown in section 6. Finally, in sections 7 and 8 a discussion about results and the conclusions are presented.

2. EEG Databases

In this work, we have used two different databases, each one with diverse mental tasks.

2.1. Math-Imagine database

This database was collected in a previous work (Diez & Pi Marti, 2006) in the Laboratory of Digital Electronics, Faculty of Engineering, National University of San Juan (Argentina). EEG signals from the scalp of six healthy subjects (4 males and 2 females, 28±2 years) were acquired while they performed three different mental tasks, namely: *(a) Relax task:* the subjects close his eyes and try to relax and think in nothing in particular; *(b) Math Task:* the subjects make a regressive count from 3 to 3 beginning in 30, i.e. 30, 27, 24,...3, 0. The subjects were asked to begin the count once again and try to not verbalize; and *(c) Imagine task:* the subjects have to imagine an incandescent lamp at the moment that it is turn on.

For each subject, the EEG signals were acquired using six electrodes of Ag/AgCL in positions F_3, F_4, C_3, C_4, P_3 and P_4 according to the 10-20 positioning system. With this electrodes were configured 4 bipolar channels of measurement (ch1: F_3-C_3; ch2:F_4-C_4; ch3:P_3-C_3; ch4: P_4-C_4). Each channel is composed by an instrumentation amplifier with gain 7000 and CMRR greater than 90dB, a bandpass analogical filter set at 0.1-45Hz and an analogical to digital converter ADC121S101 of 12 bits accuracy with a sampling rate of 150Hz.

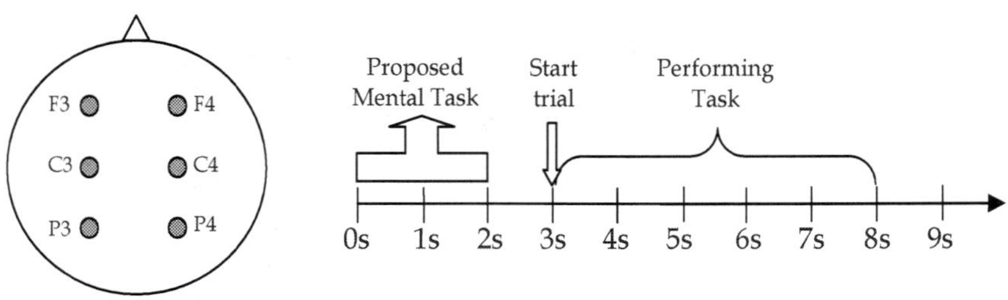

Fig. 1. Electrodes position indicated by grey circles (left), on F_3, F_4, C_3, C_4, P_3 and P_4 according to 10-20 positioning system. The acquisition protocol is presented on the right.

The subjects were trained to keep the maximal concentration while perform the mental tasks. Each mental task has a duration of 5s (750 samples) with 3s between them. The subjects were seated comfortably, with dim lighting, in front of a PC monitor. In which, were presented to subjects the proposed mental tasks (0-2s), the start signal to begin the trial (3s) and the final of the trial (8s), in according with the protocol illustrated in Figure 1. No feedback was presented to subjects during the trials. Every session had 15 trials for each mental task, i.e., 45 trials in total. Two subjects (Subj#1 and Subj#2) performed 3 sessions; the others performed only 2 sessions, i.e., two subjects had 135 trials and the rest 90 trials.
The EEG of this database were digitally filtered using a Butterworth bi-directional bandpass filter, order 10, with 6 and 40Hz as lower and upper cut-off frequencies respectively.

2.2. Motor-Imagery database

This database was acquired in the Department of Medical Informatics, Institute for Biomedical Engineering, University of Technology Graz (Austria) and it is available free on-line from http://ida.first.fraunhofer.de/projects/bci/competition_iii/ (BCI-Competition III web page). It was recorded from a normal subject (female, 25 years) during a feedback session. The subject sat in a relaxing chair with armrests. The task was to control a feedback bar by means of *(a) imagery left hand* and *(b) imagery right hand* movements. The order of left and right cues was random. The experiment consists of 140 trials, conducted on the same day.
Each trial had the first 2s in silence, at t=2s an acoustic stimulus indicates the beginning of the trial and a "+" was displayed for 1s; then at t=3s, an arrow (left or right) was displayed as cue. At the same time the subject was asked to move a bar into the direction of the arrow (Figure 2). Similar acquisition protocols were implemented in several studies (Schlögl *et al.*, 1997); (Neuper *et al.*, 1999). The recording was made using a G.tec amplifier and Ag/AgCl electrodes. Three bipolar EEG channels (anterior '+', posterior '-') were measured over C_3, C_z and C_4. The EEG was sampled with 128 Hz and analogically filtered between 0.5 and 30 Hz. The feedback was based on AAR parameters of channel over C_3 and C_4, the AAR parameters were combined with a discriminate analysis into one output parameter.
Each EEG record of the motor-imagery database was digitally filtered using a Butterworth filter, order 8, with 6 and 30 Hz as lower and upper cut-off frequencies respectively.

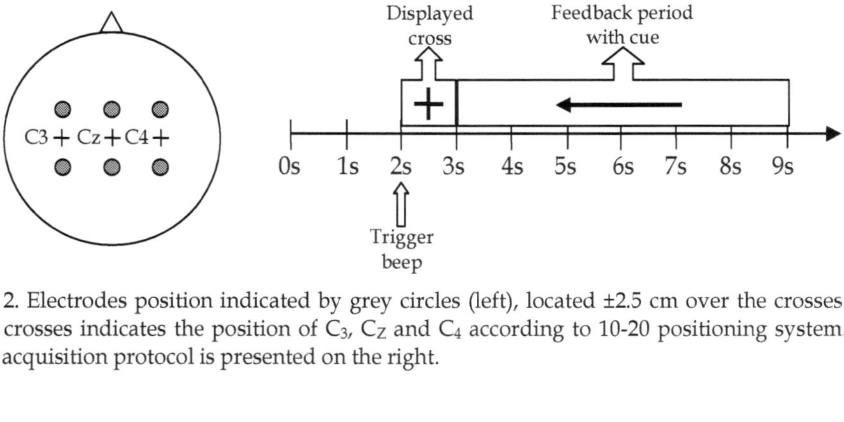

Fig. 2. Electrodes position indicated by grey circles (left), located ±2.5 cm over the crosses. The crosses indicates the position of C_3, C_Z and C_4 according to 10-20 positioning system. The acquisition protocol is presented on the right.

3. Spectral Analysis

EEG signals were processed in order to estimate the signal Power Spectral Density (PSD), this section explain the different PSD estimation methods regardless the database used. The three analysed techniques were: (a) standard periodogram, (b) Welch periodogram and (c) Burg method.

3.1. Standard Periodogram

The periodogram is considered as a non-parametric spectral analysis since no parametric assumptions about the signal are incorporated.

This technique was introduced at an early stage in the processing of EEG signals and it is based in the Fourier Transform. Considering that EEG rhythms are essentially oscillatory signals, its decomposition in terms of sine and cosine, was found useful (Sörnmo & Laguna, 2005). Basically, the Fourier spectral analysis correlates the signal with sines and cosines of diverse frequencies and produces a set of coefficients that defines the spectral content of the analyzed signal. The Fourier Transform computed in the discrete field is known as Discrete Time Fourier Transform (DTFT).

Thus, the periodogram is an estimation of the PSD based on DTFT of the signal $x[n]$ and it is defined by the following equation:

$$\hat{S}_P(f) = \frac{T_s}{N}\left|\sum_{n=1}^{N} x[n]e^{-j2\pi fnT_s}\right|^2 \tag{1}$$

where $S_P(f)$ is the periodogram, T_S is the sampling period, N is the number of samples of the signal and f is the frequency. Hence, the periodogram is estimated as the squared magnitude of the N points DTFT of $x[n]$. The DTFT is easily computed through the Fast Fourier Transform (FFT) algorithm and, therefore, also the periodogram.

A variation of the periodogram is the windowed periodogram, i.e., we apply a window, in the process of computing periodogram. Each kind of window has specific characteristics. There are many types of windows, such as triangular windows (like Bartlett's), gaussian windows (like Hanning's) and others kinds. These windows are used to deal with the problem of smearing and leakage, due to the presence of main lobe and side lobes. For more details see (Sörnmo & Laguna, 2005).

In the standard periodogram, no window is used (although no using window is the same as using a rectangular window).

In Figure 3, it is presented two periodograms (computed with a 1024 points FFT) of EEG signals from Motor-Imagery database, where an Event Related Desynchronization (ERD) is observed (Pfurtscheller & Lopes da Silva, 1999). That means, in channel 1 over C_3 (left figure) the mean power in µ-band (8 to 12 Hz) is higher than the other one in channel 2 over C_4 (right figure), i.e., in this trial, it is observed easily that subject imagines a left motor task.

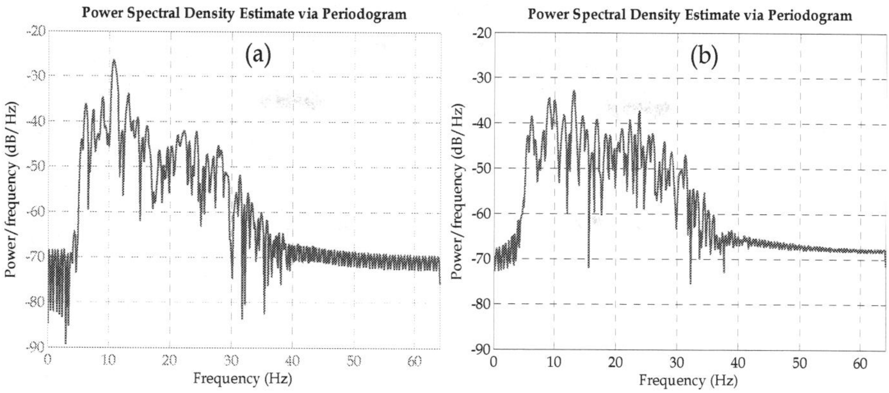

Fig. 3. Standard Periodograms from Motor-Imagery database, trial n°1, between 4 to 6 s; from (a) channel 1 (over C_3) and (b) from channel 2 (over C_4). In this trial the subject imagines a left motor task, then the mean power in μ-band over C_4 is lower than C_3. Both periodograms were estimated with a 1024 points FFT. EEG signals were previously filtered between 6 and 30 Hz.

3.2. Welch Periodogram

Welch periodogram is a version modified of the periodogram, it can use windowing or not, but the principal feature of this method is the averaging periodogram. The consequence of this averaging is the reduction of the variance of the spectrum, at the expense of a reduction of spectral resolution

The Welch periodogram can be computed performing the following steps:

1. Split the signal in M overlapped segments of D samples length each.
2. Calculates the periodogram for each segment $S_P(f)^{(m)}$. Each segment had applied a window.
3. Hence, the Welch periodogram $S_W(f)$ is calculated as:

$$\hat{S}_W(f) = \frac{1}{M}\sum_{m=1}^{M}\hat{S}_P(f)^{(m)} \tag{2}$$

The quantity of segments M could be calculated as:

$$M = \frac{N-D}{L} + 1 \tag{3}$$

where N is the number of samples of the signal and L is the number of samples overlapping between the segments. In this work, the overlapping was selected in 50% in all cases, which is the standard value in computation of Welch periodogram.

The resolution R depends on the length of segment D according to:

$$R = \frac{1}{D T_S} \tag{4}$$

Hence, high values of D (higher than 75 %, approximately, of the number of samples of the signal N) obtain a PSD similar to the standard periodogram. On the contrary, with small values of D the periodogram is smoothed. This fact can be observed in the Figure 4, where several Welch periodogram are shown, for different Hamming window lengths (16, 32, 64 and 128 points).

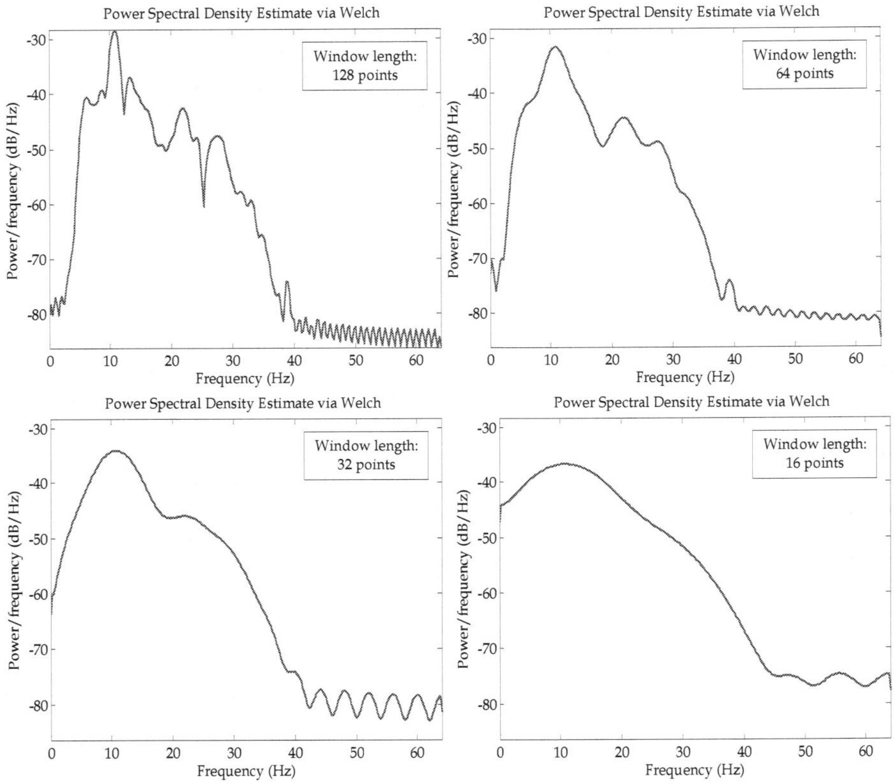

Fig. 4. Welch periodogram computed with a 512 points FFT, for different window length (128, 64, 32 and 16 points), from Motor-Imagery database, trial nº1, between 4 to 6 s; from channel 1 (over C_3). The periodogram is smoothed when decreasing the window length. A Hamming window was applied in all cases. The EEG signal was filtered between 6 to 30 Hz.

3.3. Burg method

If consider the EEG like a linear stochastic signal, the EEG can be modelled as an autoregressive (AR) model, i.e., the estimation of PSD becomes a problem of system identification.

An AR modelling is, as depicted in Figure 5, based on white noise $v_{(n)}$ feeding a filter $H_{(z)}$, thus we obtain the signal $x_{(n)}$. The white noise is considered as zero-mean and variance σ_v^2. The filter $H_{(z)}$ is expressed as:

$$H_{(z)} = \frac{1}{A_{(z)}} = \frac{1}{1 + a_1 z^{-1} + a_2 z^{-2} + \cdots + a_p z^{-p}} \qquad (5)$$

where $A_{(z)}$ is a polynomial of order p with coefficients a_p. Those can be estimated through different methods, such as autocorrelation (Yule-Walker), covariance, modified covariance and Burg method. In this work, the Burg method was utilized.

Once we are estimated the coefficients a_p, the PSD is calculated as:

$$S(f) = \frac{T_s \sigma^2}{\left| 1 + \sum_{p=1}^{P} a_p \, e^{-j2\pi f T_s p} \right|^2} \qquad (6)$$

where σ is the variance of the input signal and P is the order of the AR model.

The Burg method is a technique to estimate the coefficients a_p of the AR model. This method joint the minimization of the forward and backward prediction error variances using the Levinson-Durbin recursion in the minimization process. The prediction error filter is estimated using a lattice structure; afterwards, the parameters are transformed into direct form FIR predictor parameters. Thus, the PSD can be calculated using (6). The Burg description algorithm is beyond of the scope of this work, for mathematical concerns see (Sörnmo & Laguna, 2005).

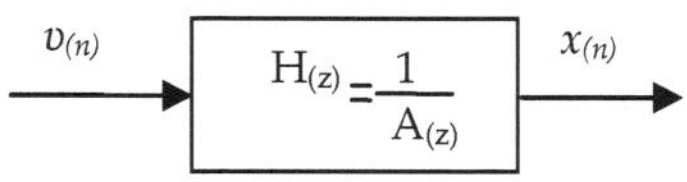

Fig. 5. Autoregressive modeling: Modeled signal $x_{(n)}$ obtained through filtering white noise $v_{(n)}$ with filter $H_{(z)}$.

3.3.1. Model order

An issue in parametric PSD is choosing the model order, since it influences the shape of estimated PSD. A low order means a smooth spectrum and, on the other hand, a high order results in a PSD with spurious peaks. One more pair of roots of polynomial $A_{(z)}$, i.e., increase the model order in two, force another peak in the estimated spectrum.

There are a few criteria to estimate "the best order" of the model. These criteria penalises the complexity of the model when increasing the model order. The most known criteria are the

Final Prediction Error (FPE), Akaike and modified Akaike (minimum description length of Rissanen).
For a signal of length N, the penalty function of each criterion is:

$$FPE_{(p)} = \frac{N+p}{N-p}\sigma_e^2 \tag{7}$$

$$AIC_{(p)} = N\ln\sigma_e^2 + 2p \tag{8}$$

$$AIC_{Modif(p)} = N\ln\sigma_e^2 + p\ln N \tag{9}$$

where σ_e^2 is the prediction error variance.
Figure 6 illustrates the penalty function of the different criteria and it is indicated the best order found for each method. It was observed, generally, that Akaike and FPE methods provide the same order of AR model, whereas the modified Akaike criterion does not. Besides, Akaike and FPE usually overvalue the order of AR model, therefore, it would be preferable to use the modified Akaike criterion.
In this work, the three criteria were tested, unfortunately, no reliable results were found. This is, the optimal order varies for each method, also varies for every acquisition channel, and for data of the same mental task. Hence, the Burg method was analyzed for several orders on each database, regardless of the order determined by the mentioned criteria.

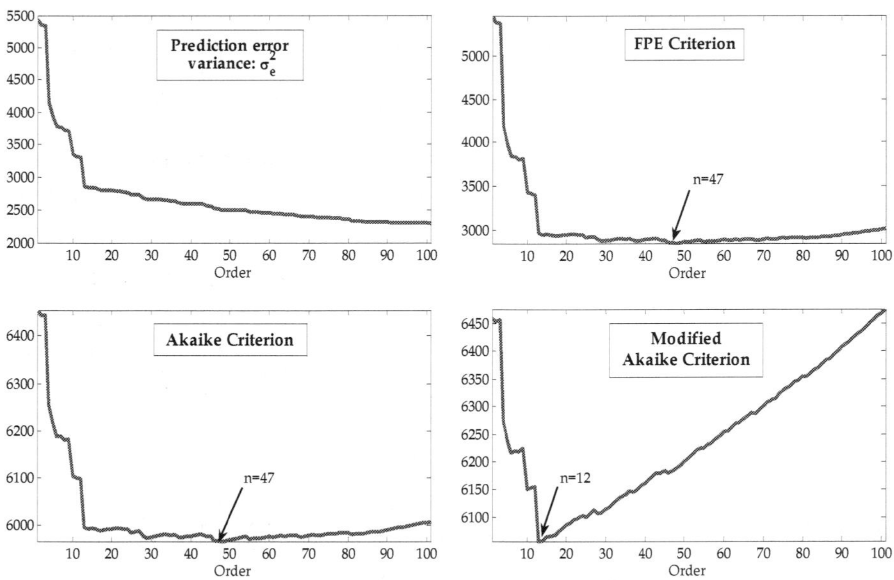

Fig. 6. Penalty functions of the different criteria (σ_e^2, FPE, Akaike and Modified Akaike), analyzed on Math-Imagery database, channel 2 in first trial.

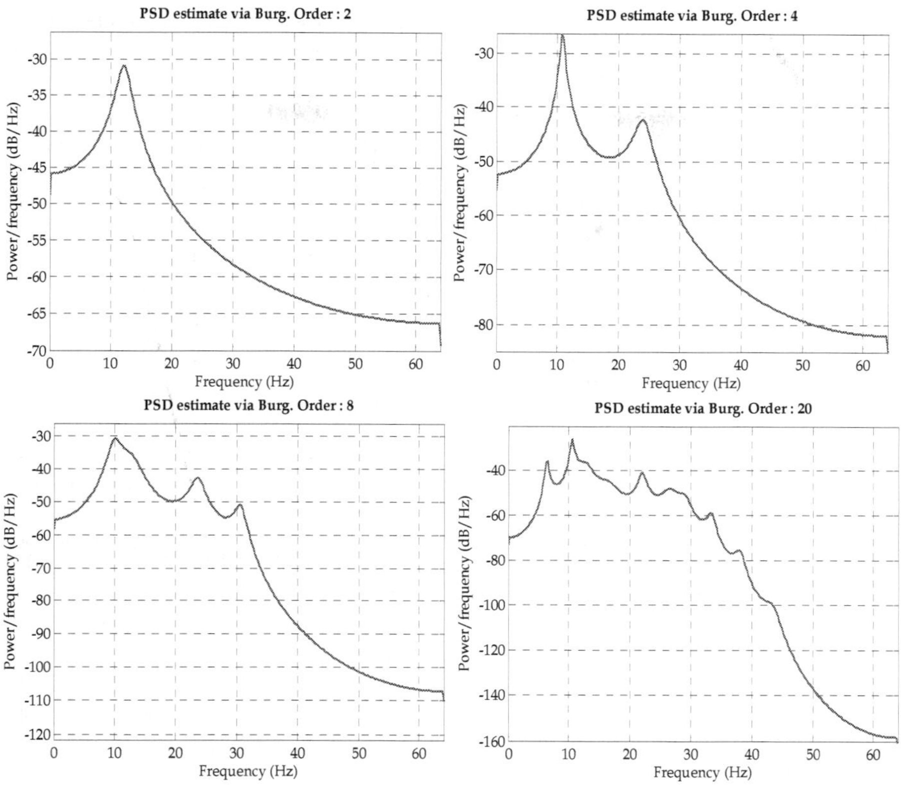

Fig. 7. PSD estimated under Burg method for different order of AR model (2, 4 8 and 20). The spectrum has more peaks when increase the order, according to *n° of peaks= AR model order/2*.

4. Features Extraction

Although, the three proposed PSD estimation methods were apply on both databases, special concerns need to be considered for each database. In this section, it is presented an explanation on the way that each PSD method was applied on each database.

4.1. Features extraction on Math-Imagery database

As was explained in section 2, the signals of this database were filtered between 6 and 40 Hz. The range of frequencies utilized includes the bands α (8 to12Hz), β (12 to 27 Hz), γ (> 27 Hz) and a part of θ-band (6 to 8Hz). The γ-band is utilized due to the improvement results shown in (Palaniappan, 2006).

For this database, we proposed a little different division of the EEG bands. The periodograms were split in bands and sub-bands according to Table I. Due to the shape of

the EEG spectrum (for higher frequencies, lower amplitudes), each sub-band is wider than precedent sub-band. This is with the intention of compensation on the values of parameters calculated.
The standard periodogram was calculated using a 1024 points FFT with zero padding, allowing a frequency resolution of 0.147 Hz. The Welch periodogram, for our 750 samples signal, was computed using a Hamming window of lengths *D=300, D=100* and *D=50,* with 50% overlapping. The Burg method was computed for various orders of the AR model, ranging from 5 to 50.
The PSD estimation methods were computed using the complete duration of trial after cue signal, i.e., a signal of 5 s.

Bands	Frequency (Hz)
Pre-α	6 to 8
α	8 to 12
β1	12 to 14
β2	14 to 18
β3	18 to 25
γ1	25 to 32
γ2	32 to 40

Table 1. Bands and sub-bands in which the PSD estimation methods were divided when applied on the Math-Imagery database. The pre-α band, is just the half of θ band.

4.2. Features extraction on Motor-Imagery database

This database was digitally filtered, as explained in section 2, between 6 and 30 Hz. In this case, the μ (8 to 12 Hz) and β (14 to 30 Hz) bands are on focus, since we tracking the Event Related Synchronization/Desyncronization (ERS/ERD) related with Motor-Imagery (Pfurtscheller & Lopes da Silva, 1999).
The subjects performed the mental task over a period of 6 s (see Figure 2), but the different PSD estimation were computed over a period of 2 s included between 4 s to 6 s. This is performed in this way due to the best results were found over this period of time (Ferreira *et al.*, 2008).
The standard periodogram was calculated using 1024 points FFT with zero padding, allowing a frequency resolution of 0.125 Hz.
For the computing of Welch periodogram were utilized Hamming windows of 128, 64, 32 and 16 points length, always with a 50% overlapping and with 512 points FFT.
The Burg method was computed using several orders of the AR model, between 4 up to 20 in steps of 2.

4.3. Spectral parameters

For the proposed bands in each database, two parameters were computed: the mean Power (P_m) and the Root Mean Square (RMS) of the signal, both evaluated in frequency domain. They are calculated as:

$$P_m = \sum_{k=L}^{H} S(k) \tag{10}$$

$$RMS = \sqrt{\sum_{k=L}^{H} S(k)} \tag{11}$$

where $S(k)$ are the sampled values of the periodogram $S(f)$, L and H are the indexes corresponding to the higher and lower sampled frequency values for each analyzed sub-band.

4.4. Feature Vector

The feature vector is the input vector presented to the classifier. There were two configuration of the input vector:

- Using the P_m of the frequency bands.
- Using the RMS of the frequency bands.

These configurations were used with the three estimation methods of the PSD.

5. Classification

The classification was conducted with some different classifier for each database in order to the results were unbiased by the classifier.

For the Math-Imagery database the classifiers used were: a Linear Discriminate Analysis (LDA), a Learning Vector Quantization (LVQ). This classification was performed for the three mental tasks at the same time. To validate the results the Leave-One-Out Cross-Validation method was utilized.

For the motor-imagery dataset were implemented a LDA, a Multilayer Perceptron (MLP) and a Support Vector Machine (SVM).

For a comparison of most used classifiers algorithms in BCI see (Lotte *et al.*, 2007). Following a briefly description of each method used in this work:

5.1. Linear Discriminate Analysis

Basically, the LDA is a linear combination of variables, on the form:

$$y_{km} = u_0 + u_1 X_{1km} + u_2 X_{2km} + \cdots + u_p X_{pkm} \tag{12}$$

where y_{km} is the value of the discriminate function for the case m on the group k, X_{ikm} is the discriminate variable X_i for the case m on the group k, u_i are the required coefficients (with $i=1, 2, \ldots, p$).

The number of discriminate functions is determined by the number of considered groups. Thus, the values of all discriminate functions (needed to separate all groups between them) determine the belonging group of the considered case. For more detailed concerns see the specific bibliography (Tinsley & Brown, 2000);(Gil *et al.*, 2001).

5.2. Learning Vector Quantization

The LVQ is essentially a kind of neural network; it was based in the self-organizing map (Kohonen, 1990) as first layer and a second layer of linear perceptrons. The first layer is trained with a competitive algorithm with the concept of neighbouring. The linear layer transforms the competitive layer's classes into the target classifications. For more detailed explanation of LVQ see (Kohonen, 1990) and (Haykin, 1999).

The LVQ was used, only, to classify the mental tasks on Math-Imagery database. The architecture was 50 neurons on competitive layer and 3 neurons in second layer. This layer is the output layer and each neurons represents a different mental task, i.e., only one neuron can be active at time.

The LVQ was trained by 300 epochs, this value was determined in a preliminary experiment using a subset of the entire data. The same procedure was implemented to determine the number of neurons in the competitive layer.

5.3. Multilayer Perceptron

Possibly, this may be the more spread used neural network in general applications. The MLP was composed with an input layer, two hidden layers and an output layer. The input layer has the same size of the input feature vector, the output layer has many neurons as classes to classify and the neurons in hidden layers are determined empirically. In this case, 10 and 5 neurons are placed in the first and second hidden layer, respectively.

The training algorithm utilized was the Levenberg-Marquardt backpropagation with an early-stopping method (Haykin, 1999).

5.4. Support Vector Machine

SVM is another tool used BCI for the classification of EEG. The SVM maps input vectors into a higher dimensional space where the classification can be easily. Then SVM finds a linear separating hyperplane with the maximal margin in this higher dimensional space.

Given a training set of instance-label pairs $(x_i; y_i)$; i = 1, ..., l where $x_i \in \Re^n$ and $y \in \Re^l$ such that $y_i \in \{1, -1\}$, the SVM require the solution of the following optimization problem:

$$
\begin{aligned}
\min_{w,b,\xi} \quad & \frac{1}{2} w^T w + C \sum_{i=1}^{l} \xi_i \\
\text{subject to} \quad & y_i \left(w^T \phi(x_i) + b \right) \geq 1 - \xi_i \\
& \xi_i \geq 0
\end{aligned}
\tag{13}
$$

where C is the penalty parameter of the error term ξ_i. The kernel function used in this work is a radial basis function on the form:

$$K(x_i, x_j) \equiv \phi(x_i)^T \phi(x_j) = e^{-\gamma \|x_i - x_j\|^2}, \gamma > 0 \tag{14}$$

Therefore, for the implementation of a SVM is needed to determine the parameters C and γ. The searching of C and γ is conducted through a grid-search using cross-validation (Hsu *et al.*, 2008). The SVM used in this work is the one implemented in LIBSVM (Chang & Lin, 2008). Finally, it was implemented two cross-validation schemes nested, an inner loop cross-validation in order to determine the parameters C and γ and an outer cross-validation in order to evaluate the performance of the SVM.

6. Results

In this section we present the results obtained in this work. In the case of Math-Imagery database, the results were obtained using a Leave-one-out-cross-validation scheme and in the case of Motor-Imagery dataset, the presented results were attained using a 10-fold-cross-validation repeated over 10 times, i.e., a 10x10-fold-CV (this is performed in order to achieve a more accuracy results).

Figure 8 and 9 show the results obtained with the standard periodogram on Math-Imagery and motor-imagery databases, respectively. In Figure 8, the accuracy achieved by the LDA is better than LVQ (except in S2) and RMS feature allows obtaining better results. In Figure 9, the performances of classifiers are similar, but once again RMS presents better results than P_m.

The results obtained with Welch periodogram on Math-Imagery database are presented in Figure 10, forthe different chosen window length. The optimal window length varies for each subject. The difference between P_m and RMS is not so clear, but still remains a little superiority of RMS. In Figure 11, are presented the results on motor-imagery dataset, we can see a superiority of RMS over P_m. The performance of LDA and MLP are similar, but the SVM are a little inferior.

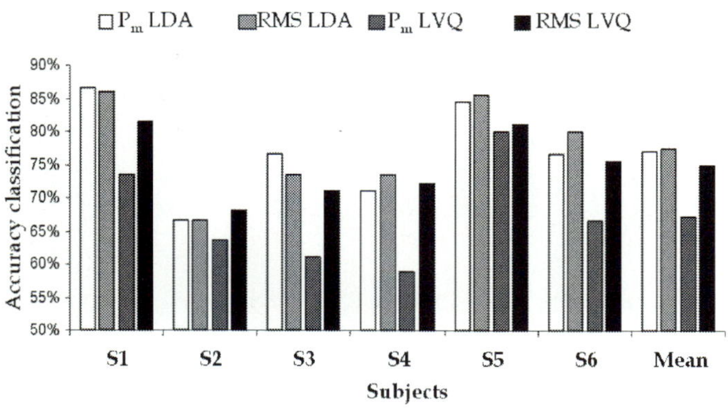

Fig. 8. Results attained with the standard periodogram, the bars represent the accuracy obtained using the Pm and RMD of bands with LDA and LVQ evaluated in the non-traditional database.

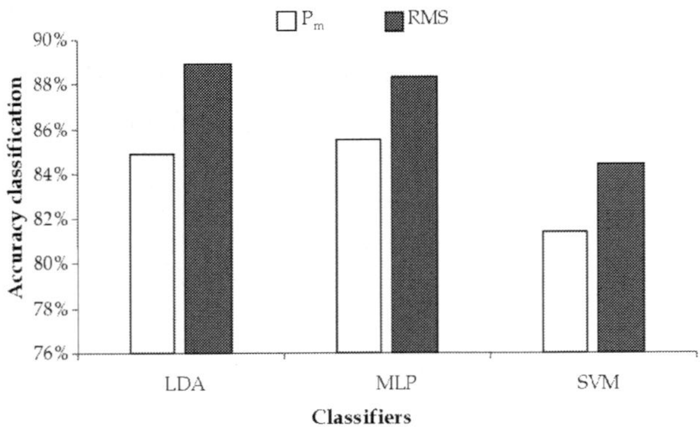

Fig. 9. Accuracy classification on motor-imagery dataset using standard periodogram for three proposed classifiers.

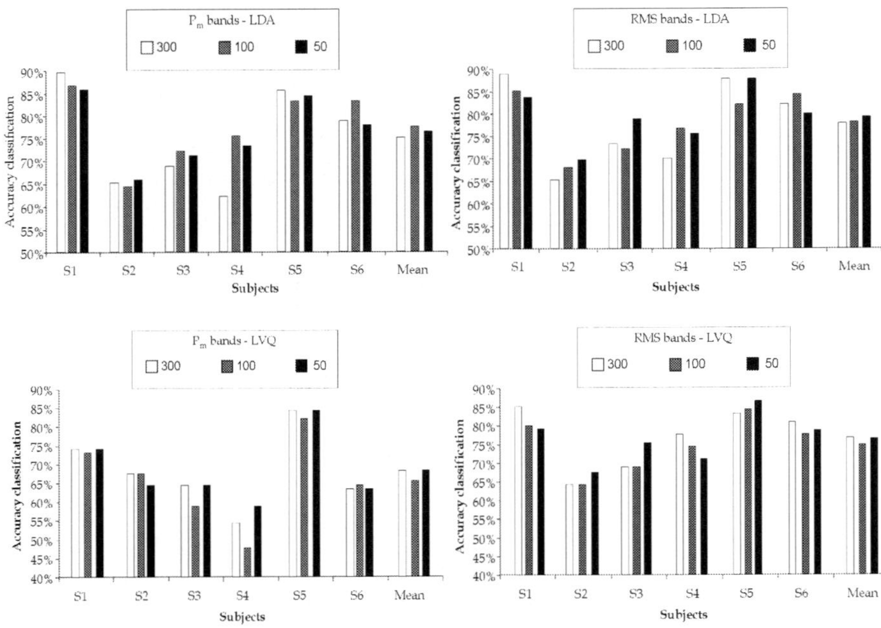

Fig. 10. Results obtained using LDA with Welch periodogram, for different window lengths. The length were 300, 100 and 50 all with 50% overlapping, for a signal of 750 samples duration

With Burg method, the results are presented in Figure 12 for the motor-imagery dataset and for the Math-Imagery database the values of accuracy classification are shown in Table 2 and Table 3. The order of AR model that allows the better accuracy classification is different for each subject, but generally the RMS performance is better than P_m.

Finally, a comparison of the best results attained with each PSD estimation method is presented in Figures 13 and 14. For the Math-Imagery dataset, it is observed in Figure 13 that the best results are obtained using Welch periodogram or Burg method. Similar results are obtained using LDA or using LVQ.
For the motor-imagery dataset, in Figure 14, it is shown the best results obtained for each classifier proposed for this dataset.

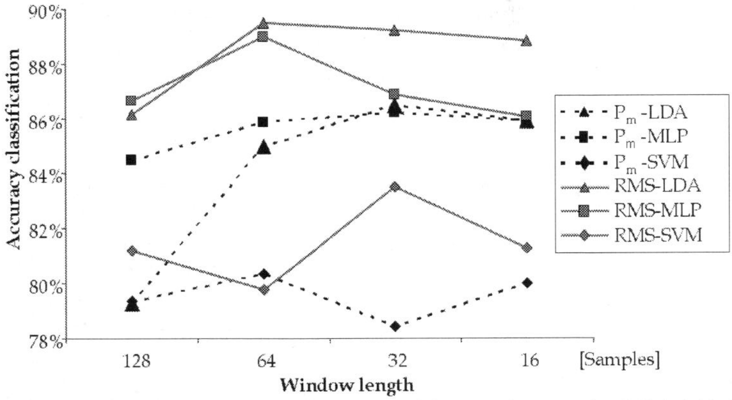

Fig. 11. Accuracy classification obtained with Welch periodogram for LDA (▲), MLP (■) and SVM (♦). The features are calculated using the Pm (dashed black line) and RMS features (continuous grey line).

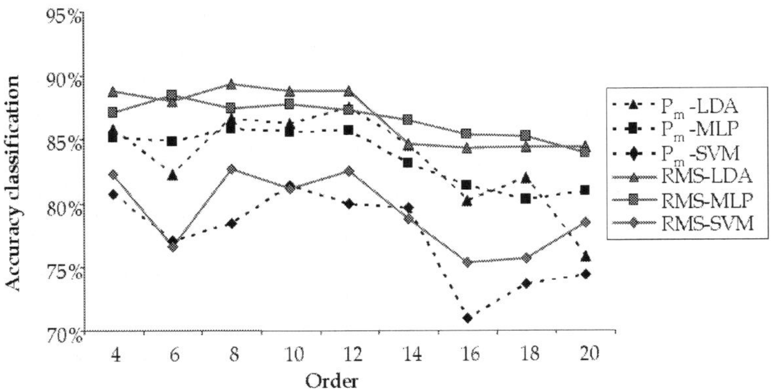

Fig. 12. Accuracy classification obtained with Burg method on motor-imagery dataset for different order of AR model with LDA (▲), MLP (■) and SVM (♦). The features are calculated using the mean power (dashed black line) and RMS (continuous grey line).

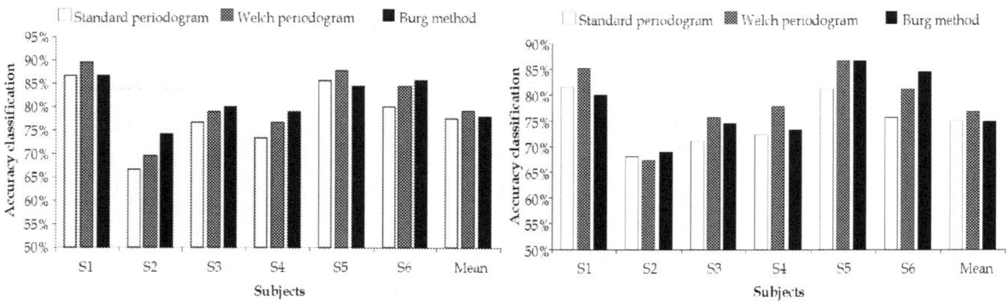

Fig. 13. Best accuracy classification obtained with each PSD estimation method proposed with the LDA (left) and LVQ (right) on Math-Imagery database.

	Order	S1	S2	S3	S4	S5	S6	Mean	Std.
P_m	5	80,0%	74,1%	80,0%	70,0%	78,9%	80,0%	**77,2%**	4,2%
	10	84,4%	67,4%	67,8%	68,9%	81,1%	77,8%	**74,6%**	7,5%
	15	82,2%	66,7%	72,2%	73,3%	80,0%	80,0%	**75,7%**	6,0%
	20	84,4%	64,4%	72,2%	75,6%	78,9%	77,8%	**75,6%**	6,8%
	30	85,2%	65,2%	71,1%	77,8%	75,6%	77,8%	**75,5%**	6,8%
	40	77,0%	61,5%	65,6%	71,1%	82,2%	78,9%	**72,7%**	8,1%
	50	81,5%	61,5%	68,9%	75,6%	76,7%	76,7%	**73,5%**	7,1%
RMS	5	80,0%	72,6%	75,6%	67,8%	81,1%	83,3%	**76,7%**	5,9%
	10	85,2%	63,0%	71,1%	73,3%	80,0%	83,3%	**76,0%**	8,4%
	15	85,2%	66,7%	74,4%	75,6%	80,0%	85,6%	**77,9%**	7,2%
	20	84,4%	63,7%	74,4%	78,9%	84,4%	82,2%	**78,0%**	8,0%
	30	84,4%	68,9%	73,3%	77,8%	80,0%	81,1%	**77,6%**	5,6%
	40	85,2%	69,6%	71,1%	74,4%	83,3%	81,1%	**77,5%**	6,6%
	50	86,7%	68,1%	70,0%	76,7%	82,2%	82,2%	**77,7%**	7,4%

Table 2. Accuracy classification obtained with Burg method and LDA on Math-Imagery database. The higher values for each subject are shaded.

	Orden	S1	S2	S3	S4	S5	S6	Media	Std.
P_m	5	68,2%	64,4%	67,8%	58,9%	80,0%	67,8%	**67,8%**	6,9%
	10	70,4%	65,9%	63,3%	50,0%	83,3%	66,7%	**66,6%**	10,7%
	15	73,3%	62,2%	58,9%	54,4%	82,2%	64,4%	**65,9%**	10,1%
	20	70,4%	62,2%	58,9%	48,9%	76,7%	65,6%	**63,8%**	9,6%
	30	72,6%	64,4%	58,9%	58,9%	80,0%	66,7%	**66,9%**	8,2%
	40	74,1%	66,7%	62,2%	60,0%	83,3%	61,1%	**67,9%**	9,15
	50	71,9%	61,5%	65,6%	50,0%	84,4%	64,4%	**66,3%**	11,4%
RMS	5	73,3%	66,7%	68,9%	72,2%	85,6%	76,7%	**73,9%**	6,6%
	10	80,0%	62,2%	74,4%	67,8%	86,7%	75,6%	**74,4%**	8,6%
	15	79,3%	62,9%	68,9%	68,9%	83,3%	77,8%	**73,5%**	7,7%
	20	77,1%	66,7%	66,7%	67,8%	86,7%	80,0%	**74,1%**	8,3%
	30	79,3%	65,2%	67,8%	72,2%	83,3%	75,6%	**73,9%**	6,8%
	40	78,5%	68,9%	66,7%	67,8%	82,2%	84,4%	**74,8%**	7,9%
	50	79,3%	64,4%	66,7%	73,3%	86,7%	77,8%	**74,7%**	8,3%

Table 3. Accuracy classification obtained with Burg method and LVQ on Math-Imagery database. The higher values for each subject are shaded.

7. Discussion

Although the standard periodogram is the simplest method and does not need to chose parameters for its implementation (except the points of FFT), generally, it not presents the best accuracy achieved in the classification on each database.

In the other hand, the Welch periodogram and Burg method obtain better results than standard periodogram, but these methods present the difficulty of having to choose some parameters for its implementation. The window length parameter in Welch method is more intuitive to choose, since it represents the smoothing in the periodogram, i.e. with smaller window length more smoothed periodogram. For Burg method, the chosen of order of AR model is more difficult, since it exists a relationship between AR model order and the number of PSD peaks (number of peaks=AR model/2), which a-priori are unknown. This fact can be observed in Figure 7.

In Math-Imagery database, the results for the Welch periodogram show that the best results were obtained using the RMS parameter, except for Subj#1. Also, it can observed that D=100 and D=50 are the best choice for the window's length. The mean values shows that RMS obtained with D=100 has the best classification (81.78%), but the RMS obtained with D=50 is just a little bit lower (81.73%). In the case of Burg method, it is not easy to select the optimal order, due to this value varies for each subject. According to the obtained results the optimal order appears between 5 and 30, for higher orders the classification results are worse. The RMS parameter do not obtained always the best results, in some cases, the P_m performed better. However, the RMS seems to be the least affected with the order of AR model. The mean values present the RMS as the superior values, except for order 5.

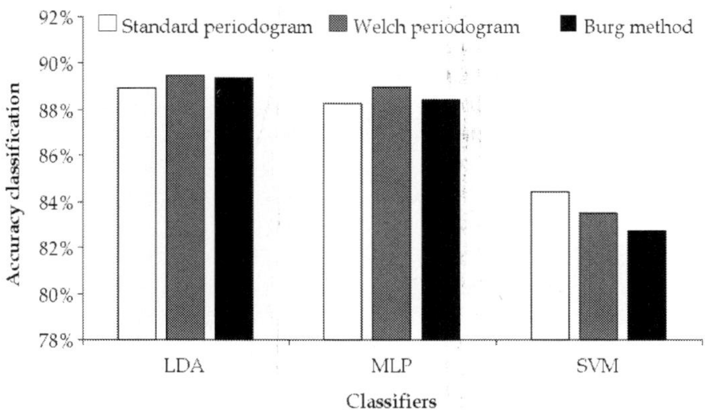

Fig. 14. Best accuracy classification obtained with each PSD estimation method proposed with the LDA, MLP and SVM.

In Figure 13, the advantages of use the Welch periodogram and the Burg method to estimate the PSD periodogram over the standard periodogram are shown. The standard periodogram obtain the worst results, except in S5 where Burg method performance is worse. Welch periodogram has better results in subjects S2 and S5 and the Burg method in the other subjects.

The mean value does not show big differences between these methods, i.e., standard periodogram, Welch periodogram and Burg method achieve 77.5%, 79.3% and 78% of accuracy classification over all subjects, respectively. In the same Figure, using the LVQ, similar results and conclusion are achieved; but with LVQ lower results are reached.
For the motor-imagery database, the RMS obtains better performances than P_m with the standard periodogram (see Figure 9) using any classifier. For Welch, the best results are reached with a window length of 64 and 32, i.e., a periodogram no so smoothed. Again the RMS presents higher values. In Burg method case, do not seem to be an optimal chose for AR model order. However, orders higher than 12 present a tendency to inferior results with any classifier and in the other side, the lower orders seems do not affect seriously the results. But with order lower than 6 it is expected that the periodogram do not describe accurately the EEG properties.
In Figure 14, the Welch periodogram present the best results using LDA and MLP. With SVM the best result is achieved by standard periodogram, but there is not a great difference between these values.
Although, out of the scope of this work, is presented a briefly comparison of the difference classifiers used in this work. The LDA present, almost in every case, good results, the MLP has a similar performance. The LVQ, do not obtain good results. The SVM obtain always lower values than LDA and MLP, but the difference is short. In the related bibliography, generally, the SVM achieve better results than other classification techniques. The poor results achieved in this work, are due possibly to the two nested cross-validation loops implemented in SVM training. This was made in order to obtain better future generalization performance and may be the results obtained with LDA and MLP are overvalued (Dornhege *et al.*, 2007).

8. Conclusions

In this work, parametric (Burg) and non parametric (standard and Welch) spectral methods were utilized in order to estimate the spectral content of EEG signals for different mental tasks. Two parameters were utilized to analyze the behaviour of every spectral estimation methods: the P_m and the RMS of different frequency bands. These methods were tested in two different databases.
We found that the use of the RMS allows higher classification accuracies with any spectral estimation technique. The Welch periodogram and Burg method are preferable in front of the standard periodogram. The use of Welch or Burg methods seems to be indistinct due to they performed similar, although in some subjects performed better one than other.

9. Acknowledgments

The authors want to thanks to Graz research group to make the motor-imagery dataset available and to Department of Computer Science National Taiwan University for development of LIBSVM. The first three authors are supported by Consejo Nacional de Investigaciones Científicas y tecnicas (CONICET), Argentina.

10. References

Akin, M. & Kiymik, M. K. (2000). Application of Periodogram and AR Spectral Analysis to EEG Signals. *Journal of Medical Systems,* Vol. 24, No. 4, (August, 2000), pp. 247-256, ISSN 0148-5598.

Bufalari, S.; Mattia, D.; Babiloni, F.; Mattiocco, M.; Marciani, M. G. & Cincotti, F. (2006). Autoregressive spectral analysis in Brain Computer Interface context, *Proceedings of the 28th IEEE EMBS Annual International Conference,* pp. 3736-3739, ISBN 1-4244-0032-5, New York, USA, Aug 30-Sept 3, 2006. IEEE press.

Chang, Chih-C. & Lin, Chih-J. (2008). LIBSVM: a Library for Support Vector Machines. Department of Computer Science National Taiwan University, Taiwan. Software available at http://www.csie.ntu.edu.tw/~cjlin/libsvm. Last updated: May 13, 2008

Diez, P. & Pi Marti, J. E. (2006). *Development of a classifier of electroencephalographic signals based on a microcontroller* (In Spanish) - Grade Thesis (May, 2006). pp. 22-57. Facultad de Ingeniería – Universidad Nacional de San Juan.

Dornhege, G.; Millán J. del R.; Hinterberger, T.; McFarland, D. J. & Müller, K-R. (2007) *Toward Brain-Computer Interfacing,* MIT Press. ISBN 978-0-262-04244-4. USA.

Ferreira, A.; Freire Bastos-Filho T. & Sarcinelli-Filho M.; Martín Sánchez, J.L.; García García J.C. & Mazo Quintas M. (2008) Evaluation of PSD components and AAR parameter as input features for a SVM classifier applied to a Robotic Wheelchair. *IBERDISCAP 2008.* Cartagena de Indias, Colombia. November 24-26, 2008.

Gil Flores, J.; García Giménez, E. & Rodríguez Gomez, G. (2001). *Books of Statistics N°12: Discriminate Analysis* (in Spanish). Ed. La Muralla S.A. and Ed. Hespérides S.I. 2001. ISBN 84-7133-704-5. Spain.

Haykin, S. (1999). *Neural Networks A Comprehensive Foundation* , 2 Edition. 1999 - Ed. Pretince Hall. ISBN 0-13-273350-1. New Jersey, USA.

Hsu, Chih-W.; Chang, Chih-C. & Lin, Chih-J. (2008). A Practical Guide to Support Vector Classification. Department of Computer Science National Taiwan University, Taiwan http://www.csie.ntu.edu.tw/~cjlin/papers/guide/guide.pdf Last updated: May 21, 2008

Krusienski, D. J.; McFarland D. J. & Wolpaw J. R. (2006). An Evaluation of Autoregressive Spectral Estimation Model Order for Brain-Computer Interface Applications. *Proceedings of the 28th IEEE EMBS Annual International Conference,* pp.1323-1326, ISBN 1-4244-0032-5, New York USA, Aug 30-Sept 3, 2006. IEEE press.

Krusienski, D. J.; Schalk, G.; McFarland, D. J. & Wolpaw, J. R. (2007). A μ-Rhythm Matched Filter for Continuous Control of Brain-Computer Interface. *IEEE Trans. on Biomedical Engineering,* Vol.54, No.2, (Feb. 2007), pp. 273-280, ISSN 0018-9294.

Lotte, F.; Congedo, M.; Lécuyer, A.; Lamarche, F. & Arnaldi B. (2007). A review of classification algorithms for EEG-based brain-computer interfaces. *Journal of Neural Engineering,*Vol. 4, No.2, (January, 2007) pp. R1-R13, IOP Publishing, ISSN 1741-2560.

Kohonen, T. (1990). The Self-Organizing Map. *Procedings of IEEE,* Vol. 78, No. 9, (September, 1990) pp. 1464-1480, ISSN 0018-9219.

Mason, S. G. & Birch, G. E. (2003) A General Framework for Brain-Computer Interface Design. *IEEE Trans. on Neural systems and Rehabilitation Engineering,* Vol.11, No. 1, (March 2003), pp. 70-85, ISSN 1534-4320.

McFarland, D. J.; Anderson, C. W.; Müller, K.-R.; Schlögl, A. & Krusienski, D. J. (2006). BCI Meeting 2005—Workshop on BCI Signal Processing: Feature Extraction and Translation. *IEEE Trans. on Neural Systems and Rehabilitation Engineering,* Vol. 14, No. 2, (June 2006) pp. 135-138, ISSN 1534-4320.

Millán del R., J.; Mouriño, J.; Franzé, M.; Cincotti, F.; Varsta, M.; Heikkonen, J. & Babiloni, F. (2002). A Local Neural Classifier for the Recognition of EEG Patterns Associated to Mental Tasks. *IEEE Trans. on Neural Networks,* Vol.13, No. 3, (May 2002), pp. 678-686, ISSN 1045-9227.

Millán del R., J.; Renkens, F.; Mourino, J. & Gerstner, W. (2004) Brainactuated interaction. *Artif. Intel.,* vol. 159, no. 1–2 (Nov.2004), pp. 241–259. ISSN 0004-3702

Neuper, C.; Schlögl, A. & Pfurtscheller, G. (1999). Enhancement of left-right sensorimotor EEG differences during feedback-regulated motor imagery. *J. Clin Neurophysiol.* Vol. 16, No.4, (July ,1999), pp. 373-382, ISSN 0736-0258.

Palaniappan, R. (2006). Utilizing Gamma Band to Improve Mental Task Based Brain-Computer Interface Design. *IEEE Trans. on Neural Systems and Rehabilitation Engineering,* vol. 14, no. 3, (September, 2006), pp. 299-303, ISSN 1534-4320.

Pfurtscheller, G.; Lopes da Silva, F.H. (1999). Event-related EEG/MEG synchronization and desynchronization: basic principles. *Clinical Neurophysiology,* vol. 110, No.11, pp 1842-1857, ISSN 1388-2457.

Pfurtscheller, G.; Neuper, C.; Schlögl, A. & Lugger K. (1998). Separability of EEG signals recorded during right and left motor imagery using adaptive autoregressive parameters. *IEEE Trans Rehabil Eng.* Vol. 6, No. 3, (September, 1998), pp 316-325. ISSN 1063-6528.

Schlögl, A.; Lugger, K. & Pfurtscheller, G. (1997). Using Adaptive Autoregressive Parameters for a Brain-Computer-Interface Experiment, *Proceedings of the IEEE EMBS 19th Annual International Conference,* ISBN 0-7803-4262-3, pp.1533-1535, Chicago, IL, Oct 30-Sept 2, 1997, IEEE press.

Sörnmo, L. & Laguna, P. (2005) *Bioelectrical Signal Processing in Cardiac and Neurological Applications,* Elsevier Academic Press. ISBN 0-12-437552-9. USA.

Tinsley, H. E. A. & Brown, S. D. (2000). *Handbook of Applied Multivariate Statistics and Mathematical Modeling* 1st edition. Elsevier Academic Press, ISBN 0-12-691360-9.

Wolpaw, J. R.; Birbaumer, N.; McFarland, D. J.; Pfurtscheller, G. & Vaughan, T.M. (2002) Brain-computer interfaces for communication and control. *Clin. Neurophysiol.,* vol. 113, pp. 767–791, ISSN 1388-2457.

16

On-site measurement, data process and wavelet analysis techniques for recognizing daily physiological states

Yoshitsugu Yasui
NTT DoCoMo, Advanced Technology Research
Japan

1. Introduction

The human body autonomously controls its physiological states in order to protect and sustain its life. Recently, it has become possible to track daily cyclical characteristics of the physiological states and understand its system and effects (Haro & Panda, 2006). In order to observe the daily physiological changes in normal life, the ability to acquire long-term stable measurements is crucial, but without interfering with daily life activities. Also, in real life situations where there are a variety of interruptions and extraneous noise sources, data must be extracted and processed with a high degree of fidelity to be meaningful. The challenges are to develop wearable measurement instrumentation and data analysis techniques to extract daily changes in physiological state. Recent advancements in semiconductor technology allow for small and light-weight sensors to be attached to the body without any interference to daily function. Commercially available mobile devices, such as cell phones, are advanced enough to provide on-site computational power and data storage. Body temperature and heart rate are the two chosen attributes for measurement since both exhibit daily changes for clinical measurements (Burger et al, 1999), (Simpson & Galbraith, 1905), (Sandra & Hanneman, 2001). On the other hand, the study of cyclical physiological mechanisms, such as biological clock (Mendlewicz & van Praag, 1983) becomes applicable only when being monitored over periods of time. Noise elimination, range filtering and techniques to recover damaged data are utilized to handle the existence of several types of noise, interference and other constraints of daily life. For data analysis, observed physiological state change is subtle and may not be represented by a series of sinusoidal oscillations. Traditional frequency decomposition techniques such as Fast Fourier Transform (FFT) or low pass filtering can cause data to be misinterpreted. Therefore, a wavelet approach is applied to handle this issue since it is a time and frequency shift algorithm that conforms its wave form into observed changes. Test results are presented, which clearly exhibits the daily changes. A wearable device, stable measurement techniques and responsible analysis make it possible to continuously monitor and hear the whispers of our body's physiological states essential for human life.

2. Physiological Data Collection

Physiological states are induced and controlled by the activities of the sympathetic and parasympathetic nervous systems. These nerves work autonomously, rarely drawing attention to their presence. However, they are certainly exhibiting changes in heart rate, body temperature or other characteristics with subtle signals, detectable with clinical measurements. The primary purpose of this investigation is to ascertain the physiological attributes in daily life by using long-term on-site monitoring methodology and meaningful data extraction techniques.

To monitor normal physiological states of the human body, and especially the daily cyclical changes, it is necessary to use a compact, lightweight and wearable mobile device.

It also requires data processing and storage functionality associated with data acquisition in order to ensure continuous monitoring that can adapt to a wide range of life situations and environments.

Cellular phones fit this bill perfectly since they have become a convenient fixture in daily life, carried by a majority of the population at all times.

Additionally, noninvasive measurement techniques are required when being applied to subjects so as not to create discomfort or distractions. With current technologies, these techniques include measuring heart rate, body temperature, brainwave activity, galvanic skin response, and the like. Body temperature and heart rate are two good candidates to be measured since both exhibit measurable changes daily (Burger et al., 1999), (Simpson & Galbraith, 1905).

Recent advancement of semiconductor technologies realizes highly accurate, small and light-weight sensors. However, even when using such advanced sensors, there are considerable constraints for achieving stable and accurate readings when they are applied to the human body exposed to multiple factors encountered in daily life. Moreover, while compact and lightweight instrumentation is important, the capability to perform measurements on an extended basis is imperative for achieving the measurement objectives.

Suppose that time historical data contains subtle signals which exhibit certain physiological state characteristics, even though masked by noise. For body temperature, the following description can be referenced from available literature (Sandra & Hanneman, 2001). "In humans, a diurnal variation has been observed lowest at 11 p.m. to 3 a.m. and peaking at 10 a.m. to 6 p.m., which are dependent on the periods of rest and activity." In general, about 1 degree Celsius deviation is considered normal diurnal change. Heart rate is another example, where circadian change is observed with dozens of heart rate fluctuations per minute between day and night.

On the other hand, the study of cyclical physiological mechanisms, such as a biological clock, becomes applicable and meaningful only when monitored over long duration of normal life.

Since data measurements need to be gathered under normal living conditions, this approach is not immune from providing erroneous data interpretation, especially when data have been corrupted due to sensor detachment or contamination from ambient noise. Body temperature and heart rate can also be affected by factors such as physical activity and other situations. Activities which require the removal of clothes or removal of sensors, such as bathing or changing clothes, may temporarily disrupt the ability to capture the data in measurements. Therefore, measured data may not be a complete series of day-long profiles to show circadian changes first hand (Philippa et al., 1986).

The assumption is that even after experiencing a number of fluctuations and interruptions induced by a variety of reasons, the overall profile of diurnal change can be distilled through robust measurement techniques, data processing and analytical methods. Therefore, an analysis which can evaluate data incompleteness and quality must also be incorporated. Next, data processing techniques that can segregate corrupt portions of data and recover meaningful measurements, in conjunction with noise filtering, should be employed to alleviate negative influence on data before executing the diurnal analysis.
The measurement and compensation techniques for degraded data are discussed in the following sections.

3. Instrumentation and Measurement

One of the project objectives is to determine whether ubiquitous devices can perform the role of detecting valuable biorhythmic information without causing undue discomfort to the user.
By collecting data on a continuous basis, it is difficult not to encounter anomalies in instrument readings due to system noise, environmental interference, physical constraints, or the need to interrupt the measurement process for unforeseeable reasons. Therefore, in addition to requiring a high-degree of measurement resilience associated with accurate sensors, adequate pre-data processing techniques are expected without deteriorating the measured data before proceeding to extract physiological parameters.
We examine below incidents and conditions that may cause degradation in data accuracy.

3.1 Anomalies

Because of the extended periods needed to extract physiological state measurements, the sensors themselves must not be invasive. Normally, sensors are attached to the skin, and they can provide erroneous data if detached for any reason. For heart monitors, this can be easily detected when sensor feedback returns a pulse of zero. It is more difficult to quickly determine whether a temperature sensor becomes detached, when data points show a surrounding temperature reading similar to that of the subject. The ambient temperature should be measured for providing reference information. When ambient temperature and expected body temperature ranges are known, the data can be segregated.
We can categorize two anomalous conditions for temperature measurement, 1) a loose fitting sensor and 2) a detached sensor. The first will cause data intermittency for an actual body temperature acquisition or show intermediate temperatures between body and ambient. It is difficult to detect this symptom and shall be dealt with as noise. If the denoising process works well, this erroneous data will be filtered out. The detail is discussed in the wavelet analysis section. Meanwhile, the sensor loose fitting may yield a sensor detachment. The sensor detachment is detected by monitoring the temperatures including the surrounding during entire test period, which yields catastrophic measurement errors. This is handled through range filtering by detecting body temperature changes over extended periods with distinct characteristics.

3.2 Noise

Every electronic device emits system noise. In a Gaussian noise profile, a data averaging approach can provide adequate noise suppression. However, other sources of disturbance are convoluted in the data. The environment produces noise that degrades data quality. For a heart rate sensor, activities of short duration which induce changes, such as walking up stairs, or stress propagated by individual incidents, is categorized as noise for our purpose since such a fast heartbeat does not indicate a normal physiological state. Rather than simply applying an averaging process, we examined the data using wavelet decomposition associated with a denoising technique to filter out such data fluctuations.

For temperature sensors, in addition to physical activities, ambient temperatures may be erroneously captured instead of body temperature. Therefore, it is also crucial to examine the noise characteristics of the data for recognizing the state of the measurement.

3.3 Physical Constraint

There are times, such as for battery replacement or recharging, when data collection needs to be temporarily interrupted. Problems attributed to the system, and intentional but temporary system terminations are also realistic conditions when measuring for long durations. An analytical data recovery procedure for missing data becomes essential. This process is also necessary since the placement of even small sensors can interfere with showering and other daily activities, and may require sensors to be detached from the skin. Discontinuities in data series are inevitable when measuring for entire days, even without anomalies or heavy noise.

3.4 Measurement System Configuration

To minimize concerns, we have chosen the chest and inside upper arm areas for the heart rate and body temperature sensor locations, respectively. Data transmission to the mobile phone, located at the waist, is done with a reliable and proven wireless connection such as Bluetooth. Other less power robust wireless systems can be reasonable alternatives. The system configuration is shown in Fig. 1.

Communication capabilities of the cell phone are ideal for providing connectivity to the database to compute and interact with other systems. In our case, analysis was performed at a remote server. Depending on resources and computational ability of the mobile handset, on-site analysis may be an alternative option. Moreover, this convenient cell phone based configuration provided additional benefits such as system monitoring, notification messages, alarms and access control.

If an ambient temperature is that of the subject, it is more difficult to detect a sensor detachment or reading error of the actual body temperature. Therefore, an ancillary sensor is implemented to measure ambient temperature for providing reference information.

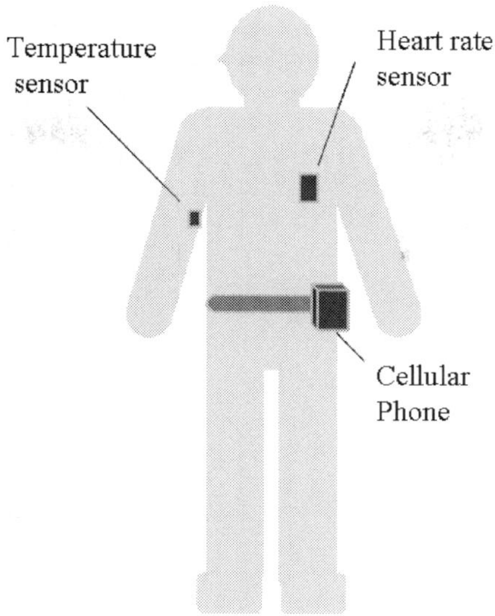

Fig. 1. Measurement System Configuration

4. Wavelet Analysis

Wavelet analysis is an excellent method for extracting signals caused by a change in state with arbitrary time and frequency.

In order to extract day-long physiological state change information, data decomposition and filtering is a straightforward approach. However, the observed changes of heart rate and body temperature are subtle and do not have any theoretical basis that can be represented by a series of sinusoidal oscillations. Therefore, traditional frequency decomposition techniques such as Fast Fourier Transform (FFT) or low pass filtering methods can cause data to be misinterpreted.

The applicability of wavelet analysis was examined in conjunction with related numerical data processing techniques.

Firstly, we focused on the noise suppression capability of the wavelet method. The term denoising refers to the process of extracting and eliminating overlaid noise from meaningful information (Misiti et.al., 2002). Several methods are proposed and available (Qi et.al., 2002), (Donoho & Johnstone, 1998), (Strang & Nguyen, 1996). To recognize noise characteristics in the measurement, the denoising of wavelet coefficients is applied in conjunction with decomposition to determine data validity.

The physiological data is normally benign and can be limited to within a certain range corresponding to known biological activity. Therefore, range filtering and data prediction techniques are applicable to the process. Data intentionally terminated or otherwise missing is recovered by using proximity data and cyclical characteristics to predict what is absent.

In wavelet analysis, the border extension technique was proposed to accommodate data points to the analysis. We note that existing border extension methods were referenced but are not adequate for this purpose (Rout & Bell, 2004). Rather than extending data to cover missing ranges, we predict missing data based on data continuity. A boundary constraint recovery approach was proposed and tested since the corrupted areas are found mid-stream, and can be recovered by using boundary information preceding and subsequent data of the corrupted region.

After these elimination and recovery processes are applied to the raw data, wavelet data decomposition techniques are executed to extract steady physiological characteristics over periods of hours and days. Since the improvement heavily depends on data characteristics, we examined the optimal strategy for each data using different scaling factors and mother wavelet.

In order to apply wavelet analysis for detecting long-term pattern changes from the readings, as explained in the previous section, the followings concerns are addressed.

1) Recovery of missing or corrupted data caused by interruptions in the data gathering process to create necessary data points.

2) Appropriate handling of data noise acquired during the measuring process to provide statistically valid data representative.

3) Selection of a proper wavelet methodology depending on data characteristics, since the objective is not to find a specific waveform but to recognize a circadian profile of state change.

4.1 Data Recovery

As mentioned in the former section, if fluctuating data are detected and determined to be corrupt, those portions must be eliminated and recreated in order to perform a wavelet analysis on the entire range of data. Since wavelet decomposition generally requires a constant interval, missing data must be recreated for the sampling purpose. The border extension method was developed for this reason to avoid border distortion of finite length of data. However, this is not directly applicable to missing data found mid-stream which we handle here. If data is corrupted due to sensor detachment or other anomaly, these points must be eliminated and recreated with the remaining data to ensure the continuity required for wavelet analysis.

In this experiment, data points are in abundance, and show only minor changes throughout the day. Therefore, we can predict and recreate the missing data using the preceding and subsequent data of the affected area.

The boundary constraint recovery approach named in the former section, the proposed method, assumes that the preceding and subsequent regions of missing data have nearly identical information in terms of data continuity. From this theory, the algorithms of periodic prediction based on the Spline interpolation method are employed, as explained in Fig 2.

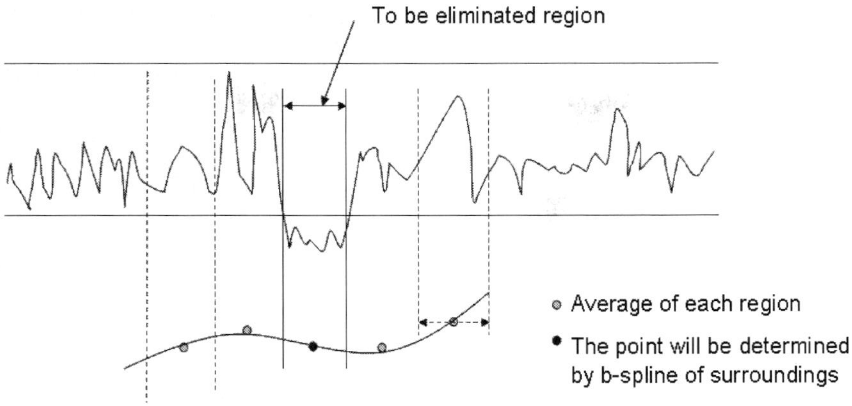

Fig. 2. Interpolation Technique for Corrupted Area

Beside anomaly or intentional detachment, corrupted data specific to heart rate includes changes in pace when placed under stress or during increased activity on a temporal or unexpected basis. For heart rate, short-range fluctuations during specific occasions have a continuous profile. Therefore, wavelet technique is also applicable to detect this region at the data filtering pre-process.

On the other hand, body temperature measurements are vulnerable to disruptions caused by sensor detachment or misreading from surrounding thermal sources.

Fluctuations beyond +/- 1 degree Celsius from the normal temperature can be eliminated as anomalous events or erroneous data theoretically as mentioned in the section 2. Such narrow band range filtering technique is applied and tested for body temperature.

Other divergent data, such as zeroes and overflows, if they are observed, must also be eliminated. Data must be recreated without deteriorating the signatures we wish to detect.

4.2 Noise filtering

Sensors are vulnerable to noise emanating from not only the environment but also the device itself. Unlike theoretically captured anomalous out-of-range data or instrument anomalies identified at the pre-process and recovery, noises are generally difficult to segregate. Wavelet denoising technique is applied at the pre-process to examine the baseline data. Since the denoising method is for shrinkage of the wavelet coefficients, this process is used for recognizing the noise characteristics of the measured data before detecting physiological state change. The purpose here is pre-process and noise assessment. The fixed hard threshold is applied here as a simple approach for the data evaluation. The detail and extended techniques are explained in the reference (Misiti, et al., 2002). Noise under electric fields generally has random distributions, which are handled using an averaging technique, but also through a wavelet denoising process that suppresses the non-dominant contribution to the wave form.

It should be noted that the pre-process provides three categories of information; the anomaly markers, the actual body condition driven by daily activities, and the noise distribution of the system in order to ensure a stable physiological state detection.

5. Measurement and Evaluations

For tracking heart rate, the sensor produces four data points per minute, which are then converted to beats per minute, of which 5760 are measured over a 24-hour period.

Once reconfigured through the aforementioned data evaluation and recovery process, it is subjected to the wavelet analysis with a proper level. The 12th power of two (2^{12} =4096) is the maximum resolution level for the 24 hours of measurements captured. The 13th order is 8192 about 34 hrs. Figure 3 illustrates a range of about 8200 data points. Since wavelet analysis is coordinated using binary systems, actual measurements may not precisely match the data extraction and specific data sampling intervals.

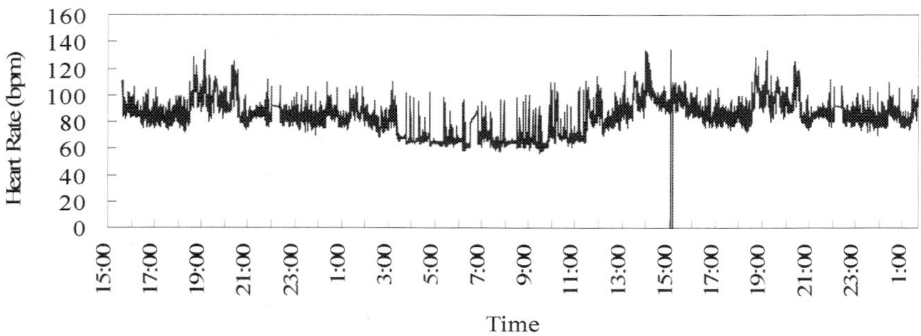

Fig. 3. Heart Rate Measured Raw Data

To accommodate the required number of data points from available data, the aforementioned border extension method can also be applied. However, this padded data can exaggerate the data characteristics since there is no theoretical validation that data have either periodic or symmetric or other specific profile at that region. It has the potential to conceal the state change and thus hinder our primary objective. Therefore, data prediction using time shift interpolation for the required interval was applied and compared with the extension methods. The method is similar to the data recovery of the eliminated portion, but the linear interpolation based on the continuity between the adjacent two points.

By assuming data characteristics, the border extension methods are executed, which can create data points to proceed directly to the wavelet analysis. We examined their effects as a comparison with the proposed interpolation technique. It is noted that for direct comparison, the decomposition for each analysis was the same as the decomposition level of 10. The comparisons with the extensions were provided in Fig. 4. In testing, a border was extended from 24hrs. to 34hrs. to create binary data points for wavelet analysis. In Fig. 4, the Periodic Boundary Extension means that the extended 10 hours was copied from the prior data between 14hrs. and 24hrs. to retain periodic characteristics of the data that yields a standard periodic extension. The Recursive Boundary Extension means that the extended data was created by copying the initial 10 hours of data into the period after 24hrs. that is assuming data repetition of a 24hr. cycle. Although they can also provide circadian profiles, the extended area beyond 24hrs. is less accurate and may lead to some misinterpretation. The 10 hour extension is rather large and may not be realistic for actual data adjustments, but it should be noted that in any case, these techniques implicitly include the assumption that data must be periodic or diurnal. Therefore, we propose that data should be processed within 24 hrs. on a daily basis and adjusted to create binary data points by interpolation for wavelet analysis. For comparison, the proposed interpolation approach of the existing data was presented, which created the same number of data points within 24hrs. to fit a wavelet analysis. It showed better circadian characteristics.

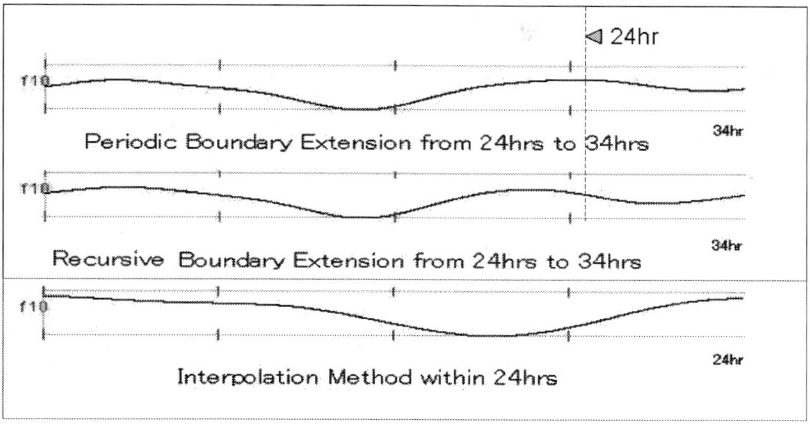

Fig. 4. Comparison with Boundary Extension Methods and Interpolation

For body temperature, the data were captured every second, and is presented in Fig.5. The data fluctuated due to much noise and interruptions. Realistically, body temperature does not need to be captured every few seconds. However, before proceeding to averaging, interpolating or wavelet denoising, the corrupted data is assessed and eliminated and recovered by the proposed process. Otherwise, the data contaminated due to sensor detachment or reading error will be convoluted into the analysis stage.

There was large corrupted period around from 21:00 to 0:00. This is suspected as a sensor detachment since it shows a temperature similar to the ambient one. The period after 12:00 was also corrupted since they showed beyond the range filtering criteria of the normal temperature, which is supposedly caused by a sensor loose fitting. The large noise shown between 18:00 and 19:00 is supposed to be an electric interference noise, since they are distributed around the average temperature. After coming back from the corrupted period from 21:00 to 0:00, the random noise level became slightly higher than the preceding period except for between 18:00 and 19:00. There may be a choice to execute a short time averaging to filter out these random noises. In this case, however, we didn't execute an averaging as a pre-process in order to examine the capability of the wavelet analysis. The range filtering criteria was set slightly wider to +/- 1.5 degrees Celsius to capture a sufficient number of data reflecting the data noise level.

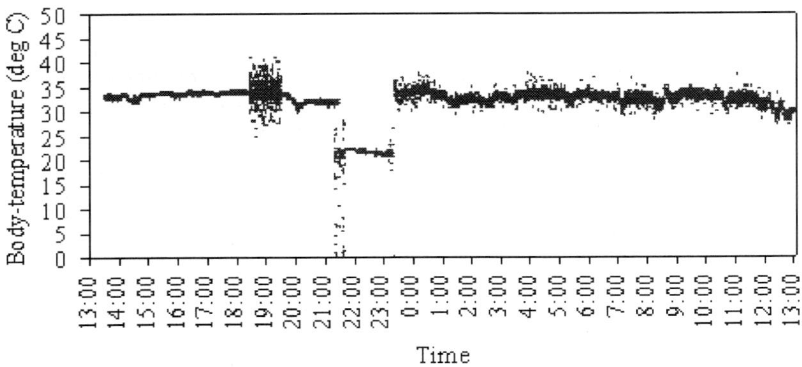

Fig. 5. Body Temperature Measured Raw Data

Figure 6 shows the result of the decomposition up to the level 10 for heart rate for the 24 hours of data. The decomposed residual profile represented by f10 in Fig.6 shows the diurnal change clearly. It should be noted that the profile has neither a 24hours cycle sinusoidal shape nor a state change having two separate stages. We collected almost similar data profiles over different days. The comparison of day to day changes and their physiological meanings are not addressed here, which must be conducted by accumulating a series of test data over several days and consulting with medical professionals. It is also difficult to reproduce a diurnal profile change, such as body clock shifts, artificially for simulation purpose. Such investigation is beyond the scope of this work.

There may be a concern regarding the effects of routine works that are repeated everyday. The large fluctuations observed around from 19:00 to 21:00 in Fig. 3 are suspected to be such activities, since they are observed repeatedly in the next day. This can be interpreted as a 24hrs. cycle even it is not produced by a physiological state but by actual life activity. Therefore, to avoid this confusion, data should be processed with each 24hrs. period. The wavelet decomposition can separate these effects if they are short-term events. The residual profile didn't indicate any effect from such activities, as shown in Fig 6.

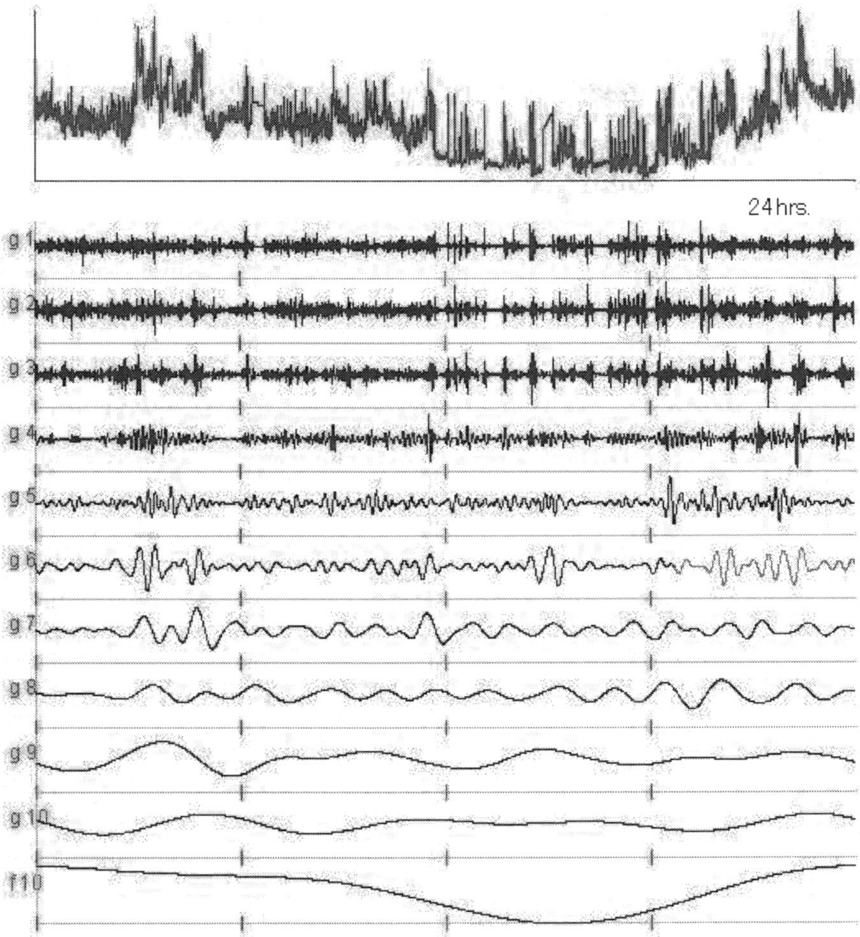

Fig. 6. Wavelet Decomposition Result for Heart Rate

Figure 7 reveals the decomposition results of body temperature. Although it is subjected to much higher noise and interruption than those of heart rate, range filtering/recreation and interpolation techniques can detect the daily state change as shown in Fig.7. A 24hr. block of data from 13:00 to 13:00 was chosen for analysis from the raw data shown in Fig.5. The large corrupted periods from 21:00 to 0:00 and after 12:00 were handled before the wavelet decomposition. The recovery procedure was applied to these areas to recreate the data.

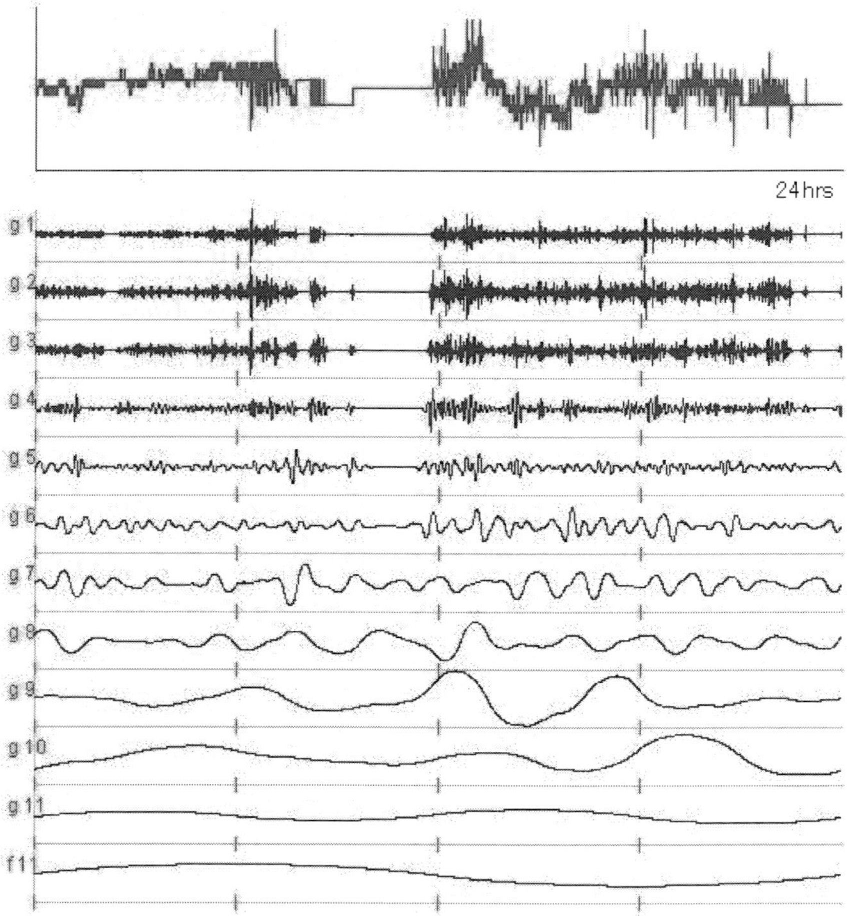

Fig. 7. Wavelet Decomposition Result for Body Temperature

The recovery process also worked for areas other than these large areas of damage when detecting data beyond the range filtering criteria. To examine the capability of the wavelet approach, we didn't execute any averaging process prior to the wavelet analysis, but employed the interpolation using the adjacent two points to create binary data points required for wavelet analysis. It is also applicable to use averaging process prior to the wavelet analysis by examining the noise floor characteristics of the sensor and electronics system. Averaging process is commonly implemented in temperature sensors for health care or medical use to garner a stable measurement. Since the application inherently assumes heavy data fluctuations, averaging should be executed sparingly so as not to convolute erroneous data into the analysis.

5.1 Body State Change

For physiological body response, the sleep and awake states are assumed to be important and are the focuses here. Medical research shows that heart rate slows during sleep, with periodical REM (Rapid Eye Movement) sleep activity inducing faster heart rates. To identify sleep disorders or to monitor the level of attention or drowsiness, cyclical body data can be helpful if significant circadian profile change is observed. Body temperature fluctuations are also a signature of the sleep state.

In the data presented, the subject who is a college graduate student aged 25 normally sleeps from 2AM to 10AM. The measurements were taken during normal days at college. When tracking physiological signatures, there are time differentials experienced. For this example, when entering sleep, the heart rate dropped first, followed significantly later by the body temperature. Each individual will respond differently. It requires more subjects and measurements to understand the relation between heart rate and body temperature in terms of physiological state recognition. To verify which changes in state are authentic, continuous monitoring is required to extract patterns. Therefore, it is important to recognize a pattern of each person by routinely measuring and evaluating the state on daily basis.

5.2 Evaluation with Wavelet

Although heart rates and body temperatures show certain changes between the two states, profiling can be complicated, exacerbated by daily activities, sleep state changes including REM or other elements. The shape neither follows a specific waveform, nor is there a sudden change among states. Extracting physiological state information is inherently slow and usually does not show a specific waveform or frequency.

Assuming that the purpose is to differentiate state changes by applying wavelet analysis, residual profiling by eliminating short-term changes and noise is essential. It is noted that there is no specific selection of mother wavelet and decomposition levels to extract circadian profile. For example, if a profile exhibits steep step changes, the extraction of a step stage change profile with existing mother wavelets is difficult. Wavelet analysis for the typical function profile is investigated in Matlab Wavelet Toolbox User's Guide (Misiti et al., 2002).

The techniques introduced here aim to eliminate misleading or false artifacts when handling data being measured during daily life to identify daily physiological profile changes. The evaluation shall be proceeding step by step. Using the denoising process, wavelet distribution can be better clarified without being submerged by the noise. In the process of extracting a diurnal profile, different decomposition levels or mother wavelets can be tested within the framework of theoretical limits mentioned above. If remaining signature represents physiological significance, further investigation will be applied.

6. Conclusion

The study addressed herein focused primarily on the instruments and data processing techniques used on a human body to monitor physiological states during normal daily life (Yasui et al., 2008). Heart rate and body temperature were the two attributes measured for this study. The physiological or medical implications from this measurement and analysis are only discussed within the change of state during daily cycles. However, it was shown that the wearable electronics and wavelet computational techniques presented can extract physiological state from data points throughout the day. This gives us positive initial proof for the use of cybernetics in gathering physiological information towards developing a non-invasive daily health tracker to better grasp the general well-being of individuals. We suppose real-life monitoring is no less important than clinical diagnosis, when aiming to find a physiological signature, such as biological clock or sleeping disorder, derived from a personal attributes and experiences. Inherent difficulties and constraints with continuous around-the-clock monitoring are tackled by the techniques proposed associated with the wavelet data handling methods. The method is able to show obvious physiological changes, even when significant noise is present and data interruptions occur while taking measurements. Cybernetics for physiological understanding will further be developed in conjunction with the advancement of consumer electronics.

7. Acknowledgement

The author would like to extend his gratitude to all joint project members at the Information, Production and System Research Center of Waseda University, NTT DoCoMo Advanced Technology Research for test support, and Mr. Kevin Williams for editing this manuscript.

8. References

Donoho, DL. & Johnstone, IM.(1998). Minimax estimation via wavelet shrinkage, *Ann. Statist.* Vol. 26, No. 3, (879-921).

Haro, LD. & Panda, S. (2006). Systems Biology of Circadian Rhythms: An Outlook, *Journal of Biological Rhythms*, Vol. 21, (507 - 518).

Li, Q.; Li, T.; Zhu, S. & Kambhamettu, C. (2002). How well can wavelet denoising improve the accuracy of computing fundamental matrices? *Motion and Video Computing, 2002. Proceedings.* , 5-6 Dec. 2002 (247 - 252)

Mendlewicz, J. & van Praag, H.M. (1983), Biological Rhythms and Behavior, *Advances in Biological Psychiatry*, Vol. 11, ISSN 0378-7354

Microsoft® Encarta® Online Encyclopedia (2008). "Biological Clocks,", "REM Sleep", http://encarta.msn.com © 1997-2008 Microsoft Corporation. All Rights Reserved.

Misiti, M.; Misiti, Y.; Oppenheim, G. & Poggi, JM. (2002). Wavelet Toolbox User's Guide, July 2002 Online only Revised (Release 13) Version 2.2

Philippa, H.; Gander, L J.; Connell R. & Graeber, C. (1986). Masking of the Circadian Rhythms of Heart Rate and Core Temperature by the Rest-Activity Cycle in Man, *Journal of Biological Rhythms*, Vol. 1, No. 2, (119-135)

Rout, S. & Bell, A.E. (2004), Narrowing the performance gap between orthogonal and biorthogonal wavelets, *Signals, Systems and Computers*, 2004. Conference Record of the Thirty-Eighth Asilomar Conference on Voi. 2, Issue, 7-10 Nov., (1757 - 1761).

Sandra, K. & Hanneman, RN. (2001). Measuring Circadian Temperature Rhythm, *Biological Research For Nursing*, Vol. 2, No. 4, (236-248).

Simpson, S. & Galbraith, J.J. (1905). "An investigation into the diurnal variation of the body temperature of nocturnal and other birds, and a few mammals", *The Journal of Physiology* Online, http://jp.physoc.org/cgi/reprint/33/3/225.pdf

Strang, G. & Nguyen, T. (1996). Wavelets and filter banks, Wellesley- Cambridge Press.

Yasui, Y.; Tian, Q. & Yamauchi, N. (2008) A data process and wavelet analysis method used for monitoring daily physiological attributes, *The proceedings of IEEE Engineering in Medicine and Biology Conference*, Vancouver (1447-1450).

17

Survey of Recent Volumetric Medical Image Segmentation Techniques

Hu[1], Grossberg[2] and Mageras[1]
[1]*Memorial Sloan-Kettering Cancer Center, New York*
[2]*City College of New York, New York*
USA

1. Introduction

The goal of medical image segmentation is to partition a volumetric medical image into separate regions, usually anatomic structures (tissue types) that are meaningful for a specific task. In many medical applications, such as diagnosis, surgery planning, and radiation treatment planning, determination of the volume and position of an anatomic structure is required and plays a critical role in the treatment outcome.

1.1 Problem domain

Volumetric medical images are obtained from medical imaging acquisition technology, such as CT, MRI, and PET, and are represented by a stack of 2D image slices in 3D space. The tissue type surrounding the voxel determines its value. Within a volumetric medical image, the variations in tissue type give rise to varying intensity. Typically this intensity is a quantized scalar value also known as a gray level. While it is possible to consider more general cases such as vector or tensor values, we will confine our discussion to the scalar case. The segmentation problem is essentially a classification problem. A label representing the region to which an image voxel belongs is assigned to each voxel. The assignment is, however, subject to some constraints, such as piecewise continuity and smoothness; thus, classification is difficult due to image acquisition artifacts.

1.2 Survey outline

This survey includes several fundamental image segmentation techniques that are widely used in the area of computer vision with application to medical images. It also includes recent developments over the last ten years that are based on these techniques. In particular, this survey focuses on the general techniques that are not specific to certain anatomic organ structure, techniques that are easily expandable to 3D, and techniques that can flexibly make use of statistical information.

In this survey, segmentation techniques are broadly categorized into four groups (Fig. **1**), according to the use of image features: region-based, boundary-based, hybrid, and atlas-based. Typically, region-based and boundary-based techniques exploit within-region

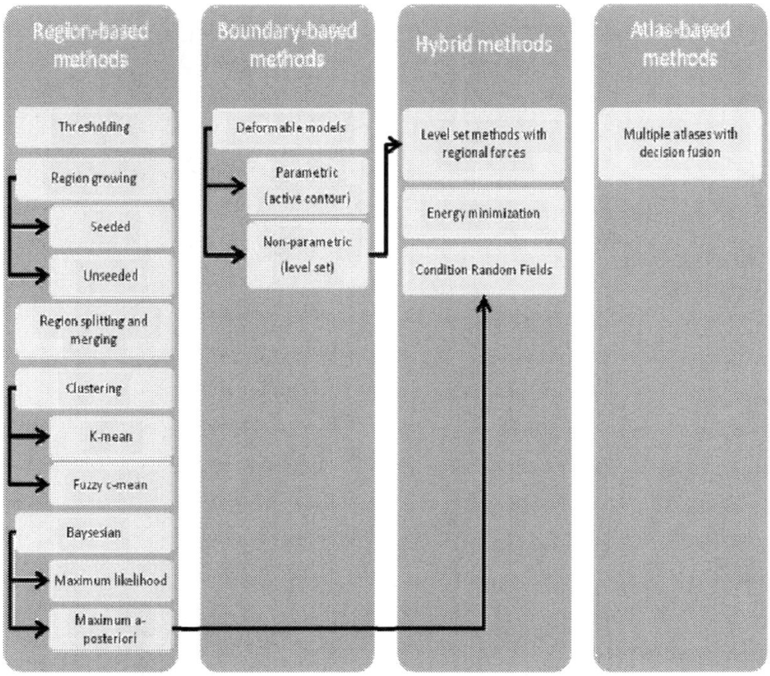

Fig. 1. The four categories of medical image segmentation techniques and their selected methods discussed in this survey.

similarities and between-region differences, respectively, whereas hybrid techniques use both region and boundary-image features, and atlas-based techniques involve image registration between an atlas and the image to be segmented. These four groups of techniques are discussed in detail in sections 2, 3, 4, and 5. Many of these methods use optimization techniques and partial differential equations (PDE). The optimization methods and the solutions to PDEs, however, are beyond the scope of this survey. Finally, the advantages and disadvantages of various types of techniques are discussed in section 6.

1.3 Notations

The following notations are used throughout the entire survey. An image f is defined over its discrete image domain Ω as

$$f(x) \in \Re, x \in \Omega \subset \Re^3. \tag{1}$$

Let r_i, $i = 1,\ldots,K$, be the labels representing K regions in the image. A segmentation g is defined over the image domain as

$$g(x) \in \{r_i \mid i = 1,\ldots,K\}. \tag{2}$$

Finally, $R_i = \{ x \mid g(x) = r_i \}$, $i = 1, \ldots, K$ are the K regions.

2. Region-based methods

In region-based methods, a region can be defined by a predicate function P based on some homogeneous property such that all voxels in a region satisfy the homogeneity criteria, that is:

$$P(R_i) = \text{true}, i = 1,\ldots,K . \tag{3}$$

Segmentation is the partition of an image Ω into K disjoint regions such that the following conditions are satisfied:

$$\Omega = \bigcup_{i=1}^{K} R_i, \tag{4}$$

$$R_i \cap R_j = \{\}, i \neq j, \tag{5}$$

$$P(R_i \cup R_j) = \text{false}, \ i \neq j. \tag{6}$$

Eq. (6) states that the predicted outcome is different for any two different regions. Region-based methods can be further categorized into five groups based on how the rules of prediction are carried out: thresholding, region growing, region splitting and merging, and classification.

2.1 Thresholding

Thresholding is the simplest and fastest region-based method. A region label is assigned to a voxel by comparing its gray-level value to one or multiple thresholds. Thresholding can be global, when a constant threshold is applied to whole image, or local or dynamic, when a different threshold is used for different regions in the image. For simplicity and without loss of generality, we assume a global single threshold θ is used to segment the image into two regions: 0:*foreground* and 1:*background* (when applicable, this two-class assumption will be applied to other methods discussed in this survey).
A predicate function P can be defined as follows:

$$\begin{aligned} P(R_0) &= \textbf{true, if } \forall x \in R_0, f(x) \geq \theta, \\ P(R_1) &= \textbf{true, if } \forall x \in R_1, f(x) < \theta. \end{aligned} \tag{7}$$

Thus, the following rules are used for segmentation:

$$g(x) = \begin{cases} r_0 & \text{if } f(x) \geq \theta, \\ r_1 & \text{otherwise.} \end{cases} \tag{8}$$

2.2 Choosing thresholds

The key factor that affects the segmentation result is the choice of threshold value. Thresholds are usually determined by consulting a histogram. For a medical image, a threshold can be obtained from a priori knowledge. In the case of CT images, voxel intensities are given in Hounsfield Units (HU), and the ranges of HU for certain tissue types are known (Table 1). For example, air is -1000, water is 0, and bone is usually larger than 250.

	Hounsfield Unit	
Tissue	Low	high
Air	-1000	-1000
Water	0	0
Fat	-150	-10
Muscle	10	50
Bone	250	1000
Lung	-100	-1000
Liver	40	60
Kidney	30	50

Table 1. Hounsfield unit range for various tissue types

Thresholds can also be chosen automatically. The automatic approaches can be further separated into two groups. One group selects the threshold based on analyzing the shape of the histogram. The other group finds the optimal thresholds by minimizing or maximizing some merit function.

2.2.1 Based on analyzing peaks and valleys of the histogram

Assuming that the distribution is a bi-modal histogram, one can find the threshold by finding its peaks and valleys. Rosenfeld and Torre (1983) analyze concavities by constructing a convex hull of the histogram and calculating the difference between the histogram and its convex hull. The threshold is chosen by locating the maximum difference (Fig. **2**). It can be described as follows:

$$\theta_{concavity} = \arg\max_{\theta}\{|\,h(\theta) - h^{hull}(\theta)\,|\}\,, \tag{9}$$

where h is the intensity histogram of the image.

Sezan (1990) carried out peak analysis by convolving the histogram with a smoothing kernel for reducing sensitivity to noise and a differencing kernel for locating the peaks. The kernel operation produces the peak detection signal. The start of a peak is indicated as the gray level at which the detection signal has a zero-crossing to negative values represented by s_i, and the end of peak e_i is defined to be the gray level at which the detection signal attains its the local maximum between the starts of the two adjacent peaks. The thresholds can be set anywhere between the two adjacent peaks, that is:

$$T_{sezan} = \{\theta_t \mid \theta_t = \lambda e_i + (1-\lambda)s_{i+1}, i = i,\ldots,K, 0 \le \lambda \le 1\}\,. \tag{10}$$

Variations on this theme that apply to MR brain image segmentation are provided by Aboutanos et al. (1999), who obtain a smoothed histogram via a Gaussian kernel followed by curvature analysis of the presence of both valleys and sharp curvature points corresponding to gray and white matters.

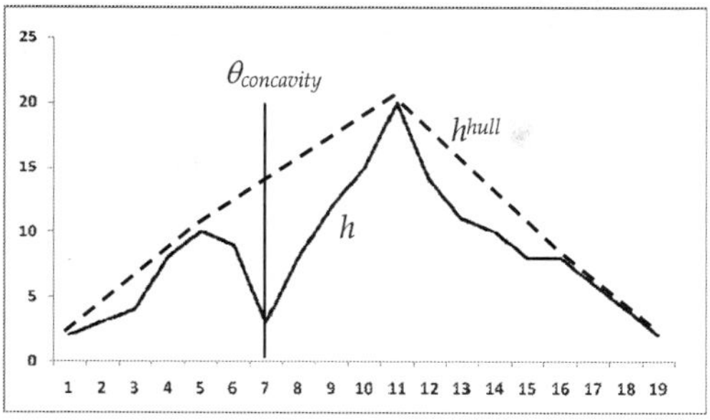

Fig. 2. A histogram h and its convex hull h^{hull}. The optimal threshold $\theta_{concavity}$ is chosen as the point at which the distance between the histogram and its convex hull is maximal.

2.2.2 Optimal thresholding

When the threshold is chosen automatically, it is usually done so by applying some measure of merit or objective function on the resulting partition. A special case of this is to apply the measure of merit on the division of the image histogram resulting from the threshold. Otsu (1979) minimizes within-class variance, which is equivalent to maximizing between-class variance:

$$\begin{aligned} \sigma_B^2(\theta) &= \sigma^2 - \sigma_W^2(\theta) \\ &= \sum_{k<\theta} p(k)(\mu_0 - \mu)^2 + \sum_{k\geq\theta} p(k)(\mu_1 - \mu)^2, \\ \theta_{Otsu} &= \arg\max_{\theta}\{\sigma_B^2(\theta)\} \end{aligned} \tag{11}$$

where probability density $p(k)$ is obtained from the histogram, and μ_1, μ_2, and μ are the mean of the two classes ($k < \theta$ and $k \geq \theta$) and the global mean, respectively. In some forms of medical images, like CT and MR, the gray levels are discrete and finite, and therefore the optimal threshold can be found by evaluating all the bins of the histogram. Kapur et al. (1985) maximized the sum of the two classes of Shannon entropies:

$$\theta_{Kapur} = \arg\max_{\theta}\{-\sum_{i\leq\theta} \frac{p(i)}{\sum_{i<\theta} p(i)} \log(\frac{p(i)}{\sum_{i<\theta} p(i)}) - \sum_{i>\theta} \frac{p(i)}{\sum_{i\geq\theta} p(i)} \log(\frac{p(i)}{\sum_{i\geq\theta} p(i)})\}, \tag{12}$$

Ridler and Calvard (1978) introduced an iterative method that finds the optimal threshold such that the threshold is equidistant to the two class means. The iterative algorithm is described below:

Algorithm: Ridler & Calvard iterative method

1. Given an initial θ^0. For example, $f_{\max}/2$.
2. At iteration i, compute the 2 class means and threshold

$$\mu_0^{(i)} = mean\{f(x) \mid f(x) < \theta^{(i)}\},\ \mu_1^{(i)} = mean\{f(x) \mid f(x) \geq \theta^{(i)}\}$$

$$\theta^{(i+1)} = \left(\mu_0^{(i)} + \mu_1^{(i)}\right)/2$$

3. repeat 2 until $|\theta^{(i+1)} - \theta^{(i)}|$ become suffciently small.

This algorithm is quite similar to the procedure used in K-means clustering, but as applied to the image histogram. Clustering methods are discussed in section 2.5.

2.3 Summary of thresholding methods

The simplicity of thresholding methods leads to implementations that are extremely fast and can even be implemented in hardware. The thresholds can be chosen using prior knowledge or analyzing the shape of the histogram, or by finding optimal ones based on clustering. If the threshold is chosen using only the image histogram then the method will not be senstive to volume preserving transformations. However, it is sensitive to image artifacts that alter the true intensity distribution. For more complete information about threshold selection, readers are referred to Sezgin and Sankur (2004).

2.4 Region growing

Region growing starts with seeds on the images. Each seed represents a region. The region grows by successively adding neighboring voxels based on the homogeneity predicate. A generic region growing algorithm for one region is given below:

Algorithm: Region Growing

RegionGrow(*seed*)

1. region $r = \{seed\}$
2. while $r.neighbors \neq \{\}$

   for each voxel x in $r.neighbors$, if $P(x,r) =$ true then $r.add(x)$.

   end while
3. return r

In seeded region growing, seed selection is decisive and is often done manually in medical image applications. The difference between the many seeded region-growing methods lies in the definition of the homogeneity criteria. Adam and Bischof (1994) use the distance between the voxel value and the region's mean value. Thus, they define a predicate as

$$P(x,r) = |f(x) - \mu_r| < T, \tag{13}$$

where T is a threshold that can also be chosen manually or even interactively, since the mean can be calculated very quickly. Instead of growing a single region, Adam's seeded region growing also examines the situation of growing multiple disjoint regions. A set of boundary voxels can be defined as

$$B = \{x \mid x \notin \bigcup_i R_i, N(x) \cap \bigcup_i R_i \neq \phi\}, \tag{14}$$

where $N(x)$ is neighbors of voxel x. During the growing steps, a voxel is chosen from B and added to the region r if the distance measure $|f(x) - \mu_r|$ as defined in Eq. (13) is the smallest among all regions.

Unseeded region growing was proposed by Lin et al. (2001), and their method does not need region seed point initialization. The method starts with an arbitrary voxel and assigns it to a region and grows the region using the generic region growing algorithm. If a neighboring voxel does not meet the homogeneity criteria for the region, then the method uses Adam's method to add the voxel to another region that has the minimum distance to the voxel while maintaining the homogeneity criteria for that region. If such a region does not exist, then a new region is created for the voxel and the new region starts growing as well. The solution found might not be the optimal one, because a voxel might not be added to the most closely related region if that region is created after the voxel was visited. It may be necessary to re-evaluate the neighborhood of any newly created region.

2.5 Region splitting and merging

A different approach to region growing is region splitting and merging. The method was presented by Horowitz and Pavlidis (1974). An image is initially split into four sub-images (eight in 3D) if it does not meet some homogeneity criteria, e.g., in their method, $|\max f_R(x) - \min f_R(x)| < T$. The sub-image relationships can be represented as a quadtree (or octree in 3D). When a new region (sub-image) is created, it is checked to determine whether it can be merged with its siblings if they have the same homogeneity properties. This is done recursively on each sub-image until splitting and merging is no longer possible. The final step merges adjacent regions across parent nodes that meet the uniformity criteria. The resulting algorithm is presented below:

Algorithm: Region Splitting and Merging

RegionSplitMerge(R)

1. Split R into four (or eight in 3D) sub-regions if it does not meet the homogeneity criteria. Merge children sub regions of the same parent node that meet these criteria. If no splitting and merging possible, then return.
2. For each sub region R_i, RegionSplitMerge(R_i).
3. If $R=\Omega$ (finished for the whole image), check adjacent regions in the quadtree (octree) across parent nodes and merge those that meet the homogeneity criteria.

2.6 Summary of region growing and splitting and merging

These methods are less sensitive to image noise then thresholding methods because of the use of regional properties and the resulting segmentation is piece-wise continuous. Some region homogeneity criteria involve thresholds as well. However, if the region mean is used as the homogeneity measure, since it can be calculated efficiently, the threshold can be

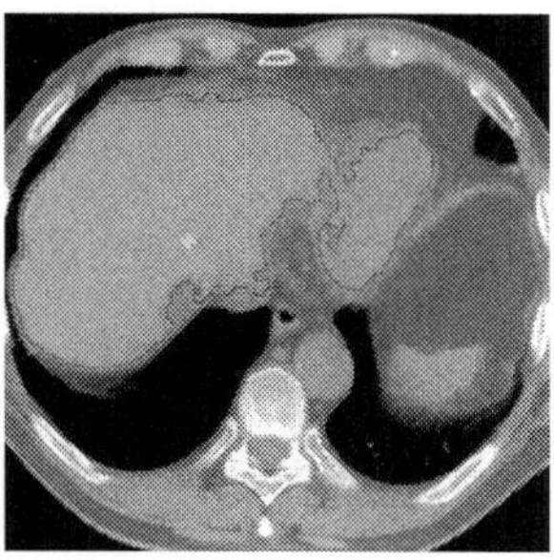

Fig. 3. CT liver segmentation using region growing shows boundary leakage. The seed point is marked as a cross.

selected interactively to obtain suitable segmentation. These methods perform quite well when segmenting organs, such as lungs or bony structures, that have well-defined boundaries. Boundary leakage remains problematic for these methods with structures having blurred boundaries (**Fig. 3**.) Type of splitting used and initial seed points are factors to the results. The results need not be translation or rotation independent. With these methods it is hard to state clearly what objective function or measure of merit the final result minimizes.

2.7 Classification methods

This section describes a number of common techniques used for pattern recognition. It does not cover all classification techniques, but rather focuses on techniques widely used in medical image segmentation. This includes unsupervised clustering algorithms, such as *K-means* and *fuzzy c-means*, and supervised Bayesian methods, such as maximum likelihood and Markov random fields.

2.7.1 Clustering

Similar to image segmentation, clustering involves dividing a set of objects into groups (clusters) so that objects from the same group are more similar to each other than objects from different groups. Often, similarity is determined by a distance measure, such as the Euclidean distance or Mahalanobis distance. Given a known number of clusters K and number of data points N, the matrix

$$U_{K\times N} = [u_{ki}],\ k = 1,\dots,K \text{ and } i = 1,\dots,N\ , \tag{15}$$

represents the partitions of the data set, where u_{ki} describes the membership of data point x_i in cluster c_k. The clustering is considered *hard* if u_{ki} is either 1 (is a member of) or 0 (is not a member of) and is determined by Boolean membership functions; or as *fuzzy* if partial membership is allowed with continuous membership functions. Let v_k be the centroid of cluster c_k. Then v_k can be calculated from

$$v_k = \sum_{i=1}^{N} u_{ki} x_i \Big/ \sum_{i=1}^{N} u_{ki}\, ,\ k = 1,\dots,K\, . \tag{16}$$

2.7.1.1 K-means

K-means is also called hard c-means. The membership value u_{ki} must satisfy

$$\forall k, \forall i, u_{ki} = \{0,1\}, \forall i,\ \sum_{k=1}^{K} u_{ki} = 1, \text{ and } \forall k, 0 < \sum_{i=1}^{N} u_{ki} < N. \tag{17}$$

By defining a distance function d_{ki}, for example, the Euclidean distance is

$$d_{ki} = \|x_i - v_k\|\ , \tag{18}$$

then the task is to find U that satisfies the membership constraints in (16) and minimizes

$$J(U,v) = \sum_{k=1}^{K} \sum_{x_i \in c_k} {d_{ki}}^2\, . \tag{19}$$

A common way to find U is by using the iterative method was proposed by Lloyd (1982). The algorithm is described below:

Algorithm: *K*-means clustering

1. Given number of clusters K, initialize centroid v_k for each cluster k randomly or heuristically.
2. Calculate each u_{ki} in membership matrix U. $u_{ki} = 1$ if x_i is closest to cluster k based on the selected distance measure d (e.g. Eq. 18), otherwise $u_{ki} = 0$.
3. Recalculate cluster centroids from U using Eq. 16.
4. Repeat 2-3 until all cluster centroids (or matrix U) are unchanged since the last iteration.

2.7.1.2 Fuzzy c-means

Fuzzy c-means (FCM) is a generalization of k-means. Unlike hard membership in k-means, it allows the data points to be partially associated with more than one cluster , showing a certain degree of membership to each cluster. The membership value u_{ki} must satisfy:

$$\forall k, \forall i, 0 \le u_{ki} \le 1, \forall i, \sum_{k=1}^{K} u_{ki} = 1, \text{and } \forall k, 0 < \sum_{i=1}^{N} u_{ki} < N. \tag{20}$$

Note that these conditions only differ from k-means' in the first condition.

One of the most widely used FCM algorithms was proposed by Bezdek (1981). In this algorithm, the objective function to be minimized is

$$J_m(U,v) = \sum_{k=1}^{K} \sum_{x_i \in c_i} u_{ki}{}^m d_{ki}{}^2 . \tag{20}$$

where $m \ge 1$ controls the degree of fuzziness. The larger the m, the fuzzier the membership assignments. If m is close to 1, then the cluster with centroid closest to the point is given more weight than the other clusters. Unlike hard membership in k-means, the membership value and centroid are calculated as follows:

$$u_{ki} = \sum_{j=1}^{K} \left(\frac{d_{ki}}{d_{ji}} \right)^{-2/(m-1)} , \tag{21}$$

$$v_k = \sum_{i=1}^{N} u_{ki}{}^m x_i \Big/ \sum_{i=1}^{N} u_{ki}{}^m . \tag{22}$$

The iterative algorithm is similar to the k-means algorithm in 2.7.1.1, except that Eqs. (21) and (22) are used for calculating U and the centroids, and the algorithm stops when

$$\max\left(\left| u_{ki}{}^{(n)} - u_{ki}{}^{(n-1)} \right| \right) < \varepsilon, \text{ for some constant } \varepsilon . \tag{23}$$

For medical image segmentation, some spatial constraints may be needed in order to generate regions that have piecewise continuity. Fig. 4 shows the comparison of segmentations of noisy brain images using fuzzy c-means with and without spatial information.

Several approaches address this problem. Pham (2002) added a penalty term in Eq. 20 for inconsistency assignments in the local neighborhood of a voxel. If voxel i is assigned to cluster k, the penalty term is the sum of the voxel i's neighbors' membership values of clusters other than cluster k, as defined below

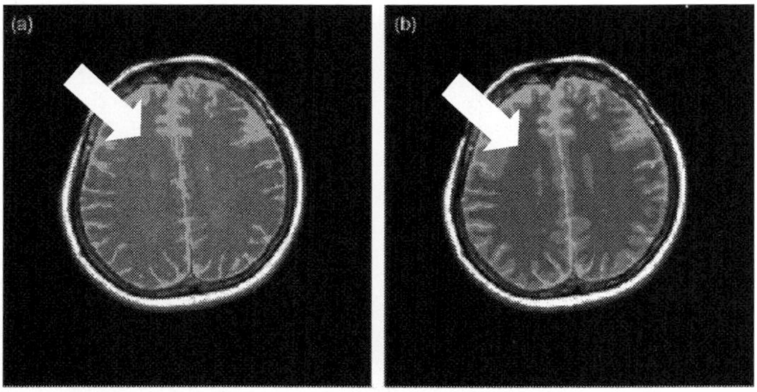

Fig. 4. (a) fuzzy c-mean segmentation without a spatial constraint (b) with a spatial constraint to preserve the piecewise continuity (arrows). Reprint from Chuang et al. (2006) with permission from Elsevier.

$$\frac{\beta}{2}\sum_{i=1}^{N}\sum_{k=1}^{K}u_{ki}{}^{m}\sum_{j\in N_i}\sum_{q\in Q_k}u_{qj}{}^{m}, \text{ where } Q_k=\{1,\ldots,K\}\setminus\{k\}\,. \tag{24}$$

Mohamed et al. (1999) modified the distance measure by incorporating the cluster assignments of neighboring voxels weighted by the distance between the reference voxel and its neighbor. The distance measure is defined below:

$$d_{ki}=d_{ki}(1-\alpha\sum_{j\in N_i}u_{kj}p_{ij}\,/\sum_{j\in N_i}p_{ij}), \text{ where } p_{ij}=\left|x_i-x_j\right|. \tag{25}$$

With this distance measure, the total effect of the neighboring pixels pulls their neighbor toward the same class.

2.7.1.3 Summary of clustering methods

Clustering methods are suitable for segmenting a site where the means of the intensity distributions of the tissue types are well separated. A common application is MRI brain image segmentation. The centers of T1-T2 intensity clusters of white matte (W), gray matter (G), cerebrospinal fluid (C), air (A) and fat (F) are shown in Fig. 5. In addition, a spatial constraint is needed to overcome the noise artifact. Since the data is grouped by positions in a feature space, there is no guarantee that points on the same cluster need to be close spatially. It is possible to add position into the feature space but this introduces the requirement of specifying a prior to balance continuity in feature space (homogeneity) with continuity in space (proximity.)

2.7.2 Bayesian

Bayesian approaches treat the class assignment of the voxels as random variables and rely on probability to derive probabilistic models for images. Usually, Bayesian decision theory is the tool for classification. Here we slightly change the notation. Let x_i be the random

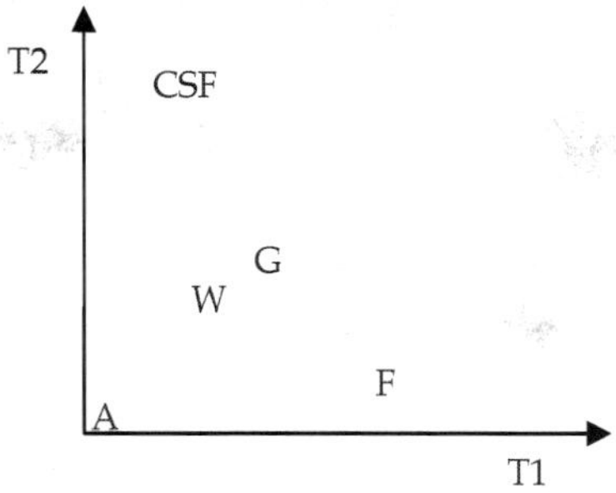

Fig. 5. Centers of clusters of T1-T2 intensity of various tissue types in an MRI brain image.

variable for class assignment of voxel i, let y_i be the random variable for an image feature (e.g., intensities) at voxel i, and let w_k represent the class k, $k = 1,\ldots,K$.

2.7.2.1 Maximum Likelihood (ML) and Expectation Maximization (EM)

Maximum likelihood methods assume that the voxel intensities are independent samples from a mixture of probability distributions of classes. For a Gaussian mixture model, the set of class parameters are

$$\theta = \{\theta_k \mid \theta_k = (\mu_k, \sigma_k, P(\omega_k)), k = 1,\ldots,K\}, \tag{26}$$

where μ_k is the mean, σ_k is the standard deviation and $P(\omega_k)$ is the prior for class k.
The maximum likelihood estimation problem is, given some observed data y, find the θ that makes the data most likely, that is

$$\theta^* = \arg\max_{\theta} P(Y = y \mid \theta). \tag{27}$$

The likelihood function is given by

$$L(\theta) = p(y \mid \theta) = \prod_{i}^{N} p(y_i \mid \theta) = \prod_{i=1}^{N} \sum_{k=1}^{K} p(y_i \mid w_k, \theta_k) p(w_k) \tag{28}$$

Since y is the observed data and is fixed, the likelihood function is viewed as a function of θ. When estimating the mixture model parameters, a good method is the EM algorithm discussed by Dempster et al. (1977). The algorithm is an iterative procedure:

Algorithm: EM algorithm for maximum likelihood estimation of Gaussian mixture model

1. Initial θ, $p(y_i \mid w_k, \theta_k)$ and $p(w_k)$, $k = 1,..,K$, are given from training data or obtained from a histogram.
2. *E-Step*
   Calculate $p(w_k \mid y_i, \theta)$ based on Bayes' rule:
   $$p(w_k \mid y_i, \theta) = \frac{p(y_i \mid w_k, \theta) p(w_k)}{\sum_{j=1}^{K} p(y_i \mid w_j, \theta_j) p(w_j)}$$
3. *M-Step*

Let $f_{ki} = p(w_k \mid y_i, \theta)$ obtained in *E-step* . Calculate new $P(w_k), \mu_k, \sigma_k$ as follows:

$$p(w_k) = \frac{1}{N}\sum_{i=1}^{N} f_{ki},\ \mu_k = \frac{\sum_{i=1}^{N} y_i f_{ki}}{\sum_{i=1}^{N} f_{ki}},\ \text{and}\ \sigma_k = \frac{\sum_{i=1}^{N} (y_i - \mu_k)^2 f_{ki}}{\sum_{i=1}^{N} f_{ki}}$$

4. Repeat *E-Step* and *M-Step* until θ does not change.

2.7.2.2 Maximum a posteriori (MAP) and Markov Random Field (MRF)

Using Bayes's rule, the a posteriori probability is given as

$$p(x \mid y) = \frac{p(y \mid x)p(x)}{p(y)}. \tag{29}$$

Since y is observed and fixed, we get

$$p(x \mid y) \propto p(y \mid x)p(x). \tag{29}$$

Maximizing the a posteriori (MAP) estimation is equivalent to maximizing $p(y \mid x)p(x)$. Again, if independence between voxels is assumed, the optimal segmentation is obtained by

$$x^* = \arg\max_x \sum_{i=1}^{N} \log(p(y_i \mid x_i)) + \log(p(x)). \tag{30}$$

The prior $p(x)$ can be modeled by an undirected graphical model-Markov Random Field (MRF) (Basag 1986; Geman and Geman 1984; Grieg et al. 1989). By the Hammersley-Clifford theorem, the prior can be written as a product of *clique potential functions* as follows:

$$p(x) = \frac{1}{Z}\prod_c \psi_c(x_c). \tag{31}$$

where c are the maximum cliques in the graph, and ψ_c is strictly positive. Thus, it is usually expressed as an exponential:

$$\psi_c(x_c) = \exp(-E(x_c)). \tag{32}$$

where E is called an energy function.

Considering the image domain based on the lattice structure with a four-connected (2D) (Fig. 6) or six-connected (3D) neighborhood system, by definition, the maximum clique consists of two neighboring voxels. Thus, we can define an energy function for the clique at each voxel i in terms of functions φ_1 and φ_2:

$$E(x_i) = \alpha\varphi_1(x_i) + \beta \sum_{j \in N_i} \varphi_2(x_i, x_j). \tag{33}$$

For simplicity, we set α to 0. Finally, we can rewrite Eq. (30) as

$$x^* = \arg\max_x \sum_{i=1}^{N} \log(p(y_i \mid x_i)) - \beta \sum_{i=1}^{N} \sum_{j \in N_i} \varphi_2(x_i, x_j). \tag{34}$$

To achieve the piecewise continuity preferred in the segmentation, φ_2 can be simply defined as a delta function to penalize the discontinuity:

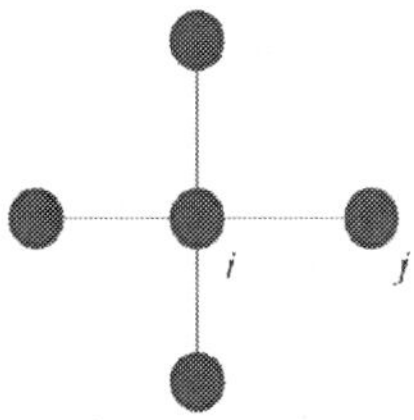

Fig. 6. Sub-graph at node i in the 2D lattice image. Each pair of {i, j}, $j \in N_i$, is a maximum clique.

$$\varphi_2(x_i,x_j) = \delta(x_i,x_j) = \begin{cases} 1 & \text{, if } x_i \neq x_j \\ 0 & \text{, otherwise.} \end{cases} \quad (35)$$

The maximization is usually done by *simulated annealing* or the *iterated conditional modes* (ICM) algorithm (Basag 1986). However, if the segmentation is a two-class problem, it can be done using a graph *min s-t cut* algorithm (Greig et al. 1989). A graph with N+2 nodes is constructed from an image grid. The additional two nodes *s* and *t* represent the two classes. Each node is connected to *s* and *t* and its neighbors with edges. The cost of each edge is assigned based on the first term and second term defined in Eq. (34). Fig. 7 shows the edge cost assignment. The maximization can then be obtained by finding the min s-t cut; and the nodes are partitioned into two groups, with one group remaining connected *s* representing a class and the other group remaining connected to *t* representing the other class. Kolmogorov and Zabih (2004) studied the energy functions that can be minimized using a graph cut.

3. Boundary-based methods

In this section, the survey focuses on deformable models that are widely used and studied in medical image segmentation because of their contour connectivity.

Deformable models are curves or surfaces defined in an image domain that change their shape under the influence of force. The forces are usually *internal*, from the curve or surface itself, or *external*, from the image data. Boundary-based methods can be divided into two groups, depending on how the curve and surface are defined: the parametric (explicit) deformable model, which is also called active contour; and the non-parametric (implicit) deformable model, which is also called level set or geometric active contour.

3.1 Parametric deformable model (active contour)

Active contours, also known as "snakes" (Kass et al. 1988), are parametric curves represented by $c(s) = (x(s), y(s))$, $0 \le s \le 1$, in the 2D image domain (for simplicity). The model is active because it always minimizes the following energy function as the shape of the contour changes

$$E(c) = \int_0^1 E_{in}(c(s)) + \lambda E_{ex}(c(s))ds \,. \quad (36)$$

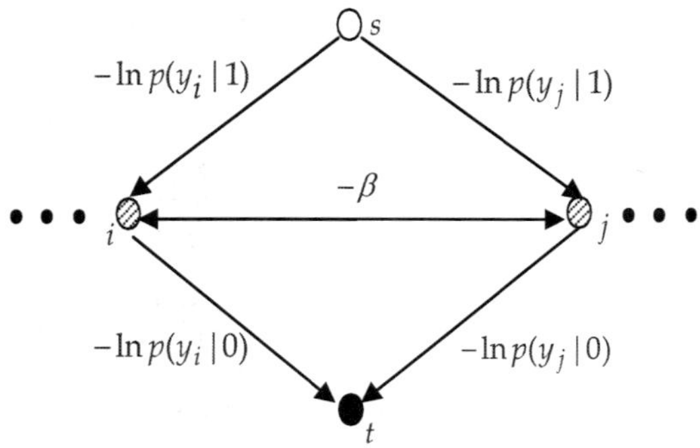

Fig. 7. Edge cost assignment for the graph cut based segmentation. Finding the minimum cost of its *s*-*t* cut is equivalent to maximizing the objective function in Eq. (34).

Here, E_{in} is the internal energy due to the bending of the contour, and E_{ex} is the external energy from the image data and external constraints. λ is a weighted constant. E_{in} can be written:

$$E_{in} = \left(\alpha(s)|c'(s)|^2 + \beta(s)|c''(s)|^2 \right)/2 . \tag{37}$$

The internal energy is meant to enforce the smoothness of the curve and is composed of a first-order term c' controlled by $\alpha(s)$ and a second-order term c'' controlled by $\beta(s)$. The second-order term causes the snake to act like a thin-plate. Setting a point to zero allows the snake to build up a corner around the point. In practice, $\alpha(s)$ and $\beta(s)$ are often chosen to be constants. The external energy can be the image force that attracts the contour toward some image features, like edges, as defined below:

$$E_{ex} = -|\nabla f| . \tag{38}$$

To reduce the noise artifacts and extend the range of the image force, we can use edges on an image smoothed with a Gaussian kernel:

$$E_{ex} = -|\nabla (G_\sigma * f)| . \tag{39}$$

The problem of finding a curve c that minimizes Eq. (36) is known as the calculus of variation problem. The curve must satisfy the following Euler-Lagrange equation:

$$\alpha c''(s) + \beta c''''(s) - \lambda \frac{dE_{ex}}{dc} = 0 . \tag{40}$$

One much discussed point about snakes is their inability to find the boundary when the initial contour is placed too far away from the actual boundary location. One solution is increasing σ in Eq. (39) to allow the snake to come to equilibrium from a longer range at coarse scale and then slowly reducing σ to allow tracking of the boundary at a finer scale.

Another solution proposed by Xu and Prince (1997) is a gradient vector field (GVF), which is a diffusion of image edge map. Let e be the edge map of image f. The GVF v=(u, v) is the vector field that minimizes the following energy function:

$$E = \int\int \mu(u_x{}^2 + u_x{}^2 + u_x{}^2 + u_x{}^2) + |\nabla e|^2 |\mathrm{v} - \nabla e|^2 \, dxdy \tag{41}$$

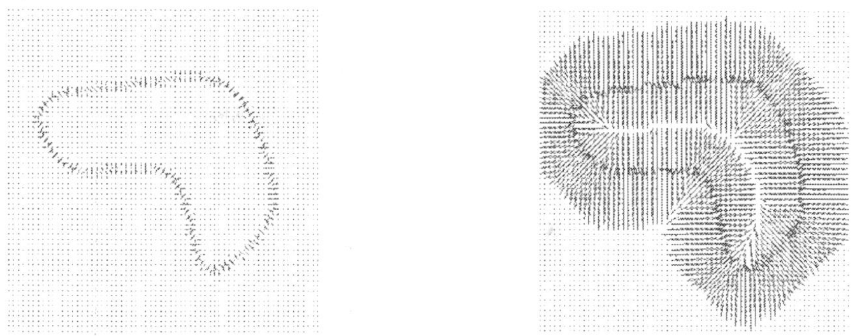

Fig. 8. An edge map (left) and its gradient vector field (right). Gradient vector field basically is the diffusion of the edge map. This allows the contour points to be pulled to the edge from longer distance.

Thus, even in the homogeneous regions of the image, the GVF has vectors that vary smoothly and point toward edges. This diffused field replaces the $-\nabla E_{ex}$ in Eq. (40) to guide the positioning of the snake. Fig. 8 shows an example of an original map and its gradient vector field.

The snake is always attracted to the strong edge in the above external image forces. However, this may not be good behavior for medical image segmentation. For example, the active contour for the lower contrast boundary may be attracted to the nearby higher contrast structures (Fig. 9). To solve this problem, Fenster and Kender (2001) used a statistical image energy function. The statistical term measures the distance between the distributions of the intensities and gradients along the contour sector's normal direction and the distributions from training data. Let the two image features defined in this method be

$$\begin{aligned} f_c &= f(c(s)) \\ \nabla f_{c^\perp} &= c^\perp(s) \cdot \nabla f(c(s)). \end{aligned} \tag{42}$$

Assume that the distributions of the two image features are normal: $N(\mu_1, \sigma_1)$ and $N(\mu_2, \sigma_2)$. Here μ and σ are given and obtained from the training contours. Then, the external energy of the active contour is defined as

$$E_{ex} = \int \frac{(f_c - \mu_1)^2}{{\sigma_{1_c}}^2} + \frac{(\nabla f_{c^\perp} - \mu_2)^2}{{\sigma_2}^2} ds. \tag{43}$$

3.2 Non-parametric deformable model (level set, geometric active contour)

The parametric deformable model has difficulty handling the change in topology of the unknown object to be segmented. Non-parametric deformable models are based on curve convolution theory and level set methods (Osher and Sethian 1988, Sethian 1999.) The curve is represented implicitly as a level set function with the extra dimension of time. The evolution of curve and surface is independent of parameterization and, therefore, the topological changes can be handled automatically.

Given a level set function with the moving curve u as its zero level set at any time t, we have

$$\phi(u(t), t) = 0. \tag{44}$$

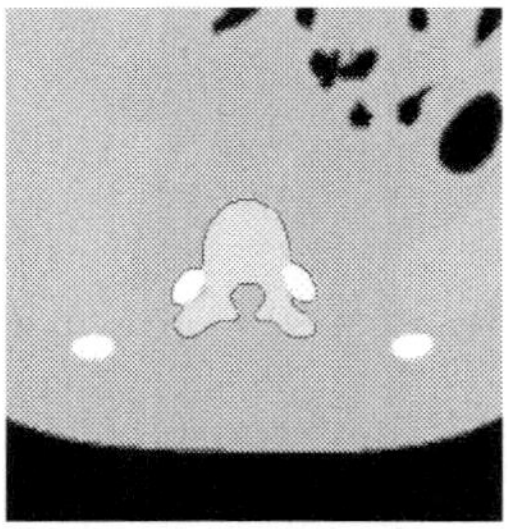

Fig. 9. Active contour to segment a phantom's spine is attracted by the stronger edges of the surrounding bones.

Using the chain rule, we have

$$\frac{\partial \phi}{\partial t} + \nabla \phi \cdot \frac{\partial u}{\partial t} = 0. \tag{45}$$

In contour evolution theory, the evolution of the contour along its normal direction can be characterized by the following equation:

$$\frac{\partial u}{\partial t} \cdot n = F \tag{46}$$

where n is an inward unit normal and F is a speed function that determines the speed of the moving curve. Assuming that $\phi < 0$ inside the zero level set curve and $\phi > 0$ outside, the inward unit normal to the level set curve is given by

$$n = -\frac{\nabla \phi}{|\nabla \phi|} \tag{47}$$

With Eq. (45) and Eq. (46), Eq. (47) can be converted into the following final *curve evolution equation*:

$$\frac{\partial \phi}{\partial t} = F|\nabla \phi| \tag{47}$$

The two most common and most-studied deformations in curve evolution theory are curvature deformation and constant deformation. Their respective speed functions are given by:

$$F = \varepsilon k, \text{ where } \varepsilon \text{ is a positive constant and } k \text{ is the curvature, and} \tag{48}$$

$$F = V_0, \text{ where } V_0 \text{ is a constant.} \tag{49}$$

The curvature k at zero level set is given by

$$k = \nabla \cdot \frac{\nabla \phi}{|\nabla \phi|} = \frac{\phi_{xx}\phi_y^2 - 2\phi_x\phi_y\phi_{xy} + \phi_{yy}\phi_x^2}{\left(\phi_x^2 + \phi_y^2\right)^{3/2}}. \tag{50}$$

In the application of image segmentation, most non-parametric deformable model methods allow the curve evolution equation to be modified in two ways: changing the speed function F and adding additional constraints. A good survey of these methods is provided by Suri et al. (2002). Some methods that include regional terms will be reviewed in the next section.

Caselles et al. (1993) and Malladi et al. (1995) independently proposed a geometric active-contour model based on the following curve evolution equation:

$$\frac{\partial \phi}{\partial t} = c(x)(k + V_0)|\nabla \phi| \,. \tag{51}$$

Here $c(x)$ is

$$c(x) = \frac{1}{1 + |\nabla(G_\sigma(x) * f(x)|} \,. \tag{52}$$

$c(x)$ can be viewed as a stopping force based on the edge image feature. This multiplicative term slows down the moving curve when the curve is near the boundary. A problem with this model is that if the boundary has gaps or is blurry the curve passes the boundary and will not be pulled back to the correct boundary. Caselles et al. (1997) and Yezzi et al. (1997) add an additional term in the equation that allows the curve to be pulled back:

$$\frac{\partial \phi}{\partial t} = c(x)(k + V_0)|\nabla \phi| + \nabla c \cdot \nabla \phi \,. \tag{53}$$

Note that $\nabla c = - | \nabla G_\sigma * f|$ behaves like the external force of active contour model in Eq. (39). It attracts the curve to the boundary and is projected onto the normal direction of the contour propagation front so that the curve can be pulled back if it passes the boundary. Fig. **10** illustrates this idea.

3.3 Summary for boundary based methods

The advantage of boundary based methods, in particular, the contour evolution methods, is the piece-wise continuity. Active contour methods are quite sensitive to the initial conditions and cannot handle changes in contour topology. Level set methods, on the other hand, handle the topology problem naturally through the implicit zero level set function. They, however, are more computationally expensive due to the iterative optimization methods for solving complex PDE. With the increasing energy or force terms introduced in these methods, users need to specify the parameters used in these terms that are not easily understandable. This makes the algorithms unintuitive to users in clinical practice.

4. Hybrid methods

Hybrid methods use both boundary and regional information for image segmentation. Many of them are the deformable models discussed in previous sections with extensions that include regional information level set methods with regional forces (4.1). Recently developed methods view image segmentation as a graph partition problem that minimizes an energy function (4.2) and is coupled with a purely statistical framework (4.3).

4.1 Level set methods with regional forces

These algorithms modify the propagation speed V_0 in the original level set segmentation to include a regional force. An elegant example is provided by Baillard et al. (2000). In this approach, probability density functions inside and outside the structure are responsible for creating a pull/push force on the propagating front.

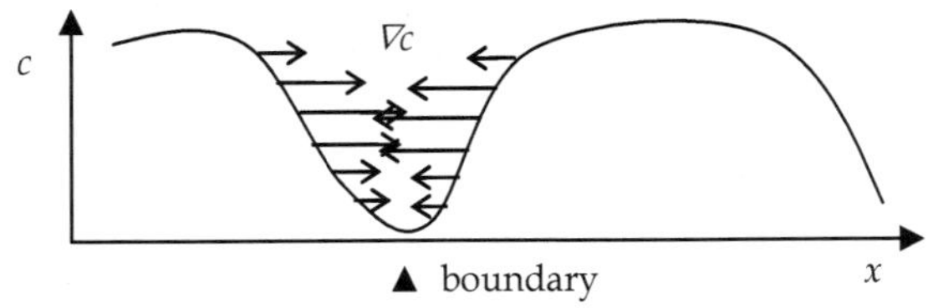

Fig. 10. Pull back force. The arrows show the gradient of c in Eq (53).

Let $g(x) \in$ {in, out} be the two classes of regions, let $p_{in}(y)$ be the probability density function of gray-level y to be estimated inside the curve, and $p_{out}(y)$ be the probability density function outside the curve. The bi-directional propagation force is estimated as

$$V_0 = sign\{\alpha p_{in}(y) - (1-\alpha) p_{out}(y)\} . \tag{54}$$

Here, $sign(z) = 1$ if $z \geq 0$, otherwise $sign(z) = -1$. This determines the moving direction of a voxel on the propagation front based on the probability that it belongs to the outside or the inside region. The stopping force $c(x)$ in Eq. (51) is also modified to be

$$c(x) = t(P_T(x \mid f, g)), \tag{55}$$

where,

$$t(p) = \begin{cases} 1-4p^3 & \text{if } p < 0.5 \\ 4(1-p)^3 & \text{otherwise} \end{cases}, \text{ and} \tag{56}$$

$$P_T(x \mid f, g) = \begin{cases} \dfrac{(1-\alpha) p_{in}(f(x))}{\alpha p_{out}(f(x)) + (1-\alpha) p_{in}(f(x))}, & \text{if } g(x) = \text{out} \\ \dfrac{\alpha p_{out}(f(x))}{\alpha p_{out}(f(x)) + (1-\alpha) p_{in}(f(x))}, & \text{if } g(x) = \text{in} \end{cases} . \tag{57}$$

P_T is called the transitional probability. This stopping term can be understood in the following way: if x on the propagation front is outside the curve and the transitional probability shows that it is likely inside the region, then the curve is crossing the boundary. Therefore, the evolution speed will slow down at x. Note that the parameters of probability density functions are estimated adaptively by stochastic-EM (SEM) without the need for training data. The method has shown impressive results for brain image segmentation.

4.2 Graph cut methods that minimize an energy function with both regional and boundary terms

Motivated by Greig's MAP-MRF formulation (1989) of an energy function with regional information and an MRF-shaped smoothness prior, Boykov and Jolly (2001) replace the smoothness term φ_2 in Eq. (34) with a boundary term:

$$E = -\sum_{i=1}^{N} \log(p(y_i \mid x_i)) + \lambda \sum_{i=1}^{N} \sum_{j \in N_i} B_{ij} \delta(x_i, x_j) , \tag{58}$$

where B_{ij} is

$$B_{ij} = \exp\left(-\frac{\left|y_i - y_j\right|^2}{2\sigma^2}\right) \cdot \frac{1}{dist(i,j)} . \tag{59}$$

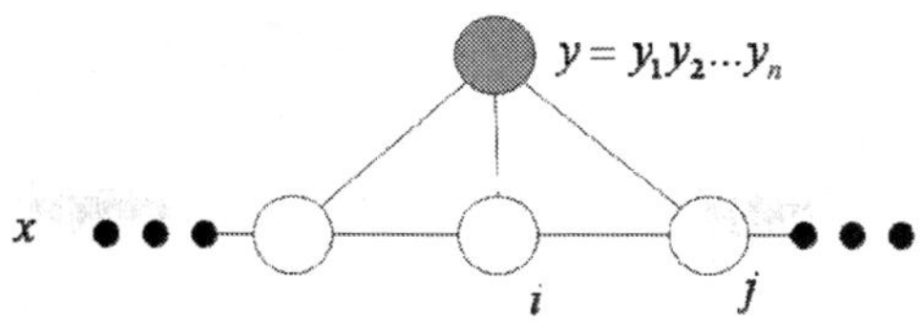

Fig. 11. Graphical model of Conditional Random Fields. Each tuple (y, x_i, x_j) is a maximum clique.

This boundary term encourages strong edges of the target region, that is, if the contrast of intensity between neighboring voxel i and j is high, they are more likely to be assigned to two different classes.

This energy function can be minimized by graph min-s-t cut as well for target object and background two-class segmentation as described in section 2.7.2.2. The method uses an interactive tool to specify the hard constraints via paintbrushes that identify the voxels inside the target region and those outside. Colorization utilizes a similar idea (Levin and Lischinski 2004). For the target or background "seed" voxels specified by the user, a high cost is assigned to the edges connecting those nodes to the class node s or t so that these nodes cannot be partitioned to the other class.

Freedman and Zhang (2005) adopted a similar approach that includes a regional term derived from the probabilistic atlas as a shape prior. The position of the voxel is included as the image feature and is used to estimate the probability of where the voxel resides as the target or background region from the probabilistic atlas in the training data.

4.3 Condition Random Fields

The major drawback of using MRF as a model for labeling voxels (unknown data) is the difficulty of using intensity information (observed data) around the voxel's neighbors. To make use of the information, independence assumptions about the observation samples must be modeled. The problem is addressed by Lafferty et al. (2001) with the formation of a formal extension of MRF called Conditional Random Field (CRF).

CRF is an MRF, but globally conditioned by the observed image y. This is accomplished by including y in the undirected graphical model and connecting y to all the unknown random variables of x in the random field (Fig. **11**). Thus, each tuple of $\{(y, x_i, x_j) \mid i \neq j, j \in N_i\}$ is a maximum clique. Similar to Eq. (31) and (32) in MRF, using the Hammersley-Clifford theorem, we have

$$p(x \mid y) = \frac{1}{Z} \prod_{c} \psi_c(x_c, y), \tag{60}$$

and

$$\psi_c(x_c, y) = \exp(-E(x_c, y)), \tag{61}$$

The maximum a posterior (MAP) estimation of Eq. (60) is equivalent to minimizing the energy function

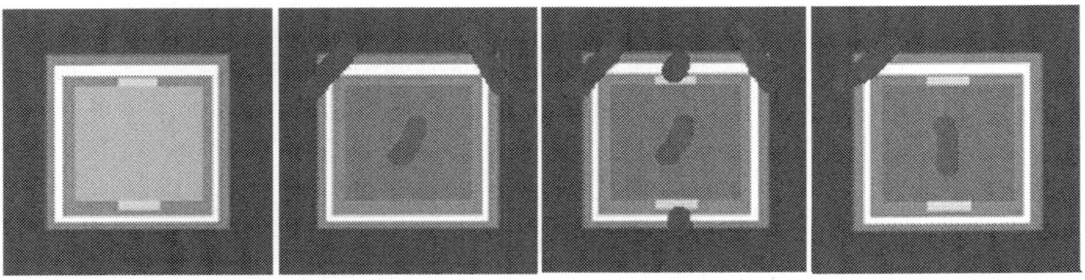

Fig. 12. Synthetic image for comparison of Boykov's method and Hu's method. The target is the inner rectangle. The second image shows that Boykov's method is meant to attract high contrast boundaries and thus mis-segment the regions (the two small rectangles.) Additional brush strokes are needed to remove the mis-segmented regions (the third image.) Hu's method correctly segments the target region once the boundary statistics are trained (the fourth image.)

$$E(x,y) = \sum_{c} E(x_c, y)\,, \tag{62}$$

Similar to Eq. (33), the energy function can then be defined over the clique with respect to voxel i as

$$E(x,y) = \sum_{i=1}^{N} \varphi_1(x_i, y) + \beta \sum_{i=1}^{N} \sum_{j \in N_i} \varphi_2(x_i, x_j, y)\,, \tag{63}$$

With this formation, also motivated by Greig et al. and Boykov et al., Hu et al. (2008) define the following potential functions using the framework of CRF:

$$\begin{aligned} \varphi_1(x_i, y) &= -\ln p(y_i \mid x_i) \\ \varphi_2(x_i, x_j, y) &= -\ln p(y_i, y_j \mid x_i \neq x_j) \end{aligned} \tag{64}$$

Note that φ_1 in the above equation is identical to the regional term in Grieg's and Boykov's energy function, whereas φ_2 can be viewed as a boundary term that describes the probability that neighboring voxels i and j belong to different regions. Those probabilities can be estimated from training data locally during the segmentation process.

With Eq. (64), CRFs become a purely statistical framework for image segmentation. This addresses the problem of Boykov's method using contrast as the boundary term that is sensitive to noise and tends to segment the target object boundary along a high contrast edge (Fig. 12.) This heuristic boundary term is usually not suitable for medical applications.

5. Atlas-based methods

Deformable atlases are adaptable templates that reflect the anatomy of new subjects and thus allow automated segmentation of the structures in new scans. Model-driven methods (e.g., the active shape model) build explicitly geometric models that are parameterized. Segmentation is achieved by adjusting the poses and parameters for controlled deformation in the target image. Intensity driven methods, on the other hand, involve image registration techniques to compute an anatomically correct coordinate transformation between a target image and an already segmented image. We will discuss these two approaches in general in the following two sections.

5.1 Atlas as average shape: active shape model/active appearance model

The active shape model (Cootes and Taylor 1992) constructs a shape prior model to enhance the performance of deformable models. By aligning training shapes in the same model space and using principal component analysis (PCA), any shape Y (set of landmark points) in the training set can be approximated by

$$Y \approx \widetilde{Y} + Pb^T , \tag{65}$$

where P is the matrix of the first m eigenvectors and $b=(b_1, b_2, ..., b_m)$ is the weighting vector – the shape parameters. Initially, the mean shape $\widetilde{Y}$ is used as the initial curve in the new scan. The deformation is computed using the standard deformable models described in Section 3. At each iteration, the displacement from the curve in the previous iteration is used to calculate the corresponding pose (rotation, translation, and scale), as well as the shape parameters, to obtain a new curve to be deformed in the next iteration. In this way, only deformations that are similar to the shapes in the training set are allowed. The iterations stop when the changes of poses and shape parameters are not significant.

The active appearance model (Cootes at al. 1998) extends this paradigm to incorporate the image intensity prior along with the shape prior, i.e.,

$$g \approx \widetilde{g} + P_g b_g{}^T . \tag{66}$$

To obtain these intensity parameters, image registration between the training data is needed. Further, PCA is applied to the combined shape and intensity parameters.
Instead of using a set of landmark points on the surface of the target object as the representation of the shape, Pizer et al. (2003) used a medial axis shape representation. The shape is represented by a set of "atoms" on the medial axis (sheet in 3D), with arms extended to control the surface formation. Instead of calculating the pose and parameters of the shape as in the active shape model, the pose and parameters of the atoms are calculated. The major advantage of this shape representation is scalability of the surface mesh. Thus, multi-scale deformation is possible.

5.2 Atlas as individual image

In this approach, an atlas is a spatial map of anatomical structures, which is usually derived from a reference image by manual segmentation. The automatic segmentation is generated by registering an image to an atlas, that is, by computing a correct coordinate mapping between the two. Then the voxels can be labeled according to the transformation mapping.

An intensity similarity measure is chosen, such as cross correlation or the more robust mutual information (MI) (Maes et al. 1997), for the registration. The displacement field is obtained by minimizing the differences between the two images based on the similarity measure with some smoothness constraints on the displacement field. The smoothness constraints can be determined using a Gaussian or an elastic model, such as thin-plate and viscous-fluid. Image registration itself is a subject of active research. Pluim and Fitzpatrick (2003) give a review of image registration methods.

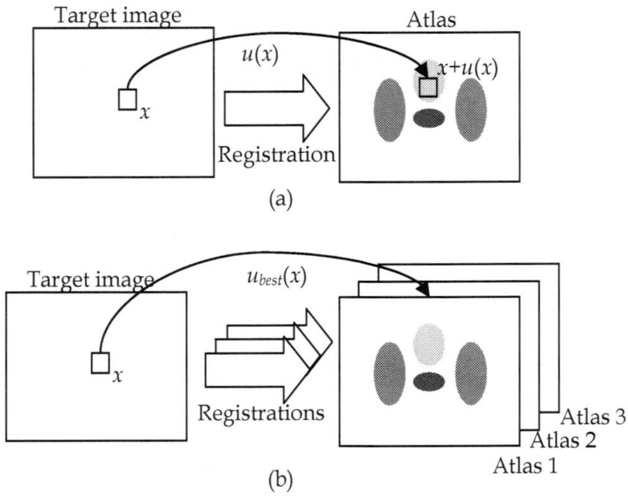

Fig. 13. (a) Atlas-based segmentation using a single atlas. Each voxel is displaced into the atlas based on the displacement field u from the registration and labeled accordingly. (b) Using multiple atlases, one registration is done for each atlas. The best registration is used to label the voxel.

The most straightforward strategy for selection of an atlas is to use a segmented image from a single (model) individual (Fig. **13**(a)). The strategy could be random or based on such heuristic criteria such as image quality or normality of the subject. One can also use multiple individual atlases to register the target image one by one and choose the best atlas for segmentation (Fig. **13** (b)). Usually, the accessible number is the final value of the registration criterion or image similarity measure.

In the pattern recognition community, multiple independent classifiers can be combined and together consistently achieve classification accuracy. Rohlfing and Maurer (2004) use the same concept to combine the results from multiple atlases to obtain the final segmentation. The coordinate transformation of registration is continuous and does not map grid points of the image to grid points in the atlas. Therefore, interpolation is required. The simplest interpolation is nearest-neighbor interpolation. A more sophisticated technique used to label data is partial volume (PV) interpolation, originally proposed by Meas et al. to generate histograms used for MI. The voxel is labeled based on a frequency histogram of labels from multiple atlases displaced within the voxel's volume. Let H_x be the frequency histogram for the labels of voxel x on the target image, for a registration u; the histogram is updated as follows

$$\begin{aligned} &H_x(L_k(x+u(x))) = H_x(L_k(x+u(x))) + w_k, k = 1,2,3,4 \text{ for 2D} \\ &w_k = d_k \Big/ \sum_{i=1}^{4} d_i, \end{aligned} \tag{67}$$

where L_k is the label of the four (2D) voxels forming the cell that contains $x+u(x)$, and d_k is the distance from $x+u(x)$ to these voxels. The best label for a voxel is the label that has highest frequency.

6. Discussion

No single method can best handle all the anatomic structures in medical image segmentation. Typically, methods discussed in this survey are modified to segment a particular structure; or a method can take advantage of other methods to serve an intermediate purpose.

Threshold-based methods are the fastest, simplest, and easiest to implement, so they are still indispensable in modern commercial software. They are useful for segmenting structures that have separated intensity distribution from the other structures. Such structures are the outer body, lung, and bone. The drawback of thresholding is that it does not guarantee piecewise continuity and is sensitive to the artifacts mentioned in section 1. However, it can be used as a starting point for other methods, such as seed points for region growing.

Region-growing methods are also fast if the mean intensity is used in the region homogeneity predicate, and therefore an interactive tool can be implemented. Region-growing methods also guarantee piecewise continuity, work quite well in finding high-contrast boundaries, and are less sensitive to noise then thresholding. The major problem is leakage if the boundary is blurred, and they are sensitive to start point position.

Cluster-based methods are easy to implement and perform well with a spatial constraint, especially for MR brain image segmentation. They may not work on CT images, since the intensity distributions of many organs overlap (Table 1.) Just like thresholding, clustering-based methods could also be used as a starting point for other techniques, such as generating an initial contour for a deformable model.

Deformable model-based methods are very popular in medical imaging. These methods also guarantee piecewise continuity, and with level set methods, the topology changes are handled naturally. Deformable model-based methods incorporating statistical regional information show promising results. However, many of them require tuning the parameters; and there is a trade-off between convergence speed and stability under the iterative optimization scheme.

Graph cut-based methods that minimize an energy function are fast and guarantee that one will find a global optimum for two-class segmentation. The results show the advantages (Hu et al. 2008) of using a probabilistic framework, such as conditional random fields (CRFs), with both statistical regional and boundary potentials. Unfortunately, multiple region segmentation using graph cut (K-cut) is NP hard (recently, Grady (2006) used a random walker for multiple region segmentation based on graph cut theory). However, multiple region segmentation can be done recursively by the two-class segmentation. This framework can also incorporate other methods, such as an atlas for additional regional properties.

Model-driven, atlas-based methods are not prone to noise and leakage because of the shape constraints from the training set. The major drawbacks are that the intensive labor for building the training set and matching the model to the image can be time-consuming, especially for complex structures that require many shape and intensity parameters to be calculated. The image registration-based atlas method is straightforward. However, it is based on image similarity and can be adversely affected when structures, such as air cavities, surgical implants, or surgically removed structures, differ between target and study images. The best application of these methods is intra-patient segmentation, such as in 4D CT images. One can segment the anatomic structures in the image set at one respiration phase, then propagate the segmentations by registration to the images at other phases (Pevsner et al. 2006). This procedure is extremely useful for studying organ or tumor motion and deformation during the treatment session.

In conclusion, the fundamental aspects of medical images -- the modalities of image acquisition, complexity of anatomical structures, the non-rigid nature of organ motion and deformation -- and increasing information from advanced modern imaging techniques make the segmentation difficult and challenging. It may not be possible to delineate certain structures without some degree of anatomical knowledge by a human, let alone with a computer. Hybrid methods, with both regional and boundary features, that utilize statistical information and are guided by expert users should shape the future of automatic medical image segmentation.

7. References

Aboutanos, G.B.; Nikanne, J.; Watkins, N. & Dawan, B.M. (1999). Model creation and deformation for the automatic segmentation of the brain in MR images. *IEEE Trans on Biomedical Engineering*, Vol. 46, Issue 11, Nov. 1999, 1346 – 1356, ISSN: 0018-9294.

Adams, R. & Bischof, L. (1994). Seeded region growing. *IEEE Trans. on Pattern Analysis and Machine Intelligence*, Vol. 16, Issue 6, June 1994, 41-647, 1994, ISSN: 0162-8828.

Baillard, C.; Hellier, P & Barillot, C. (2000). Segmentation of 3-D Brain Structures Using Level Sets. *Research Report 1291, IRISA*, Rennes Cedex, France, 16 pages, Jan. 2000.

Besag, J. (1986). On statistical analysis of dirty pictures. *J. of the Royal Statistical Society*. Series B, vol. 48, no.3, 1986, 259-302, ISSN: 1369-7412.

Bezdek, J.C. (1981). *Pattern Recognition with Fuzzy Objective Function Algorithms*. Plenum Press, New York, 1981, ISBN: 0-3064-0671-3.

Boykov, Y. & Jolly, M.P. (2001). Interactive graph cuts for optimal boundary & region segmentation of objects in N-D images. *Proc. of Int. Conf. Computer Vision*, pp. 105-112, 2001.

Caselles, V.; Catte, F.; Coll, T. & Dibos, F. (1993). A geometric model for active contours, *Numerische Mathematik*, Vol. 66, No. 1, 1993, 1-31, ISSN: 0029-599X.

Caselles, V.; Kimmel, R. & Shapiro, G. (1997). Geodesic Active Contours, *Int. J. of Computer Vision*, Vol. 22, No. 1, 1997, 61-79, ISSN: 0920-5691.

Chuang, K.S.; Tzeng, H-L; Chen, S.; Wu, J. & Chen, T-J. (2006). Fuzzy c-means clustering with spatial information for image segmentation, *Computerized Medical Imaging and Graphics*, Vol. 30, No. 1, Jan. 2006, 9-15, ISSN: 0895-6111.

Dempster, A.; Laird N. & Rubin, D. (1977). Maximum likelihood from incomplete data via the EM algorithm. *J. of the Royal Statistical Society*, Series B, Vol. 49, No. 1, 1977, 1-38, ISSN: 1369-7412.

Fenster, S.D. & Kender, J.R. (2001). Sectored snakes: evaluating learned-energy segmentations. *IEEE Trans. on Pattern Analysis and Machine Intelligence,* Vol. 23, Issue 9, Sept. 2001, 1028–1034, ISSN: 0162-8828.

Freedman, D. & Zhang T. (2005). Interactive graph cut based segmentation with shape priors. *Computer Vision and Pattern Recognition, 2005, IEEE Computer Society Conf. on,* Vol. 1, 20-25 June 2005, pp.755 - 762.

Geman, S. & Geman, D. (1984). Stochastic relaxation, Gibbs distributions, and the Bayesian restoration of images. *IEEE Trans. on Pattern Analysis and Machine Intelligence,* Vol. 6, No.6, June 1984, 721-741, ISSN: 0162-8828.

Grady, L. (2006). Random walker for image segmentation. *IEEE Trans. on Pattern Analysis And Machine Intelligence,* Vol. 28, No. 11, Nov. 2006, 1768-1783, ISSN: 0162-8828.

Greig, D.; Porteous, B. & Seheult, A. (1989). Exact maximum a posteriori estimation for binary images. *J. of the Royal Statistical Society,* Series B, Vol. 51, 1989, 271-279, ISSN: 1369-7412.

Horowitz, S.L. & Pavlidis, T. (1974). Picture segmentation by a directed split-and-merge procedure. *Proceedings of the 2nd Int. Joint Conf. on Pattern Recognition.* 1974, pp. 424-433.

Hu, Y.C.; Grossberg, M. D. & Mageras, G. S. (2008). Semi-automatic medical image segmentation with adaptive local statistics in Conditional Random Fields framework. *Proceeding of 30th Annual Int. Conf. of Engineering in Medicine and Biology Society,* Aug. 2008, pp. 3099-3102.

Kapur, J.N.; Sahoo, P.K. & Wong A.K.C. (1985). A new method for gray-level picture thresholding using the entropy of the histogram. *Computer Vision, Graphics, and Image Processing* , Vol. 29, 1985, 273–285, ISSN: 0734-189X.

Kass, M.; Witkin, A. & Terzopoulos, D. (1988). Snakes: active contour models. *Int. J. of Computer Vision,* Vol. 1, 1988, 321-331, ISSN: 0920-5691.

Kolmogorov, V. & Zabih, R. (2004). What energy functions can be minimized via graph cuts? *IEEE Trans. on Pattern Analysis and Machine Intelligence,* Vol. 26, Issue 2, Feb. 2004, 147-159, ISSN: 0162-8828.

Lafferty, J.; McCallum, A. & Pereira, F. (2001). Conditional random fields: Probabilistic models for segmenting and labeling sequence data. *Proceeding of 18th Int. Conf. on Machine Learning,* 2001, pp.282–289.

Levin, A.; Lischinski, D. & Weiss, Y. (2004). Colorization using optimization. *ACM SIGGRAPH 2004,* 2004, pp.689-694.

Lin, Z.; Jin, J. & Talbot, H. (2001). Unseeded region growing for 3D image segmentation. *ACM Int. Conf. Proceeding Series; Vol. 9, Selected papers from Pan-Sydney Workshop on Visual Information Processing,* Sydney, Australia, 2001, pp. 31-37.

Lloyd, S. (1982). Least squares quantization in PCM. Special issue on quantization, *IEEE Trans. Information Theory,* Vol. 28, Issue 2, Mar. 1982, 129–137, ISSN: 0018-9448.

Maes, F.; Collignon, A.; Vandermeulen, D.; Marchal, G & Suetens, P. (1997). Multimodality image registration by maximization of mutual information, *IEEE Trans on Medical Imaging,* Vol. 16, Issue 2, April 1997, 187-198, ISSN: 0278-0062

Malladi, R.; Sethian, J. & Vemuri, B.C. (1995). Shape modeling with front propagation: A level set approach. *IEEE Trans on Pattern Analysis and Machine Intelligence,* Vol. 17, Issue. 2, Jan. 1995, 158-175, ISSN: 0162-8828.

Mohamed, N.A.; Ahmed, M.N. & Farag, A. (1999). Modified fuzzy c-mean in medical image segmentation. *In Proceeding IEEE Int. Conf. on Acoustics, Speech, and Signal Processing 1999,* Vol. 6, Mar. 1999, pp.3429-3432.

Osher, S. & Sethian, J.A. (1988). Fronts propagating with curvature-dependent speed: Algorithms based on Hamilton-Jacobi formulations. *J. of Computational Physics*, Vol. 79, 1988, 12-49, ISSN: 0021-9991.

Otsu, N. (1979). A threshold selection method from grey-level histograms. *IEEE Trans. on Systems, Man, and Cybernetics*, Vol. 9, Issue 1, Jan 1979 , 62–66, ISSN: 0018-9472.

Pevsner, A.; Davis, B.; Joshi, S.; Hertanto, A., Mechalakos, J.; Yorke, E.; Rosenzweig, K.; Nehmeh, S.; Erdi, Y.E.; Humm, J.L.; Larson, S.; Ling, C.C. & Mageras, G.S. (2006). Evaluation of an automated deformable image matching method for quantifying lung motion in respiration-correlated CT images. *Medical Physics*, Vol. 33, No. 2, Feb. 2006, 369-376, ISSN: 0094-2405.

Pham, D.L. (2002). Fuzzy clustering with spatial constraints. *In Proceedings of the IEEE Int. Conf. on Image Processing*, New York, USA, August, 2002, pp.65-68.

Pizer, S.M.; Fletcher, P.T.; Joshi, S.C.; Thall, A.; Chen, J.Z.; Fridman, Y.; Fritsch, D.S.; Gash, A.G.; Glotzer, J.M.; Jiroutek, M.R.; Lu, C.; Muller, K.E.; Tracton, G.; Yushkevich, P.A. & Chaney, E.L. (2003). Deformable M-Reps for 3D Medical Image Segmentation. *Int. J. of Computer Vision*, Vol. 55, Issue 2-3, Nov.-Dec. 2003, 85-106, ISSN: 0278-0062.

Pluim, J.P.W. & Fitzpatrick, J.M. (2003). Image registration. *IEEE Trans on Medical Imaging*, Vol. 22, Issue 11, Nov. 2003, 1341-1343, ISSN: 0278-0062.

Ridler, T. & Calvard, S. (1978). Picture thresholding using an iterative selection method. *IEEE Trans. on Systems, Man, and Cybernetics*. Vol. 8, 629–632, ISSN: 0018-9472.

Rohlfing, T. & Maurer, C.R. Jr. (2004). Multi-classifier framework for atlas-based image segmentation. *Computer Vision and Pattern Recognition, 2004, IEEE Computer Society Conf. on*, Vol. 1, 27 June-2 July 2004, 255-260.

Rosenfeld, A. & Torre, P.D.L. (1983). Histogram concavity analysis as an aid in threshold selection, *IEEE Trans. on Systems, Man, and Cybernetics*, Vol. 13, 1983, 231–235, ISSN: 0018-9472.

Sethian, J.A. (1999). *Level Set Methods and Fast Marching Methods*. Cambridge University Press, 2nd edition, 1999, ISBN: 0-5216-4557-3.

Sezan, M.I. (1990). A Peak detection algorithm and its application to histogram-based image data reduction. *Computer Vision, Graphics, and Image Processing*, Vol. 49, 1990, 36-51, ISSN: 0734-189X.

Sezgin, M. & Sankur, B. (2004) Survey over image thresholding techniques and quantitative performance evaluation. *J.of Electronic Imaging*, Vol. 13, No. 1, 2004, 146-168, ISSN: 1017-9909.

Sonka, M. & Fitzpatrick, J.M. Eds. (2000). *Handbook of Medical Imaging. Vol. 2. Medical image Processing and Analysis*. SPIE press, 2000, ISBN: 0-8194-3622-4

Suri, J.S.; Liu, K.; Singh, S.; Laxminarayan, S.N.; Zeng, X. & Reden, L. (2002). Shape recovery algorithms using level sets in 2-D/3-D medical imagery: A state-of-the-art review. IEEE *Trans. on Information Technology in Biomedicine*, Vol. 6, Issue 1, March 2002, 8 – 28, ISSN: 1089-7771.

Xu, C. & Prince, J.L. (1997). Gradient vector flow: A new external force for snakes. *Computer Vision and Pattern Recognition 1997, IEEE Computer Society Conf. on*, 1997, pp. 66-71.

Yezzi, A.; Kichenassamy, S.; Kumar, A.; Olver, P. & Tannenbaum, A. (1997). A geometric snake model for segmentation of medical imagery, *IEEE Trans on Medical Imaging*, Vol. 16, Issue 2, April 1997, 199-209, ISSN: 0278-0062.

Fuzzy-based kernel regression approaches for free form deformation and elastic registration of medical images

Edoardo Ardizzone, Roberto Gallea, Orazio Gambino and Roberto Pirrone
DINFO – Dipartimento di Ingegneria Informatica - Università degli Studi di Palermo Italy

1. Introduction

In modern medicine, a largely diffused method for gathering knowledge about organs and tissues is obtained by means of merging information from several datasets. Such data are provided from multimodal or sequential acquisitions. As a consequence, a pre-processing step that is called "image registration" is required to achieve data integration.

Image registration aims to obtain the best possible spatial correspondence between misaligned datasets. This procedure is also useful to correct distortions induced by magnetic interferences with the acquisition equipment signals or the ones due patient's involuntary movements such as heartbeat or breathing.

The problem can be regarded as finding the transformation, generally defined by a set of parameters, that best maps one dataset (namely the input or floating image) onto the other (namely the target or base image). At the end of the process, corresponding pixels/voxels will have the same positions in both images/volumes.

This chapter starts presenting a brief taxonomy of literature registration methods. Then, an excursus of novel registration methods is presented after a more detailed explanation of the Thin-Plate Spline approach (Bookstein, 1989), which is a milestone in the field. All of these schemes use a "fuzzy kernel-based" approach able to cope with many types of deformations. The described procedures are examples of landmark-based approaches that rely on a set of a priori known control points, even though the same concepts could be extended to area-based approaches where no control points need to be detected.

All of the methods use fuzzy membership maps in a probabilistic discriminative model, which is based on kernel regression. Such techniques are based on concepts derived by Fuzzy c-means clustering process (Dunn, 1973 and Bezdek, 1981). However, no clustering algorithm needs to be performed at all.

The framework uses several measures, both quantitative and qualitative to evaluate the performance of the method.

In all of the presented approaches the global mapping function is recovered as a continuous and smooth composition of local mappings. This philosophy allows dealing with subtle local deformations without the need of using extremely time consuming complex models.

The methods were extensively tested and validated and the experimental results are reported. Final considerations and future work are then discussed.

2. Methods for image registration

Even though image registration is used for a large variety of applicative contexts, applications can be divided in four categories, depending on the image acquisition strategy:

- *Different viewpoints (or multi-view analysis)*: The same object or scene is acquired from different viewpoints: the goal is to obtain a larger view or a 3d representation of the object.
- *Different times (or multi-temporal analysis)*: Images of the same object are acquired in different times, perhaps under different conditions. The aim is to evaluate differences between two or more acquisitions.
- *Different sensors (or multimodal analysis)*: Images of the same object are acquired by different sensors, for example magnetic resonance (MR), computer tomography (CT), positron emission tomography (PET), etc.
- *Scene to model registration*: images of a real scene and its model are registered. The model can be a synthetic representation or another scene with similar content. The purpose of this method is to find the acquired image in the model and compare them.

Since there exists a lot of image types, it is impossible to design a universal method suitable for all application purposes. Each method should take into account the objects to be registered and the characteristics of the deformations to be recovered. Furthermore, even more elements such as noise corruption should be considered too. Generally, a distinction between *feature-based* and *area-based* approaches is operated, depending on how much information is used for the registration task, in the first case just a sparse information subset (the features) is used for recovering the mapping, in the latter all of the images information is taken into account. Nonetheless, every strategy generally uses four steps, with the exception of the first one. These steps are the following:

- *Feature detection*: salient and unambiguous objects such as corners, intersections, contours, etc., are manually or automatically detected in both the input and reference image. This step is omitted in area-based strategies.
- *Feature matching*: the correspondences between the images are found by means of matching the previously detected features. For this purpose, there exist several feature descriptors and similarity measures based on features appearance or informative content. Since area-based strategies use all of the image information; such methods use a dense features map simply defined by all of the pixels/voxels in the images.
- *Transform model estimation*: after the features are matched, this information is used to recover a transformation function, which defines the deformation needed to map every pixel/voxel of the input image onto every pixel/voxel of the reference image. Such a function is determined by choosing its type and defining the value of its set of parameters.
- *Image resampling and transformation*: once the deformation estimation is achieved, the mapping function is applied on the input image. Since this mapping generally brings the pixels/voxels in non-integer coordinates, proper interpolation techniques need to be used in order to avoid or limit resampling artefacts.

Each of the steps has its intrinsic problems, so each of them has to be developed taking into account the properties of the objects that have to be registered. For example the presence of noise can affect feature detection. So, if noise is assumed to be present, the detection procedure should be robust. A potential problem in feature matching is the different appearance of corresponding features due to illumination conditions or to sensors spectral sensitivity; in this case the similarity measure adopted needs to take into account these factors.
In literature there exists a large variety of approaches that had been used to deal with the registration problem. As mentioned, there not exist a unique solution since each one has its specific applicative context. Global mapping models use bivariate low-degree polynomials as mapping function. This strategy is often not suited for real cases due to the presence of local deformations in the images; however, it is used frequently as a starting point for other methods. Local mapping models overcome these limitations by registering locally the different areas of the image. Radial basis functions such as Thin-Plate spline (Bookstein, 1989) or Wendland's functions (Wendland 1995, Fornefett et al. 1999) are also used, and they are able to deal with local deformations, even if they could be considered as global mapping models. Another approach, which does not require the use of any parametric function is to model complex deformations by considering the image as a tensile material (Bajcsy R. and Kovacic S., 1989) or a viscous fluid (Bro-Nielsen and Gramkow, 1996) deformed by external and internal forces subject to constraints. Registration is achieved by the iterative minimization of an energy functional.

2.1 A classical approach: the Thin Plate Spline

One of the classical approaches to image registration is the Thin Plate Spline (TPS). The name is derived from the physical analogy, which involves the bending of a thin metal sheet. In the context of spatial coordinates transformation and image registration, lifting the plate corresponds to displace the image in one direction (i.e. x, y or z axis). The Thin Plate Spline is a parametric interpolation function which is defined by $D(K+3)$ parameters, where D is the number of spatial dimensions of the datasets and K is the number of the given landmark points where the displacement values are known. The function is a composition of an affine part, defined by 3 parameters, and K radial basis functions, defined by an equal number of parameters. In 2d its analytic form is defined as:

$$g(\mathbf{p}) = ax + by + d + \sum_{i=1}^{K} \rho\left(\left\|\mathbf{p} - \mathbf{c}_i\right\|^2\right) w_i; \quad \mathbf{p} = \begin{bmatrix} x \\ y \end{bmatrix}; \quad \mathbf{c}_i = \begin{bmatrix} c_x \\ c_y \end{bmatrix}, \tag{1}$$

where $\mathbf{p}$ is the input point, $\mathbf{c}_i$ are the landmark points and the radial basis function $\rho(r)$ is given by:

$$\rho(r) = \frac{1}{2} r^2 \log r^2, \tag{2}$$

All of the TPS parameters are computed solving a linear system defined by a closed-form minimization of the bending energy functional. Such functional is given by:

$$E_{tps} = \sum_{i=1}^{K} \left\| y_i - g\left(\mathbf{p}_i\right) \right\| + \lambda \iint \left[\left(\frac{\partial^2 g}{\partial x^2} \right)^2 + 2 \left(\frac{\partial^2 g}{\partial xy} \right)^2 + \left(\frac{\partial^2 g}{\partial y^2} \right)^2 \right] dxdy. \tag{3}$$

The functional is composed by two terms: the data term and the regularization term. The former minimizes the difference between known and recovered displacements at landmark points, the latter minimizes the bending energy of the recovered function, i.e. maximises its smoothness and it is weighted by the parameter λ. As mentioned before, for this expression a closed-form analytical solution exists, from which is possible to recover all of the required spline function parameters. The main characteristic of this function is that it exhibits minimum curvature properties.

3. Registration with fuzzy-based kernel regression

In our study we developed a class of registration algorithms, which exploit kernel regression model to recover the mapping functions. The classic kernel regression is enhanced by fuzzy related techniques, in particular the C-means clustering algorithm.
The registration schemes proposed are similar as regards the theoretical concepts they rely on, while they differ in their application. Two strategies are discussed: the former is a simple landmark-based registration approach (Ardizzone et al., 2009-1) that is described to explain how the fuzzy kernel regression concepts can be applied to elastic registration. In this scheme the global transformation function is recovered directly from the landmarks displacements. The latter strategy (Ardizzone et al., 2009-2) differs from the previous one in that the regression is used to obtain a smooth composition of affine transformations recovered from the triangulation of landmark points. Both techniques do not need to perform neither iterative nor analytic minimization procedures.

3.1 Kernel regression

In pattern recognition, there exists a class of techniques, which uses data points or a subset of them not just in the training phase, but also in the prediction phase. These are called *memory-based* methods. Linear parametric models that can be re-cast into equivalent dual representations where the predictions are given by linear combinations of a *kernel function* evaluated at the training data points are known as kernel regression methods. Kernel functions are symmetric in their argument and are defined by training data points. Kernels, which depend only on the magnitude of the distance of the argument from the training points, are known as *homogeneous* kernels or *radial basis functions.*
For our registration purpose we will use the derivation of kernel regression from the scheme known as the Nadaraya-Watson model (Nadaraya, 1964 and Watson, 1964). Assuming we have a training set $\{x_n, t_n\}$. Then, using a Parzen density estimator, the joint distribution $p(x, t)$ is modeled as

$$p(x,t)=\frac{1}{N}\sum_{n=1}^{N} f(x-x_n,t-t_n) \tag{4}$$

where $f(x, t)$ is the component density function, and there is a component centered on each data point. The regression function $y(x)$, corresponding to the conditional average of the target variable conditioned on the input variable, is given by:

$$y(x)=E[t\mid x]=\int_{-\infty}^{+\infty} tp(t\mid x)dt=\frac{\int tp(x,t)dt}{\int p(x,t)dt}=$$
$$=\frac{\sum_n \int tf(x-x_n,t-t_n)dt}{\sum_m \int f(x-x_m,t-t_m)dt} \tag{5}$$

Assuming that the component density functions have zero mean so that

$$\int_{-\infty}^{+\infty} f(x,t)dt=0 \tag{6}$$

for all values of x, then, operating a change of variable we get

$$y(x)=\frac{\sum_n g(x-x_n)t_n}{\sum_m g(x-x_m)}=\sum_n k(x,x_n)t_n \tag{7}$$

where the kernel function $k(x, x_n)$ is defined as

$$k(x,x_n)=\frac{g(x-x_n)}{\sum_m g(x-x_m)} \tag{8}$$

and

$$g(x)=\int_{-\infty}^{+\infty} f(x,t)dt \tag{9}$$

This form (7) represents the *Nadaraya-Watson* model, for localized kernel function. It has the property of weighting more the data points x_n close to x than the other ones. The kernel (8) satisfies the summation constraint

$$\sum_{n=1}^{N} k(x, x_n) = 1 \tag{10}$$

This result points out that the prediction for the value of a data point x is given by a linear combination of the training data points values and the kernel functions. Such kernel functions can have different forms, provided that (10) is satisfied.

3.2 Fuzzy c-means

Before explaining how kernel regression can be applied to the registration task, it is necessary to describe the Fuzzy c-means clustering technique (Bezdek, 1981) that is a powerful and efficient data clustering method.

Each data sample, represented by some feature values in a suitable space, is associated to each cluster by assigning a membership degree. Each cluster is identified by its centroid, a special point where the feature values are representative for its own class. The original algorithm is based on the minimization of the following objective function:

$$J_S = \sum_{j=1}^{m} \sum_{i=1}^{k} \left(u_{ij}\right)^s d\left(x_i, c_j\right)^2, \qquad 1 \leq s \leq \infty \tag{11}$$

where $d(x_i, c_j)$ is a distance function between each observation vector x_j and the cluster centroid c_j, s is a parameter which determines the amount of clustering fuzziness, m is the number of clusters, which should be chosen a priori, k is the number of observations and u_{ij} is the membership degree of the sample x_i belonging to cluster centroid c_j.

An additional constraint is that the membership degrees should be positive and structured such that $u_{i1} + u_{i2} + \ldots + u_{im} = 1$. The method advances as an iterative procedure where, given the membership matrix $U = [u_{ij}]$ of size k by m, the new positions of the centroids are updated as:

$$c_j = \frac{\sum_{i=1}^{k} \left(u_{ij}\right)^s x_i}{\sum_{i=1}^{k} \left(u_{ij}\right)^s} \tag{12}$$

The algorithm ends after a fixed number of iterations or when the overall variation of the centroids displacements over a single iteration falls below a given threshold. The new membership values are given by the following equation:

$$u_{ij} = \frac{1}{\sum_{l=1}^{m} \left(\frac{d\left(x_i, c_j\right)}{d\left(x_i, c_l\right)} \right)^{\frac{2}{s-1}}} \tag{13}$$

To better understand the whole process a one-dimensional example is reported (i.e. each data point is represented by just one value).
Twenty random data points and three clusters are used to initialize the procedure and compute the initial matrix U. Note that the cluster starting positions, represented by vertical lines), are randomly chosen. Fig. 1 shows the membership values for each data point relative to each cluster; their colour is assigned on the basis of the closest cluster to the data point.

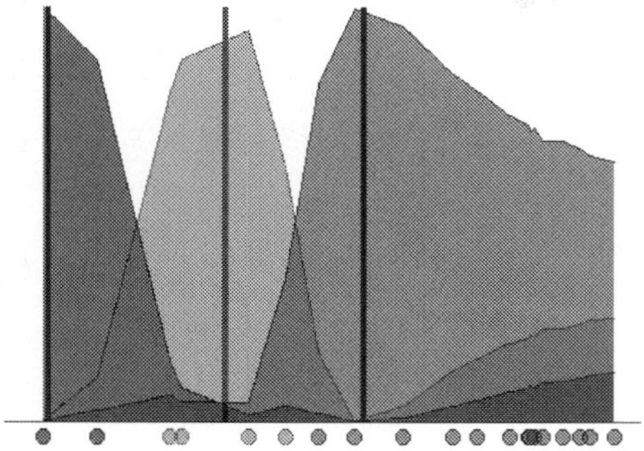

Fig. 1. Fuzzy C-means example: initial membership value assignation.

After running the algorithm, the minimization is performed and the cluster centroids are shifted, the final membership matrix U can be computed. The resulting membership functions are depicted in Fig. 2

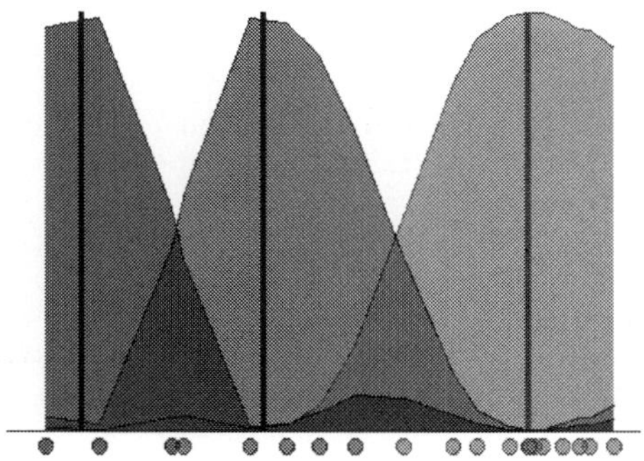

Fig. 2. Fuzzy C-means example: final membership value assignation and cluster centres positions.

3.3 Fuzzy kernel regression

Merging the results of the previous discussion it turns out that Fuzzy C-means membership functions can be used as kernels for regression in the Nadaraya-Watson model because they

satisfy the summation constraint. In the scenario of image registration, the input variables populate the feature space by means of the spatial coordinates of the pixels/voxels and cluster centroids are represented by relevant points in the images, whose spatial displacement is known. The landmark points where correspondences are known between input and reference image can be used for this purpose.
As a result of such setting there is no need to execute any minimization of the Bezdek functional, since image points are already supposed to be clustered around the landmark points (or equivalent representative points). Fuzzy C-means is used just as a starting point for the registration procedure. Once the relevant points are known, a single FCM step is performed to construct Fuzzy kernels by means of computing membership functions. For this purpose the distance measure used in (13) is the simple Euclidean distance, since just spatial closeness is required to determine how much any point is influenced by surrounding relevant points. Such membership functions are then used to recover the displacement for any pixel/voxel in the image using the following formula:

$$y(x) = \sum_{n} u(x, x_n) t_n \tag{14}$$

where $u(x,x_n)$ is the membership value for the current pixel/voxel with regard to the relevant point x_n, and t_n is a 2d/3d vector or function representing its known xy or xyz displacement. This will result in continuous and smooth displacement surfaces, which interpolate relevant points.
Even if the registration framework is unique, it can be applied in several ways, depending on the choice of the target variable, i.e. what is assumed to be the prior information in terms of relevant points and their known displacement. In the following paragraphs two different applications of the proposed framework will be described.

3.4 Simple landmark based elastic registration

A first application arises naturally from the described framework. It is very simple and is meant to demonstrate the actual use of the fuzzy kernel regression. However since it is effective notwithstanding its simplicity, it could be used for actual registration tasks.
Basically, it consists in considering the landmark points themselves directly as the relevant points representing the cluster centroids for the FCM step, and their displacements vectors directly as the target variables. Each pixel/voxel is then subjected to a displacement contribute from each landmark point. Such contribute is high for closer points and gets smaller while relative distances between the input points and the landmarks increase. The final displacement vector for any input point will consequently be a weighted sum of the landmarks points.
To better understand this technique an example of the procedure is explained: a pattern image showing four landmark points is depicted in Fig. 3a. An input point P is considered, and its distances from the four landmarks are shown. After the procedure is applied with a fuzziness value s set to 1.6, the point P results to have the following membership values for the four landmarks:

$$u_{ij} = [0.0371, 0.0106, 0.9339, 0.0183] \tag{15}$$

This means that it will receive the greatest part of the displacement contribute from the bottom-left landmark, and just a marginal contribute from the other three. The results are confirmed in Fig. 3b, where the point has been moved according to a displacement vector that is mostly similar to the displacement of the third landmark. Anyway, other landmarks give small influences too.

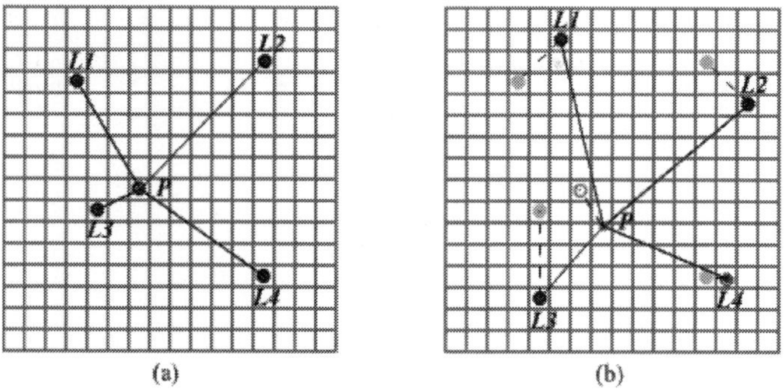

Fig. 3. Example of single point registration using four landmarks.

Repeating the same procedure for the points in the whole image, complete dense displacement surfaces are recovered, one for each spatial dimension. Such surfaces have continuity and smoothness properties.
As a first example, visual results for conventional images are shown in Fig. 4.

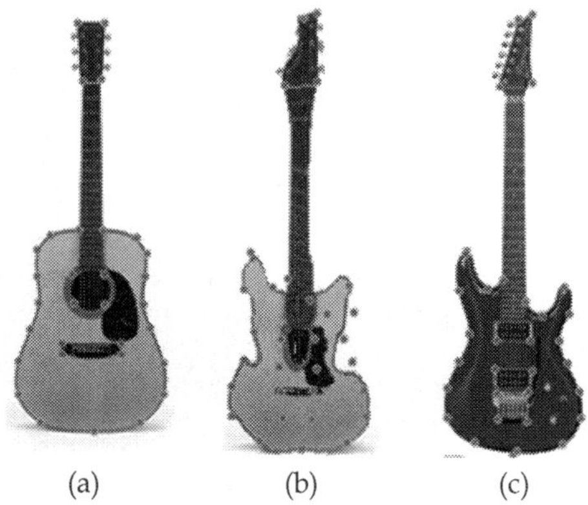

Fig. 4. Example of registration of conventional images. Input image (a), registered image (b) and target image (c). In this example 31 landmark points were used with the fuzziness s value set to 1.6

In Fig. 5 are shown the recovered displacement surfaces for x (a) and y (b) values respectively.

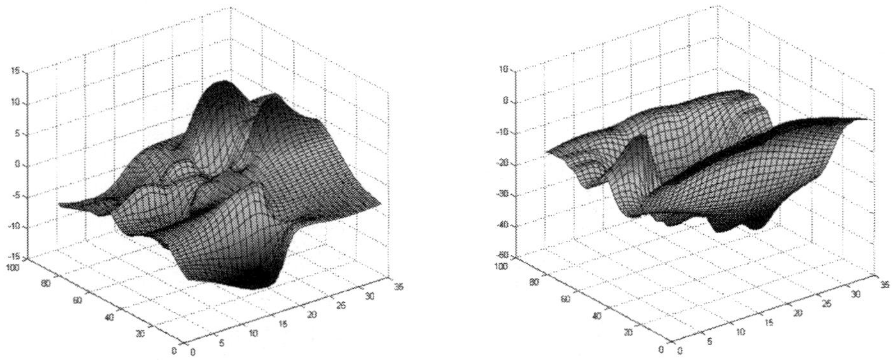

(a) (b)

Fig. 5. Displacement surfaces recovered for x (a) and y (b) values.

3.5 Improved landmarks based elastic registration

Although the simple method previously described is effective and can be useful for simple registration tasks, it does not result suitable for many applications in that it does not take properly into account relations between neighbouring landmark points. In other words, considering a single point displacement vector to represent the deformation of the image in different areas is not enough. Thus, it is necessary to find an effective way for estimating such zones. Given some landmark points, a simple way to subdivide the image space in regions is the application of the classic Delaunay triangulation procedure (Delaunay, 1934), which is the optimal way of recovering a tessellation of triangles, starting from a set of vertices. It is optimal in the sense that it maximizes the minimum angle among all of the triangles in the generated triangulation. Starting from the landmark points and their correspondences, such triangulation produces a most useful triangles set along their relative vertices correspondences. An example of Delaunay triangulation is depicted in Fig. 6.

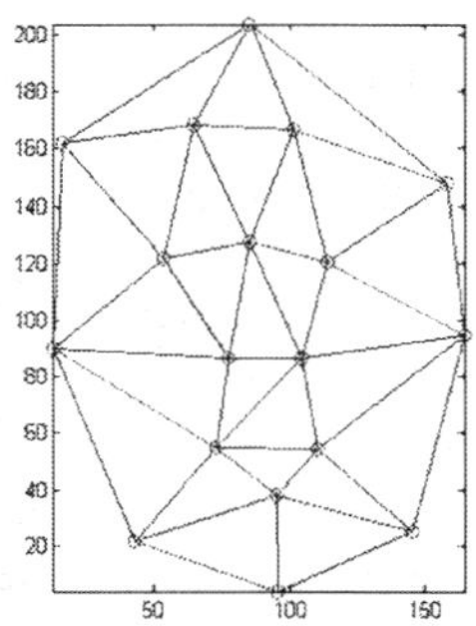

Fig. 6. Example of Delaunay triangulation.

Once we have such triangle tessellation whose vertices are known as well as their displacements, it is possible to recover the local transformations, which map each triangle of the input image onto its respective counterpart in the target image. Such transformation can be recovered in several ways; basically an affine transformation can be used. In 2d space affine transforms are determined by six parameters. Writing down the transformation equation (16) for three points a linear system of six equations to recover such parameters can be obtained. Similar considerations hold for the three-dimensional case.

$$\begin{bmatrix} x \\ y \\ 1 \end{bmatrix} = \begin{bmatrix} a & b & c \\ d & e & f \\ 0 & 0 & 1 \end{bmatrix} \begin{bmatrix} x_{0,n} \\ y_{0,n} \\ 1 \end{bmatrix} = \begin{bmatrix} ax_0 + by_0 + c \\ dx_0 + ey_0 + f \\ 1 \end{bmatrix} \Rightarrow \begin{cases} x_1 = ax_{0,1} + by_{0,1} + c \\ y_1 = dx_{0,1} + ey_{0,1} + f \\ x_2 = ax_{0,2} + by_{0,2} + c \\ y_2 = dx_{0,2} + ey_{0,2} + f \\ x_3 = ax_{0,3} + by_{0,3} + c \\ y_3 = dx_{0,3} + ey_{0,3} + f \end{cases} \tag{16}$$

Each transformation is recovered from a triangle pair correspondence, and the composition of all the transformations allows the full reconstruction of the image. Anyway, this direct composition it is not sufficient per se, since it presents crisp edges because transition between two different areas of the image are not smooth even if the recovered displacement surfaces are continuous due to the adjacency of the triangles edges. This can lead to severe artefacts in the registered image, especially for points outside of the convex hull defined by the control points (Fig. 7c and Fig. 7d), where no transformation information is determined. To better understand this problem an example of registration along the recovered surfaces plot are shown respectively in Fig. 7 and Fig. 8.

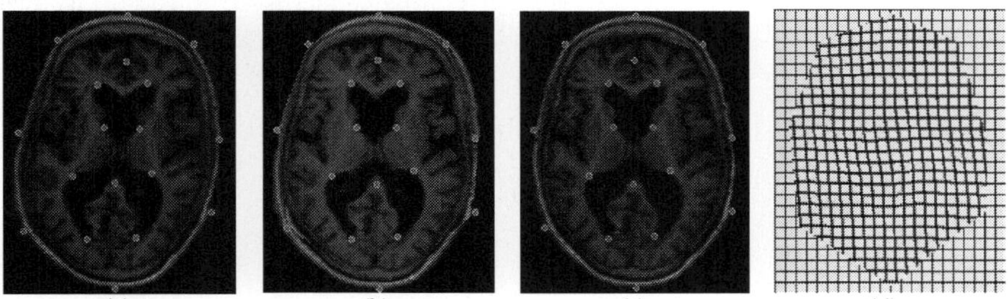

(a) (b) (c) (d)

Fig. 7. Example of MRI image registration with direct composition of affine transformations. Input image (a), registered image (b) and target image (c). Deformed grid in (d). In this example 18 landmark points were used.

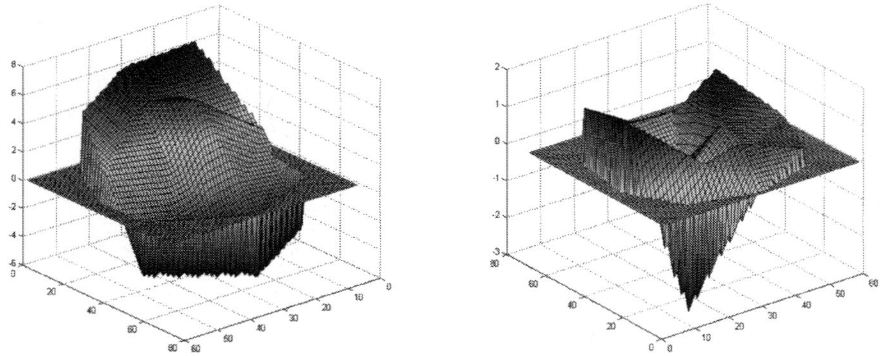

(a) (b)

Fig. 8. Displacement surfaces recovered for x (a) and y (b) values with direct affine transformation composition.

Fuzzy kernel regression technique can be used to overcome this drawback. To apply the method, relevant points acting as cluster centroids must be chosen. Since our prior displacement information is no more about landmark points, but about triangles, they cannot be chosen as relevant points anymore. Thus, we have to choose some other representative points for each triangle. For this purpose, centres of mass are used as relevant points, and their relative triangle affine transformation matrix is the target variable. In this way, after recovering the membership functions and using them as kernels for regression, final displacement for each pixel/voxel is given by the weighted sum of the displacements given by all of the affine matrices. In this way the whole image information is taken into account. The final location of each pixel/voxel is then obtained as follows (2d case):

$$\begin{bmatrix} x \\ y \\ 1 \end{bmatrix} = \sum_n \left(u_n(x,y) \begin{bmatrix} a_n & b_n & c_n \\ d_n & e_n & f_n \\ 0 & 0 & 1 \end{bmatrix} \begin{bmatrix} x_0 \\ y_0 \\ 1 \end{bmatrix} \right) \tag{17}$$

In this way there are no more displacement values that change sharply when crossing triangle edges, but variations are smooth according to the choice of the fuzziness parameter s. In Fig. 9. and Fig. 10 registration results and deformation surfaces for the previous examples are shown. Note that there are no more sharp edges in the surface plots and a displacement value is recovered also outside of the convex hull defined by the landmarks points.

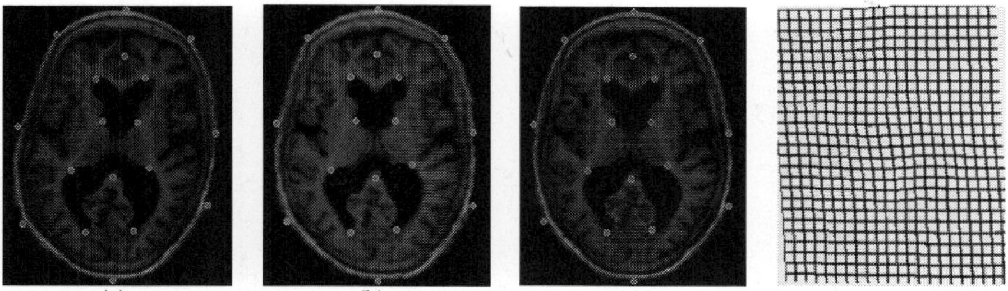

(a) (b) (c) (d)

Fig. 9. Example of MRI image registration with fuzzy kernel regression affine transformations composition. Input image (a), registered image (b) and target image (c). Deformed grid in (d). In this example 18 landmark points were used.

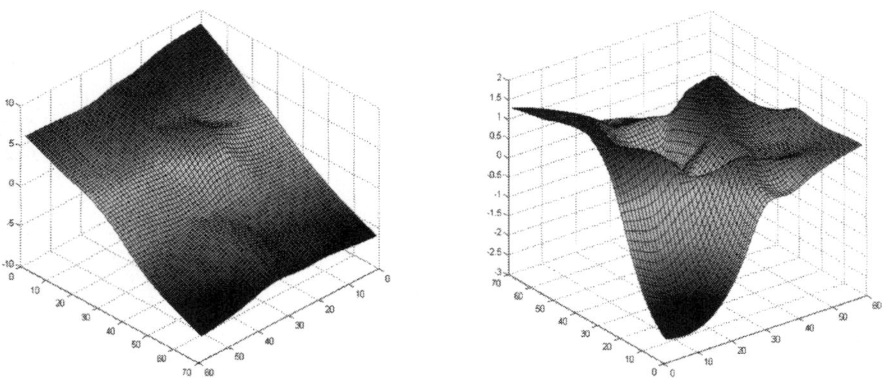

(a) (b)

Fig. 10. Displacement surfaces recovered for x (a) and y (b) values with fuzzy kernel regression affine transformation composition.

3.6 Image resampling and transformation

Once the mapping functions have been determined, the actual pixels/voxels transformation has to be realized. Such transformation can be operated in a forward or backward manner. In the forward or direct approach (Fig. 11a), each pixel of the input image can be directly transformed using the mapping function. This method presents a strong drawback, in that it can produce holes and/or overlaps in the output image due to discretization or rounding errors. With backward mapping (Fig. 11b), each point of the result image is mapped back onto the input image using the inverse of the transformation function. Such mapping generally produces non-integer pixel/voxel coordinates, so resampling via proper interpolation methods is necessary even though neither holes nor overlaps are produced.

Such interpolation is generally produced using a convolution of the image with an interpolation kernel.

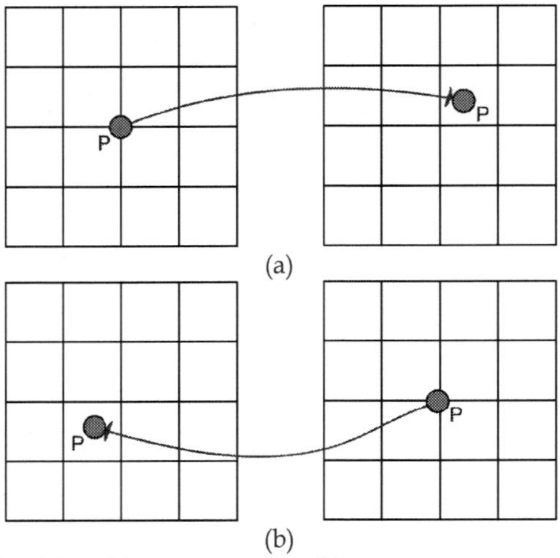

Fig. 11. Direct mapping (a) and inverse mapping (b).

The optimal interpolating kernel, the *sinc* function, is hard to implement due to its infinite support extent. Thus, several simpler kernels with limited support have been proposed in literature. Among them, some of most common are nearest neighbour (Fig. 12a), linear (Fig. 12b) and cubic (Fig. 12c) functions, Gaussians (Fig. 12d) and Hamming-windowed sinc (Fig. 12e). In Table 1 are reported the expressions for such interpolators.
Interpolating with the nearest neighbour technique consists in convolving the image with a rectangular window. Such operation is equivalent to apply a poor sinc-shaped low-pass filter in the frequency domain. In addition it causes the resampled image to be shifted with respect to the original image by an amount equal to the difference between the positions of the coordinate locations. This means that such interpolator is suitable neither for sub-pixel accuracy nor for large magnifications, since it just replicates pixels/voxels.
A slightly better interpolator is the linear kernel, which operates a good low-pass filtering in the frequency domain, even though causes the attenuation of the frequencies near the cut-off frequency, determining smoothing of the image. Similar, though better results are achieved using a Gaussian kernel.

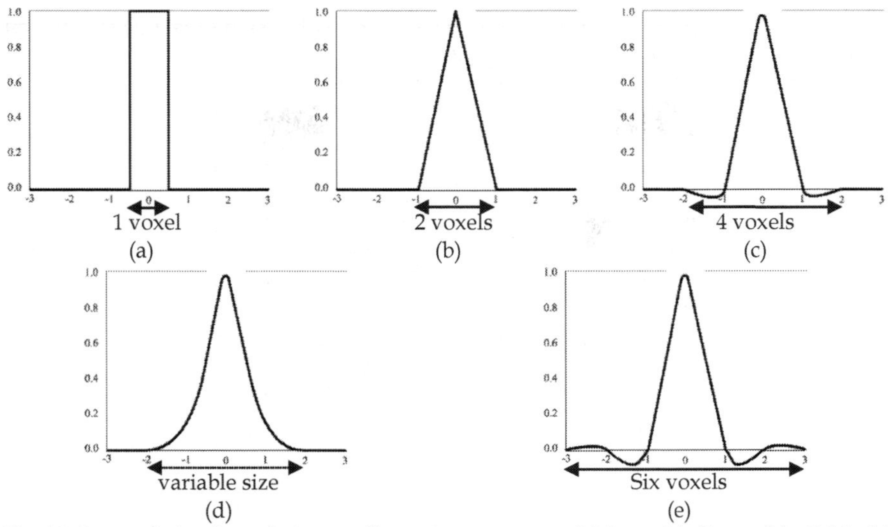

Fig. 12. Interpolation kernels in one dimension: nearest neighbour (a), linear (b), Cubic (c), Gaussian (d) and Hamming-windowed sinc (e). Width of the support is shown below (pixel/voxel number).

INTERPOLATOR	FORMULA FOR INTERPOLATED INTENSITY
Nearest Neighbour	$= \begin{cases} n_0 & \text{if } x < 0.5 \\ n_1 & \text{otherwise} \end{cases}$
Linear	$= (1-x)n_0 + xn_1$
Cubic Spline	$= \begin{cases} (a+2)x^3 - (a+3)x^2 + 1 & \text{if } 0 \le x \le 1 \\ ax^3 - 5ax^2 + 8ax - 4a & \text{if } 1 < x \le 2 \end{cases}$
Gaussian	$= \frac{1}{\sigma\sqrt{2\pi}} e^{\frac{(x-\mu)^2}{2\sigma^2}} \quad ; \sigma > 0$
Hamming-sinc	$= \sum_{i=-2}^{3} w_i n_i \Big/ \sum_{i=-2}^{3} w_i$ where $w_i = \left(0.54 + 0.46\cos\left(\frac{\pi(x-i)}{3}\right)\right)\left(\frac{\sin(\pi(x-i))}{\pi(x-i)}\right)$

Table 1. Analytic expression for several interpolators in one dimension.

Cubic Interpolator are generally obtained by means of spline functions, constrained to pass from points (0, 1), (1, 0) and (2,0), and to have continuity properties in 0 and 1; in addition the slope in 0 and 2 should be 0, and approaching 1 both form left and right, it must be the same. Since a cubic spline has eight degrees of freedom, using these seven constraints, the function is defined up to a constant a. Investigated choice of the a parameter are 1, -3/4, and 1/2 (Simon, 1975).
Due to the problems of using an ideal sinc function, several approximation schemes have been investigated. Direct truncation of the function is not possible because cutting the lobes generates the ringing phenomenon. A more performing alternative is to use a non-squared window, such as Hamming's raised cosine window.

4. Experimental results and discussion

Simple Fuzzy Regression (SFR) and Fuzzy Regression Affine Composition (FRAC) have been extensively tested with quantitative and qualitative criteria using both real and synthetic datasets (Cocosco et al., 1997, Kwan et al., 1996-1999, Collins et al., 1998). The first type of tests consists in the registration of a manually deformed image onto its original version. The test image is warped using a known transformation, which is recovered operating the registration. The method performance is then evaluated using several similarity metrics: sum of squared difference (SSD), mean squared error (MSE) and mutual information (MI) as objective measures, Structural Similarity (SSIM) as the subjective one (Wang et al., 2004). The algorithm was ran using different fuzziness values s, visual results for the proposed method are depicted in Fig. 13 and Fig. 14 and measures are summarized in Table 2 and Table 3. Comparisons with Thin-Plate Spline approach are also presented.

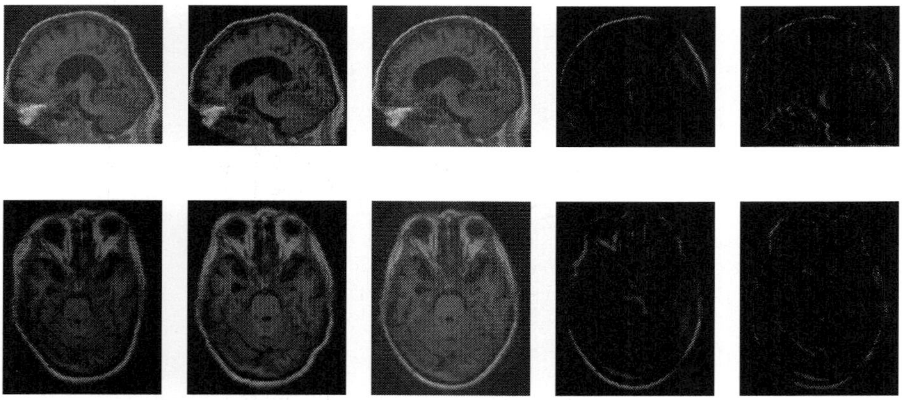

Fig. 13. Example of registration results with simple fuzzy kernel regression. From left to right: input image, registered image, target image, initial image difference, final image difference.

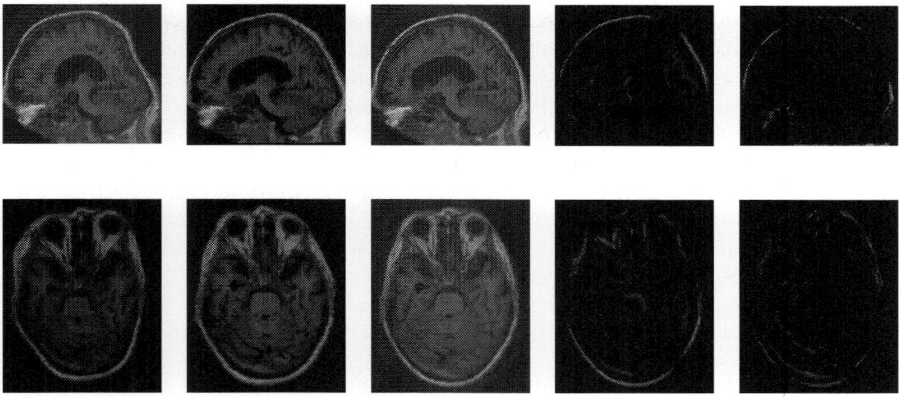

Fig. 14. Example of registration results with fuzzy kernel regression affine transformation composition. From left to right: input image, registered image, target image, initial image difference, final image difference.

	Simple Fuzzy Regression				Thin Plate Spline			
s	MSE	SSD	MI	SSIM	MSE	SSD	MI	SSIM
1.2	0.0287	1049	1.0570	0.6753				
1.4	0.0254	929	1.0945	0.6893				
1.6	0.0251	917	1.0519	0.6552				
1.8	0.0282	1033	1.0090	0.6225	0.0243	903	1.0856	0.6759
2.0	0.0361	1322	0.9563	0.5877				
2.2	0.0426	1560	0.8970	0.5534				
2.4	0.0486	1779	0.8489	0.5250				

Table 2. Comparison of similarity measures between Simple Fuzzy Regression and Thin Plate Spline approaches. Best results are underlined.

	Fuzzy Regression Affine Composition				Thin Plate Spline			
s	MSE	SSD	MI	SSIM	MSE	SSD	MI	SSIM
1.2	0.0112	410	1.1666	0.7389				
1.4	0.0101	369	1.1811	0.7435				
1.6	0.0111	408	1.1834	0.7385				
1.8	0.0133	486	1.1329	0.7037	0.0115	412	1.1654	0.7294
2.0	0.0201	736	1.0044	0.6257				
2.2	0.0277	1015	0.8985	0.5590				
2.4	0.0370	1355	0.8158	0.5115				

Table 3. Comparison of similarity measures between Fuzzy Regression Affine Composition and Thin Plate Spline approaches. Best results underlined.

From the previous tables it results that the obtained similarity measures are comparable to the Thin Plate Spline in the case of SFR registration, and better for FRAC Registration, so the proposed methods are a valid alternative from an effectiveness point of view.
From an efficiency perspective, different considerations hold. All of the tests were conducted on a AMD Phenom Quad-core running Matlab 7.5 on Windows XP. Timing performance exhibited a large speed up for both of the presented algorithms in respect of TPS: using 22 landmark points on 208x176 images, mean execution time for SFR registration is 30,32% of TPS, while for FRAC registration it is 49,65%. Such difference is due to the fact that TPS requires the solution of a linear system composed by an high number of equations, this task is not needed for the proposed methods which reduce just to distance measures and weighted sums for SFR and FRAC, the latter is a bit more expensive since the affine transformation parameters have to be recovered from simple six equations systems (2d case).
Last considerations are for memory consumption. Comparing the size of data structures, it can be seen that for SFR algorithm DxM values need to be stored for landmarks displacements, where D is the dimensionality of the images and M the number of control points, and M values are needed for the membership degrees of each point. However, once every single pixel/voxel has been transformed, its membership degrees can be dropped, so the total data structure is $M(D+1)$ large. TPS approximation has a little more compact structure, in fact it needs just to maintain the $D(M+3)$ surface coefficients (M for the non-linear part and 3 for the linear one). FRAC has the largest descriptor, it is variable since it depends on the number of triangles in which the image is subdivided, and anyway it is in the order of $2M$. Since each affine transformation is defined by $D(D+1)$ parameters and membership degrees require $2M$ additional values (i.e. one for each triangle) the whole registration function descriptor is in the order of $2M[D(D+1)+1]$. In conclusion, the storing complexity is $O(M)$ for both methods, i.e. linear in the number of landmarks used, and thus equivalent.

4.1 Choosing the *s* parameter

As resulted from the discussion of the registration methods, both techniques require the parameter s, the fuzziness value, to be assigned. Even though there exists the problem of tuning this term, experiments shown that each of the considered similarity measures is a convex (or concave) function of the s parameter and that the optimal value generally lies in 1.7±0.3. Furthermore, in this range results are very similar. Anyway, if a fine-tuning is required, a few mono-dimensional search attempts (3-4 trials on average) are enough to find the optimum solution using bisectional strategies such as golden ratio thus keeping the method still more efficient than Thin Plane Spline.

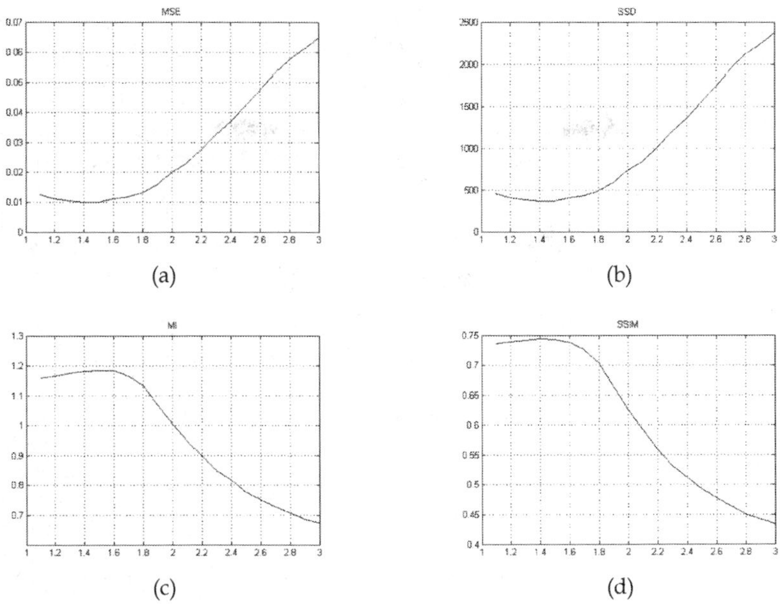

Fig. 15. Example of plot of the similarity measures versus the s parameters: MSE (a), SSD (b), MI (c) and SSIM (d).

4.2 Interpolation performance

The interpolation schemes described provide different visual results exhibiting different quality performances. Fig. 16 depicts the visual results achieved by the described interpolators. However, especially when dealing with 3d volumes, computational burden may be eccessive compared to the quality of the resampled images. Table 4 shows the average computational time normalized with respect to nearest neighbour performance.

INTERPOLATOR	TIMING PERFORMANCE
Nearest Neighbour	1
Linear	2.8534
Cubic Spline	4.1328
Gaussian	2.7913
Hamming-sinc	4.9586

Table 4. Timing performance for resampling kernels.

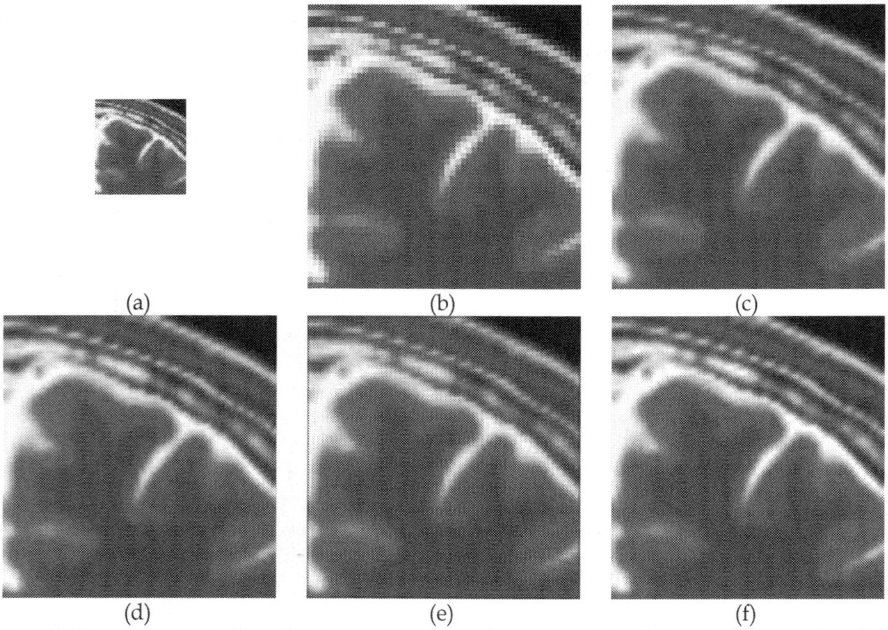

Fig. 16. Results with different interpolating kernels: original detail (a), 300% magnification with box-shaped kernel (b), triangular-shaped kernel (c), cubic kernel (d), gaussian kernel (e) and hamming sinc kernel (f).

Additionally, even if the subject goes beyond the purpose of this work, it is worth to remark that image resampling is not involved just in image reconstruction, but is also a critical matter in area-based registration techniques based on maximization of some similarity function. The choice of the interpolation method has relevant influence on the shape of such function, so a proper interpolation technique must be chosen to avoid the formation of local minima in the curve to optimize. In turn, such technique can be different from the one that provides us with the best visual results. For further reading on this topic, an interesting analysis was conducted by Liang et al. (2003).

5. Conclusion and future works

Image registration has become a fundamental pre-processing step for a large variety of modern medicine imaging tasks useful to support the experts' diagnosis. It allows to fuse information provided by sequential or multi-modality acquisitions in order to gather useful knowledge about tissues and anatomical parts. It can be used to correct the acquisition distortion due to low quality equipments or involuntary movements.

Over the last years, the work by a number of research groups has introduced a wide variety of methods for image registration. The problem to find the transformation function that best maps the input dataset onto the target one has been addressed by a large variety of techniques which span from feature-based to area-based approaches depending on the amount of information used in the process.

A new framework for image registration has been introduced. It relies on kernel-based regression technique, using fuzzy membership functions as equivalent kernels. Such framework is presented in a formal fashion, which arises from the application and extension of the *Nadaraya-Watson* model.

The theoretic core has then been applied to two different landmark-based elastic registration schemes. The former simply predicts the pixels displacement after constructing the regression function starting from the known displacements of the landmarks. The latter, after a space subdivision of the dataset into triangles, computes the affine transformations that maps each triangle into the input image onto its correspondent in the target image. Such affine transformations are then composed to create a deformation surface, which exhibits crisp edges at the triangles junctions. In this case the regression function acts as a smoother for such surfaces; each point displacement is conditioned by the influence of the affine transformations of every surrounding zone of the image, receiving a larger contribute from closer areas.

Both the proposed registration algorithms have been extensively tested and some of the results have been reported. Comparisons with thin-plate spline literature method show that quality performances are generally better. At the same time timing performance is improved due to the absence of any optimization processes. The only drawback with the proposed methods is the size of the displacement function descriptor, which is bigger than TPS parameters vector, even though it keeps linear in the number of used landmarks.

Additional analysis were conducted on the resampling process involved in image registration. Several interpolation kernels have been described and analyzed.

As future work it is possible to extend the application of this framework towards a fully automatic area based registration with no needs of setting landmark points. For this purpose, new interpolation techniques will be designed to keep into account both image reconstruction quality and suppression of local minima in the optimization function.

According to the point-wise nature of these methods, it is possible to exploit the possibilities given by parallel computing, in particular with the use of GPU cluster-enhanced algorithms which will dramatically improve the process performance.

6. References

Ardizzone E., Gallea R, Gambino O. and Pirrone R. (2009). Fuzzy C-Means Inspired Free Form Deformation Technique for Registration. *WILF, International Workshop on Fuzzy Logic and Applications*. 2009.

Ardizzone E., Gallea R, Gambino O. and Pirrone R. (2009). Fuzzy Smoothed Composition of Local Mapping Transformations for Non-Rigid Image Registration. *ICIAP, International Conference on Image Analysis and Processing*. 2009

Bajcsy R., Kovacic S. (1989). Multiresolution elastic matching. *Computer Vision, Graphics, and Image Processing*, Vol. 46, No. 1. (April 1989), pp. 1-21.

Bezdek J. C. (1981): Pattern Recognition with Fuzzy Objective Function Algoritms, Plenum Press, New York.

Bookstein F.L. (1989). Principal Warps: Thin-Plate Splines and the Decomposition of Deformations, *IEEE Transactions on Pattern Analysis and Machine Intelligence*, vol. 11, no. 6, pp. 567-585, June, 1989.

Bro-Nielsen, M., Gramkow, C. (1996). Fast Fluid Registration of Medical Images. *Proceedings of the 4th international Conference on Visualization in Biomedical Computing* (September 22 - 25, 1996). K. H. Höhne and R. Kikinis, Eds. Lecture Notes In Computer Science, vol. 1131. Springer-Verlag, London, 267-276.

Cocosco C.A. , Kollokian V., Kwan R.K.-S.,Evans A.C. (1997). BrainWeb: Online Interface to a 3D MRI Simulated Brain Database. NeuroImage, vol.5, no.4, part 2/4, S425, 1997 -- *Proceedings of 3-rd International Conference on Functional Mapping of the Human Brain*, Copenhagen, May 1997.

Collins D.L., Zijdenbos A.P., Kollokian V., Sled J.G., Kabani N.J., Holmes C.J., Evans A.C. (1998). Design and Construction of a Realistic Digital Brain Phantom. *IEEE Transactions on Medical Imaging*, vol.17, No.3, p.463--468, June 1998.

Delaunay B.N. (1934). Sur la sph`ere vide. Bulletin of Academy of Sciences of the USSR, (6):793–800, 1934.

Dunn J. C. (1973). A Fuzzy Relative of the ISODATA Process and Its Use in Detecting Compact Well-Separated Clusters, *Journal of Cybernetics* 3: 32-57.

Fornefett M., Rohr K., Stiehl H.S. (1999). Elastic Registration of Medical Images Using Radial Basis Functions with Compact Support, *Computer Vision and Pattern Recognition, IEEE Computer Society Conference on*, vol. 1, pp. 1402, 1999 IEEE Computer Society Conference on Computer Vision and Pattern Recognition (CVPR'99) - Volume 1.

Kwan R.K.-S., Evans A.C., Pike G.B. (1996). An Extensible MRI Simulator for Post-Processing Evaluation. *Visualization in Biomedical Computing (VBC'96). Lecture Notes in Computer Science*, vol. 1131. Springer-Verlag, 1996. 135-140.

Kwan R.K.-S., Evans A.C., Pike G.B. (1999). MRI simulation-based evaluation of image-processing and classification methods. *IEEE Transactions on Medical Imaging.* 18(11):1085-97, Nov 1999.

Liang Z.P., Ji, J.X and Pan, H. (2003). Further analysis of interpolation effects in mutual information-based image registration, *Medical Imaging, IEEE Transactions on*, vol.22, no. 9, pp. 1131-1140, Sept. 2003

Nadaraya E. (1964). On estimating regression, Theory of Prob. and Appl., vol. 9, pp. 141–142, 1964.

Simon K.W. (1975), Digital image reconstruction and resampling for geometric manipulation, *Proceedings of IEEE Symposium on Machine Processing of Remotely Sensed Data*, 1975, pp. 3A-1-3A-11.

Wang Z., Bovik A.C., Sheikh H.R., Simoncelli E.P. (2004). Image quality assessment: From error visibility to structural similarity. *IEEE Transactions on Image Processing*, 13:600–612, 2004.

Watson G.S. (1964). Smooth regression analysis, Sankhya, Series A, vol. 26, pp. 359 - 372, 1964.

Wendland H. (1995). Piecewise polynomial, positive definite and compactly supported radial functions of minimal degree. Adv. Comput. Math. 4, p. 389.

ICA applied to microcalcification clusters CAD in mammograms

C.J. García-Orellana, R. Gallardo-Caballero, H.M. González-Velasco, A. García-Manso, M. Macías-Macías
CAPI Research group, University of Extremadura, Spain

1. Introduction

The incidence of breast cancer in western women varies from 40 to 75 per 100,000, being the most frequent tumour among the feminine population. Latest statistics published by Cancer Research UK (Cancer Research, 2006) for year 2006 show 44,091 new cases of breast cancer diagnosed in the UK, being 99% of them detected in women. The importance of the problem in the European countries can be observed in Figure 1 where the the highest incidence rate appears in Belgium with more than 135 cases per 100,000 and a mortality rate of more than 30 per 100,000.

These pessimistic statistics illustrate the problem magnitude. Although some risk factors have been identified, **effective prevention measures or specific and effective treatments are unknown**.

The graph in Figure 2 (Cancer Research, 2006), allows to see that breast cancer treatment in an early stage of development can increment considerably the patient's survival chance. In fact, early breast cancer detection increases possibilities to allow for a conservative surgery instead to mastectomy, the only solution in advanced breast cancers (Haty et al., 1991).

The absence of a clear risk factor, different from the age, with high significance in disease's appearance makes difficult to establish any effective measure in breast cancer prevention. Nowadays, early detection of breast cancer constitutes the most effective step in this battle.

To improve early detection of breast cancer, all the health systems of developed countries perform what are known as "screening programs". In these screening programs, a review of all women at risk age is performed with a given periodicity. The most common test for the studies is mammography.

Like any other radiological test, mammography should be reviewed by expert radiologists, looking for abnormalities (asymmetry, masses, spicular lesions and clusters of microcalcifications or MCCs, mainly), being the mammography one of the more complex plates to analyze due to its high resolution and the type of abnormalities to look for.

Among the abnormalities discussed above, MCCs (groups of 3 or more calcifications per cm^2) can be one of the first signs of a developing cancer.

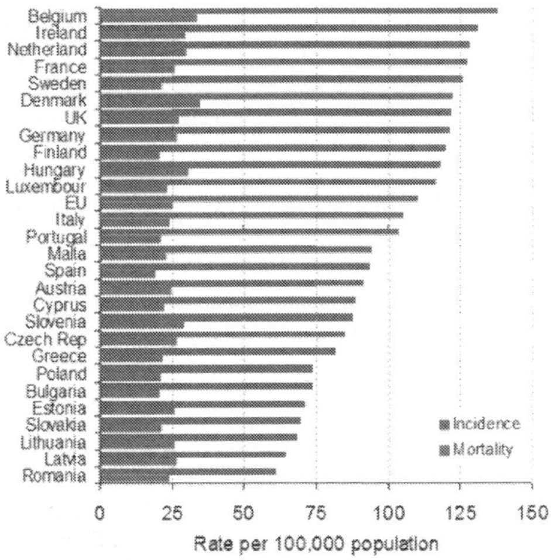

Fig. 1. Age standardized (European) incidence and mortality rates, female breast cancer in EU countries.

A microcalcification is a very small structure (typically lower than 1 millimetre), and, when they appear grouped in some characteristic shapes (microcalcification cluster, MCC) usually indicates the presence of a growing abnormality.

The detection of such structures sometimes presents an important degree of difficulty . Microcalcifications are relatively small and sometimes appear in low contrast areas, so that they must be detected by a human expert, who can be fatigued or can have variations in his attention level. This later reason makes very interesting the possibility to use a Computer Aided Diagnostic system (CAD) as a way to reduce the possibilities of misdetection of a developing breast cancer.

In order to provide a trusted helping tool for the radiologists, a CAD system must have a high sensitivity, but also a low rate of false positives per image (FPi). A too alarmist CAD system (ie, with a rather high FPi rate), is of no value in screening because it either causes the radiologist to distrust, or generates a great number of biopsies, making unfeasible the screening program. Approximately 6 in every 1,000 screening tests (0.6%) indicate the presence of cancer. Currently there are several CAD systems for mammography, some of them commercial and approved by the FDA. However, there are independent studies which indicate that their use does not provide clear benefits. In many cases, the performance of these systems is not known clearly enough, in part because results are given over their own databases, making very complicated an objective validation and comparison.

The studies by (Taylor et al., 2005) and (Gilbert et al., 2006) are performed in the context of the British Health Service. Those by (Taylor et al., 2005) do not use a great quantity of mammograms, but however, the study by (Gilbert et al., 2006) is developed with 10.267 mammograms, with a proportion of cancer similar to what can be found in screening. These studies try to evaluate the difference in performance between a "double reading" strategy and a "simple reading plus CAD".

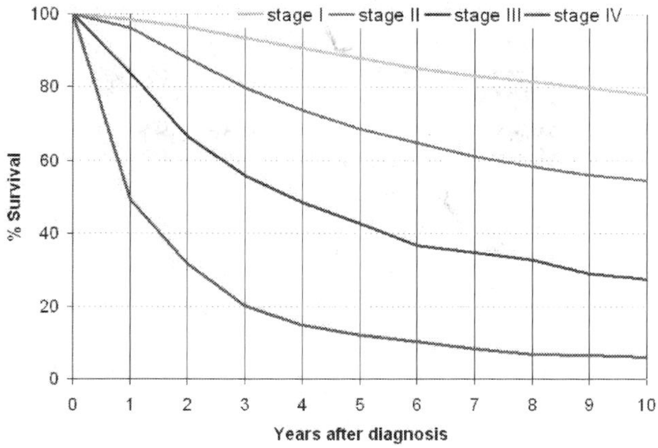

Fig. 2. 0-10 year relative survival for cases of breast cancer by stage diagnosed in the West Midlands 1985-1989 followed up to the end of 1999, as at January 2002

The studies by (Taylor et al., 2005) indicate that there is no significant improvement neither in sensitivity nor in specificity (they even talk about an increase in the cost), indicating that it should be due to the low specificity of the system. They conclude that the subject must be studied in deep before adopting.

On the other hand, the study by (Gilbert et al., 2006) conclude that there is obtained an improvement on the sensitivity, but also an increase in the recall rate, when CAD is used. The final conclusion is that the system must be evaluated better, an that a successfully implantation of the CADe system depends on its specificity (i.e., on reducing the number of FP).

Another interesting study is by (Fenton et al., 2007). This study is different from the other two, it is a statistical analysis of the screening data from 43 centers, between 1998 and 2002. They compare the results of the centers using CAD with those centers that do not. The final conclusion is that the CAD usage reduces the precision when interpreting mammograms while the number of biopsies increases (and, therefore, the "positive prediction value" (PPV)).

PPV has three different variants depending on different diagnostic stages. When referred exclusively to screening it is named as PPV1. This value provides the percentage of all positive screening examinations that result in a tissue diagnosis of cancer within one year. The two other kinds of parameters provide information about cases recommended for biopsy or patients with clinical signs of the disease. PPV1 values recommended by Agency for Health Policy and Research rely on the range 5 to 10% (ACR, 2003). Few studies provide values for this parameter, being more common to provide sensitivity and specificity or false positive rate as outcome measures.

Although screening can be useful to detect different signs of malignancy (good defined or circumscribed lesions, stellate lesions, structural distortion, breast asymmetry, etc), the clearest sign to detect early breast cancer is the presence of microcalcification clusters (MCCs) (Lanyi, 1985). Indeed, from 30 to 50% mammographic detected cancers present

MCCs (Chan et al., 1988; Dhawan and Royer, 1988); and 60–80% of breast carcinomas reveal MCCs upon histological examinations (Sickles, 1986).
Even nowadays, the automatic interpretation of microcalcifications remains very difficult. It is mainly due to their fuzzy nature, low contrast and low distinguishability from their surroundings. One microcalcification is very small, its size varies between 0.1 and 1.0 mm, being the average size 0.3 mm. Those smaller than 0.1 mm are very difficult to distinguish from the high frequency noise present in the mammogram. Besides, they present different size, form and distribution, and therefore it is not possible to fit a template.
In this field, the different approaches range from the most simple consisting in improving the visibility of what are known *regions of suspicion* in the mammogram, in order to make easier the work of the radiologist, to proposals of complete computer aided diagnosis systems. The radiologists define a region of suspicion as that region which is more brilliant than the surrounding tissue, has a uniform density, circular shape and diffuse edges. To treat these regions, several techniques are normally used, as for instance: contrast stretching, enhancement by histogram equalization (Karssemeijer, 1993), convolution mask enhancement (Chan et al., 1987) and adaptive neighbourhood enhancement (Woods et al., 1991; Dhawan et al., 1986).
Other groups of techniques include works based on region-based enhancement (Morrow et al., 1992; Shen et al., 1994); and feature-based enhancement. In the last subgroup we can distinguish two different lines. The first one consist on increasing the contrast in suspicious areas and the other one is to remove background structures and noise according to microcalcifications features. There have been used many different techniques for contrast enhancement, as higher order statistical (HOS) (Gurcan et al., 1997); fuzzy logic (Chen et al., 1998) and multi-scale analysis (Laine et al., 1994). Among those proposals based on background removal we can find techniques as fractal modelling of the background tissue (Li et al., 1997), morphological processing (Dengler et al., 1993) or wavelet reconstruction (Wang & Karayiannis, 1998).
A higher step than enhancing is developed by different proposals to detect microcalcifications or masses based on different feature extraction methods. In the literature we can find different approaches among which we can point out:

- Individual microcalcification features. Features extracted directly from mammogram such as perimeter, area, compactness, elongation, eccentricity, etc. (Nam & Choi, 1998; Bottema & Slavotinek, 2000).
- Statistical texture features. Including different methods like Surrounding Region Dependence method (SRDM) (Kim & Park, 1999), Spatial Gray level dependence method (Ferrari et al., 1999), Gray level difference method (GLDM) (Lee et al., 1998) or Spatial Gray Scale Co-Occurrence Matrix (SGLCM) (Yang et al., 2005) for the detection of MCCs.
- Multi-scale texture features. Methods based on wavelet transform (Yu et al., 1999), Gabor filter bank (Bhangale, 2000) or Laplacian of Gaussian filter (Netsch & Peitgen, 1999).
- Fractal dimension features (Caldell et al., 1990).

The last step corresponds to the approaches which study the malignancy of the abnormalities detected in the mammograms. Normally, they use feature vectors very similar to those used in the approaches of individual calcifications detection, along with a classifier which can be neural network-type (Jiang et al., 1997), K-nearest neighbour (Zadeh et al., 2001), Bayesian networks (Bankman et al., 1994) or binary decision trees (Zheng & Chan, 2001).

Finally, we can also cite several commercial equipments as can be ImageChecker® by R2 Technology, MammoReader™ by Intelligent Systems Software or SecondLook™ by CADx. These three equipments have obtained the approval of the Federal Food and Drug Administration (FDA) for their use in medical dependencies. Nevertheless, as we commented above, there exist diverse opinions regarding their reliability, according to different studies (Taylor et al., 2005; Gilbert et al., 2006; Fenton et al., 2007; Serio & Novello, 2003).

The rest of chapter follows with the methodology that we have used in our work. Next, we describe the details of system implementation. After that, we show our results and finally we deal with the conclusions.

2. Methodology

Our work proposal is based in the use of a technique known as Independent Component Analysis (ICA), as an efficient image feature extractor which will be used in a neural classifier. Independent Component Analysis is a technique which, unlike some classic methods as variance or standard deviation, uses high order statistics. Moreover, using samples from the signal space to model, is able to infer a base which let us represent any image (signal) belonging to the space with a low number of components.

This is the same task we carry out when we decompose a signal in its Fourier components or build wavelet decomposition, in the multiresolution field. But there are important differences between the mentioned methods and ICA. First, both Fourier and wavelet decompositions use fixed bases. On the other hand, ICA bases are generated to fit as better as possible the data space to model. In addition, an ICA development builds base matrices which maximize the non gaussianity of the input data space; this means that ICA bases model the most interesting characteristics of the modelled space. And this is precisely the key fact which leads us to use ICA as a feature extractor block instead of other more extended techniques as the previously mentioned wavelet transform or principal component analysis.

The second important element in our architecture is the neural classifier. This kind of systems has characteristics which are especially interesting to broach the problem. Perhaps the most well-known can be the capability to adjust its operation by means of "samples". Colloquially, we can say they have learning capability. Moreover, these systems have another important characteristic which is known as generalization capability. Generalization in neural classifiers is the capacity to provide a right response for a completely unknown input. As can be inferred, this characteristic makes a neural classifier a great choice for a classification task like our, where input data variability is very high (contrast variations, mammography errors, artifacts, etc.).

2.1 Data source

Although nowadays digital mammography systems have become popular, up to date the main data source in research investigation tasks has been digitized mammograms. Mammographic scanners provide a high resolution level: pixel sizes ranging in tenths of micron, and grey level resolution from 11 to 16 bits (2,048 to 65,536 grey values). This gives us an idea of the precision level which can be used working with mammograms.

The current data source for our work is the mammographic database known as Digital Database for Screening Mammography (DDSM). Developed by the Island Vision Group at the University of South Florida may be the most extensive and better quality free to use database for research purposes. It comprises about 2,500 complete cases, providing the four typical views in a mammographic study (left and right cranio-caudal and medio-lateral-oblique). Furthermore, it provides useful information for the case as age, film type, scanner, etc. But the most interesting feature for our work is that it provides what is called *ground truth marks* when a breast presents a biopsy proven abnormality, specifying its type and distribution in the ACR internationally accepted nomenclature named BIRADS.

There are other databases in this field, as can be MIAS or Nijmegen; but they are unavailable or its distribution is restricted. MIAS group provides a reduced version free of charge (miniMIAS), but its low spatial and spectral resolution makes it useless for microcalcification detection problems.

2.2 Dataset prototypes generation

This was probably one of the slowest phases of this development because we propose, as a first approximation, to carry out pixel level diagnostic. So, with the help of an experienced radiologist we made a pixel labelling work using predefined classes over mammogram regions, once converted to optical density. These set of regions correspond to all ROIs defined in the DDSM database but also include some manually selected regions which contain significant mammogram structures like vascular calcifications or artifacts.

The set of classes to study includes not only microcalcifications belonging to a cluster (hence malignancy indicatives) but also benign microcalcifications, large rod-like calcifications, round calcifications, lucent-centered calcifications, healthy tissue and several kinds of artifacts.

Totally we have inserted a training set of more than 4,600 microcalcification prototypes, over 6,700 benign and more than 100,000 healthy or benign prototypes.

Due to the high number of available prototypes and foreseen the following training step, we decided to build different training sets by varying different prototypes percentages while including all malignant microcalcification prototypes. These new training sets will be used in the following training steps carried out in the project.

2.3 Independent Component Analysis (ICA)

Independent Component Analysis appears as a possible solution to the problem of blind source separation (BSS) (Jutten & Herault, 1991; Comon, 1994). Basically, the goal in BSS is to recover the signals generated by unknown sources using sensor observations which provide a number of signals supposed to be a linear mixture of independent and unknown source signals. ICA can be used to solve this problem supposing statistical independence of these sources. The problem can be stated in equation (1).

$$\mathbf{x} = \mathbf{A} \cdot \mathbf{s} \tag{1}$$

Being **x** the observed signals, **A** the mixture coefficients and **s** the unknown sources (Hyvärinen et al., 2001). To apply this technique in feature extraction on mammography, we must suppose that a region of a given size in the mammography (called 'patch') is as linear combination of a series of independent unknown sources, a priori. These unknown sources can be seen as statistical independent 'patches', and can be estimated by ICA using samples. The process provides us a base of functions (small squared images in our case) that lets us expand a given 'patch' from the mammography in terms of it. The mentioned procedure can be expressed graphically as shown in Figure 3.

Where a_i coefficients represent the features to extract and which let us characterize a region from its sources.

The use of coefficients from a linear combination as parameters to characterize patterns has been widely used, for example in wavelets transforms or Gabor filters. Nevertheless, we think that ICA value added is that the base functions are specifically created for the image space under study on the opposed to wavelet transforms.

There exist many studies that have used ICA as a feature extraction technique and in particular for image analysis (Bell & Sejnowski, 1997; Hyvärinen et al., 1998; Jenssen & Eltoft, 2003).

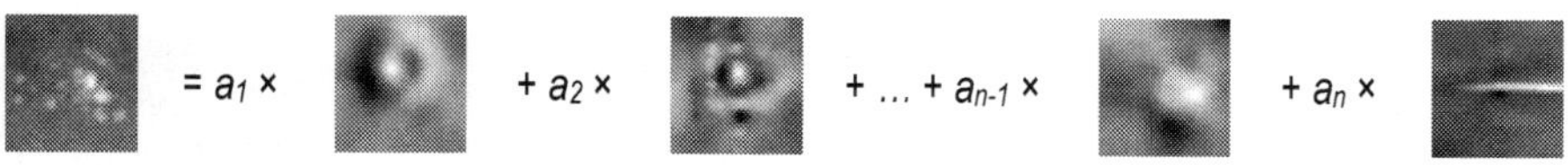

Fig. 3. ICA expansion.

The studies carried out by (Christoyianni et al., 2002) conclude that results obtained with ICA improve results obtained by different statistical parameters (GLHM and SGLDM). However, the study is carried out using only 58 regions of suspicion from the free version of the MIAS database. Ignoring the big difference in the number of cases which provide each database, the key difference between them is resolution (200µm/pixel for MIAS and 43.5µm/pixel for DDSM). This characteristic along with grey level depth can be a key factor for a successful handling of microcalcifications.

Other authors also apply ICA to extract features in mammograms. For instance, in (Campos et al., 2005) a similar scheme to (Christoyianni et al., 2002) is followed, but including the feature selection carried out by means of the forward-selection method. The work is also carried out with the mini-MIAS database.

In relation to these works and also to our previous exposition about the databases, we would like to remark that almost all the papers broach the usage of ICA to describe complete regions of interest (ROIs), scaled or centered. We think that this strategy, although may be valid with mini-MIAS and mass detection, is totally unsuitable for the DDSM database and microcalcification based approaches. A greater spatial resolution will lead to bigger ICA input for each ROI, increasing computational requirements in ICA matrices procurement phase and the number of features to obtain an effective ROI classification. We are using ICA at vicinity-of-pixel level, instead of considering complete ROIs, what means that we needed to label groups of pixels individually within each ROI.

2.4 Neural classifiers

Our work in microcalcification clusters CAD is not only centered on isolated prototypes evaluation. We have developed a complete software system to detect ROIs in mammograms and analyze its malignancy. The pattern recognition block is implemented by using a neural network with only one hidden layer. The number of neurons that includes the hidden layer is adaptable from 50 to 200. The selected training algorithm is RPROP (Riedmiller & Braun, 1992), a well known, fast converging and robust algorithm. The training system is implemented using the kernel abstraction characteristics provided by Stuttgart Neural Network Simulator (SNNS). This feature permits us to build standalone trainers which can be run in our Beowulf cluster, allowing us to study an important number of configurations and to evaluate performance dependence on ICA window size and the number of features to be used.

2.5 ROI generation

The previously described classifier provides a map of suspicious pixels for each input mammogram. This map is filtered to eliminate spurious single-pixel positives. The filtered image is further fed into a ROI builder subsystem which groups neighboring microcalcifications into zones of interest.

The first step of the ROI builder consists in an object detector that isolates microcalcifications and computes its sizes. In a second step, we carry out an object grouping phase by means of a density map. For each pixel of the mammogram we compute the number of neighbour microcalcificacions in an area of $1cm^2$. After that, we filter the density map retaining only those zones which have a density value equal to or greater than 3, following the classic definition provided in (Sickles, 1986). This procedure provides us an easy way to obtain ROIs avoiding costly region growing and merging operations because they are completely inherent to the process and don't need further calculations.

Each possible generated ROI in a mammogram, is tagged as true positive (TP) if it overlaps with the ROI provided in the DDSM database (if present). Analogously the ROI is tagged as false positive (FP) if there exist no overlapping with an actual zone of interest of the mammogram or the mammogram is healthy. On the contrary, if DDSM contains malignant ROIs for a mammogram and our system fails to find them we compute all those ROIs as false negatives (FN).

And finally, a healthy mammogram successfully diagnosed is considered as a true negative (TN). In a computerized diagnosing system, the previous four parameters are usually expressed in terms of mean values per image, being false positives per image (FPi) a common performance index. Figure 4 shows a processed mammogram which yields one TP ROI (the upper one) and four FPs. The true positive ROI includes a detailed view which shows the microcalcifications that define it.

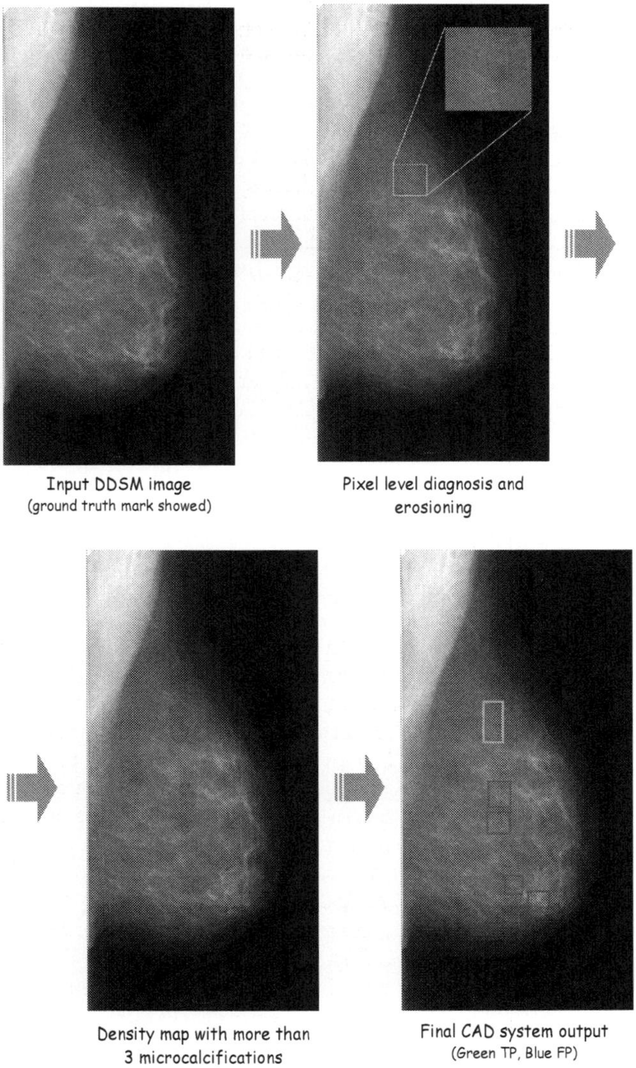

Fig. 4. Example of mammogram process (case D-4183, with 1 TP and 4 FP).

2.6 False positive correction

An automated ROI generator may lead to an excessively big region if the output of the neural network classifier provides an scattered microcalcifications distribution over the whole mammogram. Considering the previously stated evaluation criterion, large ROIs can lead to a misleading low FP rate.

In order to deal with the possibility of an excessive ROI growth, instead of using false positives per image (FPi) as a performance index, we have defined a new parameter called weighted false positive per image (WFPi). A false positive ROI increases this parameter as many times as it exceeds the maximum estimated ROI size (MRS) plus one. The MRS is the area of the largest MCC-ROI defined in DDSM database calcification subset (39.69 cm^2). Moreover, WFPi is also increased if a true positive ROI exceeds the MRS, see (2) for reference. Thus this parameter penalizes not only false positives but also unjustified true and false ROI growths.

Hence, WFPi improves common FPi confidence degree and makes it a preferable figure of merit for a completely automated system. Nevertheless, it is important to note that providing results in terms of this parameter leads to a worsening of overall results.

$$WFPi = \sum_{\text{FP \#}} \left(1 + \frac{area(FP_i)}{MRS} \right) + \sum_{\text{TP \#}} \left(\frac{area(TP_i)}{MRS} \right) \tag{2}$$

2.7 Evaluation of different sets

To test our system robustness we have defined four different database subsets with the aim of stating that the system performance depends on this choice. The four views provided for each case are used in this study. Table 1 summarizes the main characteristics of the chosen subsets and includes the total number of mammograms processed.

Firstly, we have created a big set of cases (GLOBAL) which includes an important number of clearly normal cases (all cases from normal volumes) and as much malignant MCCs cases as possible (all cancer cases from cancer volumes whose lesion type is diagnosed as a kind of microcalcification cluster). This subset should allow us to test our overall system performance on a more realistic situation than that proposed in (Heath et al., 2000), which only comprises malignant MCC cases.

Secondly, we decided to use the validation subset proposed in (Heath et al., 2000) (CALC 1) which contains all cases of the BCRP CALC 1 subset as specified by DDSM creators. It must be noted that none of this cases have been considered to train the neural classifier used in this system. Results obtained over this subset can be compared with those obtained in research works that follow the guidelines provided by DDSM authors in (Heath et al., 2000).

Furthermore, we studied a third subset (SET 1) which includes the same cases studied in (Roffilli, 2006). It is comprised of all the cases from normal volumes 8 and 10 plus all MCC cases from cancer volumes 2,7 and 12.

Finally, SET 2 is a favorable selection of cases from GLOBAL subset.

Set	Description	Mammograms
GLOBAL	Vols. normal and cancer	4,372
CALC_1	BRCP_CALC_1	200
SET_1	Vols. 8 and 10 of normal and vols. 2, 7 and 12 of cancer	408
SET_2	Selection of favourable cases	1,622

Table 1. Data included in the considered sets.

3. System Implementation

As can be deduced from the previous sections, the proposed system is very complete and somewhat complex. In this section we describe in deep the elements which constitute the system and its characteristics.

3.1 Computational infrastructure

The DDSM database provided by Island Vision Group is accessible by FTP, so we dumped it to a dedicated server with a storing capacity of 290 gigabytes where 240 gigabytes are used exclusively to store the images and configuration files which constitutes the database.
As previously mentioned, DDSM provides case information in file form. As this format is not adequate to work with this data in an intensive way, we have decided to insert this information in a SQL database server which runs in one of our Linux servers.
At the same time this database engine allows us to store some information for different project phases, letting us to centralize all needed data, both input as output, and facilitating statistics procurement task.

Some project phases require high computational resources and volatile memory requirements. Fortunately our research group owns various multiprocessor servers with important memory resources which have allowed us to carry out the project; obviously typical hardware infrastructure is insufficient to deal with a project like the proposed here.
We can point out an Opteron bi-processor server with 16 gigabytes of RAM, a second 64-bit server Athlon64 four-cores-processor with 8 gigabytes of RAM and various 32-bit bi-processor servers which hold the database engine, the distributed file system and backup.
A special mention is due to the most important computation resource of the group, a Beowulf type cluster with 45 Phenom 9850 nodes each one equipped with 4 gigabytes of RAM. This is the resource where all massive calculations are carried out and lets us reduce dramatically simulation times, thanks to its 180 CPU cores.

3.2 Management interface

A reliable image work requires developing a tool that makes easy to visualize these images and to make different operations with them like marking or correcting. The tool developed by our group is called Mamoprot and lets us to solve many different issues arisen in various development stages of the project.
Mamoprot is a modular application written in C++ and developed against the widget library QT, which runs under Linux environment. It is completely integrated with the relational database server that manages the project. This tool lets to carry out many different operations. Besides basic visualization operations (contrast adjustment, brightness, basic filtering and enhancement) working with overlays allows us to perform many interfacing operations. Specifically Mamoprot is the tool that we used to visualize and mark prototypes in overlays, and also let us to diagnose the visualized overlay with a given configuration, visualize ICA decomposition of the overlay and rebuild the image using only some components. The first module of Mamoprot was used by experts to insert training prototypes in the database.
Mamoprot is also designed to deal with mammograms, letting us to visualize them with overlapped expert marks and stored regions of interest. The application also permits us to

carry out a diagnostic of the whole mammogram, viewing pixel based classification and the possibly generated ROIs with that system configuration. Finally, this module allows us to create new overlays and to add new prototypes for interesting regions.
And finally, Mamoprot permits to insert visually new diagnostic configurations, selecting system characteristics to be studied. In Figure 5, we can see a Mamoprot snapshot for the mammogram module; particularly we show the diagnostic results for a complete mammogram. Discontinued blue rectangles mark benign auxiliary ROIs previously added to the database, red discontinuous rectangle marks the original DDSM malignant overlay, green solid line rectangle accounts for true positive finding and the blue solid border rectangle is a false positive generated by the system.

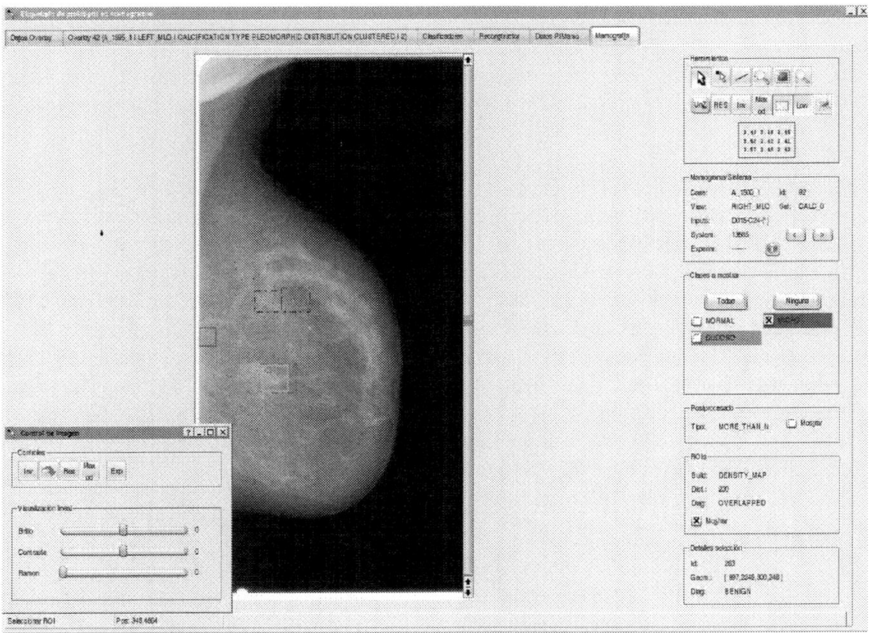

Fig. 5. Mamoprot interface.

4. Results

In our work we have trained more than 4,000 classifiers, we have evaluated more than 140,000 complete mammograms (with different classifiers and decision systems), and more than 450,000 ROIs have been generated.With these numbers, it is clear the importance of the SQL database in order to get the results in an easy way.
To evaluate complete mammogram performance we have decided to use FROC curve analysis (Free-response Receiver Operating Characteristic), as a widely accepted technique. Furthermore, we have decided to use "Weighed False Positive per Image" (WFPi) instead of "False Positive per Image" (FPi).

4.1 Global results

First, we present the results over the BCRP_CALC_0 and BCRP_CALC_1 subsets of DDSM database.

The use of WFPi instead of FPi deteriorate our results, but it is evident that it provides a more reliable vision of the overall system performance. Table 2 shows the values of these parameters for one of the best configurations obtained for global results, and Figure 6 shows FROC curves globally and for the subsets BCRP_CALC_0 and BCRP_CALC_1 (showing in every case WFPi instead of FPi). These results are obtained for a 13x13 patch size with 40 ICA components.

FPi	WFPi	Sens. (%)
0,40	0,40	24,5
2,18	2,20	54,1
2,79	2,83	63,8
3,33	4,17	84,1
2,78	4,20	88,5
2,65	4,35	90,4
3,57	6,74	97,6

Table 2. Global results.

4.2 Results over different sets

We thought that it could be interesting to compare the results obtained when we use different sets of mammograms to test the performance. As we said before, we have defined four different subsets of DDSM (Table I).

Figure 7 shows the modified FROC curves obtained for each of the subsets defined in Table 1. In the x-axis we have replaced regular FPi values with the previously defined WFPi performance index.

We can observe that modified FROC curves for GLOBAL and BCRP_CALC_1 groupings follow a similar trend. Due to we are restricting our study to MCC detection and diagnosis, and given the previous definition of BCRP_CALC_1, this behaviour seems to suggest that this set of mammograms is an adequate sample to provide results over the whole DDSM database.

On the other hand, results for subset SET 1 show a clear improvement over GLOBAL and BCRP_CALC_1 subsets; we can observe better sensitivity values for the same or even lower WFPi. However, it is evident that this subset does not reflect valid results for the whole database.

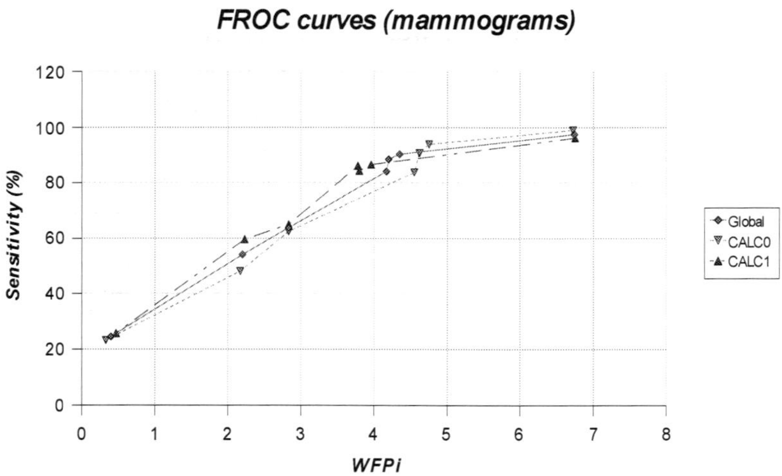

Fig. 6. FROC curves corresponding to complete mammograms.

Finally, we can observe an important improvement in the modified FROC curve for SET 2. We obtain high sensitivity values at low WFPi rates even when this subset has approximately 1,600 mammograms, a number of mammograms higher than those included in both BCRP_CALC_1 and SET 1.

Table 3 shows a WFPi and FPi comparison at a common sensitivity value of 80% for each analyzed subset. As can be seen, WFPi values are higher than the corresponding FPi. This effect is stronger in the GLOBAL subset (the most comprehensive one) where the WFPi value is a 13% higher than the associated FPi.

Set	FPi	WFPi	Sensitivity
GLOBAL	3,75	3,97	78,04 %
CALC_1	3,26	3,67	80,65 %
SET_1	2,24	2,29	81,82 %
SET_2	1,03	1,25	80,09 %

Table 3. Performance parameters for the proposed subsets.

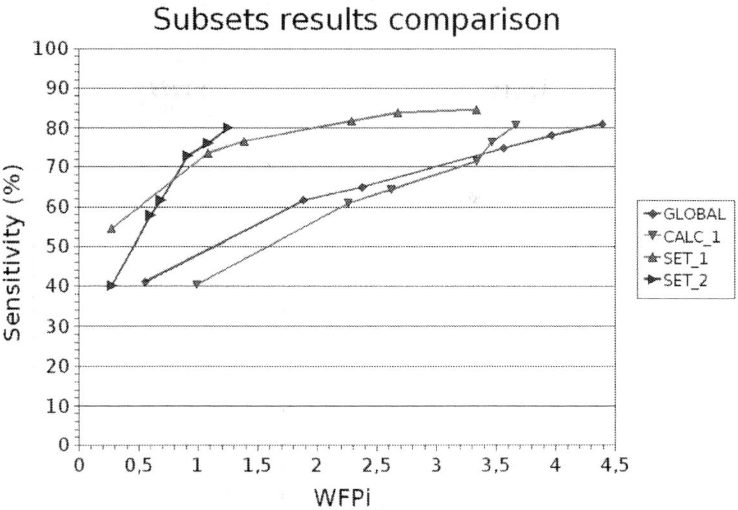

Fig. 7. FROC curves for proposed subsets.

5. Conclusions

The previously described results show that ICA lead to systems with an acceptable performance for mammograms taken from the BCRP_CALC_1 of the DDSM database.
The results showed in Figure 6 and the previous analysis let us to state that the election of the specific subset used in this research work has an important influence on the results provided by our CAD system, at least from the MCC detection and diagnosis point of view. Hence, we think that, in this particular research field, not only raw results, but also a clear specification of the set used to provide them, should be provided.
Finally, we must conclude that Independent Component Analysis is a valid technique to deal with the microcalcification detection problem. However, as a future research plan, we are studying the possibility of improving the system performance by adding new prototypes in particular zones where diagnostic results deteriorate the overall performance.

6. Acknowledgments

This work has been partly supported by the *Junta de Extremadura* and FEDER through project PRI08A092.

7. References

American Collage of Radiology (ACR). (2003) BI-RADS® - Breast Imaging Atlas - Mammography, Fourth Edition.

Bankman, I.N.; Tsai, J.; Kim, D.; Gatewood, O. & Brody, W. (1994). Detection of microcalcification clusters using neural networks. Annual International Conference of the IEEE Engineering in Medicine and Biology Society-Proceedings. Vol. 16, pp. 590-591.

Bell, A.J. & Sejnowski, T.J. (1997). The 'independent components' of natural scenes are edge filters. Vision Research, 37:3327-3338.

Bhangale, T.; Desai, U.B. & Sharma, U. (2000). An unsupervised scheme for detection of microcalcifications on mammograms. IEEE International Conference on Image Processing. September 10-13, pp. 184-187.

Bottema, M.J. & Slavotinek, J.P. (2000). Detection and classification of lobular and DCIS (small cell) microcalcifications in digital mammograms. Pattern Recognition Letters, 21; pp. 1209-1214.

Caldell, C.B.; Stapleton, S.J.; Holsworth, D.W. & Jong, R.A. (1990). Characterization of mammographic parenchymal pattern by fractal dimension. Phys. Med. Biol., 35 (2); pp. 235-247.

Campos, L.F.A.; Silva, C.A. & Barros, A.K. (2005). Diagnosis of Breast Cancer in Digital Mammograms Using Independent Component Analysis and Neural Networks. 10th Iberoamerican Congress on Pattern Recognition, CIARP 2005, Havana, Cuba, November 15-18, 2005. LNCS. Vol. 3773, pp. 460-469.

Cancer Research UK (2006). Breast Cancer Factsheet. Technical report, London. URL: http://www.cancerresearchuk.org.

Chan, H.P.; Doi, K.; Vyborny, C.J.; Lam, K.L. & Schmidt, R.A.. (1988). Computer-aided detection of microcalcifications in mammograms - methodology and preliminary clinical study. Invest. Radiol, 23 (9); pp.664-671.

Chan, H.P.; Vyborny, C.J.; McMahon, H.; Metz, C.E.; Doi, K. & Sickles, E.A. (1987). Digital mammography: ROC studies of the effects of pixel size and unsharp-mask filtering on the detection of subtle microcalcifications. Invest. Radiol. 22 (7); pp. 581-589.

Cheng, H.D.; Lui, Y.M. & Freimanis, R.I. (1998). A novel aproach to microcalcification detection using fuzzy logic technique. IEEE Trans. Med. Imag. 17 (3); pp. 442-450.

Comon, P. (1994). Independent component analysis - a new concept? Signal Processing, 36: 287-314.

Christoyianni, L.; Koutras, A.; Dermatas, E. & Kokkinakis, G. (2002). Computer aided diagnosis of breast cancer in digitized mammograms. Computerized Medical Imaging and Graphics, 26, 309-319.

Dengler, J.; Behrens, S. & Desaga, J.F. (1993). Segmentation of microcalcifications in mammograms. IEEE Trans. Med. Imag., 12 (4); pp. 634-642.

Dhawan, A.P.; Buelloni, G. & Gordon, R. (1986). Enhancement of mammographic features by optimal adaptive neighborhood image processing. IEEE Trans. Med. Imag. 5 (1); pp. 8-15.

Dhawan, A.P. & Royer, E.L. (1988). Mammographic feature enhancement by computerized image processing. Comput. Methods Programs Biomed, 27 (1); pp. 23-35.

Fenton, J.; Taplin, S.; Carney, P.; Abraham, L.; Sickles, E.; D'Orsi, C.; Berns, E.; Cutter, G.; Hendrick, E.;Barlow, W. & Elmore, J. (2007). Influence of Computer-Aided Detection on Performance of Screening Mammography. The New England Journal of Medicine (NEJM), Vol. 356 (14), 1399-1409.

Ferrari, R.J.; de Carvalho, A.C.P.; Marques, P.M.A. & Frere, A.F. (1999). Computerized classification of breast lesions: shape and texture analysis using an artificial neural network. Image Process. Appl., pp. 517-521.

Gilbert, F.; Astley, A.; McGee, M.; Gillan, M.; Boggis, C.; Griffihs, P. & Duffy, S. (2006). Single Reading with Computer-Aided Detection and Double Reading of Screening Mammograms in the United Kingdom National Breast Screening Program. Radiology. Vol. 241 (1), 47-53.

Gurcan, M.N.; Yardimci, Y.; Cetin, A.E. & Ansari, R. (1997). Detection of microcalcifications in mammograms using higher order statistics. Signal Process. Lett. 4 (8); pp 213-216.

Haty, B.G.; Kornguth, P.; Fisher, D.; Beinfield, M. & McKhann, C. (1991). Mammographically Detected Breast Cancer: Results with Conservative Surgery and Radiation Therapy. Cancer, 67; pp. 2801-2804.

Heath, M.; Bowyer, K.; Kopans, D.B.; Moore, R. & Kegelmeyer Jr., P. (2000). The digital database for screening mammography. Proceedings of the 5th International Workshop on Digital Mammography (Toronto, Canada, June 2000). Medical Physics Publishing.

Hyvärinen, A.; Karhunen, J. & Oja, E. (2001). Independent Component Analysis. John Wiley and Sons.

Hyvärinen, A.; Oja, E.; Hoyer, P. & Hurri. J. (1998). Image feature extraction by sparse coding and independent component analysis. In ICPR'98, pp. 1268-1273, Brisbane, Australia.

Jenssen, R. & Eltoft, T. (2003). Independent component analysis for texture segmentation. Pattern Recognition, 36, 2301-2315.

Jiang, Y.; Nishikawa, R.M.; Wolverton, D.E.; Metz, C.E. & Schmidt, R.A. & Doi, K. (1997). Computerized classification of malignant and benign clustered microcalcifications in mammograms. Proceedings of 19th International Conference-IEEE/EMBS, October 30 - November 2, pp. 521-523.

Jutten, C. & Herault, J., (1991). Blind separation of sources, part I: an adaptive algorithm based on neuromimetic architecture. Signal Processing, vol.24, no. 1, pp. 1-10.

Karssemeijer, N. (1993). Adaptive noise equalization and image analysis in mammography. Information Processing in Medical Imaging: 13th International Conference, AZ, USA; pp. 472-486.

Kim, J.K. & Park, H.W. (1999). Statistical textural features for detection of microcalcifications in digital mammograms. IEEE Trans. Med. Imag., 18 (3); pp. 231-238.

Laine, A.F.; Schuler, S.; Fan, J. & Huda, W. (1994). Mammographyc feature enhancement by multiscale analysis. IEEE Trans. Med. Imag., 13 (4); pp. 7250-7260.

Lanyi, M. (1985). Morphological analysis of microcalcifications. Early breast cancer: Histopathology, diagnosis & treatment. Springer Verlag.

Lee, C.S.; Kim, J.K. & Park, H.W. (1998). Computer-aided diagnostic system for breast cancer by detecting microcalcification. SPIE 3335; pp. 615-626.

Li, H.; Liu, K.J.E. & Lo, S.C.B. (1997). Fractal modeling and segmentation for the enhancement of microcalcifications in digital mammograms, IEEE Trans. Med. Imag., 16 (6); pp. 785-798.

Morrow, W.M.; Paranjape, R.B.; Rangayyan, R.M. & Desautels, J.E.L. (1992). Region-based contrast enhancement of mammograms. IEEE Trans. Med. Imag. 11 (3); pp. 392-406.

Nam, S.H. & Choi, J.Y. (1998). A method of image enhancement and fractal dimension for detection of microcalcifications in mammogram. Procceedings of the 20th Annual International Conference of the IEEE Engineering in Medicine and Biology Society, Vol. 20 (2); pp. 1009-1012.

Netsch, T.; Peitgen, H.O. (1999). Scale-space signatures for the detection of clustered microcalcifications in digital mammograms. IEEE Trans. Med. Imag., 18 (9); pp. 774-786.

Riedmiller, M. & Braun, H. (1992). RPROP - A Fast Adaptive Learning Algorithm. Technical Report (To appear in: Proc. of ISCIS VII), Universit¨at Karlsruhe.

Roffilli, M. (2006). Advanced machine learning techniques for digital mammography. Departament of Computer Science. University of Bologna. Bologna (Italy), Tech. Report.

Serio, G.V. & Novello, A.C. (2003). The advisability of the adoption of a law that would expand the definition of mammography screening to include the review of x-ray examinations by use of a computer aided detection device. Tech report.

Shen, L.; Rangayyan, R. & Desautels, J.E.L. (1994). Application of shape analysis to mammographic calcifications. IEEE Trans. Med. Imag., 13 (2); pp. 263-274.

Sickles, E.A. (1986). Mammographic features of 300 consecutive nonpalpable breast cancers. Am. J. Radiol, 146; pp. 661-665.

Taylor, P.; Champness, J.; Given-Wilson, R.; Johnston, K. & Potts, H.. (2005). Impact of computer-aided-detection prompts on the sensitivity and specificity of screening mammography. HealthTecnol Assess. Vol. 9 (6), 1-58.

Wang, T.C. & Karayiannis, N.B. (1998). Detection of microcalcifications in digital mammograms using wavelets. IEEE Trans. Med. Imag., 17 (4); pp. 498-509.

Woods, K.; Clarke, L.P. & Velthuizen, R. (1991). Enhancement of digital mammograms using a local thresholding technique. Annual International Conference of the IEEE Engineering in Medicine and Biology Society, 13 (1); pp. 114-115.

Yang, S.C.; Hsu, H.H.; Hsu, G.C.; Chung, P.C.; Guo, S.M.; Lo, C.S.; Yang, C.W.; Lee, S.K. & Chang, C.I. (2005). 3D localization of clustered microcalcifications using cranio-caudal and medio-lateral oblique views. Computerized Medical Imaging and Graphics, 29; pp. 521–532.

Yu, S.; Guan, L. & Brown, S. (1999). Automatic detection of clustered microcalcifications in digitized mammogram films. J. Electron. Imag., 8 (1); pp. 76-82.

Zadeh, H.S.; Nezhad, S.P. & Rad, F.R. (2001). Shape-based and texture-based feature extraction for classification of microcalcification in mammograms. Proc. SPIE 4322; pp. 301-310.

Zheng, L. & Chan, A.K. (2001). An artificial intelligent algorithm for tumor detection in screening mammogram. IEEE Trans. Med. Imag., 20 (17); pp. 559-567.

20

Nanomedicine in Cancer

César A González
Universidad del Ejército y Fuerza Aérea
Instituto Politécnico Nacional
México

1. Introduction

Nanotechnology is now a very important field of study in most academic institutions around the world. The industry has concentrated its efforts on nanotechnology as it has shown that investment in this field is very profitable. The development of research in the area of nanotechnology requires sophisticated equipment and techniques including: scanning electron microscopy, transmission microscopy with accessories to achieve high resolution, quantum tunneling microscopy, X-ray spectroscopy of dispersion energy, as well as electron diffraction of low energy.

The use of nanotechnology suggests that certain fields of medicine can be a revolution, specially in monitoring the disease through imaging, tissue repair, and control of the evolution of diseases, protection and improvement of biological human systems, pain relief and administration of drugs to specific cells, just to refer some of the most important applications. All these applications would be new technological advances that are promoting a new era in assistencial medicine.

Cancer is a leading cause of death throughout the world. Of the 58 million deaths that occurred in the world in 2005, 7.6 million (13%) were due to cancer. The types of cancer leading to overall mortality in humans are the lung, stomach, liver, colon and breast. Over 70% of all cancer deaths occurred in developing countries. It is expected that the global number of deaths from cancer continue to increase throughout the world and reach 9 million in 2015 and 11.4 million in 2030.

Nanomedicine has shown an important growing in the war against cancer in the last two decades. Early detection is the main limitation of the current cancer treatments. Several techniques at molecular scale have been focused on early detection and treatment of the disease by identification and selective targeted of cancer cells but their applications in the clinical practice still represent important methodological challenges. The National Cancer Institute of the United States has launched the "Alliance for Nanotechnology in Cancer", a plan that includes the development and creation of miniature tools for early detection and effective treatment of this evil affects millions of people in the world.

It is currently designing new nanoscale devices, i.e. nanodevices capable of one or more clinical features, including the detection of cancer in its earliest stages, tracking their location inside the body, or the supply of drugs specifically targeting malignant cells. This chapter is oriented to describe newer nanodevices designed to detect cancer in early stages as well as its specific location in the body. The information is presented as a contrast between the innovative value of the concept and their clinical feasibility. The main body of the content is segmented as follows: First; new nanostructures for labelling cancer cells are cited. Second; image techniques for cancer detection assisted by nanostructures are roughly reviewed. Then; an author proposal for cancer detection and monitoring through magnetic fields at multiple frequencies assisted by magnetic nanoparticles is described, including its theoretical and practical fundaments. Last; potential hazards of nanomedicine in cancer are briefly described.

2. Nanoestructures for Labelling Cancer Cells

The research in nanotechnology that is focuses on the diagnosis of cancer is currently considered in two main fronts: diagnostic based on laboratory and in vivo. This section present some representative nanostructures currently designed for labelling tumoral cells and its implication in the cancer diagnosis at both laboratory and in vivo levels.

The "nanowires" are 1-20 nm nanostructures constructed trough an array in which the silicon is coated with antibodies (bioreactivas molecules) that recognize tumor cells. The coupling of "nanowires" to regions of tissue with tumor cells produce a change in the electrical conductivity of the tissue that can be detected and measured using electronic instrumentation, which indicates the presence of a tumour in the body, the sensitivity could be up to 100 times greater than other diagnostic techniques based on normal imaging (Benerjee and Verma, 2006).

The "cantilevers" or flexible nanorods are constructed using lithographic techniques used in the semiconductor industry. These devices are formed with nanorods covered with molecules capable of binding to specific substrates such as DNA (Deoxyribonucleic Acid) or antibodies directed to a genetic sequence from tumour cells, thus allowing timely diagnosis of cancer in patients (Ziegler, 2004).

Currently have been developed a wide variety of nanoscale particles (20-400 nm) that serve as devices for the diagnosis of cancer, i.e. superparamagnetic metal nanoparticles coupled to an antibody that has the potential to serve as nanobiomarkers, useful to detect virtually any protein or nucleic acid of tumor origin, since they are produced in excess by the cell affected, this technique add much higher detection sensitivity compared with current conventional methods (Jain et al. 2005) and (Ivkov et al. 2005).

The "quantums dots" are nanocrystals of semiconductor materials such as cadmium selenium which promise to perform the diagnoses of cancer in the laboratory. The nanocrystals are coupled to specific particles and act as sources of light whose colors are dependent on the molecular size of the particle. When "quantums dots" are attached to an antibody or another molecule able to bind to a tumour protein of interest, they act as a beacon that emits light when it is coupled to an organ or tissue affected, allowing the diagnosis of cancer at early stages and with a high specificity (Tada et al. 2007).

One of the lines of development in nanomedicine is the "nanotubes", which are composed of lamellar or spherical structures of carbon atoms. These are known as bio-carriers nanodevices, which can transport drugs or molecules such as proteins or DNA directly to inside of tumour cells to be used as nanobomb, which will pop by stimuli such as light and infrared light to destroy tumour cells without affect normal cells (Kam et al. 2005).

The potential use of nanoparticles to modulate the gene expression has been recently shown; targeted human serum albumin nanoparticles loaded with antisense oligonucleotides against polo-like kinase 1 (PlK1) were developed. The coupling of the antibody trastuzumab to nanoparticles showed a specific targeting to HER2-overexpressing BT-474 cells. Authors observed a reduction of Plk1 mRNA and protein expression as well as an increased activation of Caspase 3/7. The study provides the basis of an alternative technique for tumour treatment promoting a better agents penetration into primary and metastatic target cells (Spänkuch, 2008).

Recently; some innovative groups are in the process of creating prototypes of next-generation nanodevices called "Nanobots" or nanorobots. It is intended that the nanorobots will be designed as nanostructures with 200 to 600 nm with features of auto replication and total autonomy. An example of this technology is the vehicle anti-cancer developed in the European community, which can carry anti-cancer drugs and directed specifically towards the site where the tumour, and once located the target, release a regulated drug that selectively destroy tumor cells without affecting other normal cells.

3. Image Techniques for Cancer Detection Assisted by Nanostructures

3.1 Current systems for cancer diagnosis and its limitations

Magnetic Resonance Imaging (MRI) systems provide the advantage of high spatial resolution in very well differentiated pathological tissue, in contrast; MRI shows a poor spatial differentiation of neoplasies in early stages as well as disseminated cancer during metastatic processes, and is necessary to increase the spatial resolution of the MRI systems in order to get a useful diagnosis. Other method to get images related to the diagnosis of neoplasies is the Computerized Tomography (CT). CT uses the basic principles of the conventional radiography (X-ray) to create a map of the tissue in a specific region, limitations about spatial resolution for cancer detection are similar than those reported for (MRI). Different image techniques by contrast agents have increased the resolution of MRI and CT systems; nevertheless a poor specificity still represents a technical limitation.

Tumour associated to cancer is visible on both MRI and CT. However, the diagnostic is complicated by the fact that on CT it produces low signal, which can be confused with low-signal producing edema. On MRI tumours produces a hypersignal, which may be confused with hypersignal producing edematous tissue. Specific detection and continuous monitoring of edema differenced of tumours is also important in treatment and assessment of medical condition. The technical characteristics of MRI and CT equipments, as well as the difficulties to transport and maintain patients in the MRI and CT physical spaces convert those systems as unviable equipments for continuous monitoring of the critically ill in intensive cares and emergency rooms.

Is well reported that the hypervascularisation of malignant neoplasies promotes changes in the Electrical Impedance (EI) of tissue, this conditions have suggested the use of bioimpedance measurements to detect cancer in different organ and tissues. Scharfetter and colleagues have considered the Electrical Impedance Spectroscopy (IES) as a possibility to produce information relative to abnormal conditions in tissues (Scharfetter, 1999). Some researchers as Newell and Holder have proposed the use of Electrical Impedance Tomography (EIT) as an important method to evaluate and monitor neoplasies in different organs and tissues (Newell, 1996), (Holder, 1999). EIT uses an arrangement of electrodes to inject subsensorial currents and measure the resultant voltages. Data are used to reconstruct a map of the tissue impedance. Griffiths proposed the use of bioelectrical measurements by non-invasive electromagnetic coils as a valuable alternative to monitor, without physical contact, the health status of organs and tissues (Griffiths et al., 1999) and (Griffiths, 2001). Several authors as Al-Zeiback and Korzhenevskii have concurred in the proposal of non-contact measurements for the development of alternative imaging techniques by Magnetic Induction Tomography (MIT) (Al-Zeiback et al. 1993), (Korzhenevski and Cherepenin, 1997) and (Korjenevsky and Cherepenin, 1999).

The sensibility of EIT and MIT is a function of the electrical properties of the studied organ or tissue, and the electrical conductivity provides an important contribution. The main EIT and MIT application have been focused on the detection of edema (fluid accumulation). The use of bioimpedance measurements in the detection of malignant tumors still represents a technological challenge because the electrical conductivity of tumoural tissue is poorly differentiable with respect to normal tissue. In study reported by Burdette, normal and tumoural human mama tissue represent electrical conductivities of 4 and 3.5 to 8 $mS*cm^{-1}$ respectively, both measured at 500MHz (Burdette, 1982).

3.2 Bioconjugated nanoparticles in cancer diagnosis and its limitations

Monoclonal antibodies allow the typification of tumoural cells by specific antigens recognition (bioreactive molecules in the cell´s surface). Currently is possible to develop the union of different monoclonal antibodies to magnetic nanoparticles, those nanoparticles have a preconditionated surface for the union of bioreactive molecules such as proteins or antibodies. DeNardo developed a method to design reactive bio-probes, which allow the coupling of the complex antibody-nanoparticle to the membrane of tumoural cells. Experimental results have shown the specificity of such probes when are in contact with tumoural antigens (DeNardo et al. 2005).

Some researchers e.g. Magin and Saini have developed effective contrast agents to MRI and CT based on the use of magnetic and supermagnetic nanoparticles (Magin et al. 1986) and (Saini et al. 1987). As Ito et al. explain; the objective to use those characteristical nanoparticles has been to improve the contrast between tissues decreasing the relaxation signal T2 for the case of MRI (Ito et al. 2005). The results indicate that such methods have technical viability; however its potential application in the clinical practice demands the use of expensive and complex imaging systems available in few medical facilities.

Shinkai et al. proposed the use of an impedance magnetic sensor for malignant tumor diagnosis in brain assisted by magnetic nanoparticles. The proposed diagnosis technique involves nanoparticles magnetization by a static magnetic field of 1.8T (Shinkai et al. 1998). The nanoparticles magnetic field distribution is detected by the impedance magnetic sensor with high resolution for static magnetic fields; the spatial resolution of the system is a function of the magnetization field intensity; which demands energy, large and impractical magnets as portable systems for continuous monitoring.

Current in vivo cancer diagnosis in organ and tissues based on contrast imaging techniques assisted by magnetic nanoparticles depend on the use of systems with complex and expensive technology which are available to only a small part of the prospective patient population in danger of developing cancer; therefore the whole concept of imaging assisted by nanotechnology still represents technical challenges before to be considered a portable tool for non invasive cancer diagnosis and continuous monitoring of the therapeutic response in oncology departments, rural population and medically underserved populations.

4. Magnetic Induction Spectroscopy (MIS) for Cancer Detection

The use of MIS (magnetic fields at multiple frequencies) assisted by magnetic nanoparticles has been proposed as a non invasive and inexpensive technique for cancer detection. To this end the author of this chapter has suggested that measuring induction phase shift throughout the bulk of tumoural tissue in time and over a broad range of frequencies, instead of producing an image of the tumor, could be used as an inexpensive and mobile alternative technique for cancer detection. The method includes the union of magnetic nanoparticles coupled to target cancer cells, and the effect produced by that coupling in the spectrum of inductive phase shift at multiple frequencies. The principle is based on the use of a primary magnetic field which induce a current density in tissue, those currents generate a second magnetic field which perturb the primary magnetic field, the magnitude of the perturbation is a function of the tissue electrical properties, mainly because the electrical conductivity. Selective coupling of magnetic nanoparticles to tumoural cells in a specific tissue volume increases the volumetric tissue electrical conductivity; in consequence an increase of the primary magnetic field perturbation is observed. The perturbation could be measured as a spectrum of phase shift in a second sensor coil. The magnitude and morphology of the inductive phase shift spectra determine the presence of tumoural tissue, metastasic processes and in general cancer in organ and tissues.

In order to optimize the detection technology, in recent study has been explored the possible use of a magnetron coil on the inductive volumetric phase shift of the brain in the presence of a haematoma (González et al 2007). The sensitivity of a magnetron coil with that of a circular coil has been compared. The results have shown that the magnetron coil has a somewhat greater sensitivity to the detection of a haematoma than the circular coil (González et al 2007). The effect of haematoma location in the brain on the planar magnetron and circular coil measurement, with a numerical simulation has been explored. The results reveal that the location of the haematoma has a substantial effect on the sensitivity of the magnetron and circular coils. Furthermore, we find that at certain different frequencies the various locations of the haematomas produce no volumetric phase shift. (Rojas et al 2008). Those changes in the spectra of inductive phase shift are expected to be amplified by the use of magnetic nanoparticles coupled to tumoural cells.

4.1 Theoretical fundaments of MIS assisted by magnetic nanostructures

i. Selective coupling of bioconjugated nanoparticles

The selective coupling principle of bioconjugated nanoparticles to tumoural cells is based on the union of magnetic nanoparticles to molecular ligands with affinity to specific bioreceptors in tumoural cells. Specifically the covalent union of magnetic nanoparticles to monoclonal antibodies (bioconjugated nanoparticle-antibody) has been proposed as cancer markers. To create bioconjugated nanostructures the use of magnetic nanoparticles with magnetite nucleus (Fe3O4) and polisacaride coat with functional carboxyl groups has been chosen. The typical diameters are in the order of 50 to 300 nm and have superparamagnetic properties. The ligand of the bioconjugated corresponds to monoclonal antibodies with amino functional groups activated by carbodimine. Carbodimine reacts with carboxyl groups of the magnetic nanoparticles to produce O-acilurea and amino ligand reactions. These reactions produce a covalent union that warrants a stable coupling of the magnetic nanoparticle to the antibody. Figure 1 shows schematically a representation of the principle of the covalent union by carboxyl groups of magnetic nanoparticles and its ligand given by a monoclonal antibody. The bioconjugated nanoparticle-antibody is added to the cell membrane by a non-covalent union created between the antibody and its receptor (biomarker) in the cell surface.

ii. Increment of the electrical conductivity in tumoural tissue

Different electrical circuits have been proposed to represent the electrical behaviour of cellular suspension and biological tissues as a function of its electrical properties. (Schwan, 1957), (Tregear, 1966) and (Salter, 1979). Cole and Cole proposed a general electric circuit to represent biological materials as a function of its electrical properties and frequency. Their model suggests the representation of membrane cells as capacitive elements, as well as the protein structures, intracellular and extracellular fluids as resistive elements. The simplified equivalent circuit suggests a parallel-series resistive-capacitive arrangement. The composed electrical conductivity of such model is a function of the permittivity of the membrane cell, protein content, intracellular fluids and frequency; those factors are reflected as changes in the electrical conductivity. The mathematical expression to estimate the composite electrical conductivity is given by eq. (1) (Cole and Cole, 1941), (Cole and Cole, 1942).

$$\sigma = \sigma_0 + \frac{\Delta\sigma}{1+(j\omega\tau)^{-\alpha}} \tag{1}$$

Where σ_0 represents the electrical conductivity of the material in direct current, $\Delta\sigma$ corresponds to the changes in electrical conductivity which could be associated to the presence of magnetic nanoparticles, ω is the angular frequency, τ is a temporal constant corresponding to the arraignment resistive-capacitive and α represents positive values $1 \geq \alpha \geq 0$.

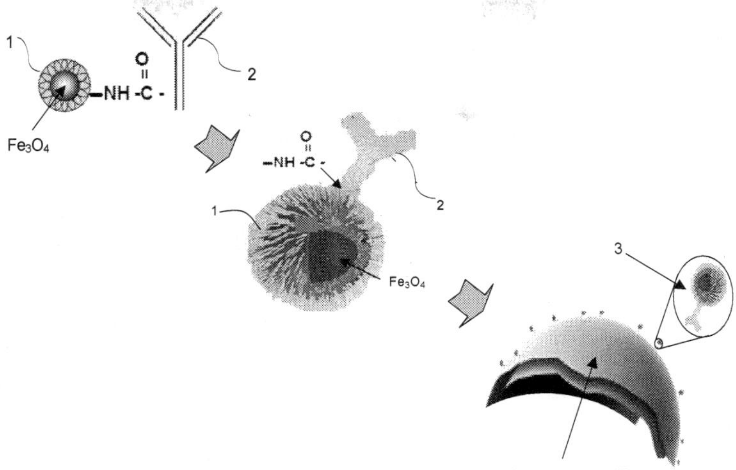

Fig. 1. Representation of the principle of a covalent union between carboxyl groups (1) of the coat of magnetic nanoparticles (Fe3O4) and specific ligand of cancer cells given by a monoclonal antibody (2). The structure conformed is known as bioconjugated "nanoparticle-antibody" (3).

iii. *The effect of electrical conductivity changes in tumoural detection by MIS*

Currents induction in conductive materials by oscillating magnetic fields is explained in the basis of the Farady induction law; which formulated in terms of the Maxwell general equations is expressed by:

$$\Delta \times E = -\partial B / \partial t \tag{2}$$

Eq. (2) indicates that a variable magnetic field **B** induces an electromotive potential **E** in a conductive media, such potential is a function of the magnetic flux and induces an electrical current flux in the medium, those currents are known as eddy currents.

Accordingly with the charge conservation law, an induced current density **J** in a conductive material is directly proportional to the induced electrical potential **E** and to the electrical conductivity σ of the material. The charge conservation law derived from the Maxwell general equations is formulated as:

$$J = \sigma E \tag{3}$$

Eq. (3) allows to argue that and increase in the electrical conductivity represents an increase of the energy absorbed by the material; then the union of bioconjugated magnetic nanoparticles to the membrane cells through selective monoclonal antibodies promotes that the electrical properties of tumoral cells change in such a way that increments in the composite electrical conductivity are observed. Those conductive increments allow that magnetic fields of different frequencies induce eddy currents selectively in the marked tumoural cells, then the perturbations of the magnetic fields are larger than those generated in healthy tissue; it means those generated without the union of magnetic nanoparticles to the membrane cells.

4.2 Practical description of how to detect cancer in vivo by MIS

In vitro cancer detection represents a promising concept for non-invasive diagnosis and monitoring. Figure 2 shows the basic concept for tumoural cells detection in suspension trough the use of MIS assisted by magnetic nanoparticles. The assumption is early cancer detection in blood trough magnetic nanoparticles coupled to specific tumoural biomarkers (i.e. Her2/neu, +hMAM or +Survivin) that are overexpressed in blood cells at the first stages of cancer. The volumetric electrical conductivity increments of tumoural cells given by the presence of magnetic nanoparticles promote increments in the perturbation of the MIS fields and the inductive phase shift spectrum.

Cancer detection by MIS at an organ or biological tissue comprising: a body or volume of biological tissue exposed to the in vivo interaction with bioconjugated magnetic nanoparticles, such organ or volume of biological tissue is positioned between a first antenna or inductive coil and a second antenna or detector coil, an injection spectrum of current variable in a wide bandwidth in the first coil or antenna, detecting the spectrum of voltage variable induced in the second coil or antenna, an estimation of the spectrum of inductive phase shift between the first and second coil or antenna, and depending on the morphological characteristics and magnitude of the spectrum of inductive phase shift detected, it could be associated to the presence of cancer cells, malignant tumours or metastases in the volume under study.

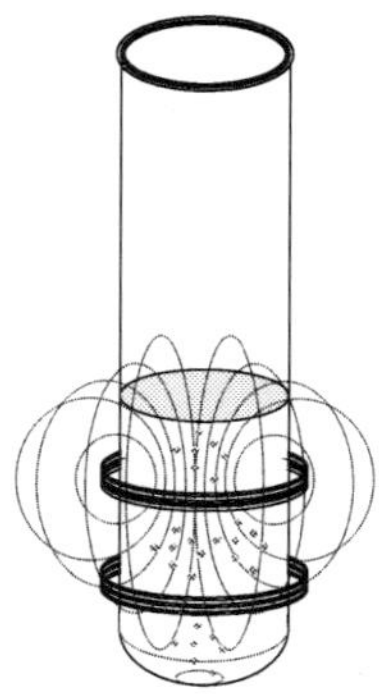

Fig. 2. Basic concept for tumoural cells detection in suspension trough the use of MIS assisted by magnetic nanoparticles. The concept is early cancer detection in blood trough magnetic nanoparticles coupled to specific tumoural biomarkers that are overexpressed in blood cells at the first stages of cancer.

The in vivo interaction of the organ or volume of biological tissue being studied with bioconjugated magnetic nanoparticles is developed trough the intravenous infusion of magnetic nanoparticles coupled to a monoclonal antibody which is characteristic of specific receptors overexpressed on the surface of target cancer cells. Figure 3 shows a general scheme about how to detect breast cancer in vivo by MIS. First; the bioconjugated nanoparticle-antibody is injected intravenously to reach the tumoural region increasing its electrical conductivity. Then; increments in the inductive phase shift associated to the presence of tumoural cells or metastatic processes are detected by MIS. The idea is to take advantage of the condition in which the electrical conductivity of the tumour is increased to amplify the magnitude of the inductive phase shift spectrum.

A general description of the electronic instrumentation involves the generation of magnetic fields through a programmable digital synthesizer connected to the first coil. The collection of signals in both coils is via a differential amplifier, the phase difference signal between the two coils is estimated through a phase detector circuit. A control system programming is done through an analog-digital converter and a dedicated microprocessor. In general; the technological proposal is a minimally invasive method for the detection of malignant tumours and metastatic processes in organs and tissues.

5. Hazards of Nanomedicne in Cancer

Nanomaterials have a unique surface contact layer with the body tissue in comparison to bulk materials, and this unique property need to be investigated from a toxicological point of view. Given the unique reactive characteristic of nanoparticles; it´s expected that nanoparticles have an impact on the toxicity but it may differ depending on the type of particles used (i.e. biological vs non-biological origin). Nanoparticles have different physico-chemical characteristics in comparison to microsize particles, those typical characteristics may result in different distributions of the particles inside the body as well as side effects. In this sense; it is expected that the nanostructural interaction in tissues and cells, as well as its potential toxicity, greatly depend on the composition of the nanoparticle.

Magnetic iron oxide nanoparticles have been used intravenously as MRI contrast fluids in the clinical practice of cancer detection; the body distribution profile of those nanoparticles has been shown to depend on size, charge and thickness of the coating (such as dextran-coating) of the nanoparticles [Chouly et al, 1996]. In addition; it has shown that new magnetic contrast agents could be compartmentalised in lysosomes, exocytosed and returned to the normal iron pool. Nanoparticle degradation was shown to be dependent on coatings more than on particle sizes [Briley Saebo,2004]. The key safety issue with these products in the clinical practice is the risk of anaphylactic reactions. In recent review about toxicology of nanoparticles used in health care products; is concluded that no deaths associated to nanosized magnetic iron oxide products had been reported [Costigan, 2006]. This report compared reactions to those reported for non-nanosized iron oxide intravenous therapeutic products as well as literature reports, and concluded that it is unclear whether the anaphylactic reactions are due to direct mediator releasing effects of iron (or dextran) or an immunological mediated mechanism. In addition; the study concludes that the toxicity information available regarding healthcare nanoparticles is limited. However, there were not identified mechanisms of toxicity that would evade conventional hazard identification testing currently required [Costigan, 2006].

In general; the nanoparticles size opens the potential for crossing the various biological barriers within the body. In the best of the cases the potential to cross the blood brain barrier may open new ways for drug delivery into the brain. The nanosize also allows for access into the cell and various cellular compartments including the nucleus. Recently; De Jong and Borm have reviewed the main application and hazards of drug delivery and nanoparticles (De Jong and Borm, 2008), their main conclusion besides the potential beneficial use is drawn to the questions how we should proceed with the safety evaluation of the nanoparticle formulations for drug delivery. In view of these specificities; investigations in pharmaco-kinetic and toxicological distribution studies of nanoparticles are warranted.

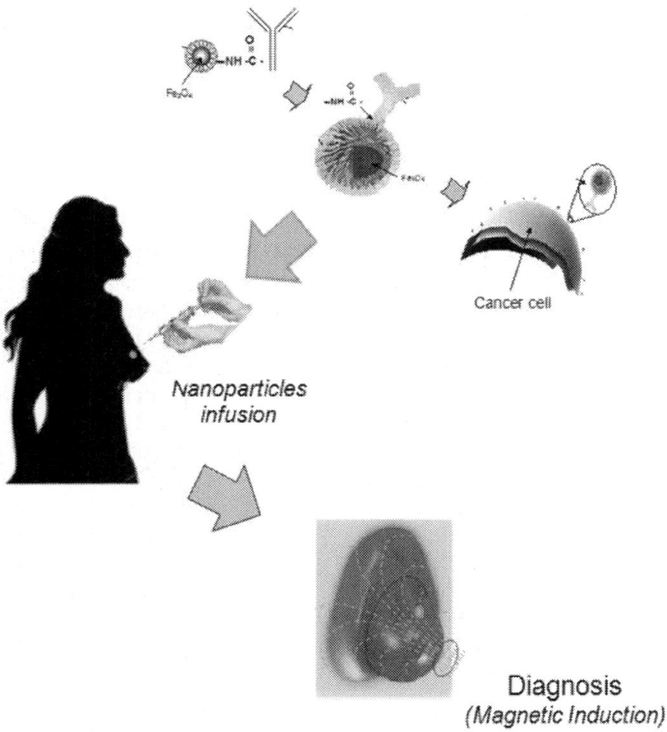

Fig. 3. General scheme to detect breast cancer in vivo by MIS assisted with magnetic nanoparticles. The bioconjugated nanoparticle-antibody is injected intravenously to reach target cells in the suspicious tumoural region and to increase its electrical conductivity. Increments in the inductive phase shift spectrum detected by MIS could be associated to the presence of tumoural cells or metastatic processes.

6. References

Al-Zeiback and Saunders NH, (1993). "A feasability study of in vivo electromagnetic imaging." *Phys. Med. Biol.* 38: 151-160.

Burdette EC, (1982). Electromagnetic and Acoustic Properties of Tissues. In Pyisical Aspects of Hyperthermia, G.H. Nussbaum (ed), *AAPM Medical Physics Monographs* No. 8, pp 105-150.

Briley Saebo K, Bjornerud A, Grant D, Ahlstrom H, Berg T, Kindberg GM, (2004). "Hepatic cellular distribution and degradation or iron oxide nanoparticles following single intravenous injection in rats: implications for magnetic resonance imaging". *Cell Tissue Res*, 316(3), 315-23

Benerjee HN and Verma M, (2006). Expert Review of Molecular Diagnostics, September 2006, Vol. 6, No. 5, Pages 679-683.

Cole KS and Cole RH, (1941). "Dispersion and absortion in dielectrics, I. Alternating current characteristics", *J. Chem Phys.* 9,341-351.

Cole KS and Cole RH, (1942) "Dispersion and absortion in dielectrics, II. Direct current characteristics", *J. Chem Phys.* 10, 98-106.

Chouly C, Pouliquen D, Lucet I, Jeune JJ, Jallet P, (1996). "Development of superparamagnetic nanoparticles for MRI: effect of particle size, charge and surface nature on biodistribution". *J microencapsul*, 3:245-255.

Costigan S, (2006). "The toxicology of nanoparticles used in health care products". Available at the website of the *Medicines and Healthcare products Regulatory Agency, Department of Health, UK*. Accessed 17 June 2009.

URL : http://www.mhra.gov.uk/home/idcplg?IdcService=SS_GET_PAGE&nodeId=996.

DeNardo SJ, DE Nardo GL, Miers LA, Natarajan A, Foreman AR, Gruettner C, Adamson GN and Ivkov R, (2005). "Development of Tumor Targeting Bioprobes (111In-Chimeric L6Monoclonal Antibody Nanoparticles) for Alternating Magnetic Field Cancer Therapy". *Clin Cancer Res*, 11(19 Suppl) 7087s-7092s.

De Jong WH and Borm PJA, (2008). "Drug delivery and nanoparticles: Applications and hazards". *Int. J Nanomedicine* 3(2):133-149.

Griffiths H, Stewart WR and Gough W, (1999). "Magnetic induction tomography - A measuring system for biological materials." *Ann NY Acad Sci*, 873: 335-345.

Griffiths H, (2001). "Magnetic Induction tomography." *Meas. Sci. Technol*, 12: 1126-31.

González CA, Rojas R and B Rubinsky (2007). "Circular and Magnetron Inductor/Sensor Coils to Detect Volumetric Brain Edema by Inductive Phase Shift Spectroscopy: A Sensitivity Simulation Study." *Proceedings of the 13th International conference on Electrical Bioimpedance and 8th Conference on Electrical Impedance Tomography* Graz, Austria: 315-319.

Holder DS, González-Correa CA, Tidswell T, Gibson A, Cusick G and Bayford RH, (1999). "Assessment and Calibration of a Low-Frequency System for Electrical Impedance Tomography (EIT), Optimized for Use in Imaging Brain Function in Ambulant Human Subjects" *Ann NY Acad Sci*, 873: 512-519.

Ivkov R, DeNardo SJ, Daum W and DeNardo GL, (2005). "Application of High Amplitude Alternating Magnetic Fields for Heat Induction of Nanoparticles Localized in Cancer". *Clin Cancer Res*, 11 (19 Suppl) 7093s-7103s.

Ito A, Shinkai M, Honda H and Kobayashi T, (2005). "Medical Application of Functionalized Magnetic Nanoparticles" *Journal of Bioscience and Bioengineering*. 100(1) 1-11.

Jain TK, Morales MA, Sahoo SK, Leslie-Pelecky DL and Labhasetwar V, (2005). "Iron Oxide Nanoparticles for Sustained Delivery of Anticancer Agents. Molecular" *Pharmaceuthics*. Vol.2, No. 3, 194-205.

Korzhenevski AV and Cherepenin A, (1997). "Magnetic induction tomography." *J. Comm. Technol. Electron.* 42(4): 469-474.

Korjenevsky AV and Cherepenin A, (1999). "Progress in Realization of Magnetic Induction Tomography." *Ann NY Acad Sci* 873: 346-352.

Kam NWS, O'Connell M, Wisdom JA and Dai H, (2005). "Carbon nanotubes as multifunctional biological transporters and near-infrared agents for selective cancer cell destruction". *Proceedings of the National Academy of Sciences of the United States of America (PNAS 2005).* August 16, Vol. 102 No. 33, 11600-11605.

Magin RL, Wright SM, Niesman MR, Chan HC and Swartz HM, (1986). "Liposome Delivery of NMR Contrast Agents for Improved Tissue", *Imaging. Magn. Reson. Med.* 3, 440-447.

Newell, J.C.; Edic, P.M.; Xiaodan Ren; Larson-Wiseman, J.L. and Danyleiko Newell, (1996). "Assessment of acute pulmonary edema in dogs by electrical impedance imaging." *IEEE Trans Biomed Eng*, 43(2): 133-8.

Rojas R, Rubinsky B and González CA (2008). "The Effect of Brain Hematoma Location on Volumetric Inductive Phase Shift Spectroscopy of the Brain with Circular and magnetron Sensor Coils: A Numerical Simulation Study." *Physiol Meas* 29: S255-S266.

Schwan HP, (1957). Electrical properties of tissue and cell suspension. In : Lawrence JH, Tobias CA (eds). *Advances in biological and medical physics*, Vol V, 147-209. Academic Press, New York.

Salter DC, (1979). Quantifying skin disease and healing in vivo using electrical impedance measurement. In: Rolfe P (ed.) *Non-invasive physiological measurement*. Vol 1. Academic Press New York.

Saini S, Stark DD, Hahn PF, Wittenberg J, Brady TJ and Ferrucci JT, (1987). "Ferrite Particles: A Superparamgnetic MR Constrast Agent for the Reticuloendothelial System". *Radiology*, 162, 211-216.

Shinkai M, Ohshima A, Yanase M, Uchiyama T, Mohri K, Wakabayashi T and Yoshida J, (1998). "Developmente of Novel Magnetic Sensing for Brain Lesion Using Functional Magnetic Particles". *Kagaku Kougaku Ronbunshu*, 24 174-178.

Scharfetter H, Ninaus W, Puswald B, Petrova GI, Kovachev D and Hutten H (1999). "Inductively Coupled Wideband Transceiver for Bioimpedance Spectroscopy (IBIS)" *Ann NY Acad Sci*, 873: 322-334.

Spänkuch B, Steinhauser I, Wartlick H, Kurunci-Csacsko E, Strebhardt K I and Langer K, (2008). "Downregulation of Plk1 Expression By Receptor-Mediated Uptake of Antisense Oligonucleotide–Loaded Nanoparticles". *Neoplasia*. 10, 223–234.

Tregear RT, (1966). Physical functions of skin. Academic press, New York.

Tada H, Higuchi H, Wanatabe TM and Ohuchi N, (2007). "In vivo Real-time Tracking of Single Quantum Dots Conjugated with Monoclonal Anti-HER2".*Cancer Res*, 67(3): 1138-1144.

Ziegler C, (2004). "Cantilever-based biosensors". *Anal Bioanal Chem*, 379:946-959.

21

Capacitive Sensing of Narrow-Band ECG and Breathing Activity of Infants through Sleepwear

Akinori Ueno, Tatsuya Imai, Daisuke Kowada and Yoshihiro Yama
Tokyo Denki University
Japan

1. Introduction

Sudden infant death syndrome (SIDS) is defined as the sudden unexpected death of an infant < 1 year of age, with onset of the fatal episode apparently occurring during sleep, that remains unexplained after a thorough investigation, including performance of a complete autopsy and review of the circumstances of death and the clinical history (Krous et al., 2004). SIDS has ranked the third leading cause of death for infants in Japan in 2007, after congenital malformations, deformations and chromosomal abnormalities, and certain conditions originating in the perinatal period (Statistics and Information Department, 2007). An apparent life threatening event (ALTE) is defined as an episode that is frightening to the observer and that is characterized by some combination of apnea (central or occasionally obstructive), color change (usually cyanotic or pallid), marked change in muscle tone, choking or gagging (Little et al., 1987). In order to prevent a recurrence of ALTE or to avoid an occurrence of SIDS, home monitoring of breathing activity and heart rate (HR) for infants may be introduced at the discretion of the doctor or the parent(s). In conventional monitors such as VitaGuard (GeTeMed GmbH, Germany) and SmartMonitor 2 (Children's Medical Ventures, USA), a conductive adhesive is used for maintaining reliable ohmic contact of electrodes with the skin. Therefore, monitoring for a long period of time using conventional methods may cause irritation and skin allergy. Besides, in some cases, adhesion of the paste was so tight for their skin that the skin was peeled off when the electrode was detached from the body surface after the long time monitoring. To relieve the potential of irritation and damage to the skin, Gramse et al. (Gramse et al., 2003) proposed special pajamas named MamaGoose (Verhaert Design and Development, Belgium), which incorporated dry electrodes and strain gauge for cardiopulmonary monitoring. Catrysse et al. (Catrysse et al., 2004) also addressed the similar problem by employing textile electrodes and a coil-shaped fabric sensor, which do not require any conductive adhesive for the measurement. The ideas of dry sensors embedded in clothing are quite rational. However, there are still some challenges to be addressed regarding direct contact of sensors with the skin, because that may provoke skin allergy and dermatitis. Moreover, repetitive use of the embedded electrode has a disadvantage in a hygiene standpoint in highly humid countries such as Japan, because they can't be washed easily.

In order to obviate these risks and the disadvantage, our research group advanced the principle of capacitive sensing and succeeded in detecting electrocardiographic potential (ECG) through commonly available cloth from the subject's limb (Ueno et al., 2004), from the dorsal surface of adult subjects (Furusawa et al., 2003, Ueno et al., 2007a, and Ueno et al., 2007b) and from that of infants (Kato et al., 2006) in a supine position. This approach eliminated direct contact of the electrodes to the skin and then enabled the interjacent cloth being changed and washed handily. Moreover, with a view to application to preventing ALTE and SIDS, our group extended the capacitive sensing technique to that capable of measuring breathing activity simultaneously with ECG (Ueno & Yama, 2008, and Yama & Ueno, 2009). In this chapter, we describe the principle of the capacitive sensing technique and present our latest advances for these capacitive sensing approaches.

2. Principle of Measurement

2.1 Principle of Capacitive Sensing of ECG

The proposed approach of capacitive sensing is an expansion of the principle of the capacitive (or insulator) electrode (Richardson et al., 1968, and Lopez & Richardson, 1969). Instead of rigid metal electrode and insulator in their coupling, the proposed coupling is composed of a conductive fabric electrode, clothes such as sleepwear and diaper, and the skin of the subject, as shown in Fig.1.

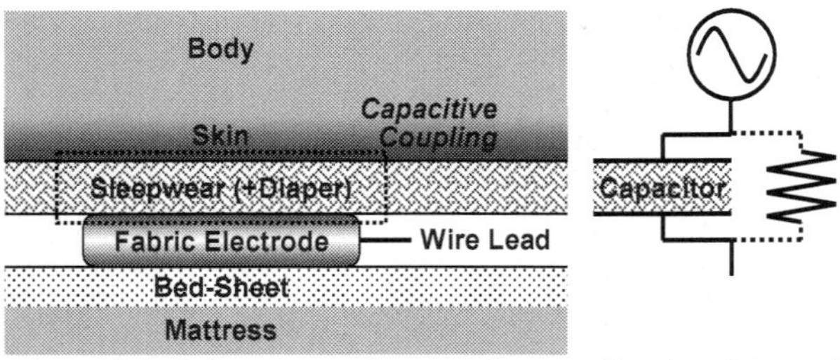

Fig. 1. A schematic model of the proposed capacitive coupling involving a fabric electrode, inserted clothes of sleepwear (plus diaper) and the skin, and its equivalent circuit elements

According to the equivalent circuit elements in Fig.1, impedance Z [Ω] of the coupling is given by

$$Z = \frac{R}{\sqrt{1+(2\pi fCR)^2}} = \frac{1}{\sqrt{1/R^2 + (2\pi fC)^2}} \tag{1}$$

where C [F] is capacitance of the coupling, R [Ω] is resistance of the inserted clothes and f [Hz] is frequency of the source signal. Since R is so high in dry condition that it can be regarded as infinity, impedance of the coupling at dry condition ($Z_{R=\infty}$) can be described as follows:

$$Z_{R=\infty} = \frac{1}{2\pi fC} \tag{2}$$

Therefore, the coupling can carry an alternating bioelectric current through the capacitance of the coupling. Since direct contact of electrode with the skin is unnecessary in this approach, the proposed method can eliminate potential causes of metal allergy and dermatitis experienced in conventional methods. Moreover, the proposed method has an advantage in enabling commonly available clothes to be inserted between electrode and the skin. In equation (2), C can be represented by the following equation (3) using coupling area S [m^2], distance d [m] between electrode and the skin, and permittivity ε [F/m] of the mediated clothes.

$$C = \varepsilon \frac{S}{d} \tag{3}$$

By putting equation (3) into equation (2), $Z_{R=\infty}$ can be expressed as

$$Z_{R=\infty} = \frac{1}{2\pi} \times \frac{d}{f\varepsilon S} \tag{4}$$

Thus, the wider the electrode area becomes (or the closer the coupling distance becomes), the smaller the coupling impedance results. However, due to smaller permittivity of the commonly available clothes than that of insulators incorporated in commercial capacitors, coupling impedance in reality is estimated to reach in the order of a few or a few tens of Giga-ohms. Accordingly, commercial electrocardiographs having input impedance around a hundred Mega-ohms are incapable of detecting ECG signal through the clothes. In the proposed method, voltage loss at the coupling is reduced by employing an impedance transformer IC having high input impedance at the front end so as to achieve reasonable signal to noise ratio (SNR).

On the other hand, once the resistance of inserted clothes is decreased, for instance, by perspiration or moisture in the atmosphere, the following inequality expression is obtained:

$$Z = \frac{1}{\sqrt{\frac{1}{R^2} + (2\pi fC)^2}} < \frac{1}{2\pi fC} \left(= Z_{R=\infty}\right) \tag{5}$$

Thus, the more the subject sweats, the higher SNR of the output signal becomes. In other words, there is no adverse effect of perspiration of the subject on the SNR of the obtained signal in this approach.

2.2 Principle of Breathing Activity Measurement

In our previous experiments, it has been revealed that the capacitive sensing is susceptible to body motion of the subject. This susceptibility is assumed because the motion alters geometric parameters S and d of the coupling in equation (3), and thereby changes capacitance and impedance of the coupling. This disadvantage can be regarded as an advantage from the other side that the capacitive sensing is highly sensitive to body motion. In fact, some of the obtained signals had contained a periodic variation involving low frequency component and had seemed to be caused by breathing chest movement. Considering all these facts, a separation filter (Asaishi et al., 2002) shown Fig. 2 is employed in the proposed measuring circuit to divide the detected signal into a high frequency component including ECG and a low frequency component containing breathing activity. In order to design a differential separation filter with high common mode rejection ratio (CMRR), mirroring technique (Pallàs-Areny & Webster, 1999) is applied to a single-ended separation filter.

Looking at a relationship between v_{in} and v_{out_High} of a single-ended filter in Fig. 2, v_{out_High} is integrated with a time constant τ and then returned negatively to v_{in}. Since the difference between v_{in} and the integrated value of v_{out_High} is amplified with an amplification factor A to obtain v_{out_High}, transfer function $G_{High}(s)$ between v_{in} and v_{out_High} is given by

$$G_{High}(s) = \frac{v_{out\_High}}{v_{in}} = \frac{\tau s}{1 + \frac{\tau}{A} s} \tag{6}$$

Equation (6) represents a trasfer function of 1st-order high-pass Butterworth filter. On the other hand, v_{out_Low} is produced by the integration of v_{out_High}, and then transfer function $G_{Low}(s)$ between v_{in} and v_{out_Low} is

$$G_{Low}(s) = G_{High}(s) \cdot \frac{1}{\tau s} = \frac{1}{1 + \frac{\tau}{A} s} \tag{7}$$

Equation (7) means a transfer function of 1st-order low-pass Butterworth filter. In the present study, the amplification factor A and the time constat τ are set to 1 v/v and 0.16 sec respectively, so as to achieve a corner frequency f_c of 1 Hz.

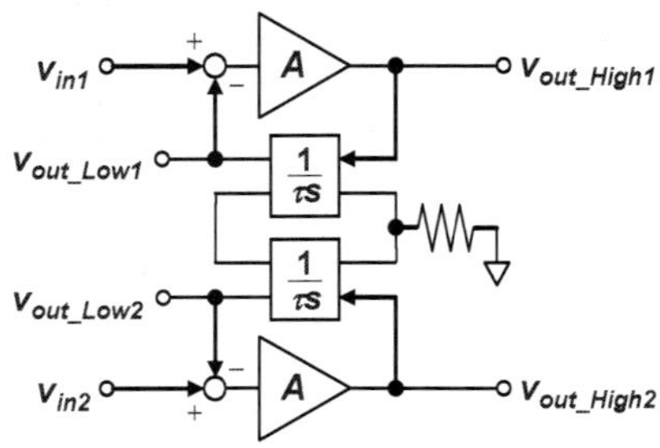

Fig. 2. A block diagram of the differential separation filter

3. Materials and Methods

3.1 Bed-sheet Electrode Unit

Both ECG and breathing activity signals were picked up by a common bed-sheet electrode unit placed on a mattress. The unit was composed of a commercial cotton bed sheet and carbon-coated conductive fabrics with conductive adhesive (Kitagawa Industries, CSTK). The rectangular fabrics having 20 or 25 mm width were used as lead electrodes and a rectangular fabric with 40 or 50 mm width was used as a reference electrode. These fabrics were stuck to the bed-sheet with the adhesive in a horizontal-striped pattern at even intervals, as shown in Fig. 3. Convex terminals for lead wire connection were mounted in each fabric on both sides.

Vertical position of the sheet was adjusted so that the reference electrode was placed beneath the breech of the subject lying in a supine position. Two fabrics which were located respectively under the scapulae and the lumbar region were manually selected for the lead electrodes. Capacitive coupling involving skin, sleepwear and electrode was held by the subject's weight on the sleepwear and by repulsive force from the mattress. The electrodes were connected to a measuring device, as described in the next section, by shielded wires.

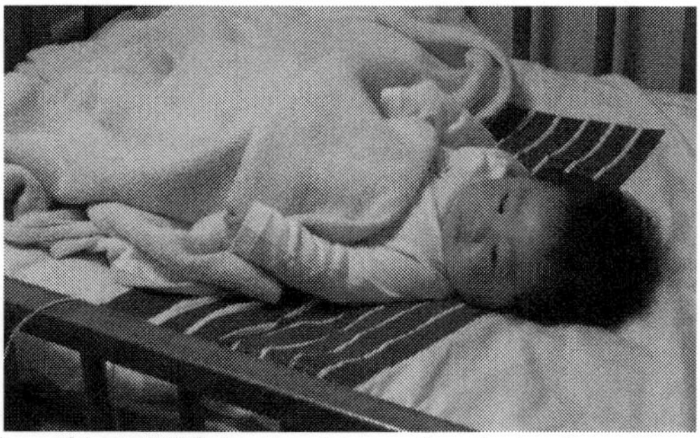

Fig. 3. An image of the subject #10 lying supine on the electrode unit

3.2 Pilot Measuring Device

The pilot measuring device with filtering and amplification circuitry was manufactured according to a block diagram in Fig. 4. The device consisted of a common part and independent parts for sensing ECG signal and breathing activity respectively. The device was powered by regulated batteries to obviate the possibility of electric shock.

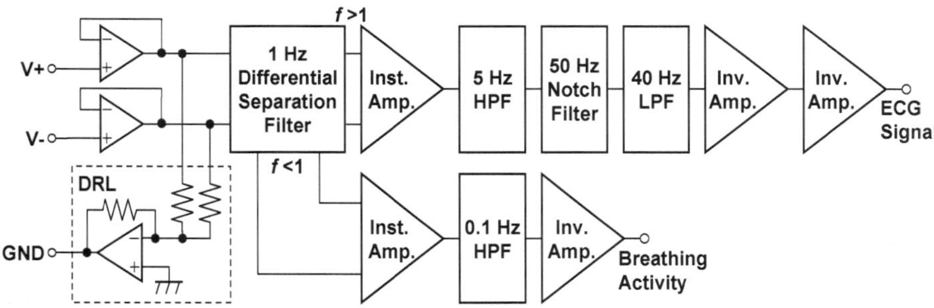

Fig. 4. A block diagram of the developed measuring device

The common part was composed of two buffers, the differential separation filter described in the subsection 2.2 and a driven-right-leg (DRL) circuit. Each buffer functioned as an impedance matching circuit to mediate the high impedance of the capacitive coupling with low impedance required by the subsequent circuitry. Operational amplifier ICs with high input resistance (National Semiconductor, LF356, 1TΩ according to the specification sheet) were used in the present study. The differential separation filter separated the input signal into high frequency component containing ECG signal (>1 Hz) and low frequency component including breathing activity (<1 Hz). The separation filter was constructed of two sets of subtracters, amplifiers and integrators according to Fig. 2. The block diagram in Fig. 2 is a modification of a so called DC suppression circuit (Spinelli et al., 2004). The DRL circuit was employed in order to reduce common mode noise mainly due to power line interference (Spinelli et al., 1999, and Kim et al. 2005). CMRR of the device at 10, 20 and 30 Hz were 61, 61 and 59 dB respectively.

The independent part for sensing ECG signal consisted of an instrumentation amplifier, a high-pass filter (HPF), a notch filter, a low-pass filter (LPF) and two inverting amplifiers as shown in Fig. 4. The circuit elements of the HPF and the LPF were determined in order to obtain a cutoff frequency of 5 and 40 Hz, respectively. The notch filter was used to reduce 50-Hz interference. Although electrocardiograph for diagnostic purpose requires a bandwidth from 0.01 to 100 Hz, we narrowed the bandwidth of the developed device to improve a tolerance for the body motion. Another independent part for obtaining breathing activity consisted of an instrumentation amplifier, a HPF and an inverting amplifier. The HPF was introduced to avoid saturation due to DC offset voltage. Frequency-gain response of the developed device is shown in Fig. 5.

Both output signals from the device were digitized at 1 kHz by an analog-to-digital converter with 16-bit resolution and stored in a personal computer using a data acquisition system (Biopac Systems, MP-150 system). Obtained breathing activity signal was filtered off-line with a digital LPF (IIR, f_c=1 Hz, Q=0.707).

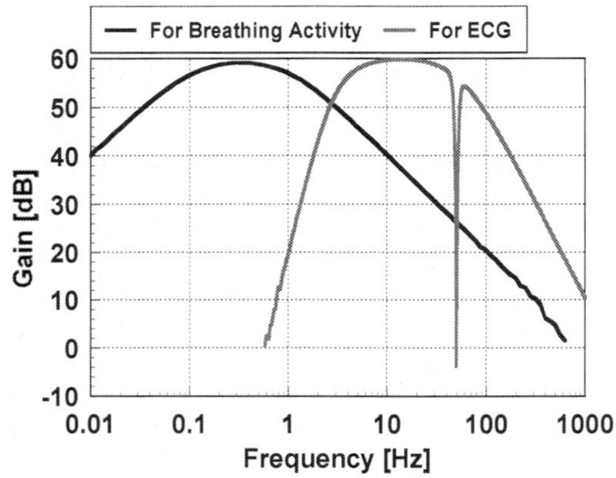

Fig. 5. Frequency-gain responses of the developed circuit for measuring breathing activity and for measuring narrow-band ECG

3.3 Comparison of Breathing Activity with Respiratory Air Flow in Adult Subjects

In order to evaluate breathing activity signal obtained with the developed device, simultaneous measurement with respiratory air flow was conducted using a commercial pneumotachograph (Biopac Systems, TSD107). Considering load of wearing a mask on the subject's face, the experiments were conducted for adult subjects instead of infant subjects. Four adult males from whom informed consents were previously obtained participated to the experiment. A bed-sheet electrode unit which we had specified and fabricated for adult subjects in previous study (Ueno et al., 2007b) was employed for the measurement. Each subject was instructed to wear the face mask which was connected to the pneumotachograph and to lie on the bed-sheet electrode unit which was linked with the developed device. As the 1st experiment, the subjects were requested to cease their breathing for about 10 sec after natural breathing. In the 2nd experiment, the subjects were instructed to breathe along to a rhythm of metronome that was set preliminary at a certain speed ranging from 7 to 26 repeat/min. Respiratory rates were calculated respectively from the two signals measured simultaneously with the pneumotachograph and with the developed device. The calculation was conducted automatically using a peak-detection function implemented in software (Biopac Systems, Acknowledge 3.9.0) supplied with the data acquisition system. Preparatory filtering with a digital band-pass filter (IIR, 0.1-0.6 Hz, Q=0.707) was applied off-line to both signals before the calculation.

3.4 Simultaneous Measurement of Narrow-Band ECG and Breathing Activity in Infants

Ten infants, aged 53 to 187 days, experienced the experiment (see Table 1). Four of the ten infants partook in the experiment more than once on different age in day. Totally sixteen subjects participated to the experiment. Each subject wearing cotton sleepwear was laid in a supine on the bed-sheet electrode unit. Both high frequency and low frequency components were measured using the developed system from the dorsum of the subject through the sleepwear (and a diaper at the reference electrode). As a reference signal, a directly measured ECG was wirelessly monitored using a commercial bioamplifier (Teac Instruments, BA1104CC) and a commercial telemeter unit (Teac Instruments, TU-4). Two disposable lead electrodes were attached directly to the right and the left flank, and a reference electrode was placed on the frontal surface of the subject's abdomen. To measure another reference signal, a commercial photoplethysmographic sensor (Biopac Systems, TSD200A) was applied to the right or the left earlobe. A special bioamplifier (Biopac Systems, PPG100C) involving a 0.5-100 Hz band-pass filter (BPF) was used for amplifying the sensor signal. Photoplethysmogram (PPG) was measured only from a part of the subjects because the sensor unit was introduced in the later experiments. The output signals from the developed device (i.e. breathing activity and narrow-band ECG), the reference ECG and the reference PPG were simultaneously measured using the data acquisition system. Preparatory filtering with a digital LPF (IIR, f_c=40 Hz, Q=0.707) was applied to PPG signal to reduce power line interference. Since it is known that breathing activity overlaps with baseline of the PPG (Nakajima et al., 1993), filtering operation using a digital BPF (IIR, 0.1-0.6 Hz) was doubly applied to the preprocessed PPG signal to extract the breathing activity for the third reference signal.

Subject ID	Age in day	Weight [kg]	Gender	Thickness of the clothes [μm]	Reference signal
#1_1st	65	5.4	male	1083+diaper	ECG
#1_2nd	121	6.5	male	540+diaper	ECG
#1_3rd	185	7.4	male	540+diaper	ECG
#2	187	6.8	male	540+diaper	ECG
#3_1st	64	4.9	female	540+diaper	ECG
#3_2nd	133	6.7	female	780+diaper	ECG
#3_3rd	167	7.0	female	680+diaper	ECG, PPG
#4_1st	68	7.1	male	610+diaper	ECG
#4_2nd	132	8.5	male	680+diaper	ECG, PPG
#5	178	8.0	male	565+diaper	ECG
#6	69	5.1	female	730+diaper	ECG
#7_1st	123	7.2	female	730+diaper	ECG
#7_2nd	178	7.7	female	670+diaper	ECG, PPG
#8	130	6.2	female	570+diaper	ECG, PPG
#9	53	4.5	female	707+diaper	ECG, PPG
#10	75	6.3	male	600+diaper	ECG, PPG

Table 1. Subject information and measured references

3.5 Comparison of R-R Intervals using Bland-Altman Plot

In order to evaluate accuracy of the signal obtained with the developed device, R-R intervals were calculated respectively from the narrow-band ECG signal, the PPG signal and the reference ECG signal, that were measured simultaneously in the subsection 3.4. Each R-R interval was computed automatically using the peak-detection function in the software. Data section with 1-minute length where the triple signals were commonly stable was selected for the analysis for five subjects of #3_3rd, #4_2nd, #8, #9 and #10. Preparatory filtering with a digital BPF (IIR, 0.5-40 Hz, Q=0.707) was applied to the all selected data. To develop Bland-Altman Plots (Bland & Altman, 1986) between the narrow-band ECG and the reference ECG, and also between the PPG and the reference ECG, difference of R-R intervals as well as mean R-R intervals was calculated for corresponding set of R-R intervals in each subject.

3.6 Comparison of Spectral Powers of Heart Rate Variability

In order to discuss the effect of detection accuracy of R-R intervals, HR variability (HRV) was analyzed for the triple R-R intervals described in the subsection 3.5. A function of HRV analysis installed in the data acquisition software (Biopac Systems, Acknowledge 3.9.0) was used. Data section of the subject #9 with 90-sec length where the triple signals were commonly stable was selected for the analysis. Preparatory filtering with a digital BPF (IIR, 0.5-40 Hz, Q=0.707) was applied to the selected data. Frequency of HRV from DC to 3 Hz was analyzed. The spectral power of very low frequency (VLF: DC-0.04 Hz), low frequency (LF: 0.04-0.15 Hz), high frequency (HF: 0.15-0.40 Hz) and very high frequency (VHF: 0.40-3.00 Hz) were computed respectively.

4. Results and Discussions

4.1 Comparison of Breathing Activity with Respiratory Air Flow in Adult Subjects

As can be seen in Fig. 6, output signal from the low frequency part of the developed device (Fig. 6(a)) fairly captured characteristics of air flow signal measured with the commercial pneumotachograph (Fig. 6(b)). We could see a synchronization of both signals in the former part of the recordings and could easily recognize an onset of breath-holding at the beginning of the latter part. These visual synchronization and breath-holding were observed in all 4 subjects. Moreover, respiratory rate calculated from the breathing activities of 4 subjects presented a high correlation (r=0.995) and was consistent with that calculated from the respiratory air flow, as shown in Fig. 7. Since the chest movements for breathing were observed not only in adults but also in infants in our previous experiments, it is expected that the proposed device is capable of sensing breathing activity in infants with high sensitivity as well. Cause of a subtle error in respiratory rate in Fig. 7 was assumed due to shallow breathing and body motion. Increase in filter order of the HPF or the differential filter in the future is considered to improve the accuracy of the device, because a spectral power from 0.2 to 0.5 Hz, which was mainly originating from motion artifacts, was a certain level in the obtained recordings.

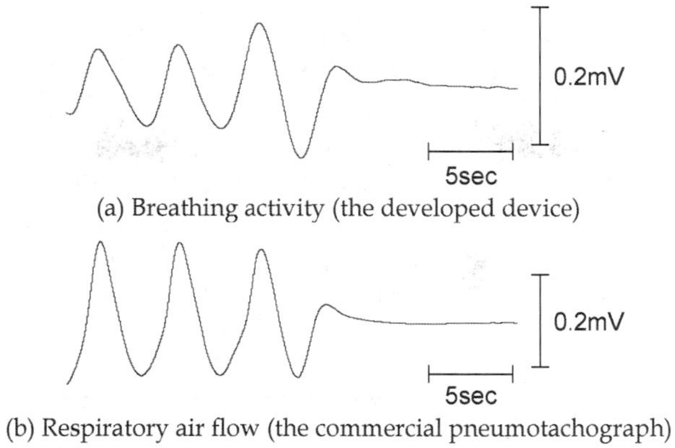

Fig. 6. Recordings of (a) breathing activity obtained from low frequency part of the developed device, and (b) respiratory air flow measured with the commercial pneumotachograph

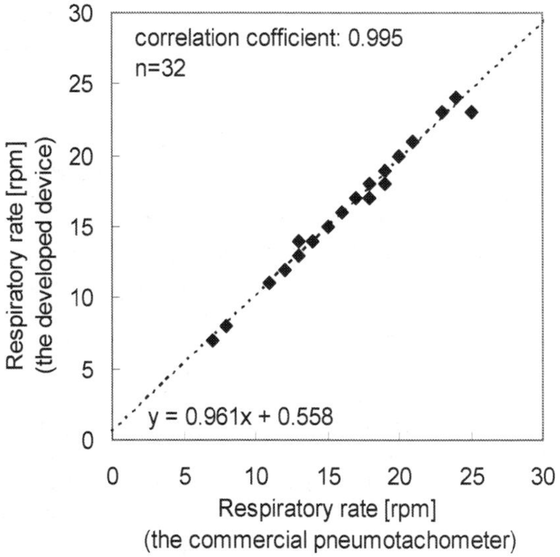

Fig. 7. Correlation of respiration rates between the pneumotachograph and the developed device

4.2 Simultaneous Measurement of Narrow-Band ECG and Breathing Activity in Infants

Fig. 8 shows recordings typical of those obtained while subject #4_2nd was sleeping. Variation of the signal measured with the low frequency part of the developed device (Fig.

8(a)) was consistent with that of the breathing activity (Fig. 8(b)) derived from the PPG recording in Fig. 8(e). Although a slight phase lag due to mechanical delay of the vessel or to an algorithm of the digital filter was observed in the breathing activity from PPG, this consistency was confirmed in 4 of 6 subjects from whom PPG had been measured as the reference signal. Additionally, synchronizations of sleep-breath sound and signal fluctuation detected with our system were auditory confirmed in 8 of the rest 10 subjects.

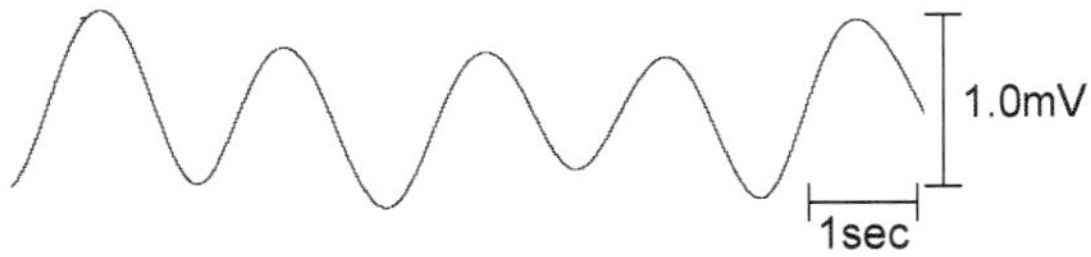

(a) Breathing activity measured with the developed device

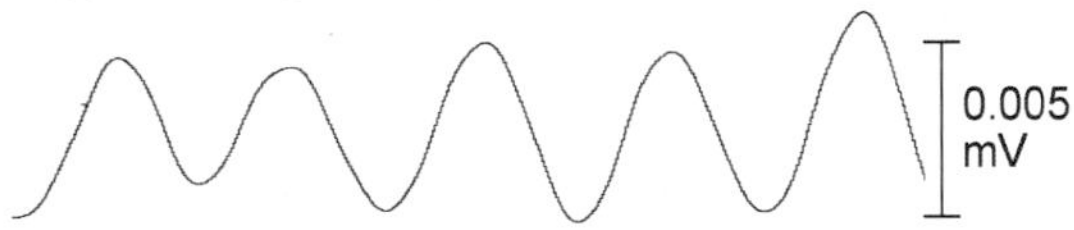

(b) Breathing activity extracted from PPG recording

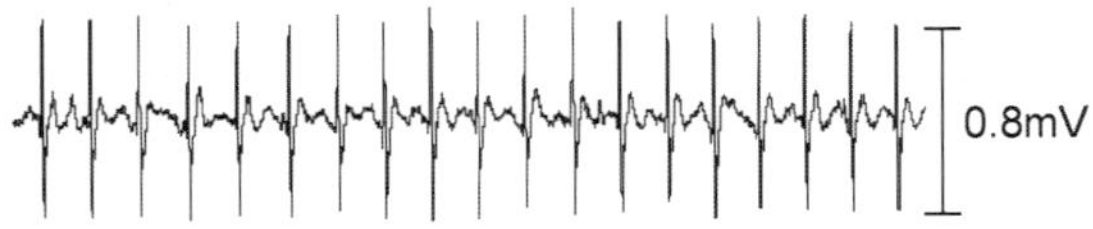

(c) Narrow-band ECG measured with the developed device

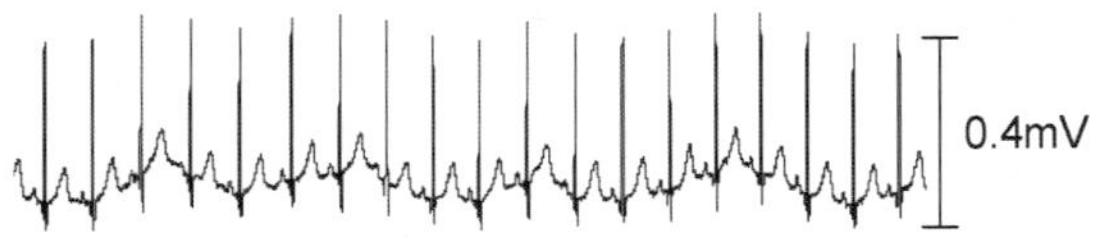

(d) Reference ECG measured with the commercial telemeter

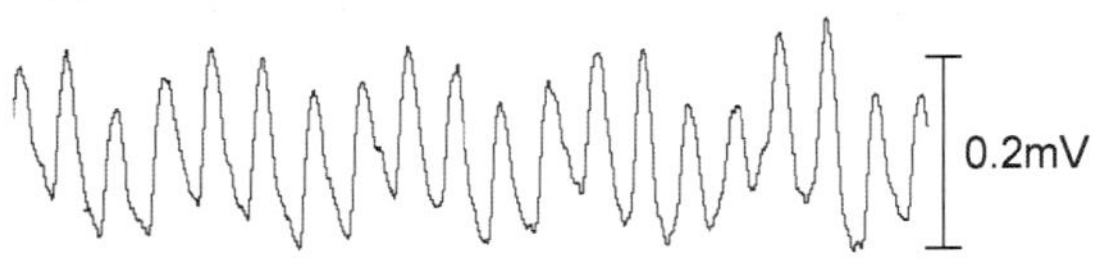

(e) PPG recording measured with the commercial photoplethysmograph

Fig. 8. Typical recordings of (a) breathing activity measured with the low frequency part of the developed device, (b) breathing activity extracted from the PPG recording in Fig. 8(e) using a digital 0.1-0.6 Hz BPF, (c) narrow-band ECG measured with the high frequency part of the developed device, (d) reference ECG measured with the commercial telemeter, (e) PPG recording measured with the commercial photoplethysmograph (subject #4_2nd)

For the subjects of #1_1st and #7_2nd, the developed system failed to measure breathing activity as well as narrow-band ECG because they continued thrashing their limbs with certain intensity throughout the measurement. In the case of subject #1_2nd and subject #3_3rd, moderate motions of limbs were generated throughout the measurement, and then only breathing activity couldn't be detected. Since time constant of the HPF in the low frequency part (i.e. recovery time against each motion) was longer than that in the high frequency part of the developed device, the moderate motions might lead the failure only for breathing activity measurement in these two subjects. As another cause of the failure, it was considered that the order of HPF was primary. Therefore, shortening of the time constant and increasing of the filter order seemed necessary to improve stability of the system against body motion.

As for heart activity, narrow-band ECG obtained with the high frequency part of the proposed system (Fig. 8(c)) presented periodical spikes synchronized with the reference ECG in Fig. 8(d) and with PPG recording in Fig. 8(e). The synchronization with at least one reference was observed in 14 of 16 subjects. In the subjects of #1_1st and #7_2nd, stable output signals couldn't be measured for the reason noted above.

These results demonstrate that the proposed system is capable of sensing breathing activity and narrow-band ECG simultaneously whenever the subject is sleeping or in a resting state even wearing a diaper and a sleepwear. Although there is still room for improvement in terms of its practical use, the proposed system appears promising for application to infant monitor to sense breathing activity and HR without attaching any sensors directly on their skins. As for susceptibility of the system to body motion, there are considered two ways of approaching. One is the improvement of stability of the system against the body motion, as previously stated. Another is active utilization of the susceptibility for detection of defective arousal reaction in infants. The defective arousal reaction has been implicated in the development of SIDS (Sawaguchi & Tedsuka, 1999). Franco et al. reported that risk factors such as "exposure to cigarette smoking" and "prone position" decreased arousals in infants (Franco, 1998, 1999, 2004, and Groswasser, 2001). Therefore alternative use of the low frequency part of the developed device for detecting breathing activity or body motion caused by defective arousal reaction would be beneficial for a preventive SIDS monitor.

4.3 Comparison of R-R Intervals using Bland-Altman Plot

It is known that scattering plots in Bland-Altman plot with small dependency on horizontal axis and with small vertical deviation from the zero line indicate preciseness of the method under consideration compared with another referencing method. As can be seen, distribution of plots in Fig. 9(a) was independent of the horizontal axis and was obviously narrower along with a horizontal zero line than that in Fig. 9(b). Corresponding to the distributions, 95% confidence interval between the reference ECG and narrow-band ECG in Fig. 9(a) was more than 30 times smaller than that between the reference ECG and PPG in Fig. 9(b). Since accuracy of R-R interval in narrow-band ECG was within ±2 ms and more than 30 times higher than that in PPG, the developed device can be used not only for monitoring ECG but also for measuring precise HR instantaneously.

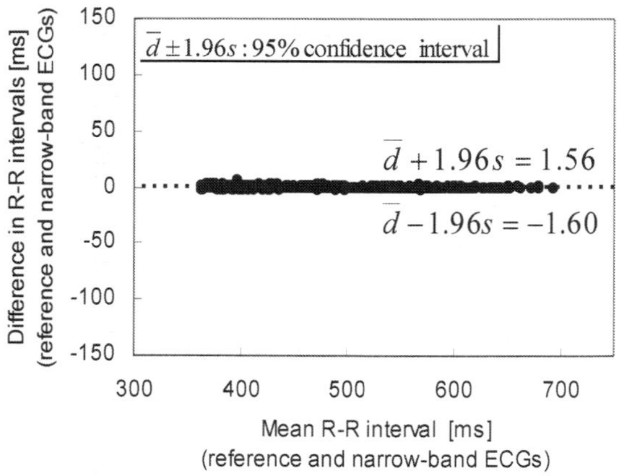

(a) between reference ECG and narrow-band ECG

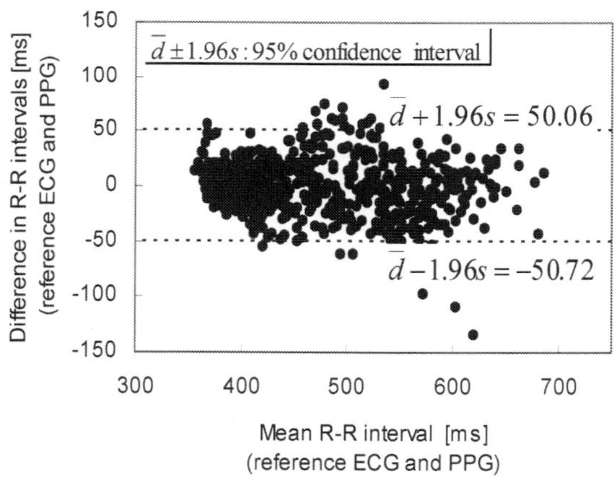

(b) between reference ECG and PPG

Fig. 9. Comparison of R-R intervals using Bland-Altman plot among the reference ECG, narrow-band ECG measured the developed device and PPG

4.4 Comparison of Spectral Powers of Heart Rate Variability

High accuracy of HR calculated from narrow-band ECG can be recognized also in Table 2. In accordance with the results of Fig. 9, powers of HRV in the frequency bands of VLF, LF and HF that were analyzed from narrow-band ECG were identical respectively to those from the reference ECG. In contrast, the powers obtained from the PPG contained errors more than 0.50% in above all frequency bands even though a short-time data section with 90sec length was used for the analysis. In addition, the power in VHF band obtained from the narrow-band ECG was 100 times more accurate than that from the PPG. Thus, the results in Table 2 also support that the developed device has an advantage in measuring accurate HR for a long time.

This advantage of our system may be utilized in other applications, for instance, in detecting seizures in the newborn. Greene (Greene et al., 2007) proposed a method for the detection of seizures in the newborn using heartbeat timing interval features. Seizures occur in 6-13 % of low birth weight infants and 1-2 per 1000 infants born at term (Rennie, 1997). Clinical evidence suggests that neonates with seizures have poor health outcomes, with morbidity in 50 % of survivors, and a high (30%) probability of death (Tharp, 2002). Therefore, it seems a critical issue to increase performance of our system so as to be utilized in NICU (neonatal intensive care unit). Another example is an application to adult (particularly elderly) subjects. Since it is reported that autonomic nervous system dysfunction, estimated by high HR and low HRV, may be associated with the development of diabetes in healthy adults (Carnethon, 2003), our system would be suitable for an awareness-free HR monitor in daily use for health management.

Frequency band [Hz]	Power of HRV [s^2]		
	Reference ECG	PPG	Narrow-band ECG
VLF: DC-0.04	0.118	0.117 (0.78%)	0.118 (0.00%)
LF: 0.04-0.15	0.858	0.853 (0.50%)	0.858 (0.00%)
HF: 0.15-0.40	0.432	0.435 (0.71%)	0.432 (0.00%)
VHF: 0.40-3.00	0.235	0.221 (5.75%)	0.234 (0.05%)

*Values in ( ) indicate error rate against the power obtained from the reference ECG

Table 2. Comparison of spectrum powers of HRV among the reference ECG, the reference PPG, and the narrow-band ECG measured with the developed device

5. Conclusion and Future Prospects

We proposed an approach for obtaining narrow-band ECG as well as breathing activity simultaneously from an infant who wears a diaper and a sleepwear, and lies supine on a bed-sheet electrode unit. We manufactured a pilot measuring device based on the approach and performed verification experiments for 4 adults and for 16 infant subjects. The measurement yielded the following results.

- We could see an onset of breath-holding and synchronized variations in breathing activity signal measured with the low frequency part of the developed device for 4 adult subjects, compared with respiratory air flow signal measured with a commercial pneumotachograph.
- Respiratory rate calculated from the breathing activity was highly correlated (r=0.995) and consistent with that calculated from the respiratory air flow.
- The proposed system was capable of sensing breathing activity and narrow-band ECG simultaneously whenever the infant subject was sleeping or in a resting state even wearing a diaper and a sleepwear.
- Since accuracy of R-R interval in narrow-band ECG was within ±2 ms and more than 30 times higher than that in PPG, the developed device can be used not only for monitoring ECG but also for measuring precise HR.

- High accuracy of HR calculated from narrow-band ECG could be recognized also in the spectral powers of HRV.

Although the system is susceptible to body motions when the subject is alive and thus there is still room for improvement in terms of its practical use, the proposed system appears promising for application to infant monitor to sense breathing activity and accurate HR without attaching any sensors directly on their skins.
Future issues to be addressed are as follows: (1) improvement of stability of the system against body motions, (2) combination with software for detecting life threatening events of infants, (3) bandwidth extension of the part for ECG measurement so as to derive time domain parameters such as QT interval, (4) application to aged subjects with a view to use in home healthcare.

6. Acknowledgment

This study was supported in part by Academic Frontier Project for Private Universities: matching fund subsidy from MEXT (Ministry of Education, Culture, Sports, Science and Technology), 2003-2004, in part by Industrial Technology Research Grant Program in 2005-2008 from NEDO (New Energy and Industrial Technology Development Organization of Japan), and in part by Grant-in-Aid for Young Scientists (B) in 2009 (21 700512).

7. References

Asaishi, T.; Ueno, A.; Hoshino, H.; Mitani, H. & Ishiyama, Y. (2002). Measurement of sympathetic skin response by using DC servo circuit -Detection of DC and AC components, and an application for estimating the nerve's conduction velocity-, *Life Support*, Vol. 14, No. 3, 10-15, 1341-9455

Bland, J.M. & Altman, D.G. (1986). Statistical methods for assessing agreement between two methods of clinical measurement, *The Lancet*, Vol.1, 307–310, 0140-6736

Carnethon, M.R.; Golden, S.H.; Folsom, A.R.; Haskell, W. & Liao, D. (2003). Prospective investigation of autonomic nervous system function and the development of type 2 diabetes: The atherosclerosis risk in communities study 1987-1998, *American Heart Journal*, Vol. 107, 2190-2195, 0002 - 8703

Catrysse, M.; Puers, R.; Hertleer, C.; Van Langenhove, L.; Van Egmondc, H. & Matthys, D. (2004). Towards the integration of textile sensors in a wireless monitoring suit, *Sensors and Actuators A*, Vol. 114, 302–311, 0924-4247

Franco, P.; Pardou, A.; Hassid. S.; Lurquin, P.; Groswasser, J. & Kahn, A. (1998). Auditory arousal thresholds are higher when infants sleep in the prone position, *Journal of Pediatrics*, Vol. 132, 240-243, 00223476

Franco, P.; Groswasser, J.; Hassid, S.; Lanquart, J.P.; Scaillet, S. & Kahn, A. (1999). Prenatal exposure to cigarette smoking is associated with a decrease in arousal in infants, *Journal of Pediatrics*, Vol. 135, 34-38, 00223476

Franco, P.; Seret, N.; Van Hees, J.N.; Scaillet, S.; Vermeulen, F.; Groswasser, J. & Kahn, A. (2004). Decreased arousals among healthy infants after short-term sleep deprivation, *Pediatrics*, Vol. 114, 192-197, 0031-4005

Furusawa, Y.; Ueno, A.; Hoshino, H.; Kataoka, S.; Mitani H. & Ishiyama, Y. (2003). Low invasive measurement of electrocardiogram for newborns and infants, *Proceedings CD-ROM of the IEEE EMBS Asian-Pacific Conference on Biomedical Engineering*, No.022216-1, Keihanna Plaza Hotel, 0-7803-7944-6, October 2003, IEEE Publishing, Piscataway

Gramse, V.; De Groote, A. & Paiva, M. (2003). Novel concept for a noninvasive cardiopulmonary monitor for infants –A pair of pajamas with an integrated sensor module, *Annals of Biomedical Engineering*, Vol. 31, 152-158, 0090-6964

Greene, B.R.; de Chazal, P.; Boylan, G.B.; Connolly, S. & Reilly, R.B. (2007). Electrocardiogram based neonatal seizure detection, *IEEE Transactions on Biomedical Engineering*, Vol.54, No.4, 673-682, 0018-9294

Groswasser, J.; Simon, T.; Scaillet, S.; Franco, P. & Kahn, A. (2001). Reduced arousals following obstructive apneas in infants sleeping prone, *Pediatric Research*, Vol.49, 402-406, 00313998

Kato, T.; Ueno, A.; Kataoka, S.; Hoshino, H. & Ishiyama, Y. (2006). An application of capacitive electrode for detecting electrocardiogram of neonates and infants, *Proceedings of 28th Annual International Conference of the IEEE EMBS*, pp. 916-919, 1-4244-0033-3, Marriott at Times Square, Sept. 2006, IEEE Publishing, Piscataway

Kim, K.K.; Lim, Y.K. & Park, K.S. (2005). Common mode noise cancellation for electrically non-contact ECG measurement system on a chair, *Proceedings of 27th Annual International Conference of the IEEE EMBS*, pp. 5881-5883, 0-7803-8740-6, Shanghai International Convention Center, Sept. 2005, IEEE Publishing, Piscataway

Krous, H.F.; Beckwith, J.B.; Byard, R.W.; Rognum, T.O.; Bajanowski, T.; Corey, T.; Cutz, E.; Hanzlick, R.; Keens, T.G. & Mitchell, E.A. (2004). Sudden infant death syndrome and unclassified sudden infant deaths: A definitional and diagnostic approach, *Pediatrics*, Vol. 114, No. 1, 234-238, 1098-4275

Little, G.A.; Ballard, R.A.; Brooks, JG et al. (1987). National Institutes of Health consensus development conference on infantile apnea and home monitoring, Sept 29 to Oct 1, 1986, *Pediatrics*, Vol. 79, No. 2, pp. 292-299, 0031-4005

Lopez, J.A. & Richardson, P.C. (1969). Capacitive electrocardiographic and bioelectric electrodes, *IEEE Transactions on Biomedical Engineering*, Vol.BME-16, 99, 0018-9294

Nakajima, K.; Tamura, T. & Miike, H. (1993). Heart and respiratory rates monitor using digital filters. *Japanese Journal of Medical Electronics and Biological Engineering*, Vol. 31, No. 4, 360-366, 00213292

Richardson, P. C.; Coombs, F.K. & Adams, R.M. (1968). Some new electrode techniques for long term physiologic monitoring, *Aerospace Medicine*, Vol.39, 745-750, 0001-9402

Pallàs-Areny, R. & Webster, J.G. (1999). 7.1.6 Differential Filters, In: *Analog Signal Processing*, 333-337, John Wiley & Sons, 978-0471125280, U.S.A.

Rennie, J.M. (1997). Neonatal seizures, *European Journal of Pediatrics*, Vol. 156, 83–87, 1432-1076

Sawaguchi, T. & Tedsuka, Y. (1999). The physiological definition of the arousal reaction in infants in reference to the hypothesis of defective arousal reaction in SIDS, *Research and Practice in Forensic Medicine*, Vol. 42, 341-346, 0289-0755

Spinelli, E.M.; Martínez, N.H. & Mayosky, M.A. (1999). A transconductance driven-right-leg circuit, *IEEE Transactions on Biomedical Engineering*, Vol. 46, No. 12, 1466–1470, 0018-9294

Spinelli, E.M.; Martínez, N; Mayosky, M.A. & Pallàs-Areny, R. (2004). A novel fully differential biopotential amplifier with DC suppression, *IEEE Transactions on Biomedical Engineering*, Vol. 51, No. 8, 1444–1448, 0018-9294

Statistics and Information Department, Ministry of Health, Labour and Welfare, Japan (2007). *Vital Statistics Japan*, http://www.mhlw.go.jp/toukei/saikin/hw/jinkou/suii07/deth8.html

Tharp, B.R. (2002). Neonatal seizures and syndromes. *Epilepsia*, Vol. 43, 2-10, 0013-9580

Ueno, A.; Furusawa, Y.; Hoshino, H. & Ishiyama, Y. (2004). Detection of electrocardiogram by electrodes with fabrics using capacitive coupling, *IEEJ Transactions on Electronics, Information and Systems*, Vol. 124, No. 9, 1664-1671, 0385-4221

Ueno, A.; Akabane, Y.; Kato, T.; Hoshino, H.; Kataoka, S. & Ishiyama, Y. (2007a). Capacitive sensing of electrocardiographic potential through cloth from the dorsal surface of the body in a supine position -A preliminary study, *IEEE Transactions on Biomedical Engineering*, Vol. 54, No. 4, 759-766, 0018-9294

Ueno, A.; Shiogai, Y. & Ishiyama, Y. (2007b). A primary study of indirect ECG monitor embedded in a bed for Home Health Care, *IEEJ Transactions on Electronics, Information and Systems*, Vol. 127, No. 10, 1792-1799, 0385-4221

Ueno, A. & Yama, Y. (2008). Unconstrained monitoring of ECG and respiratory variation in infants with underwear during sleep using a bed-sheet electrode unit, *Proceedings of 30th Annual International Conference of the IEEE EMBS*, pp. 2329-2332, 978-1-4244-1815-2, Vancouver Convention & Exhibition Centre, Aug. 2008, IEEE Publishing, Piscataway

Yama, Y. & Ueno, A. (2009). Unrestrained facile measurement of narrow-band ECG and respiratory variation in infants with a capacitive sheet-type sensor, *Transactions of Japanese Society for Medical and Biological Engineering*, Vol. 47, No. 1, 42-50, 1347-443X

EEG-Based Personal Identification

Hideaki Touyama
Toyama Prefectural University
Japan

1. Introduction

In recent years, there have been many discussions about a new interaction technique which directly connects a human brain and a machine. A brain-computer interface (BCI) is a communication channel which enables us to send commands to external devices only by using brain activities (Wolpaw et al., 2002). As one of the candidates for noninvasive and compact BCI systems, an electroencephalography (EEG) has been investigated. A variety of brain activities have been reported in the context of the BCI based on EEG; for instance, motor imageries (Pfurtscheller & Neuper, 1997; Blankertz et al., 2006), visual evoked potentials (VEP) (Middendorf et al., 2000; Cheng et al., 2002), P300 evoked potentials (Farewell & Donchin, 1988; Bayliss, 2003), etc. With such brain activities, many applications have been developed in laboratories such as a virtual keyboard or computer mouse.

The technique to extract the human brain information provides and has driven a new research paradigm; the EEG-based biometry (or biometrics). The concept of the biometry has lately been more and more emerging (Fig. 1). For example, face, fingerprint, and iris have been considered and the part of those has been in practical use. By using human brain activities as a new modality, we have several advantages (Marcel et al., 2007). It is confidential, very difficult to mimic, and almost impossible to steal, and furthermore easy to change on purpose the 'password' according to the users mental tasks or intentions.

In spite of the expected use, there has been little work on the EEG-based biometry. Paranjape et al. studied on the EEG signals recorded from the subjects with eyes open and closed (Paranjape et al., 2001). They examined EEG trials from 40 subjects, and the classification accuracy of about 80 percent was achieved. Poulos et al. investigated one-channel EEG on occipital site to extract the four major EEG rhythms (alpha, beta, delta and theta) during closed eyes, where the classification performance of 95 percent was obtained involving four subjects and more than 250 EEG patterns (Poulos et al., 1999). Palaniappan et al. reported the VEP-based biometry (Palaniappan et al., 2007). Marcel et al. studied the person authentication based on motor imageries and word generation tasks (Marcel et al., 2007). Thorpe et al. proposed the concept of 'pass-thought' (Thorpe et al., 2006) using P300 evoked potentials based on oddball paradigm with flashing letters on a computer monitor. These works revealed the feasibility of the EEG-based biometry. However, it would be difficult to change the EEG signals (password) on purpose, except for the method using P300 responses.

Biometrics	Behavioral	Voice
		Keystroke
		Signature
	Physiological	Face
		Fingerprint
		Vein
		Iris
		DNA

Fig. 1. A variety of biometrics. There are two main classes. One is behavioral and the other is physiological one. In behavioral class, behavior of a person such as voice, keystroke, signature etc. is used. In physiological class, the shape of the body is used such as face, fingerprint, vein, iris, DNA etc. The EEG is a new modality of the biometry.

In this book chapter, we investigate the possibility of EEG activities during photo retrieval to perform the personal identification extracting the P300 evoked potentials. In particular, the use of non-target photo images is focused in order to improve the identification performances. By using photo retrieval tasks, there is a remarkable advantage mentioned above; it is easy to change the pass-thought based on the scheme of the oddball paradigm. Furthermore, the photo retrieval is very familiar with people and easy to achieve with no training. The identification performances will be examined by using Principal Component Analysis (PCA) with a variety of conditions of EEG averaging.
This chapter is structured as follows: In section 2, the experimental methods will be explained. The analysis protocols and the results of the personal identification will be shown in section 3 and 4, respectively. Finally, the discussions and conclusions will be mentioned including our considerations on future works.

2. Experimental Methods

Five normal volunteers (denoted as s1-s5) with normal vision participated in the experiments as subjects (males, range from 23 and 36 yr). The subjects were naïve for the EEG measurement in this study and comfortably sitting on an arm-chair facing a screen in the electromagnetically shielded room.

2.1 EEG Recordings

To address the performance of the personal identification, a modular EEG cap system was applied for scalp recordings. Only one-channel EEG signals were analyzed from Cz according to the international 10/20 system (Fig. 2). A body-earth and a reference electrode were on a forehead and on a left ear lobe, respectively. The analogue EEG signals were amplified at a multi-channel bio-signal amplifier (MEG-6116, NIHON KOHDEN Inc. Japan). The amplified signals were band-pass filtered between 0.5 and 30 Hz and sampled at 128 Hz by using a standard A/D converter. The digitized EEG data was stored in a personal computer.

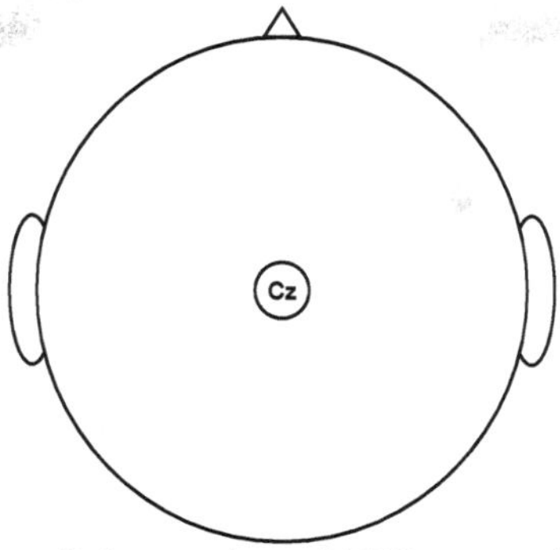

Fig. 2. The electrode montage. Only one-channel EEG was analyzed using a modular EEG cap system according to the international 10/20 system.

2.2 Experimental Tasks

The experimental task sequence was shown in Fig. 3. Nine photo images were randomly projected one by one from backside every 0.5 sec on the screen with about 11.4 degrees of visual angle. Earlier 2 sec was for eye-fixation and the following 4.5 sec included one-time presentation of each photo. The 20-time repetitions were performed to construct 1 session (for 130 sec = 6.5 sec x 20 times). For each subject, the session was repeated at most 5 times to collect the datasets.

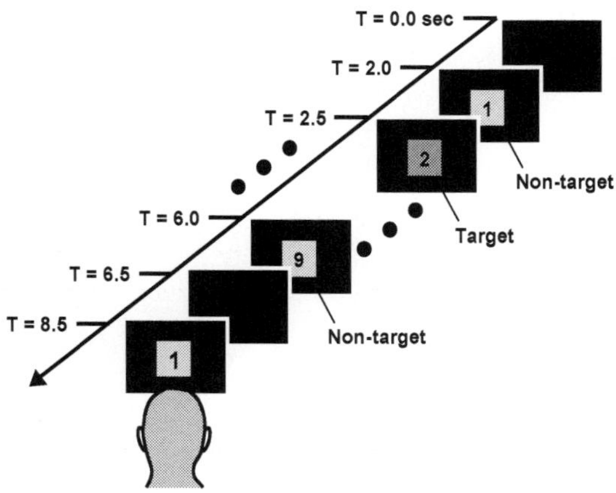

Fig. 3. The experimental task sequence. The subject focused attention on the centre of the interested photo images silently counting the number of times the images were presented.

Photo Number	Photo images
1	Face of a familiar man
2	Female bust with a bikini
3	Face of a baby
4	Face of a puppy
5	Girl's COSPLAY
6	Kiss of men
7	Broken buildings
8	Corpse of a bird (fake)
9	Dolls buried in mud

Table 1. Contents of Photo Images
The contents of photo images used in this study. These photo images were selected in advance by the author.

The task was to focus attention on one or more photo images in which the subject was interested and silently count the number of times that the target photos were presented (oddball tasks). These interested (target) photos were selected just before the experiment by subjects themselves and were keys for the personal identification. For non-interested (non-target) photo images, the subjects were instructed to ignore them. Most of the photo image sets were sampled by the author from a public photo archive Flickr (See the website). The contents of photo images are shown in Table 1, which includes the image of 'Face of a puppy' 'Girl's COSPLAY', and so on.

3. Analysis Protocols

To perform the personal identification focusing on the effect of non-target stimuli, the following analysis protocols were adopted.

3.1 Questionnaire

After the EEG recordings, the subjects received a brief questionnaire. A question was *"Which were your target photos?"* These results were used in the following analyses to assign the tags of 'target' and 'non-target'.

3.2 Averaging

The uniqueness of the recorded EEG activities is one of the important keys to achieve the personal identification. To check this briefly, the average waveforms both for target and for non-target photos were at first investigated for each subject.

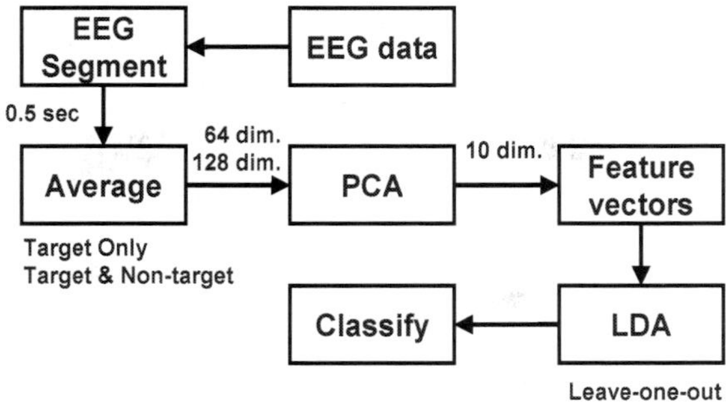

Fig. 4. The identification algorhithm. The Principal Component Analysis (PCA) was used to reduce the dimension of the feature vectors. The classification is done using Linear Discriminant Analysis (LDA).

3.3 The Identification Algorithm

For the personal identification, the EEG data both during target and non-target photo retrieval were extracted for each subject. The datasets were categorized into five according to five subjects. There were totally 1,000 single-trial target EEG datasets for all subjects.

For future applications, only one-channel EEG was investigated in the identification. To examine the use of the non-target photos, the feature vectors were constructed not only from the EEG during target photo retrieval also non-target. From one electrode site Cz, the EEG potential values were considered to have 128-dimensional feature vectors from the 0.5 sec of samples of temporal EEG signals (0.5 sec x 128Hz x 2 (target and non-target)). For target data only, half of the 128 dimensions were considered. The number of the feature dimension was reduced to 10 by applying PCA. Linear Discriminant Analysis (LDA) was used for the classification (Fig. 4). To estimate the identification performance a leave-one-out method was adopted, where only one data was used for the testing and the others were for the trainings. In our study, the number of times of averaging for the non-target photos was twice of that of target photos.

4. Results

In the questionnaire, it was found that the numbers of the selected photos were three, one, two, one and three among nine photo images for the subject s1-s5, respectively.

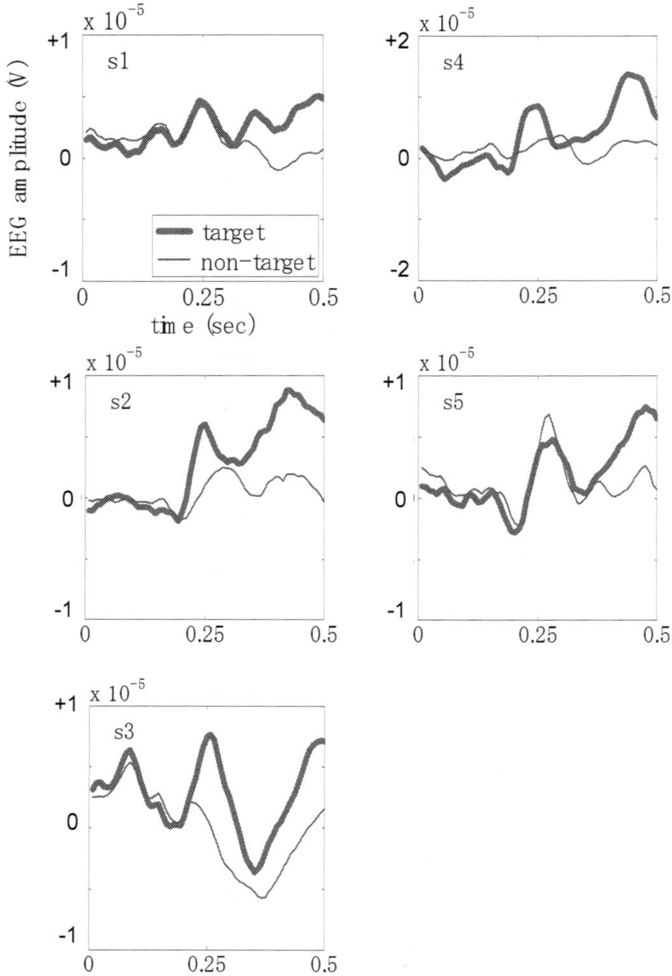

Fig. 5. Average waveforms on one electrode site Cz during target and non-target photo retrieval. The positive potentials were expressed in upper directions (y-axis).

In Fig. 5, it was clearly found that the target and non-target waveforms of each subject were very unique, which would be responsible for the personal identification. The tendency of the enhancements of the EEG amplitudes beyond 0.3sec was observed with target photo images for all subjects. The P300 evoked potentials were clearly observed for some subjects, which would be responsible for the high performance of the oddball-based BCI controls (Krusienski et al., 2007). In our previous works, the identification between target and non-target photo images could be done with 80-90% of the identification performances (Touyama & Hirose, 2008).

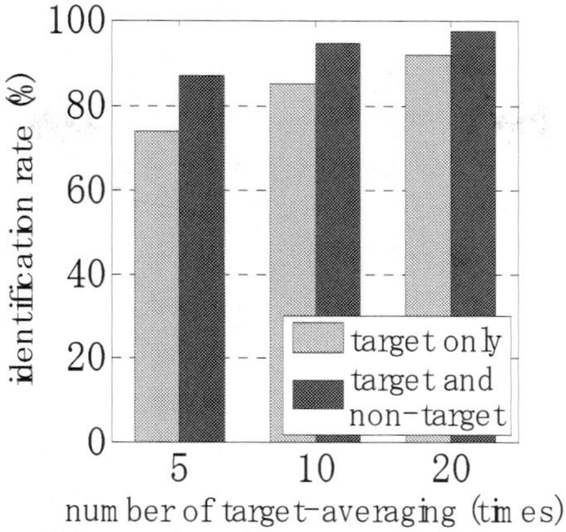

Fig. 6. The dependence of the number of target-averaging times on personal identification rates.

Fig. 6 shows the estimated personal identification rates. It was found that the performances were successfully improved if we consider both target and non-target retrieval. The rates were 87.2, 95.0 and 97.6% for 5, 10 and 20-time target-averaging, respectively. Only with target retrieval, the performances were 74.1, 85.1 and 92.2% for 5, 10 and 20-time target-averaging, respectively.

5. Discussions

In this study, by using human brain activities, the possibility of the personal identification was addressed in offline analyses. It was found that the personal identification was possible with high identification rate using only one-channel EEG signals during photo retrieval. In particular, the performance was enhanced if the system involved the EEG during non-target photo retrieval in addition to that during target photo retrieval. The enhanced performance was 95.0% with 10-time averaging. It was found that the number of averaging time more than 20 had a tendency of saturated performances.

Usually, in the oddball paradigm, the non-target stimuli are more frequently prepared and presented than target ones. Thus, we have lots of non-target stimuli. This means we have a large number of EEG averaging time for non-target stimuli, which would yield to the enhanced performance of EEG based personal identification.

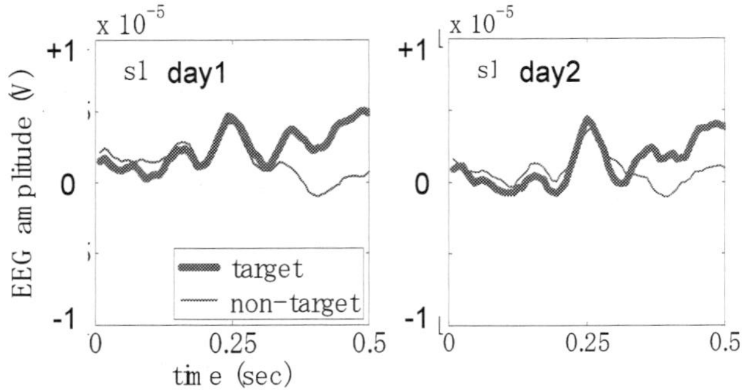

Fig. 7. EEG waveforms during target and non-target photo retrieval for different photo image sets. This result was obtained with the subject s1 over two days (left: day1, right: day2). In both cases, the number of target photos was three. The positive potentials were expressed in upper directions (y-axis).

The subjects in this study selected freely their interested photo images just before the EEG measurement. Our additional experiments revealed the reproducible waveforms if the photo image sets were exchanged to others. One of the examples was shown in Fig. 7. This result suggested the possibility to change target (or non-target) photo images ('password') on purpose, which would be one of the advantages of the EEG-based biometry in oddball paradigm. Furthermore, note that the photo retrieval tasks are easy to achieve for ordinary people.

Here, there were several points to be considered for future developments. The first one is to shorten the time during photo retrieval. According to the experimental protocols in this study, the minimum time to obtain 10-time averaging of target EEG was 15.0 sec (= 4.5 sec x 10 times / 3 photos), if the subject selected three among nine photo images. The increase of the target photo images would be one of the solutions, while the decrease of the P300 amplitudes might be accompanied by more frequent presentations of the target photo images. The second is the authentication. In our study, only the identification was addressed. But, for the practical use, the authentication is very required. In the authentication, the system must confirm and deny the identity claimed by a person (Marcel et al., 2007). The third is the number of the subjects. There is still a possibility to reduce the identification performance with many subjects (for example, more than 100 people). Then, more sophisticated classification algorithm will be investigated in future works.

To achieve higher performance within short time period, there is a possibility to combine other possible brain signals with P300 evoked potentials. For example, in our previous works on the BCI using steady-state VEP, the power spectrum density of such kind of VEP could be different between people. Thus, a variety of experimental tasks should be considered in one experimental session, which will be investigated quantitatively in future works.

The EEG-based personal identification and authentication was motivated and driven by the novel studies on the BCI. The personal identification system would serve rich controls of the BCI systems.

6. Conclusions

In this study, we investigated the feasibility of personal identification using one-channel EEG during photo retrieval in oddball paradigm. The use of non-target photo images was explained to improve the identification performances. The PCA and the LDA were applied to have the identification rates in offline. It was found that the performances were successfully improved if non-target photo retrieval was considered as well as target photo retrieval. The identification rates were 87.2, 95.0 and 97.6% for 5, 10 and 20-time target-averaging, respectively. This study revealed a future possibility of photo retrieval tasks to realize the personal identification using human brain activities, which will yield rich controls of machine for the each user of brain computer-interface.

7. Acknowledgment

This work was partly supported by Tateisi Science and Technology Foundation in Japan.

8. References

Bayliss, J.D. (2003). The use of the evoked potentials P3 component for control in a virtual apartment, *IEEE Transaction on Neural Systems and Rehabilitation Engineering,* 11 (2).

Blankertz, B.; Dornhege, G.; Krauledat, M.; Muller, K.R.; Kunzmann, V.; Losch, F. & Curio, G. (2006). The Berlin Brain-Computer Interface: EEG-based communication without subject training, *IEEE Trans Neural Syst. Rehabil. Eng, 14*(2), Jun, pp. 147-152.

Cheng, M.; Gao, X.; Gao, S. & Xu, D. (2002). Design and Implementation of a Brain-Computer Interface With High Transfer Rates, *IEEE Transactions on Biomedical Engineering, 49*(10), pp. 1181-1186.

Farwell, L.A. & Donchin, E. (1988). Taking off the top of your head: Toward a mental prothesis utilizing event-related brain potentials, *Electroenceph. Clin. Neurophysiol., 70,* pp. 510-523.

Krusienski, D.J.; Sellers, E.W.; McFarland, D.J.; Vaughan, T.M. & Wolpaw, J.R. (2008). Toward enhanced P300 speller performance, *Journal of Neuroscience Methods,* Vol. 167, Issue 1, pp. 15-21.

Marcel, S. & Millan Jose del R. (2007). Person authentication using brainwaves (EEG) and maximum a posteriori model adaptation, *IEEE Transaction on pattern analysis and machine intelligence,* Vol. 29, Issue 4, pp. 743-752.

Middendorf, M.; McMillan, G.; Calhoun, G. & Jones, K.S. (2000). Brain-Computer Interfaces Based on the Steady-State Visual-Evoked Response, *IEEE Transactions on Rehabilitation Engineering, 8*(2), pp. 211-214.

Paranjape, R. B.; Mahovsky, J.; Benedicenti, L. & Koles, Z. (2001). The Electroencephalogram as a Biometrics, *Proc. Canadian Conf. Electrical and Computer Engineering,* Vol. 2, pp. 1363-1366.

Palaniappan, R. & Mandic, D.P. (2007). Biometrics from Brain Electrical Activity: A Machine Learning Approach, *IEEE Transaction on pattern analysis and machine intelligence,* Vol. 29, No. 4, pp. 738-742.

Pfurtscheller, G. & Neuper, C. (1997). Motor imagery activates primary sensorimotor area in man, *Neurosci Lett, 239,* pp. 65-68.

Poulos, M.; Rangoussi, M.; Chrissikopoulos, V. & Evangelou, A. (1999). Parametric Person identification from the EEG Using Computational Geometry, *Proc. IEEE Int'l Conf. Electronics, Circuits, and Systems*, Vol.2, pp. 1005-1008.

See the website, http://www.flickr.com/.

Thorpe, J.; van Oorschot, P. C. & Somayaji, A. (2006). Pass-thoughts: Authenticating with Our Minds, *Proceedings of the 2005 Workshop on New Security, The Association for Computing Machinery*, New York.

Touyama, H. & Hirose, M. (2008). EEG-Based Photo Pickup, *Proceedings of 18th International Conference on Artificial Reality and Telexistence (ICAT 2008)*, pp. 277-280.

Wolpaw, J.R.; Birbaumer, N.; McFarland, D.J.; Pfurtscheller, G. & Vaughan, T.M. (2002). Brain-computer interfaces for communication and control, *Clinical Neurophysiology, 113*, pp. 767-791.

23

Skin and Non-Solid Cancer Incidence in Interventional Radiology using Biological and Physical Dosimetry Methods

M. Ramos[1], A. Montoro[2], S. Ferrer[1], J.I. Villaescusa[2], G. Verdu[1], M. Almonacid[2]
[1]Department of Chemical and Nuclear Energy. Polytechnic University of Valencia
[2]Radiation Protection Service. Hospital Universitario La Fe
Valencia (Spain)

1. Introduction

Interventional radiology has been extended during last years, increasing the necessity of developing radiation protection procedures, not only for patients, but for radiologists and radiology assistants [ICRP 2000]. In the past, radiation injuries of patients exposed to fluoroscopy and other interventional techniques have been analysed as deterministic effects of radiation exposures [Vanagunas et al. 1990, Vano and Gonzalez 2004]. However, medical staff is exposed to low levels of ionizing radiation which are fractionated in time, therefore suspicious to develop stochastic effects such as skin and non-solid cancer incidence (leukaemia, lymphomas and/or myelomas).

Factors affecting doses are dependent on exposure time, field size, technical characteristics of radiation equipment, patient size, examination type, operation mode, complication of examination or staff experience [Kottou et al. 2005]. Some indicative values for effective or equivalent dose per interventional technique found in the literature are shown in Table 1.

Interventional technique	**Effective/equivalent dose**	
	Doctor (μSv)	**Patient (mSv)**
Cardiology	0.5 - 18.8	8.3 per hour
Cerebral embolization	-	2.5 – 10.5
ERCP (Endoscopic retrograde cholangiopancreatography)	Lens (eye) - 340	7.3 (mean to whole body)
	Thyroid - 300	
	Hands - 440	
CT fluoroscopy	7-48	-
Neuro interventional procedures	3.7 ± 2.3 (mean ± SD)	11.3 (mean)

Table 1. Some indicative values for effective or equivalent dose per interventional technique

Staff (radiologists and assistants) receives doses from scattered radiation, but many are not aware of this fact, due to a lack of formation and education on radiation protection practices. In some countries, cumulative radiation doses to the hands, eyes, and thyroid may restrict the number of procedures that interventionists can undertake and there have been reports of radiation injuries to clinicians, including cataracts [Shrimali et al. 1972, Vano et al. 1998a, 1998b]. Additionally, staff doses can be considerably increased if inappropriate x-ray equipment practices or inadequate personal protection items are used (i.e. lead apron, shielding panels…) [ICRP 2000].

Biological dose estimation based on analysis of dicentric chromosomes in solid stained metaphases has provided the most reliable method, being used widely for this purpose. This methodology has been used not only to assess acute doses but also to evaluate protracted and fractionated doses like those received occupationally. For past or chronic exposures, an alternative to the conventional use of dicentrics is the analysis of AST (apparently simple traslocations). After an exposure to ionizing radiation, translocations are induced at a frequency similar but stable to that of dicentrics [Barquinero et al. 1999], whose yield remains relatively constant over time [Lloyd et al. 1998, Lindholm et al. 2002]. Translocations are chromosomic aberrations which can be detected easily by fluorescence in situ hybridization (FISH), and their analysis is a valuable tool in cases of old or longterm exposures, due to their stability [IAEA 2001, Edwards et al 2005].

The objective of this study is the estimation of stochastic effects derived from low dose and low LET dose rate in a specific population group of the Radiology Department of the Hospital La Fe (Valencia), based on physical and biological dosimetry. These subjects have been selected due to the clinical observation of radiation injuries such as aged skin, telangiectasia in nasal region or radiodermitis. Effective doses are generally absorbed in skin, lymphatic fluid and blood, and consequently there is an associated risk to induce a skin and a non-solid cancer, which must be estimated.

2. Materials and methods

2.1 Study population

The subjects under study is a group of nine radiologists from the radiology department of the Hospital La Fe (Valencia), three females and three males with ages ranging from 43 to 58 years old. The groups were exposed to direct and scattered X-ray radiation over a period of 8-28 years, being routinely monitored with film badges or thermoluminescence dosimeters (TLD's). Procedures used by the group of radiologists were endoscopic retrograde cholangiopancreatography, pneumatic dilatation, and insertion of nasoenteric tubes or prosthesis in the gastrointestinal tract.

Table 2 shows employed radiological techniques, common irradiated corporal zone, years of employment, estimated time per patient for each technique and mA - min per year for each worker.

Case	Sex	Age	Years of employment	Ionizing radiation expositions	Radiological techniques	mA·min per year
1	m	56	22	Radiology Endoscopy	Ballon angioplasty/stent Chemoembolization Biopsy TIPS Thrombolysis Aortic endoprosthesis Angioplasty	4800 8000 660 1980 528 1485 6000
2	m	43	8			
3	f	45	13			
4	f	58	25	Radiology Endoscopy	Endoscopy retrograde cholangiopancreatography (ERCP) Digestive stents dilatation	12000 54.45
5	f	57	27			
6	m	54	28	Radiology	Artrography Mielography	1625 1300

Table 2. Interventional procedures and techniques in group of study

Physically recorded doses have been obtained from film badges placed on the wrist and thermoluminescence dosimeters (TLD's) placed near the chest. Biologically recorded doses have been obtained by extrapolating the yield of translocations to their respective dose-effect curves. Chromosome aberrations were detected by fluorescence in situ hybridization (FISH). Table 3 shows a description of the group of nine radiologists and the estimation of the physical and biological effective doses, where Σ_i is the accumulated dose during all professional activity [Montoro et al 2005].

Case	Age	Years	Sex	Physical doses (mSv)				Biological doses (mSv)
				TLD		Wrist		AST
				$\bar{d}\ [d_{min}, d_{max}]$	Σ_i	$\bar{d}\ [d_{min}, d_{max}]$	Σ_i	
1	56	22	m	3.27 [0,14.8]	75.2	76.1 [0,238.1]	988.9	546 [236-940]
2	43	8	m	2.82 [0,7.1]	21.3	90.1 [60.7,122.1]	450.6	46 [0-289]
3	45	13	f	4.48 [0.3,26]	60.2	64.7 [7.8,169.9]	776.0	99 [0-376]
4	58	25	f	8.91 [0,48.7]	228.1	103.7 [49.8,152.1]	201.9	596 [73-1710]
5	57	27	f	4.67 [0,21]	115.2	25.9 [-,-]	25.9	166 [8-440]
6	54	28	m	3.69 [0.8,13.8]	105.8	9.0 [0,167.4]	216.6	441 [179-773]

Table 3. Physically and Biologically recorded Doses with 95% Confidence Limits. Estimated doses for total apparently simple translocations (AST) using the dose-effect curve: Y = (0.86 ± 0.13) x 10-2 + (6.57 ± 1.06) x 10-2 D + (4.15 ± 0.55) x 10-2 D^2

2.2 Risk of exposure induced cancers (REIC)

There are different indicators when evaluating the associated induced cancer risk to people exposed to ionizing radiation. These indicators are adequate to make comparisons and to be included in quality controls assessment. One of these estimators is the excess absolute risk for cancer incidence, EAR, defined as the excess probability of developing a cancer after an exposure to ionizing radiation, where is a set of covariates, such as sex, age-of-exposure, attained age, effective dose or latency period.

The UNSCEAR Reports present a large group of cohorts and case-control studies of risk estimates for solid and non-solid cancers after exposures to ionizing radiation. The most important source of radio-induced cancers is the Radiation Effects Research Foundation Life Span Study, which links the Japanese atomic bomb survivors and the Hiroshima and Nagasaki tumor registry data for 1958 through 1987 [UNSCEAR 2000]. However, this report includes only detailed models for risks of solid cancer mortality and incidence (except skin cancer) based on age-at-exposure and attained age.

A risk model based on average EAR per person-year-sievert (PYSv) from external low-LET exposures has been introduced for transporting risks from the Japanese population to the exposed population. Table 4 shows the average excess absolute risk (EAR) for cancer incidence in males and females.

		EAR $(10^4\ \text{PYSv})^{-1}$
		Male / Female
Solid cancer	Skin cancer	0.89 / 0.72
Non-solid cancer	Leukaemia	3.35 / 2.29
	Hodgkin's disease	0.04 / 0.04
	Non-Hodgkin's lymphoma	0.73 / -0.20[a]
	Multiple myeloma	0.26 / -0.08[a]

Table 4. Average excess absolute risk (EAR) for incidence cancer (104 PYSv)-1 from the Life Span Study cohort (UNSCEAR 2000 report)

The risk of exposure-induced cancer (*REIC*) is defined as the probability that an individual suffers a radio-induced cancer, not necessarily fatal, over all of his or her life. The REIC is estimated as

$$REIC = \left(\sum_{j=e+L}^{M} s_{1j} EAR_j \right) \tag{1}$$

where e is the age-at-exposure, L is the latency period and s_{1j} is an estimator of the survival function, that is

$$s_{1j} = \prod_{i=e}^{j} \left[1 - \lambda_{all}(i) \right] \tag{2}$$

The baseline mortality function per male and female has been obtained from INE database (www.ine.es), assuming an additive model for epidemiology from EAR of the Life Span Study cohort. The excess absolute risk has been transported to the population of the Valencian Community through the baseline mortality function λ_{all}, using the software RADRISK. This software has been developed on Matlab 7.0, based on the software SCREENRISK which is used for estimating the breast cancer incidence and mortality in the Valencian Breast Cancer Screening Program [Ramos et al. 2005].

3. Results

Effective doses obtained from the wrist dosimeter have been used for estimating the skin cancer incidence, whereas TLD's and biological doses have been employed for estimating non-solid cancer incidences.

Tables 5 and 6 show the risk of exposure-induced cancer derived from physically recorded doses and biologically recorded doses. As observed, there is an appreciable increment in the cancer incidence due to exposed radiation in some cases, especially for skin cancer and leukemia. The REIC for induced non-Hodgkin lymphomas and multiple myeloma is negligible for females, derived from the negative EAR trend from the UNSCEAR 2000 report.

Case	Sex	Age	Wrist dosimeter	TLD dosimeter			
			Skin Cancer	Leukemia	Hodgkin's disease	Non-Hodgkin's disease	Multiple myeloma
1	m	56	5.39	1.54	0.01	0.33	0.12
2	m	43	2.38	4.25	0.00	0.09	0.03
3	f	45	4.36	1.07	0.01	< 0	< 0
4	f	58	1.10	3.98	0.06	< 0	< 0
5	f	57	0.15	2.15	0.03	< 0	< 0
6	m	54	1.45	2.67	0.03	0.58	0.20

Table 5. Risk of exposure-induced cancer (REIC) per 1000 for non-solid cancer incidence derived from physically recorded doses (wrist and TLD dosimeter)

Case	Sex	Age	Leukemia	Hodgkin's disease	Non-Hodgkin's disease	Multiple myeloma
1	m	56	11.21	0.13	2.44	0.87
2	m	43	0.91	0.01	0.20	0.07
3	f	45	1.77	0.03	< 0	< 0
4	f	58	10.40	0.18	< 0	< 0
5	f	57	3.11	0.05	< 0	< 0
6	m	54	11.14	0.13	2.42	0.86

Table 6. Risk of exposure-induced cancer (REIC) per 1000 for non-solid cancer incidence derived from biologically doses

4. Discussion and conclusions

The discrepancies observed between the physically recorded doses and the biologically estimated doses due to that physical dosimetry is low estimated because of radiologists did not always wear their dosimeters or that the dosimeters were not always in the radiation field, which implies a possible partial-body exposure.

These results are in accordance with DIMOND report which states that staff doses in interventional procedure are highly dependent on radiation protection measures taken (Peer et al 2003). Unfortunately the dosimeters are not placed on the same worker's point in every hospital (i.e. chest dosimeter is placed commonly on belt) and are not used every day by misleading for the majority of interventionists.

Suitable theoretical and practice education and training for the personnel in radiology (and cardiology) is necessary. Training in radiological protection for patients and staff should be an integral part of the education for those professionals using interventional techniques. Risks and benefits, including radiation detriment, should be taken into account when new interventional techniques are introduced.

Other non-solid cancer incidence is negligible, but it has been considered that is derived from the hypothesis of constant excess-absolute risk (EAR) over the life of the radiologist. Future work will include a more complex model for estimating EAR, based on attained age or age-at-exposure applicable to non-solid and non-melanoma skin cancer.

Despite all uncertainties transporting risks, the average radiological detriment, expressed as the risk of exposure-induced cancer (REIC) is appreciable for some cases and some cancer incidence, such as skin cancer and leukaemia.

5. Acknowledgements

This study has been approved by the Specialized Medical Safety Section of the Hospital La Fe from Valencia.

6. References

Barquinero JF et al (1999) Comparison of X-ray dose–response curves obtained by chromosome painting using conventional and PAINT nomenclatures *Int J Radiat Biol* 75 1557–1566.

Peer S et al (2003) Relevant training issues for introduction of digital radiology: results of a survey. *DIMOND Report.* Available at http://www.dimond3.org/Reports/WP%204/2-0Training%20needs%20.pdf

Edwards AA et al (2005) Review of Translocations detected by FISH for retrospective biological dosimetry *Radiat Prot Dosim* 81(2) 139-45.

IAEA (2001) Cytogenetic Analysis for Radiation Dose Assessment, A Manual. *Technical Reports Series* no. 405, International Atomic Energy Agency, Vienna

ICRP Publication 85 (2000) Avoidance of radiation injuries from medical interventional procedures

Kottou S et al. (2005) Correlation of patient and staff doses in interventional cardiology *Rad Prot Dos* 1-4

Lindholm C et al (2002) Intercomparison of translocation and dicentric frequencies between laboratories in a follow-up of the radiological accident in Estonia *Int J Radiat Biol* 78 883–890.

Lloyd DC et al (1998) Accidental intake of tritiated water: A cytogenetic follow-up case on translocation stability and dose reconstruction *Int J Radiat Biol* 73 543–547.

Montoro A et al (2005) Biological dosimetry in a group of radiologists by the analysis of dicentrics and translocations *Rad Res* 164(5) 612-17.

Ramos M et al (2005) Use of risk projection models to estimate mortality and incidence from radiation-induced breast cancer in screening programs *Phys Med Biol* 50 505-520

Shrimali R, Jain AM, Shastri KD (1972) Radiation injuries of hand of radiologists (case reports). *The Journal of the Association of Physicians of India* 20(3) 269-71

UNSCEAR (2000) Sources and Effects of Ionizing Radiation: 2000 Report. *General Assembly, Scientific Annexes.* United Nations, New York

Vanagunas A, Jacob P, Olinger E (1990) Radiation-Induced Esophageal Injury: A Spectrum from Esophagitis to Cancer *Am J Gastroenterol* 85 808-12.

Vano E, Arranz L, Sastre JM, Moro C, Ledo A, Garate M, et al (1998) Dosimetric and radiation protection considerations based on some cases of patient skin injuries in interventional cardiology *Br J Radiol* 71

Vano E, Gonzalez L, Beneytez F, Moreno F. (1998) Lens injury by occupational exposure in non-optimised interventional radiology laboratories Br J Radiol 71

Vano E and Gonzalez L (2004) Avoiding radiation injuries from interventional fluoroscopic procedures. *European Radiology Supplements* 59-65

24

Nonlinear Projective Filtering of ECG Signals

Marian Kotas
Silesian University of Technology, Institute of Electronics
Poland

1. Introduction

Since the beginnings of the noninvasive electrocardiology, development of the methods for reconstruction of the electrocardiogram (ECG) embedded in noise has stimulated the progress in the field. The predominant types of noise are baseline wander, powerline interference, electromyographic (EMG) noise and motion artifacts. Among them EMG and motion artifacts are the most difficult to be suppressed. It stems from the fact that their frequency spectra overlap that of the desired ECG, which makes the classical band-pass filtering ineffective. To mitigate the problem, the synchronized averaging was introduced. The method assumes that the ECG signal is repeatable and that the noise is additive, independent and of zero mean. Linear time-alignment (Jane et al. 1991) of the respective ECG beats and construction of an average one results in significant suppression of the noise; however, the inter-beat variability of the cardiac cycles is lost.

In many applications it is advantageous to suppress noise while preserving the variability of the desired signal morphology. In such cases, it is more advantageous to create a space of possible shapes instead of constructing an average template. This task can be accomplished with the help of principal component analysis (PCA) (Olmos et al., 1999; Kotas, 2006). In (Paul, 2000) the signal subspaces were constructed in the discrete cosine transform domain. However, modeling ECG beats with the help of the intrinsically linear PCA allows a limited success only (Kotas, 2006). In (Hu & Nenov, 2006) construction of the signal subspaces was preceded with the nonlinear alignment of ECG beats. New capabilities emerged when the method of nonlinear state-space projections (NSSP) was applied to ECG processing (Schreiber & Kaplan, 1996). Although this method also performs locally linear projections, globally the operation is nonlinear and allows more effective processing of the signal. This version of nonlinear projective filtering (NPF) was compared (Hu & Nenov, 2006) to several other sophisticated methods of ECG noise suppression and achieved the best results in EMG noise environment. NPF allows not only a kind of smoothing of ECG signals but can also be used for separation of signal components with overlapping spectra. It was successfully applied (Richter et al., 1998) to fetal ECG extraction from the maternal abdominal signals.

Although NSSP method offers so advantageous performance, its practical applications are limited by the high computational costs. In (Kotas, 2004) linear time-alignment of the ECG beats was used to decrease the number of the constructed signal subspaces. In the conditions tested, projective filtering of time-aligned ECG beats (PFTAB) was several hundreds faster than NSSP. Moreover, PFTAB appeared rather effective in EMG noise

environment. This method can be regarded as an extension of time averaging, preserving the deviations of the individual beats from the average one. However, when the length of the individual beats and the positions of the low amplitude ECG waves are highly variable, its performance can decrease. The method of dynamic time warping (Sakoe & Chiba, 1978) helped to overcome the problem. Projective filtering of time-warped ECG beats (PFTWEB) appeared much more effective in such conditions (Kotas, 2008b).
Application of nonlinear projective filtering to ECG reconstruction prior to the analysis of the ventricular repolarization significantly improves the accuracy of the measurements (Kotas, 2007a). The ability of the method to extract the fetal ECG from the maternal abdominal electric signals was demonstrated in (Kotas, 2007b).
The aim of this study is to reveal the fundamental differences among the mentioned versions of the nonlinear projective filtering and to present how these differences influence the NPF performance. In sections 2, 3 and 4 the necessary details of the compared methods operation are reminded. The differences among the methods and their applications are studied in section 5. The final conclusions are formulated in section 6.

2. Nonlinear state-space projections

The method was proposed by (Schreiber & Kaplan, 1996) as an effective tool for suppression of the wide-band electromyographic noise, contaminating the ECG signals. It forms the state-space representation of the observed noisy signal by application of the embedding operation (Schreiber & Kaplan, 1996). A point in the embedding space is a vector:

$$\mathbf{x}^{(n)} = [\, x(n), x(n+\tau), \ldots, x(n+(m-1)\tau\,]^{\mathrm{T}} \tag{1}$$

where $x(n)$ is the processed signal, τ is the time lag (τ=1 in this application), m is the embedding dimension.
For each point $\mathbf{x}^{(n)}$ a small neighborhood $\Gamma^{(n)}$ is constructed, composed of the points which are close to $\mathbf{x}^{(n)}$

$$\Gamma^{(n)} = \left\{ k : \left\| \mathbf{x}^{(k)} - \mathbf{x}^{(n)} \right\| \leq \varepsilon \right\} \tag{2}$$

where $\|.\|$ denotes the distance, ε is the radius of the neighborhood (Schreiber, 1995).
Within each neighborhood the local mean is computed (the neighborhood mass center)

$$\overline{\mathbf{x}}^{(n)} = \frac{1}{\left|\Gamma^{(n)}\right|} \sum_{k \in \Gamma^{(n)}} \mathbf{x}^{(k)} \tag{3}$$

($|\Gamma^{(n)}|$ denotes the cardinality of $\Gamma^{(n)}$) and the covariance matrix $\mathbf{C}^{(n)}$ of the neighborhood points deviations from the mass center (Schreiber & Kaplan, 1996). Then the transformed version of the covariance matrix is calculated $\mathbf{G}^{(n)}=\mathbf{R}\mathbf{C}^{(n)}\mathbf{R}$. $\mathbf{R}$ is a diagonal penalty matrix introduced to penalize the corrections of the first and the last coordinates of $\mathbf{x}^{(n)}$ ($r_{1,1} = r_{m,m} = r$, where r is large (Schreiber & Kaplan, 1996), and the other diagonal entries of $\mathbf{R}$ are equal to 1). The transformed covariance matrix undergoes eigendecomposition, and the calculated eigenvectors $\mathbf{e}_i^{(n)}$ corresponding to the largest eigenvalues are used to compose the so-called signal subspace. After constructing the subspace of the assumed dimension q ($q < m$) the point $\mathbf{x}^{(n)}$ is projected into this subspace

$$\mathbf{x}'^{(n)} = \bar{\mathbf{x}}^{(n)} + \mathbf{R}^{-1}\mathbf{E}_q^{(n)}\mathbf{E}_q^{(n)\mathrm{T}}\mathbf{R}\left(\mathbf{x}^{(n)} - \bar{\mathbf{x}}^{(n)}\right) \qquad (4)$$

where $\mathbf{E}_q^{(n)} = [\mathbf{e}_1^{(n)}, ..., \mathbf{e}_q^{(n)}]$.
The projection is performed for each trajectory point. Since each sample of the processed signal occurs in m points, its correction is a result of m individual corrections. It can be calculated as their average (Schreiber & Kaplan, 1996).

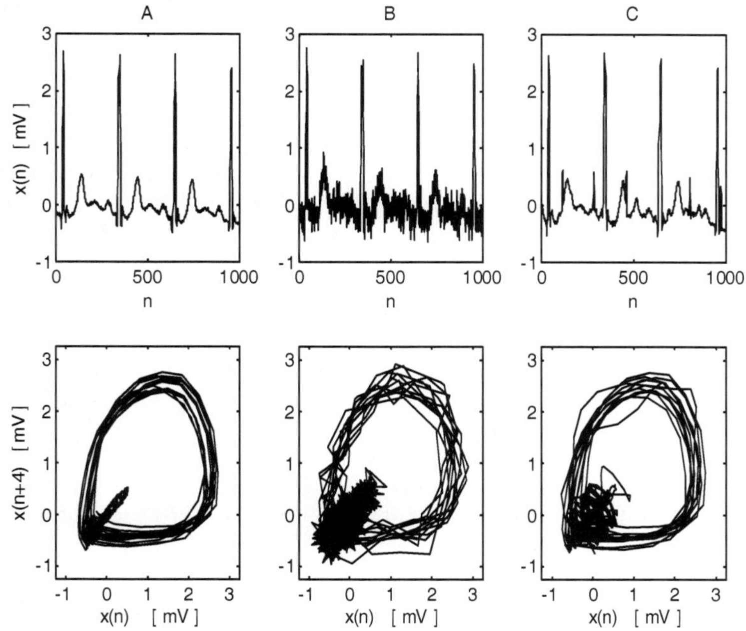

Fig. 1. Embedding space trajectories obtained for: a high quality ECG (A), the ECG with white Gaussian noise (B) and the simulated signal of a pregnant woman (C).

Since high dimensional embedding cannot be shown graphically, two-dimensional trajectories were presented in Fig.1. Although for noise reduction much higher embeddings are required, even such two-dimensional representation reveals some interesting properties of the ECG signal state-space structure. The trajectory of a high quality ECG (A) is close to a nonlinear manifold. For the same desired ECG contaminated with white Gaussian noise, the trajectory fluctuates around the "clean" one. Similarly, addition of the fetal ECG (C) results in the appearance of small loops circulating around the "clean" trajectory.

The described method (NSSP) is aimed to create locally linear signal subspaces for the respective points of the state-space trajectory. By projecting the points into these subspaces we shift the trajectory towards the "clean" one and, as a result, we suppress noise preserving the fluctuations of the desired ECG. Averaging of locally linear projections results in globally nonlinear transformation of the trajectory. Similar transformation of the trajectories obtained for the maternal abdominal signals (see Fig.1 C) results in suppression of the fetal electrocardiogram (FECG) and estimation of the maternal ECG (MECG). To extract the FECG, we simply subtract the estimated MECG from the original abdominal composite signal.

The ability of NSSP to suppress the wide-band ECG noise while preserving the desired component morphological variability and even to separate the signal components of similar spectral properties (MECG and FECG) is a great advantage. Another advantage is that the method is very general. It can be applied without a complicated adjustment of its action to processing of different signals. However, its practical applications are limited by the extremely high computational costs (resulting from the fact that for each point of the state-space trajectory we have to determine the neighborhood and to create the signal subspace individually). To reduce these computational costs, the approach preceded by ECG beats time-alignment was developed (Kotas, 2004). This operation allows limiting the number of the constructed signal subspaces to the number of different positions within a beat, and the points occupying the same position within different beats can be projected into the same subspace.

3. Projective filtering of time-aligned ECG beats

In this method, construction of signal subspaces and state-space projections are preceded (Kotas, 2004) with the following operations:

- Linear filtering for baseline wander and power line interference suppression (Wariar & Eswaran, 1991),
- QRS complex detection (Hamilton & Tompkins, 1986),
- Beats classification as either dominant or aberrant (Pahlm & Sörnmo 1987): the latter are excluded from further analysis, as well as the beats preceded or followed by aberrant ones,
- Cross-correlation function based synchronization of the detected complexes.

The last operation produces a set of fiducial marks $\{r_k \mid k=1,2,\ldots,K\}$ corresponding to the same position within the respective detected QRS complexes. Once the fiducial marks are established, the intrinsic operations of the method can be realized.

Each beat begins the assumed number of samples before its fiducial mark and ends one sample before the beginning of the next beat (Kotas, 2004). In order to facilitate construction of local signal subspaces (LSS), the respective beats are stored in an auxiliary matrix $\mathbf{T}$ (although in this method the term local refers to the position within a beat, it is also related with the points location in the embedding space). Each beat occupies one column of $\mathbf{T} = [\mathbf{t}_k]_{k=1}^{k=K}$. The number of rows (which is denoted as I) depends on the length of the longest beat ($RR_{\max}$). It must be large enough to allow construction of a signal subspace for the position $j = RR_{\max}$. Thus $I = RR_{\max}+(m\text{-}1)$, and all the beats in $\mathbf{T}$ are extended to this length - the method of zero order extension, which extends a beat by repeating its last sample (Chou, 2006), is applied.

Time-alignment of the beats enables easy determination of LSS corresponding to the respective positions within a beat. To this end, for each j $(1 \leq j \leq RR_{max})$ a submatrix of **T** is selected (Kotas, 2004)

$$\mathbf{T}^{(j)} = [\mathbf{t}_k^{(j)}]_{k=1}^{k=K} = [t_{i,k}^{(j)}]_{i,k=1}^{i=m,k=K}, \quad \text{where } t_{i,k}^{(j)} = t_{i-1+j,k} \tag{5}$$

containing the vectors $\mathbf{t}_k^{(j)}$, which correspond to the synchronized trajectory points.
To make construction of signal subspaces more robust against outliers, we form a local neighborhood $\Gamma^{(j)}$ by rejecting the assumed fraction c_R of the most distant points. After determination of the local neighborhood, the local mean $\bar{\mathbf{t}}^{(j)}$ is computed and the covariance matrix $\mathbf{C}^{(j)}$ - of the deviations from the mean. In projective filtering of time-aligned ECG beats, the concept of penalizing the corrections of the first and the last coordinates of the embedding space vectors was desisted (Kotas, 2004). A local signal subspace corresponding to the jth neighborhood is calculated by eigendecomposition of the covariance matrix $\mathbf{C}^{(j)}$.
After creating the signal subspaces for the respective positions within an ECG beat (the learning phase of PFTAB), the processing phase begins. It consists of the following steps: determination of a position j within a beat, the point under correction occupies; projecting the considered point into the corresponding signal subspace; averaging of the results of the respective points projection (Kotas, 2004).
The introduced modifications significantly decreased the computational costs of NSSP. Moreover, PFTAB appeared not only much faster, but also rather effective in processing the ECG signals disturbed by EMG noise (the influence of noise on determination of neighborhoods was cancelled). This property appeared particularly advantageous when application of projective filtering to fetal ECG extraction was studied (Kotas, 2007b). Unfortunately, high fluctuations of the cycles length and large temporal shifts of the low amplitude ECG waves can decrease PFTAB performance. Therefore a new version of nonlinear projective filtering was developed (Kotas 2008b). In this version, the method of dynamic time warping (Sakoe & Chiba, 1978) was applied to neighborhoods determination.

4. Projective Filtering of Time Warped ECG Beats

The preprocessing steps of the method are the same as in PFTAB. They produce a set of fiducial marks $\{r_k \mid k=1,2,\ldots, K\}$ corresponding to the same position within the respective detected QRS complexes. The embedding space points are divided into successive, slightly overlapping sequences of vectors whose time indices belong to the following sets

$$\Psi_k = \{a_k + l \mid l = 0,1,\ldots,N_k\}, \quad k = 1,2,\ldots,K-1 \tag{6}$$

where

$$a_k = r_k - b - \tfrac{m}{2}, \quad N_k = r_{k+1} - r_k + 2b \tag{7}$$

$b \in N$ is a small number introduced to immunize the method against small errors of the fiducial marks determination (Kotas, 2008b).

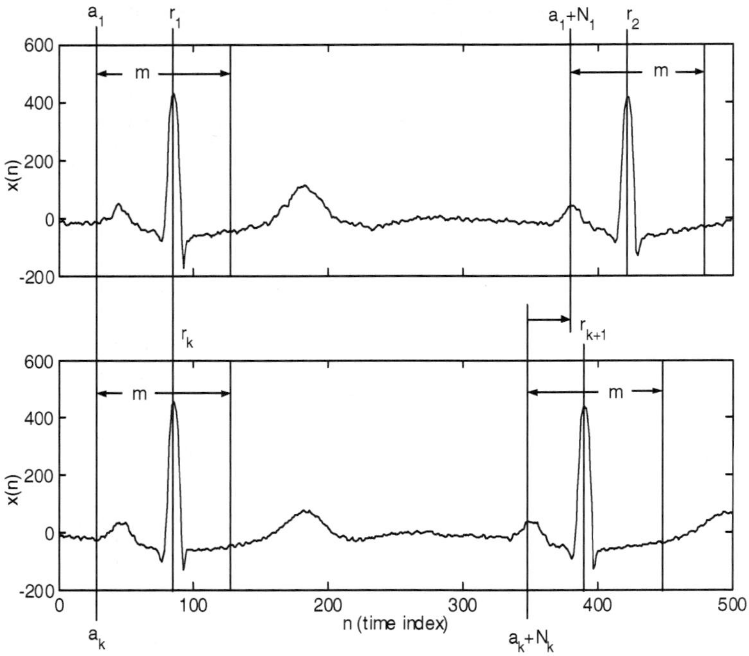

Fig. 2. The ECG signal sections containing successive QRS complexes. The presented delay windows show the first and the last state-space points of Ψ_1 and Ψ_k respectively. The kth sequence of points is time warped with respect to the first one.

The general concept (Kotas, 2008b) is to perform the nonlinear alignment of the successive sequences of vectors (Ψ_k, k = 2, 3, ... K-1) with respect to the first sequence and this way to determine the neighborhoods corresponding to the respective positions within Ψ_1.

For small b the side points $\mathbf{x}^{(a_1)}$ and $\mathbf{x}^{(a_1+N_1)}$ overlap QRS complexes (see Fig.2), and thus their neighborhoods can be determined on the basis of the preprocessing step results:

$$\Gamma^{(a_1)} = \left\{a_k \;\middle|\; k = 1,2,...,K-1\right\}$$
$$\Gamma^{(a_1+N_1)} = \left\{a_k + N_k \;\middle|\; k = 1,2,...,K-1\right\} \tag{8}$$

Determination of the neighborhoods corresponding to the respective positions within Ψ_1 is performed in the following way (Kotas, 2008b).

1) In the first step each neighborhood of a point from Ψ_1 is filled with this point only, and so the time index of this point is included in the neighborhood set

$$\Gamma^{(a_1+l)} = \{a_1 + l\}, \quad l = 0,1,...,N_1 \tag{9}$$

These points become the first mass centers of the respective neighborhoods. Then we set $k = 2$ and go to the next step.

2) The sequences of points that belong to Ψ_k are time warped with respect to the sequence of the mass centers. For this purpose, the so-called warping paths are calculated: $w_{k,l}$, $l = 0, 1, \dots, N_1$, containing the indices of the vectors $\mathbf{x}^{(a_k+w_{k,l})}$ that are aligned with the successive mass centers $\overline{\mathbf{x}}^{(a_1+l)}$. The warping path is calculated by minimizing

$$Q_k = \sum_{l=0}^{N_1} \left\| \mathbf{x}^{(a_k+w_{k,l})} - \overline{\mathbf{x}}^{(a_1+l)} \right\| \tag{10}$$

while preserving the border conditions, the monotonicity conditions and the condition restricting the number of successive points from Ψ_k that may be omitted in the warping path (Kotas, 2008a). The minimization is performed with the use of the dynamic programming (Sakoe & Chiba, 1978).

3) After the kth sequence Ψ_k has been time warped with respect to the sequence of the mass centers, the neighborhoods are supplemented with the points whose indices are stored in the warping path

$$\Gamma^{(a_1+l)} = \Gamma^{(a_1+l)} \cup \left\{ a_k + w_{k,l} \right\} \tag{11}$$

4) The mass centers of the respective neighborhoods are updated and k is incremented. If $k < K$-1 we go to step 2, otherwise we end the algorithm.

After determination of the respective neighborhoods, the corresponding signal subspaces are constructed. As in PFTAB, to make the constructed subspaces robust against outliers, in each neighborhood the assumed fraction c_R of the most distant points is rejected. Construction of signal subspaces for the respective positions within Ψ_1 ends the learning phase of PFTWEB. The processing phase, as in PFTAB, consists of state-space points projecting and introduced corrections averaging - for details see (Kotas, 2008b).

5. Results

In this section, we will first observe and analyze the differences among the compared versions of nonlinear projective filtering. Then we will study the chosen versions ability to suppress noise or to separate the signal components with overlapping spectra.

5.1 Distributions of neighborhoods points

Different approaches to neighborhoods determination result in different contents and properties of the constructed neighborhoods.

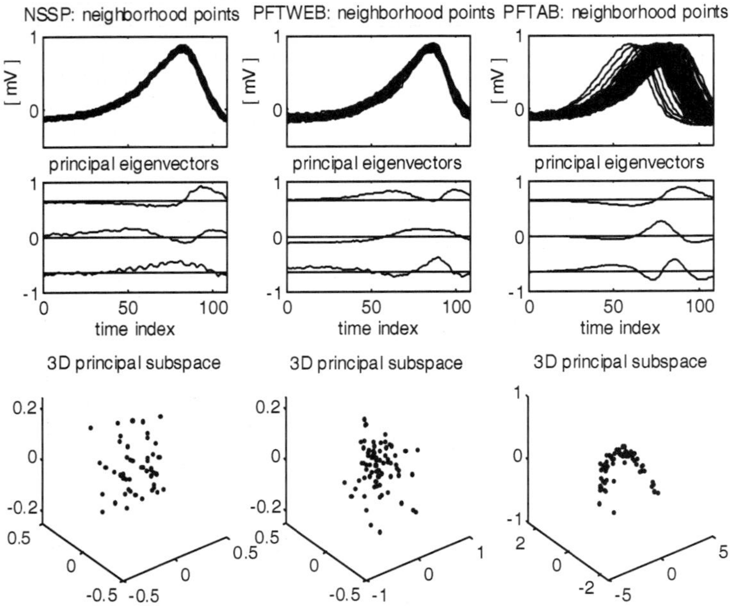

Fig. 3. The neighborhoods determined by the respective methods while processing a high quality signal with a shifting T wave. The uppermost are one-dimensional representations of the neighborhood points; below, the first three principal eigenvectors - vertically shifted; below, distributions of the neighborhoods points in 3D principal subspaces.

In Fig.3 we can see that one-dimensional representations of the points included into the neighborhood by NSSP are very close to each other. Their dispersion in the three-dimensional principal subspace is very low. The neighborhood was determined to perform reconstruction of one state-space point only. Since this point must be located close to the center of the presented cloud of points, a high precision of reconstruction is possible even for a very low dimension of the signal subspace.

The neighborhood determined by PFTAB is of much higher dispersion. It is caused by different positions of the individual T waves within the ECG beats. The characteristic structure of the points three-dimensional representation reveals nonlinear relations among them. For so low level of noise, higher variability of the desired component assured determination of very smooth principal eigenvectors. However, since many points of the neighborhood are located very far from the mass center, much higher dimension of the signal subspace is necessary for their precise reconstruction.

Applying nonlinear alignment of the sequences of state-space vectors (PFTWEB), we achieved relatively precise synchronization of the T waves. Although the dispersion of points is larger than that achieved by NSSP, it is much smaller than that obtained by PFTAB. As a result, the dimension of the signal subspace doesn't have to be so high as for PFTAB.

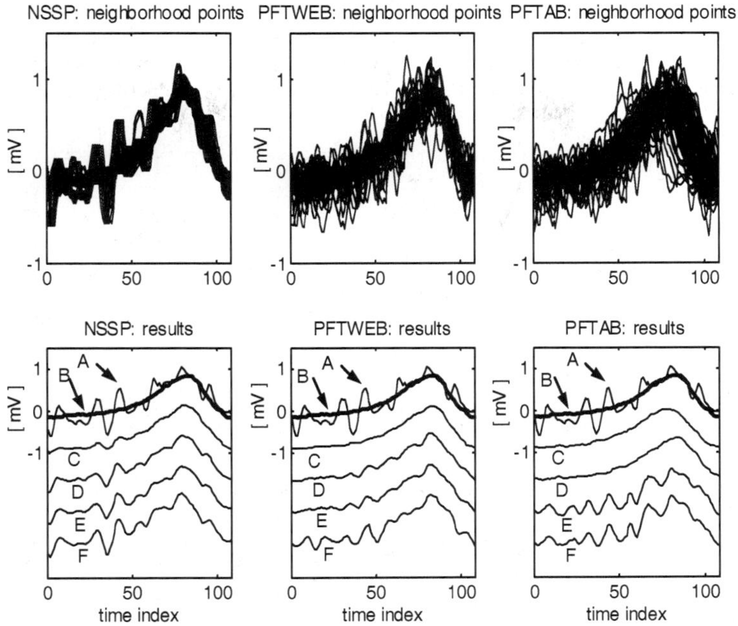

Fig. 4. Results of a state-space point reconstruction in the simulated EMG noise environment: A - the point under reconstruction; B - the desired component of A; C - the neighborhood mass center; D,E,F - results of reconstruction for the signal subspace dimension of 1, 2 and 3 respectively (C,D,E,F are vertically shifted).

The influence of real electromyographic, highly correlated noise on state-space points reconstruction was illustrated in Fig. 4. For NSSP not only the desired, but also the noise component had a great impact on neighborhood determination (the noise deviations from the desired component are well synchronized). As a result, even the neighborhood mass center (C) contains a discernible noise component. With increasing dimension of the signal subspace, suppression of noise was less and less effective.

For PFTAB the noise components of the neighborhood points are not synchronized and calculation of the mass center caused their effective suppression. Although the mass center (C) is shifted with respect to the desired component (B), for q=1 relatively precise reconstruction was achieved - with effective suppression of noise.

Application of dynamic time warping allowed more flexible determination of the neighborhood with rather low influence of noise. It improved calculation of the neighborhood mass center, which is visually free of noise and closer to the desired component (B) than the mass center constructed by PFTAB. However, for increasing q the suppression of noise was less and less effective.

Separation of the maternal and the fetal ECG is even more difficult than suppression of EMG noise. In the first stage, projective filtering is applied to suppress the fetal component and to estimate the maternal ECG. In the second stage, the estimated MECG is subtracted from the original composite signal and this way suppressed. As a result, the fetal component is extracted. However, when the estimated MECG contains some residua of the fetal QRS complexes, its subtraction causes inconvenient suppression of the fetal ECG.

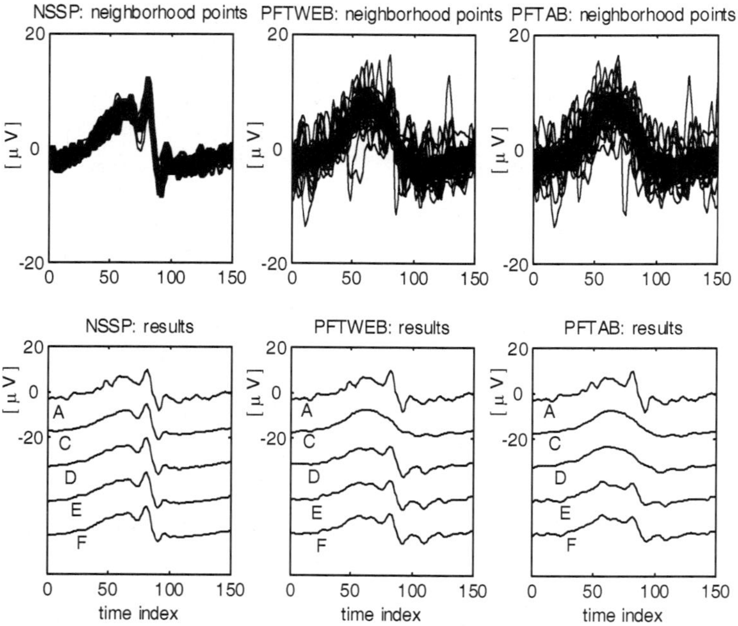

Fig. 5. Results of a state-space point reconstruction for the real maternal abdominal signal (the point corresponds to the maternal T wave with the overlapping fetal QRS complex). The further description is as in Fig.4. For this signal the desired component (B) was not available.

Reconstruction of the point corresponding to the maternal T wave with the overlapping fetal QRS complex is illustrated in Fig. 5. In this case NSSP failed. Most points of the neighborhood contained a fetal QRS complex and were synchronized with respect to it. As a result, the complex was preserved in the neighborhood mass center (C) and, consequently, the state-space projection could not have caused its suppression. For PFTWEB the complex was suppressed by calculation of the mass center. However, projections into the principal subspaces of different non-zero dimension resulted in its reconstruction. Only PFTAB allowed suppressing the fetal complex for non-zero dimension of the signal subspace.

Although many factors influence state-space points reconstruction, and in different conditions the results can be quite different, the presented cases were chosen to illustrate the most typical action of the compared methods. We can conclude that PFTWEB is most appropriate for ECG enhancement in EMG noise environment, but PFTAB allows most effective extraction of the fetal ECG.

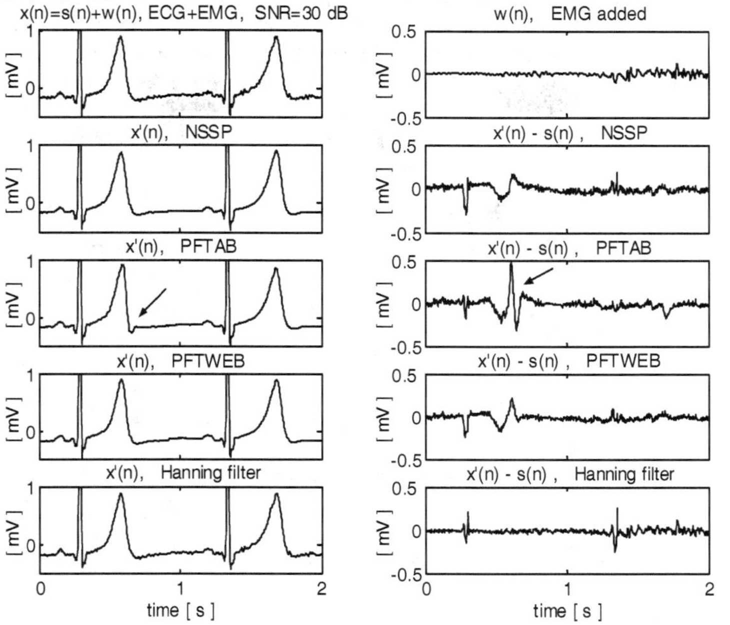

Fig. 6. Results of ECG signal filtering in a case of the significantly shifted T wave. The arrows indicate poor results obtained by PFTAB.

5.2 Suppression of noise versus precision of the desired ECG reconstruction

The most important parameters of the projective filters are: embedding dimension (m) and the dimension of signal subspaces (q). When the level of noise is low, it is crucial to assure high precision of the desired component reconstruction. To achieve it, we can either increase q or decrease m. For higher level of noise, however, it is very important to assure its effective suppression. It can be achieved by decreasing q or increasing m. In (Kotas, 2008c) the parameters balancing both requirements (for SNR=10 dB) were chosen: τ_m=500 ms and q=1 for NSSP; τ_m=200 ms and q=2 for PFTAB; τ_m=400 ms and q=2 for PFTWEB (τ_m is the embedding window width, corresponding to m, independent from the sampling frequency applied).

The precision of the desired component reconstruction, offered by the respective filters for the above parameters, is illustrated in Fig.6. For reference the results obtained by application of the low-pass Hanning filter ($H(z)=(z+2+z^{-1})/4$) are presented. The processed signal characteristic feature is high variability of the QT interval. Particularly the first T wave in the presented signal segment is considerably shifted to the left. For q=2, PFTAB was not able to reconstruct the shifted wave precisely. Much better results were achieved by both NSSP and PFTWEB.

Analyzing the residual noise ($x'(n)$-$s(n)$) obtained for NSSP and PFTWEB, we can notice that the first QRS complex was reconstructed with lower precision than the second one. It was caused by the influence of the shifted T wave of high amplitude on determination of neighborhoods for the points overlapping both the QRS complex and the T wave. For the first complex in the figure, the amplitude of the residual noise is comparable for all filters applied. However, for the second one, the Hanning filter introduces much higher disturbances than any of the three projective filters compared.

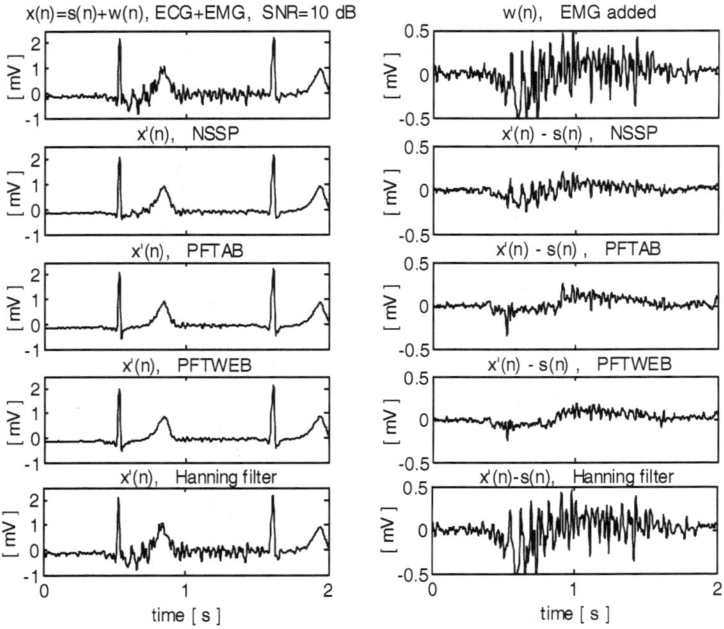

Fig. 7. Results of ECG signal filtering for a moderate level of the EMG noise.

The ability of the projective filters to suppress the EMG noise was illustrated in Fig.7. In the presented example, PFTWEB performed best, but PFTAB achieved rather comparable results. NSSP caused significant suppression of noise as well; however, for this filter energy of the residual EMG noise was clearly higher. The Hanning filter, which introduces similar distortions of the QRS complex as the projective filters (see Fig.6), caused hardly any suppression of the EMG noise. Concluding, nonlinear projective filtering allows much more effective processing of the ECG signals, with higher precision of the desired component reconstruction and better suppression of noise. Among the compared versions of NPF, the best compromise between both requirements was achieved by PFTWEB.

5.3 NPF for reliable evaluation of the repolarization duration (RD) variability

The time between depolarization and repolarization of the ventricles is covered by the QT interval (from the QRS onset to the T wave end). It is an important electrocardiographic parameter, often used to quantify the duration of ventricular repolarization (Malik, 2000).

Since precise determination of the QRS onset and the T wave end is relatively difficult, new variables were defined to evaluate the repolarization duration variability. The problem is discussed at length in (Merri et al., 1993; Tikkanen et al., 1999). According to (Tikkanen et al., 1999) the most precise measurement of RD can be obtained if the left limit of the repolarization interval is defined as the position of the R wave maximum (R) and the right limit as the position of the T wave peak (Tp). According to (Merri et al., 1993) the RTp interval is highly correlated with the actual QT interval; therefore, it can be used for the analysis of repolarization duration variability. In (Kotas 2008c) the experiments with the latest version of the nonlinear projective filtering were performed. NPF improved evaluation of RD variability both in time and frequency domain. This area of projective filtering applications is discussed in this subsection.

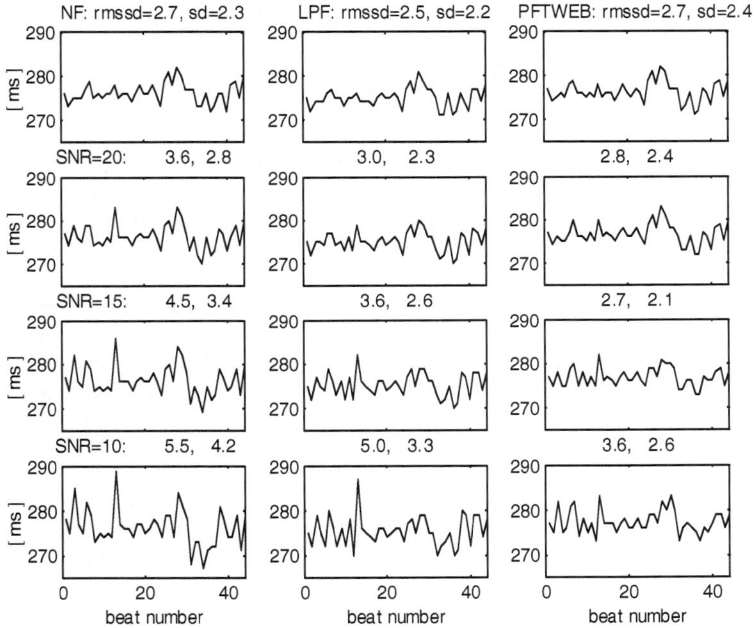

Fig. 8. The RTp series determined on the basis of a high quality ECG (the uppermost) and the ECG with EMG noise added (below). Each series is evaluated with two indices of variability: SD and RMSSD - defined by (12). The columns correspond to the filtering operations executed before the measurements (NF denotes "not filtered").

Fig.8 presents the RTp series determined on the basis of a high quality ECG from the QT database (Laguna et al., 1997) and for the signals with EMG noise added. For the localization of the T wave peak, the procedure developed by (Laguna et al., 1990) and modified by (Tikkanen et al., 1999) was used; for the precise description - see (Kotas, 2007a). The procedure was applied to the original (not filtered) signals and to the signals enhanced by different operations. Since the measurements of the repolarization duration can be performed for high quality signals only, and the precision of the desired signal reconstruction is of the primary interest, PFTWEB was applied with q=3 for τ_m=400 ms (the dimension of the signal subspaces is higher than in the previous experiments). For reference the low-pass filter with the cut-off frequency of 15 Hz, which had appeared effective in (Kotas 2008c), was employed.

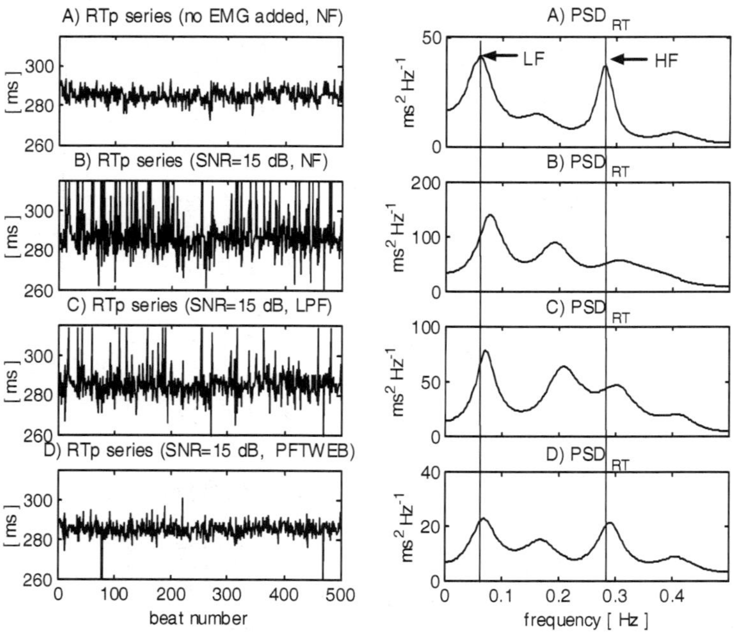

Fig. 9. Spectral analysis of RTp interval variability: A) the series obtained for a high quality ECG; B,C,D) the series obtained after different filtering operations, for the signal with EMG added. LF and HF are the low and the high frequency peaks of the true PSD (of series A).

The determined time series are evaluated with two indices of variability: the standard deviation (SD) and the root mean square of the successive differences (Tikkanen et al., 1999)

$$RMSSD_x = \sqrt{\frac{1}{N-1}\sum_{n=1}^{N-1}\left(x(n+1)-x(n)\right)^2} \qquad (12)$$

where $x(n)$, n = 1, 2, …, N is the analyzed time series.

We can notice that addition of even very weak noise (SNR=20 dB) raises the errors of the measurements performed on the original not filtered (NF) signals. Since the RD measurement errors increase the RD series variability, for the growing level of noise the variability indices grow as well. Application of low-pass filtering slightly decreased the measurement errors and the growth of the indices. However, PFTWEB allowed much more precise measurements and, as a result, most reliable evaluation of the RTp series variability in time domain.

The PFTWEB influence on spectral analysis of the RTp intervals variability was illustrated in Fig.9. The uppermost on the left is the series established on the basis of a high quality ECG signal from the QT database. When the signal was contaminated by the EMG noise of highly variable level (the average SNR=15 dB), localization of the T wave maximum failed in numerous cases. As a result, series B is rather jagged - corrupted by large measurement errors. Preceding the measurements with low-pass filtering slightly improved the measurements - the number of large errors decreased. However, application of PFTWEB caused much more significant improvement of the results. Only a few large errors of RTp interval determination occurred.

For each RTp series determined, the following operations were performed: large measurement errors were detected and replaced by the preceding values, the corrected series was resampled with the frequency of 1 Hz (by application of first order interpolation) and then filtered to remove the low frequency trend (the Butterworth high-pass filter with the cut-off frequency of 0.02 Hz was applied in forward and reverse direction). The power spectra were estimated by application of the autoregressive modeling (Lim & Oppenheim, 1988) with the model order equal to 10.

The repolarization interval series often contain the oscillatory components of low frequency (LF) - close to 0.1 Hz - related with the slow waves of the arterial pressure, and high frequency (HF) - close to 0.25 Hz - related with respiration (Lombardi et al., 1996). For series A both components are distinct. However, addition of EMG noise to the analyzed ECG signal resulted in numerous measurement errors which spoiled not only the time properties of the determined RTp series, but also deformed their power spectra. Only after projective filtering (D) the two highest spectral peaks are close to the original ones (A). Thus, nonlinear projective filtering allowed most reliable analysis of the repolarization duration variability also in the frequency domain.

5.4 NPF for fetal ECG extraction

An important area of projective filtering applications is related with processing and analysis of the maternal abdominal electric signals for extraction of the fetal component (Richter et al., 1998; Kotas, 2007b). NPF can be combined with spatial approaches to achieve FECG signal enhancement (Kotas, 2008a) or even to perform separation of the multiple FECG signals in twin pregnancies (Kotas et. al., 2008b). In this chapter, we study the influence of NPF on the results of fetal QRS complexes detection. This issue is of high significance, because the noninvasive fetal electrocardiography offers higher accuracy of fetal heart rate monitoring than the routine instrumentation based on the Doppler ultrasound technique (Jeżewski, Wrobel & Horoba, 2006). The applied detection method consists of linear band-pass filtering for noise attenuation, differentiation for QRS slopes estimation, squaring and moving window integration and, finally, comparison with the threshold for QRS peaks localization (Kotas et al, 2008a).

As it was mentioned in $5.1, separation of the maternal and the fetal ECG in a single-channel signal can be accomplished in two stages. First, projective filtering is applied to suppress the fetal component and to estimate the maternal ECG. Then, the estimated MECG is subtracted from the original composite signal and this way suppressed. As a result, the fetal component is extracted. This procedure was illustrated in Fig.10. The uppermost, on both sides of the figure, is the composite maternal abdominal signal obtained after high-pass filtering. Since fetal QRS detection was of interest, and the requirements limiting distortions of the desired component did not have to be satisfied, a relatively high cut-off frequency of 5 Hz was applied. The results of MECG enhancement by application of PFTAB (the most appropriate for FECG extraction, as we inferred in $5.1) are presented below on the left; the FECG extracted - on the right.

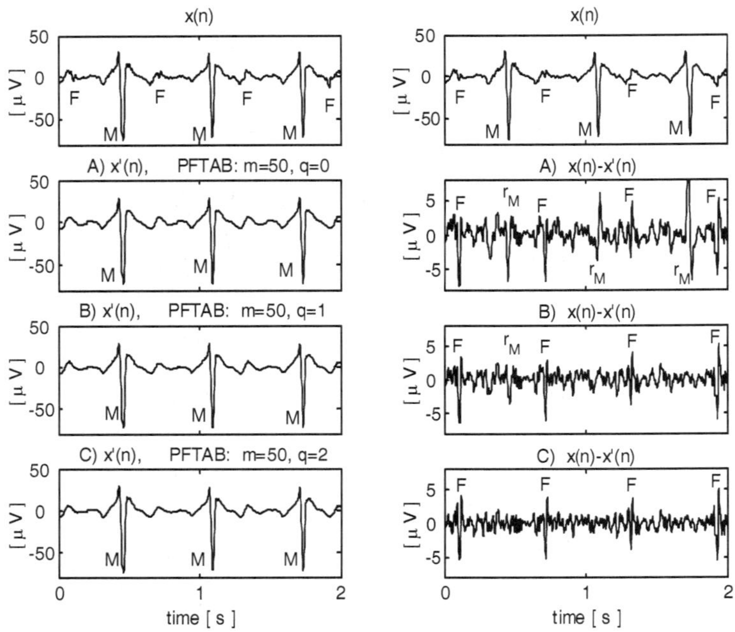

Fig. 10. The maternal abdominal signal (the uppermost on both sides of the figure) and the results of MECG enhancement (on the left) and FECG extraction (on the right): F marks the fetal QRS complexes, M-the maternal ones and r_M-residua of the latter.

The figure illustrates the influence of the dimension q of local signal subspaces on MECG enhancement and FECG extraction. For q=0, the operation of PFTAB is similar to time-averaging, and the filter is not able to preserve the morphological changes of the respective maternal QRS complexes. As a result, the operation of subtraction produced the FECG signal corrupted with the residua of these complexes. For q=1, the residua were significantly smaller, and for q=2 they almost vanished. Unfortunately, for higher values of q projective filtering preserves some residua of fetal QRS complexes in the estimated MECG signal, and the subtraction leads to inconvenient suppression of these complexes. Different dimensions of local signal subspaces can be applied for different positions within a beat to improve the results of FECG extraction (Kotas, 2007b); however, this study is limited to the basic approach, and the constant dimensions are used.

For evaluation of PFTAB influence on the results of fetal QRS detection, ten four-channel signals (five minutes long) were used. For each signal, the fetal QRS complexes locations were marked manually and stored. In the experiments, PFTAB was applied with c_R=0.25, τ_m=200 ms and q varied from 1 to 3 to FECG extraction in the respective channels of the test signals. The test detections were performed in each channel separately.
Comparing the locations of the detected complexes with the previously stored reference ones, we can establish the number of missed complexes (N_M) and the number of false alarms (N_{FA}). Results of the detection tests are evaluated with the following performance index (Hamilton & Tompkins, 1986)

$$PI = \frac{N - N_{FA} - N_M}{N} \cdot 100[\%] \quad (13)$$

The obtained indices are presented in Table. 1.

PI [%]	c1	c2	c3	c4	c1-c4
PFTAB: q=1	93.3	96.8	94.1	79.2	90.9
PFTAB: q=2	94.2	96.5	95.9	83.4	92.5
PFTAB: q=3	93.0	96.1	95.4	80.7	91.3
TS	93.3	95.8	93.0	82.4	91.1
AICF	92.1	96.3	91.5	75.9	89.0

Table 1. Performance indices obtained for different methods of MECG suppression in the respective channels of the test signals and for all channels together.

For reference the detection tests were performed in the FECG signals extracted by application of the method of template subtraction (TS) and the method based on the adaptive impulse correlated filter (AICF). TS performs maternal QRS complexes detection, synchronization, time-averaging, scaling and subtraction. Moreover, it is modified by the additional operations (e.g. subtraction of the template derivative) decreasing the MECG residua and preventing the FECG suppression in cases of the maternal and the fetal complexes coincidence (Matonia et al., 2006). The second reference method employs AICF (Laguna et al. 1992) instead of PFTAB to MECG signal enhancement and then performs the operation of subtraction for FECG extraction. Before application of this method, the test signals, originally stored with the sampling frequency of 500 Hz, were resampled with the frequency of 1000 Hz to decrease the synchronization errors. After MECG suppression, the extracted FECGs were again resampled with the original frequency.
During recording of the test signals, the repeatable arrangement of electrodes on a surface of a maternal abdomen was applied (as described in (Kotas et al., 2008a)). Analyzing Table 1, we can infer that among the recorded channels, the second one most often contained the fetal ECG of the best quality. Since for high amplitude fetal QRS complexes the very precise suppression of the maternal ones is not crucial, in this channel the similar performance indices were obtained for all compared methods of MECG suppression. The best results were achieved by PFTAB applied with q=1. In the fourth channel, however, the amplitude of the fetal complexes was most often rather low, and the precision of MECG suppression was of high significance. For this channel, the differences among the compared methods were

the greatest, and PFTAB applied with q=2 was most effective. It was also most effective in the first and the third channel. We can conclude that among the compared methods of MECG suppression, the one based on projective filtering of time-aligned beats allows most effective detection of fetal QRS complexes in the signals of poor quality. This result is of high significance, because very often the diagnostic analysis of the signals from the maternal abdominal wall is hindered by difficulty in performing successful detection of the fetal QRS complexes.

6. Conclusion

Research in the field of nonlinear dynamics resulted in development of the method of nonlinear state-space projections, which can help to solve the very crucial problems related with ECG signals processing. The method forms the multidimensional state-space representation of the processed one-dimensional signals, determines the neighborhoods of all state-space points and creates the signal subspaces for the respective of them. Each state-space point undergoes projection into its individual signal subspace. Averaging the introduced corrections leads to reconstruction of the processed signal one-dimensional representation. NSSP method allows suppressing noise whose spectrum overlaps that of the desired signal. Moreover, it can be applied to the separation of signal components that are not separable in the frequency or time domain, such as the maternal and the fetal ECG contained in the maternal abdominal signals. However, a severe shortcoming of this method is its high computational cost. It results mostly from the necessity to create the signal subspaces for each state-space point individually.

This chapter describes the modifications of the NSSP method that highly decreased its costs and adjusted its operation to the particular properties of the processed ECG signals and, as a result, increased its performance in this field of application. The modifications are based on different approaches to the determination of neighborhoods. Linear time-alignment of the ECG beats allowed constructing the signal subspaces for the successive positions within a beat only. This significantly reduced the computational costs. Moreover, the developed method (PFTAB) almost completely cancelled the influence of high energy EMG noise, or the other signal components apart from the dominant one on determination of the neighborhoods. The performed experiments have proved that projective filtering of time-aligned ECG beats can successfully be applied to fetal ECG extraction from the maternal abdominal signals for fetal heart rate determination.

Application of nonlinear alignment of the sequences of state-space points to neighborhoods determination made the method more flexible. Although projective filtering of time warped ECG beats is less immune than PFTAB to such signal components as the fetal ECG, it allows more precise reconstruction of the desired ECG embedded in EMG noise. Applied to signal enhancement prior to the analysis of the dynamic changes of the low level ECG waves, it allowed precise evaluation of the beat-to-beat variability of the repolarization duration - both in time and frequency domain. The method can also be applied prior to the measurements of other indices quantifying the ventricular repolarization. This issue will be a topic of further study.

7. Acknowledgment

The author thanks Dr Janusz Jeżewski and the staff from the Institute of Medical Technology and Equipment, ITAM, for the access to the database of the maternal abdominal ECG signals.

8. References

Chou, H. H., Chen, Y. J., Shiau, Y. C. & Kuo T. S. (2006), An Effective and Efficient Compression Algorithm for ECG Signals With Irregular Periods", *IEEE Trans. Biomed. Eng.*, Vol. 53, pp. 1198-1205, ISSN: 0018-9294.

Hu, X., Nenov, V. (2006) A Single-Lead ECG Enhancement Algorithm Using a Regularized Data-Driven Filter, *IEEE Trans. Biomed. Eng.*, Vol. 53, pp. 347-351, ISSN: 0018-9294.

Hamilton, P. S. & Tompkins, W. J. (1986) Quantitative investigation of QRS detection rules using the MIT/BIH arrhythmia database, *IEEE Trans. Biomed. Eng.*, Vol. 33, pp. 1157-1165, ISSN:0018-9294.

Jane, R.; Rix, H., Caminal, P. & Laguna, P. (1991) Alignment Methods for Averaging of High Resolution Cardiac Signals: A Comparative Study of Performance, *IEEE Trans. Biomed. Eng.*, Vol. 38, pp. 571-579, ISSN:0018-9294.

Jeżewski, J., Wrobel, J., & Horoba, K. (2006) Comparison of Doppler Ultrasound and Direct Electrocardiography Acquisition Techniques for Quantification of Fetal Heart Variability, *IEEE Trans. Biomed. Eng.*, Vol. 53, pp. 855-864.

Kotas, M. (2004) Projective Filtering of Time-Aligned ECG Beats, *IEEE Trans. Biomed. Eng.*, Vol. 51, pp. 1129-1139, ISSN:0018-9294.

Kotas M. (2006) Application of projection pursuit based robust principal component analysis to ECG enhancement, *Biomed. Signal Process. Control,* Vol. 1, pp. 289-298.

Kotas M. (2007a) Projective filtering of time-aligned ECG beats for repolarization duration measurement, *Computer Methods and Programs in Biomedicine,* Vol. 85, No. 2, pp. 115-123, ISSN:0169-2607.

Kotas M. (2007b) Projective Filtering of Time-Aligned Beats for Foetal ECG extraction, *Bulletin of the Polish Academy of Sciences, Technical Sciences*, Vol. 55, No.4,pp. 331-339.

Kotas M. (2008a) Combined Application of Independent Component Analysis and Projective Filtering to Fetal ECG Extraction, *Biocybernetics and Biomedical Engineering,* Vol. 28, No. 1, pp. 75-93.

Kotas M. (2008b) Projective filtering of time warped ECG beats, *Computers in Biology and Medicine,* Vol. 38, No. 1, pp. 127-37, ISSN:0010-4825.

Kotas M. (2008c) Robust Projective Filtering of Time Warped ECG Beats, *Computer Methods and Programs in Biomedicine,* Vol. 92, No. 10, pp. 161-172, ISSN:0169-2607

Kotas, M., Jeżewski, J., Kupka, T. & Horoba K. (2008a) Detection of low amplitude fetal QRS complexes, in Proc. of 30th IEEE/EMBS Conference, pp. 4764-4767.

Kotas, M., Jeżewski, J., Matonia, A. & Kupka T. (2008b) Separation of abdominal fetal electrocardiograms in twin pregnancy, *Journal of Medical Informatics and Technologies*, Vol. 12, pp. 83-90.

Laguna, P., Thakor, N.V., Caminal, P., Jane, R., Yoon, H. (1990) New Algorithm for QT Interval Analysis in 24 Hour Holter ECG: Performance and Applications, *Med. Biol. Eng Comp.*, Vol. 28, pp. 67-73.

Laguna, P., Jane, R., Meste, O., Poon, P. W., Caminal P., Rix, H., Thakor, N. V. (1992) Adaptive Filter for Event-Related Bioelectric Signals Using Impulse Correlated Reference Input: Comparison with Signal Averaging Techniques, *IEEE Trans. Biomed. Eng.*, Vol.39, pp. 1032-1043, ISSN: 0018-9294

Laguna, P., Mark, R.G., Goldberg, A., & Moody, G.B. (1997) A Database for Evaluation of Algorithms for Measurement of QT and Other Waveform Intervals in the ECG, *Proceedings of Int. Conf. Computers in Cardiology,* pp. 673-676, ISBN 0-7803-4445-6, Lund, Sweden, Sep. 1997.

Lim, J. S., Oppenheim, A. V. (1988) Advanced Topics in Signal Processing, Prentice Hall, ISBN: 0130131296, Englewood Cliffs, New Jersey, USA.

Lombardi, F., Sandrone, G., Porta, A., Torzillo, D., Terranova, G., Baselli, G., Cerutti, S. & Malliani, A. (1996) Spectral analysis of short term R-Tapex interval variability during sinus rhythm and fixed atrial rate, *European Heart Journal,* Vol. 17, pp. 769-778.

Malik, M., & Batchvarov, V. (2000) Measurement, Interpretation and Clinical Potential of QT Dispersion, *J. Am. Coll. Cardiol.*, Vol. 36, pp. 1749-1766.

Matonia, A., Jeżewski, J., Horoba, K., Gacek, A. (2006) The Maternal ECG Suppression Algorithm for Efficient Extraction of the Fetal ECG from Abdominal Signal, *Proc. IEEE EMBS Conf.*, New York City, USA, pp. 3106-3109.

Merri, M., Alberti, M. & Moss, A. J. (1993) Dynamic Analysis of Ventricular Repolarization Duration from 24-hour Holter recordings, *IEEE Trans. Biomed. Eng.*, Vol. 40, pp. 1219-25, ISSN: 0018-9294.

Olmos, S., Garcia, J., Jane, R. & Laguna, P. (1999) ECG signal compression plus noise filtering with truncated orthogonal expansions, *Signal Processing,* Vol. 79,pp. 97-115, ISSN:0165-1684.

Pahlm, O. & Sörnmo, L. (1987) Data Processing of Exercise ECG's, *IEEE Trans. Biomed. Eng.*, Vol. 34, pp. 158-165, ISSN: 0018-9294.

Paul, J. S., Reddy, M. R. & Kumar V. J. (2000) A transform domain SVD filter for suppression of muscle noise artefacts in exercise ECG's, *IEEE Trans. Biomed. Eng.*, Vol. 47, No.5, pp. 654-663, ISSN: 0018-9294.

Richter, M., Schreiber, T., & Kaplan, D. T. (1998) Fetal ECG extraction with nonlinear state space projections, *IEEE Trans. Biomed. Eng.*, Vol. 45, pp. 133-137, ISSN: 0018-9294.

Sakoe, H. & Chiba, S. (1978) Dynamic programming optimization for spoken word recognition, *IEEE Trans. ASSP*, Vol. ASSP-26, pp.43-49.

Schreiber T. (1995) Efficient neighbor searching in nonlinear time series analysis, *Int. J. Bifurcation and Chaos*, Vol.5, pp. 349-358.

Schreiber, T. & Kaplan, D. (1996) Nonlinear Noise Reduction for Electrocardiograms, *Chaos*, Vol. 6, pp. 87-92.

Tikkanen, P. E., Sellin, L. C., Kinnunen, H. O., & Huikuri, H. V. (1999) Using simulated noise to define optimal QT intervals for computer analysis of ambulatory ECG, *Med. Eng. Physics*, Vol. 21, pp. 15-25.

Wariar, R. & Eswaran, C. (1991) Integer coefficient bandpass filter for the simultaneous removal of baseline wander, 50 and 100 Hz interference from the ECG, *Med. Biol. Eng. Comput.* Vol. 29, pp. 333-336.

Recent developments in computer methods for fMRI data processing

Evanthia E. Tripoliti and Dimitrios I. Fotiadis
University of Ioannina
Greece

1. Introduction

Functional Magnetic Resonance Imaging (fMRI) is a relatively new procedure which uses magnetic resonance imaging to measure tiny metabolic changes which take place in an active part of the brain. It is becoming a diagnostic method for learnng how a normal, disease or injured brain performs, as well as, for assessing the potential risks of surgery or other invasive treatments on the brain. Physicians perfom fMRI to examine the anatomy of the brain, to determine precisely which part of the brain is handling critical functions, such as thinking, speech, motion and sensation, to assess the effects of stroke, trauma or degenerative diseases (such as Alzheimer's Disease) on brain function, to monitor the growth and function of brain tumors and to plan surgery, radio therapy or other surgical treatments of the brain.

After an fMRI paradigm has been designed and carried out, the resulting data must be passed through various analysis steps before the physician can obtain answers to questions about experimentally-related activations at the individual or multi-subject level and address the above matters. The goal of a computer-based fMRI analysis is to detect automaticaly, in a robust, sensitive and valid way, those parts of the brain which show increased intensity at the points in time where stimulation was applied. The fMRI analysis methods consist of three basic stages: preprocessing, signal detection - description, and extraction of the brain connectivity.

The purpose of preprocessing is to remove various kinds of artefacts and condition the data, in order to maximize the sensitivity of the next stage of analysis. Preprocessing includes spatial or temporal filtering of fMRI data and image restoration. After preprocessing, signal detection is accomplished. It aims to determine which voxels are activated by the stimulation. This can be performed by simple correlation analysis or more advanced methods. The main output of this step is an activation map which indicates those points in the image where the brain has been activated in response to the stimulus. Signal description aims at modeling the response shape by several parameters and relating these parameters to variables of the the stimulation context. Finally, connectivity analysis attempts to estimate brain networks.

The aim of this chapter is to provide an overview of the computer methods which have been developed to accomplish the above stages of the computer-based fMRI data analysis. The chapter is organised as follows: first (Section 2), some fundamental features of the fMRI modality (including what is fMRI, how does fMRI work, what does fMRI measure, what are the advantages and disadvantages of fMRI, what are the sources of noise in fMRI, what are the spatial and temporal characteristics of fMRI, etc.) are described. The next section (Section 3) provides an overview of the preprocessing methods used in fMRI analysis. Then (Section 4), a summary of the main ideas that have been proposed to model and detect the fMRI signal is presented. In the fifth section, a description of connectivity analysis mehtods is given. Finally (Section 6), the importance of fMRI studies in understanding brain function and the applications of fMRI are exposed.

2. Description of the fMRI modality

Functional Magnetic Resonance Imaging (fMRI) is a neuroimaging technique which uses the physical phenomenon of Nuclear Magnetic Resonance (NMR) and the associated technology of MRI to detect regional changes in cerebral metabolism or in blood flow, volume or oxygenation in response to task activation. It utilizes Blood Oxygen Level Dependent (BOLD) constrast which is based on the differentiation of the magnetic properties of oxygenated (diamagnetic) and deoxygenated (paramagnetic) blood. These magnetic susceptibility differences lead to small but detectable changes in susceptibility weighted MR image intensity (Jezzard et al., 2001, Lazar, 2008).

2.1 fMRI image formation

When the human brain receives a stimulus an increase in neuronal activation takes place. When neurons are activated require energy. This energy is supplied in the form of glucose and oxygen (the oxygen is carried in hemoglobin). The resulting increased need for oxygen is overcompensated by a large incerease in perfusion. As a result, the venous oxyhemoglobin concentration increases and the deoxyhemoglobin concentration decreases. As the later has paramagnetic properties, it alters the T2* weighted magnetic resonance image signal (deoxyhemoglobin is sometimes referred to as an endogenous contrast enhancing agent, and serves as the source of fMRI signal) (Jezzard & Clare, 2001). More specifically, the intensity of the fMRI image increases in the activated areas. As the conditions are alternated, the signal in the activated voxels increases and decreases according to the paradigm (Figure 1).

2.2 BOLD response

As mentioned above neural activity requires increased local blood flow to supply additional oxygen. The increased need for oxygen leads to increase in perfusion. Increasing the prefusion rate in a tissue volume element generally leads to the dilution of the venous deoxyhemoglobin, reducing the tendency of the blood to decrease the magnetic resonance signal. This incease in signal intensity is referred as the BOLD.

A schematic representation of the common features of the fMRI BOLD response to a period of neural stimulation is given in Figure 2. fMRI BOLD response is divided into three epochs: a) initial dip, b) positive BOLD response, and c) post stimulus undershoot. Immediately after electrical activity commences there may be a brief period of approximately 0.5-1sec during which the fMRI signal decreases slightly below the baseline (~0.5%). This is known as initial dip. Subsequently, the BOLD response increases, yielding a robust positive BOLD response whose peak is located 5-8sec after the stimulus is applied. Finally, upon cessation of the stimulus, there is a return of the BOLD response to baseline, often accompanied by a post stimulus undershoot, during which the response passes through baseline and remains negative for several seconds. Eventually, the response returns to baseline (Hoge & Pike, 2001).

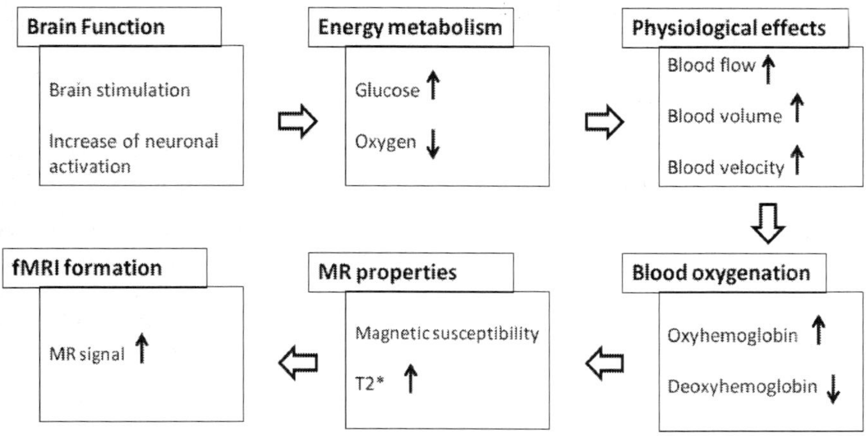

Fig. 1. Schematic representation of the fMRI formation.

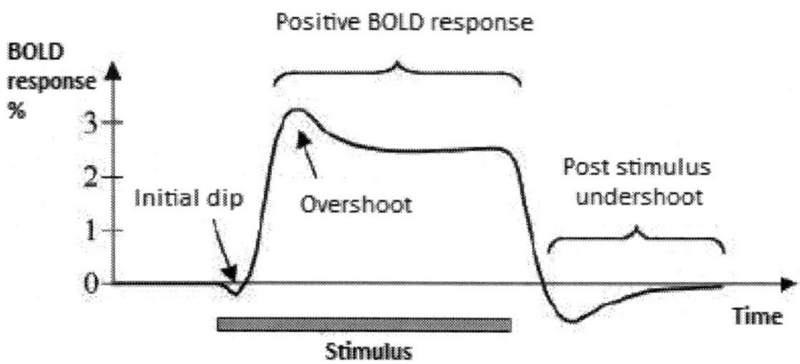

Fig. 2. Schematic representation of the BOLD response.

2.3 fMRI paradigm

During the fMRI paradigm the subject is positioned in the scanner and asked to alternatively perform several tasks or is stimulated to trigger several processes or emotions. Tne stimuli are usually audio, visual and motor, but can involve more complex functions such as memory and thought. Each of the above conditions is repeated several times and can be separated by rest periods. More specifically, there are two types of fMRI designs: a) event related designs in which stimuli of different types are intermixed, and b) block designs in which stimuli of the the same type are presented in blocks. The brain of the subject is scanned repeatedly, using Echo Planar Imaging (EPI) technique. EPI is a fast magnetic resonance imaging sequence which allows the acquisition of a brain volume in less than 3 seconds (Figure 3) (Jezzard & Clare, 2001).

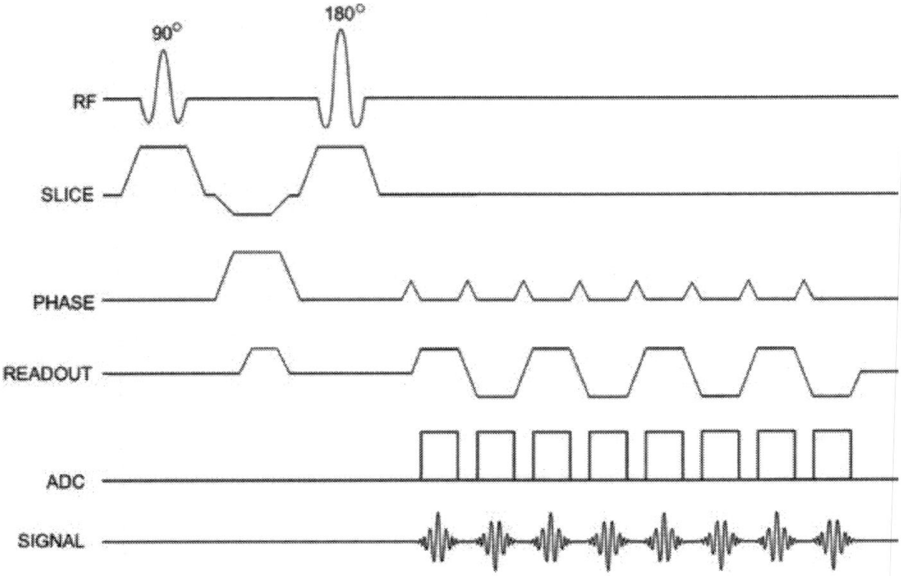

Fig. 3. Echo Planar Imaging (EPI) technique.

2.4 Advantages and disadvantages of the fMRI modality

The fMRI image volume offers several distinct advantages over other functional image modalities, such as PET and SPECT. These advantages are: a) it is considerably safer since no contrast agent is needed in order the signal to be administrated, b) the total scan time is very short, and c) it has high spatial and temporal resolution. The disadvantages of the fMRI are the following: a) it is very expensive, and b) it captures a clear image only if the patient does not move.

2.5 Spatial and temporal resolution in fMRI

One reason for the popularity of fMRI is its good spatial and temporal resolution. Spatial resolution in fMRI means the smallest activated area that can be reliably detected. It is basically limited by imaging time and by reasonable signal to noise ratio (SNR). Smaller voxels indicate smaller SNR but also improve spatial resolution by enabling the detection of smaller structures and smaller activated areas. Temporal resolution is defined as the shortest time between two stimuli in the same cortical area which produce distinguishable responses. Due to short acquisition time high temporal resolution of fMRI is possible in principle. However, it is limited by a blurred intrinsic hemodynamic response and a finite SNR (Menon & Goodyear, 2001).

2.6 fMRI time series

The functional images, as already mentioned, are T2* weighted images with lower spatial resolution than anatomical images. However, functional images are not considered as anatomical images of the object and they are not examined as those. The collection of them in a certain time rate consitutes a set of images. Each voxel's intensity value in each image of the set is called time series of the specific voxel (Figure 4).

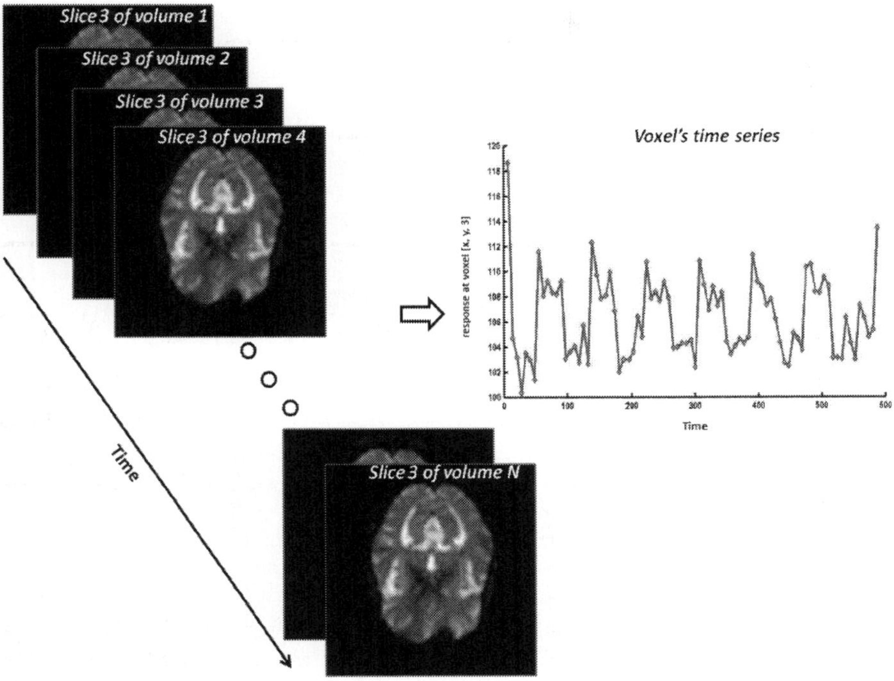

Fig. 4. fMRI time series.

2.7 Sources of noise in fMRI

fMRI time series contain not only the activity evoked by the experiment (effects of interest) but also structured and random noise. Noise in fMRI has several sources. These are: a) thermal noise arising from the subject, the receiver coil and the amplifiers, b) systematic noise arising from subject motion, c) systematic noise arising from tissue pulsation related to cardiac and respiratory cycles, and d) noise due to slow fluctuations in blood oxygenation (Lazar, 2008).

3. fMRI analysis – preprocessing stage

A successful fMRI paradigm is the one that ensures that the evoked neural activity generated by the stimulus or task constitutes a signal which can pass through all transformations which are necessary for the preprocessing and statistical analysis stages. Preprocessing is performed to remove extraneous sources of variation and isolate the fMRI signal. There are six preprocessing steps that are needed in order the confounding effects of artefacts to be removed and the SNR to be enhanced. These are: slice timing, motion correction, intensity normalization, spatial normalization, spatial and temporal filtering.

3.1 Slice timing

Functional MRI volumes are formed one slice at a time. The scan time of individual slice differs within a repetition time (TR) depending on the acquisition order. More specifically, in ascending or descending sequential acquisition, the last slice is collected almost one TR after the first slice. In interleaved acquisition (all odd slices are collected first followed by all even slices) adjacent slices are collected a TR/2 apart. A problem is that later analysis steps assume that every voxel is sampled at exactly the same time. It is desirable to correct for this time shift. Slice timing correction makes the data in each slice to correspond to the same time instant. It is achieved by phase shifting of the sines that make up the signal. Each voxles time series is transformed to the frequency domain, phase shift is applied to the data and then the inverse Fourier transform is applied to recover the corrected time series (Smith, 2001, Strother, 2006).

3.2 Motion correction

One of the strongest fMRI artefacts are the movement related ones. If the subjects move their head during the fMRI paradigm, the position of the brain within the functional images will vary over time. Consequently any voxel's time series does not refer to the same anatomical point in the brain. Since the head movement cannot completely eliminated by scanner enviromental manipulation, it is corrected afterwards through mathematical transformations. Motion correction is achieved by the spatial alignment of the voxels across the sequentially collected fMRI image volumes. Spatial alignment is perfromed by registering the whole time series of the images to a target image (usually image picked first or middle image volume). Registration is based on the fact that only rigid body movement occurs. Thus, rigid body transformation is applied where six parameters (three translations and three ratotions) are needed. For the determination of the optimal value of parameters a cost function is used. Many of the differences between registration algorithms concern the choice of the cost function and the optimization strategies which are used (Smith, 2001, Strother, 2006).

3.3 Intensity normalization

In fMRI experiment there is additional scan-to-scan variance at very low spatial frequencies that cannot be readilly accounted for by the experimental stimulus. One possible cause of changes is the scanner itself (scanner drift). Several global normalization approaches have been developed to model and control this variation. Intensity normalization refers to the rescaling of all intensities in an fMRI volume by the same amount. It is applied to each functional volume separately. A common approach for intensity normalization is the following. For each fMRI volume, the mean intensity across all voxels, which have been an intensity above a predetermined threshold, is calculated. Then all intensity values are rescaled by a constant value, so that the new mean intensity becomes a preset value. An alternative procedure is to use mean intensity value of each volume as confounding variables in later statistical analysis. Such methods present the following probelm. If the activation is strong then the activation itself will increase the mean intensity, thus, after normalization the "non-activated" parts of the volume will be negatively correlated with the stimulation, and will show up as "deactivation" in the final statistical image. Solutions to this problem, as well as, a comparison of detrending methods can be found in (Smith, 2001, Strother, 2006).

3.4 Spatial normalization

It is performed for two reasons. First, it enables to report the locations of activation according to a well know coordinate space, and second, it enables group comparisons. It is performed by a two step procedure: a) determination of an optimum 12 affine transformation (3 translations, 3 rotations, 3 zooms and 3 shears) between the template image and the image to be normalized, and b) estimation of nonlinear deformations defined by a linear combination of 3D Discrete Cosine Transform (DCT) basis functions (Smith, 2001, Strother, 2006).

3.5 Spatial smoothing

The importance of measuring and manipulating the spatial correlations of fMRI has been studied in (Poline & Mazoyer, 1995, Friston et al., 1993a, Worsley et al. 1996). Additionaly, the impact of spatial smoothing, as a preprocessing step, on signal detection of fMRI signal has been mentioned in (Skudlaski et al., 1999, Parrish et al., 2000, Lowe & Sorenson, 1997, Strother et al., 2004). There are two reasons for applying spatial filtering: a) blurring can increase SNR, and b) certain statistical theory, which may be used in later processing, requires the fMRI images to be spatially smoothed. A variety of methods for spatial filtering and a comparison of such methods have been reported in the literature (Smith, 2001, Nandy & Cordes, 2004, Sole et al., 2001, Long et al., 2004, Wink & Roerdink, 2004). The most common method for carrying out spatial smoothing is to convolve each volume with a Gaussian kernel. The width of the kernel lies between 3mm and 10mm of full width half maximum (FWHM) for fMRI. The recommended FWHM for fMRI is 2-3 times the voxel size. The convolution is performed in all three directions of the fMRI volume.

As far as it concerns temporal filtering, works on each voxel's time series instead on each spatial volume image. It aims to remove low and high frequency components without damaging the signal of interest. High pass filtering removes slow varying unwanted signals such as physiological effects (heartbeat, breathing) or scanner related drifts. High pass filtering is often achieved using finite impulse linear filters or alternatively using non linear high pass filtering procedures. Another approach is to model low frequencies in late statistical procedures instead of removing them at the preprocessing stage. Lowpass filtering attempts to reduce high frequency noise. A common way to carry out low pass filtering is the linear convolution with a Gaussian kernel (Smith, 2001, Strother, 2006). Other more sophisticated approaches use wavelet filtering, Markov random fields and local neighborhood smoothing (Kruggel et al., 1999).

4. fMRI analysis – modeling and inference stage

After the improvement of the quality of the fMR images, statistical analysis is carried out to determine which voxels are activated by the stimulation. The current section presents an overview of the methods reported in the literature concering modeling and detection of fMRI signal.

Most functional MRI studies are based on the correlation of hemodynamic response function with stimulation. Activation is then defined as stimulus-linked and time-dependent local intensity changes in the image. Strategies for fMRI data analysis, in terms of signal analysis, consist of two steps: signal description and signal detection. Signal description aims at modeling the BOLD response by parameters which describe the stimulation context. Signal detection aims to detect significantly activated areas and it is commonly achieved by applying a test statistic. A statistical parametric map is created. The value of each voxel in this map express how closely the voxel's time series is from the expected time course. Voxels with high correlation values are given high activation score while voxels with low or no correlation have low score. In case of negative activation (deactivation) voxels are given a negative score.

The fMRI analysis has generated an abundant literature. The methods can be grouped into two broad categories: a) univariate methods (hypothesis testing methods), and b) multivariate methods (exploratory methods). Univariate methods try to define which voxels can be characterized as activated given one single model. This allows the parameterization of the response and then the estimation of the model parameters. This is followed by a statistical test which assesses the signal estimation and concludes to the presence or the absence of activation. The methodological variations can be related to the estimation procedure used or the statistical method employed to assess the presence of activation. Multivariate methods extract information from the dataset, often with any prior knowledge of the experimental conditions. They generally, extract a set of meaningful patterns from the dataset. In order to achieve this, they use some structural properties, such as decorrelation, independence, similarity measures, that can discriminate between features of interest present in the data. The gap between the two families of methods tried to bridge methods which use multivariate linear models. According to the description of the two groups of methods, methods such as Generalized Linear Model and some extensions of it, Wavelet basis functions, Bayesian framework, Principal Component Analysis (PCA), Independent Component Analysis, Canonical Correlation Analysis (CCA), Clustering techniques can be used for the analysis of fMRI data.

4.1 Generalized Linear Model

One of the most common approach in fMRI statistical analysis is the construction of a model that describes the way in which the BOLD response depends on the stimulus. A widely used mathematical model for this purpose is the Generalized Linear Model (GLM) (Friston et al., 1995a). It consists of two parts: fixed effects and random error. The fixed effects are the part of the model that do not vary if the experiment is repeated. The ranodm error is the part which explains how the observations vary even if the experiments is repeated on the same subject and under the same conditions. The mathematical formula of GLM is given as:

$$\mathbf{Y} = \mathbf{X}\beta + \mathbf{e}, \tag{1}$$

where **Y** is a matrix representing the time series of all the voxels, **X** is the design matrix of the predictors, **β** are the unknown coefficients of the predictors, and **e** is the error, usually assumed to be normally distributed with zero mean and variance σ^2 (independent and identically distributed). The error **e** may have a constant or a non constant variance, as well as, nonzero covariance. The columns of the design matrix **X** reflecting how the signal is varying in active areas (stimuli presented at each time point) and can contain different types of covariates of interest including: factors which describe the experimental design, predicted hemodynamic responses and categorical covariates, such as demographics of the subject group membership and so forth.
The basic GLM is usually used under the following assumptions: a) voxels are independent, b) time points are independent, c) the error variance at each time point is the same, and d) the same model, as given by the design matrix, is appropriate for every voxel in the brain (Lazar, 2008). Under these assumptions, the estimates of **β** can be obtained through the ordinary least squares (OLS). Thus, the estimated parameters are given as:

$$\hat{\beta} = (X^T X)^{-1} X^T Y. \tag{2}$$

The estimated parameters define how well the model, described in the design matrix, fits the time series of each voxel. However, the assumptions reported previously do not hold in practice. Thus, statistical research in fMRI has focused on ways of improving and extending the generalized linear model, or it has centered on alternative analysis methods.

4.2 Extensions of the Generalized Linear Model

A great part of the fMRI literature has concentrated on the improvement of the GLM described above in order to take into account temporal correlations, spatial correlations or both.

4.2.1 Temporal correlations

The basic GLM model described above assumes that the error term has zero mean and variance $\sigma^2\mathbf{I}$. This means that the error term is independent and identically distributed. However, fMRI errors are not independent. Temporal correlations exist due to physiological effects and scanner instability. In order temporal correlations to be addressed three general methods are proposed in the literature: a) ignoring temporal correlation, b) prewhitening, and c) precolouring. Ignoring temporal correlations leads to under estimation of variance, over estimation of significance and to many false positives. Prewhitening is assumed to be a statistical optimal approach but requires the precise estimation of autocorrelation structure. Precolouring has the advantage that autocorrelation structure estimation is avoided but on the other hand is statistically insufficient.

The autocorrelation models used in the literature extend the basic GLM by modeling the error term as a stochastic process. This can be achieved using an autoregressive model (AR(1), AR(p), AR(1) + white noise model) (Friston et al., 2000a, Marchini and Ripley, 2000, Kershaw et al., 1999, Burock & Dale, 2000, Purdon et al., 2001, Purdon & Weisskoff, 1998, Worsley et al., 2002). Thus, the error term is replaced with zero mean and unknown covariance structure. The variance is given as $\sigma^2\mathbf{V}$, where $\mathbf{V}$ is a matrix whose elements depend on the autocovariance function between two time points. The matrix V is the autocorrelation matrix for the intrinsic and assumed correlations. The intrinsic correlations are described by:

$$\mathbf{V}_i = \mathbf{K}_i\mathbf{K}_i^T. \quad (3)$$

The assumed correlations are described by:

$$\mathbf{V}_a = \mathbf{K}_a\mathbf{K}_a^T. \quad (4)$$

The matrices $\mathbf{K}_i$ and $\mathbf{K}_a$ correspond to convolution matrices.

Based on this modeling of error term, a general class of procedures is obtained by multiplying the GLM by matrix $\mathbf{S}$ (Friston et al., 2000a). This yields a model of the following form:

$$\mathbf{SY} = \mathbf{SX}\beta + \mathbf{Se}, \quad (5)$$

where $\mathbf{S}$ is the applied temporal filter matrix. A variety of methods have been reported in the literature concerning the estimation of the matrix $\mathbf{S}$. These methods were developed either in the time or frequency domain. Generally, if $\mathbf{S}$ has a Toeplitz form then it can be considered as an applied (de)convolution. However, $\mathbf{S}$ can take any one of the following forms:

$$\mathbf{S} = \begin{cases} \mathbf{K}_i^{-1} & \text{"whitening"} \\ \mathbf{K}_{AR(1)}^{-1} & \text{AR(1) model} \\ \mathbf{K}_{AR(p)}^{-1} & \text{AR(p) model} \\ \mathbf{K}_{1/f}^{-1} & \text{1/f model} \\ \mathbf{I} & \text{"none"} \end{cases}. \quad (6)$$

A comparison of the methods for selecting the matrix $\mathbf{S}$ can be found in (Friston et al., 2000a).

Until know it is assumed that the correlation structure is known. However, in practice $\mathbf{V}$ is unknown and thus must be estimated. Getting the correct correlation structure is important for three reasons: a) it leads to the best estimator, b) it guides us to the best design of the experiment, and c) it leads to the correct estimator of the variance, vital for getting the correct statistics. A variety of methods have been proposed for the estimation of **V**. It must be mentioned that no simple methods exist that give best unbiased answers. The best methods all involve costly iterative calculations which are expensive to compute.

4.2.2 Spatial correlations

So far no information has been used from neighboring voxels, and all the models have been fitted independently at each voxel. If the signal extends over a certain region in space then it can be shown that signal detection is optimal if the data is simply averaged over all voxels in that region. Since the location of the region of interest is not known it is reasonable to smooth the data (spatial smoothing) with a kernel. The shape of the kernel models the assumed spatial activation patterns. Smoothing the data has been criticized because it sacrifices resolvability for detection ability. Moreover, the width of the signal to be detected should be known in advance.

Instead of smoothing the data or ignoring the spatial correlations, spatial modeling is another approach. Spatial modeling aims to analyze statistical parametric maps in order to detect those areas of the brain that were activated by the stimulus. A variety of methods has been proposed in the fMRI literature (Marchini & Presanis, 2004, Hartvig & Jensen, 2000). The most widely used methods are based on the thresholding of statistical parametric maps. The threshold value is determined using the classical approach where a null hypothesis of no activation at each voxel is postulated and then tested. The core unit of this approach is to choose a significance level for each test such that the family-wise error rate (FWE) is controlled at some pre specified level. This induces a multiple-comparisons problem which is addressed by using random field theory. Another way of spatial modeling is though Bayesian framework, more specifically spatial mixture models, or clustering techniques. These models explicitly model activated voxels in addition to the "null" distribution of non activated voxels. Benjamini & Hochberg (1995), Genovese et al. (2002) suggested that thresholds can be defined by controlling the false discovery rate (FDR). A different Bayesian analysis is described by Smith et al. (2003) and Smith & Fahrmeir (2007). Their approach is based on the basic linear model but the voxel time series is modeled as the sum of a baseline trend, an activation profile and an error. Their analysis is concentrated on the second term of the model. The application of the method to simulated and real data detected more isolated voxels than a comparable linear model-based analysis. Also the use of anatomical prior information increased the sensitivity of preserving details of activated structures.

As far as it concerns the use of clustering techniques for localization and characterization of spatial patterns of activation blurs the distinction between purely spatial and spatiotemporal models. Bowman & Patel (2004) tried to build a spatial model that does not have a temporal component. Although, their method was developed for PET images they indicate that the statistical issues are the same and the analysis can be used for fMRI as well.

4.2.3 Spatio-temporal correlations

A more natural way to handle functional neuro-imaging data is to build models that incorporate both spatial and temporal correlations. The most straightforward approach to achieve this is to apply clustering techniques to the time series data or spatial regularized approach, the so called "direct modeling". Time series clustering is a non model approach since no parametric model is specified for the spatial relations. These are clarified by the

detected clusters. With direct modeling spatial models are fitted, often with an aid of prior information provided by neuro-scientific reasoning or previous experiments.
Application of clustering techniques prerequisites an answer to the following questions: a) what should be clustered, b) what clustering algorithms should be used, c) which is the number of clusters, and d) how is the number of clusters decided. A variety of methods have been proposed in the fMRI literature to address those issues. As far as it concerns the first question there are two perspectives: a) clustering fMRI time series proposed by Baumgartner et al. (1998) and b) clustering features of fMRI time series proposed by Goutte et al. (1999). After the determination of the nature of the dataset, clustering algorithms (hierarchical clustering, k-means, fuzzy clustering) are utilized. A basic input of the clustering algorithms is the number of clusters. Methods described in (Filzmoser et al., 1999, Baumgartner et al., 1998, Balslev et al., 2002, Fadili et al., 2000) are trying to address this issue. However, the problem remains inherently difficult.
In direct modeling both temporal and spatial components are modeled explicitly (Lazar, 2008). Some authors (Solo et al., 2001, Purdon et al., 2001, Katanoda et al., 2000, Worsley et al. 2002) use a spatial regularization of the noise estimate. A potential disadvantage of these models is the adequacy of the spatial model, which is usually isotropic. Another way of spatial regularization is the use of Markov random fields (Descombes et al., 1998). The inference based on Markov random fields can be interpreted within the Bayesian framework where the prior probabilities is given by the voxel time course, while the posterior probability takes into account the contextual information carried by the neighboring voxels.

4.2.4 Estimation of parameters

An important concern in model based fMRI analysis is the ability to find unbiased estimators of the parameters. In the previous sections the least square estimation procedure is reported. Another attractive approach is the maximum likelihood framework. Least squares estimation approach yields maximum likelihood estimators under the assumption that the noise is Gaussian. This idea has been generalized in (Nan & Nowak, 1999) to deal with complex data.
In the previous sections, Bayesian framework is reported as a method for spatial or spatiotemporal modeling. However, another application of this framework in fMRI analysis is in the estimation of parameters. The main difference between maximum likelihood and the Bayesian framework is the introduction of priors in the statistical model of the data. The introduction of Bayesian concepts is in fact a way to optimize parameters in an expectation – maximization fashion. Genovese (2000) and Worsley (2000) proposed a Bayesian model for the estimation of parameters. A similar approach is previously described by Kershaw et al. (1999). They use informative priors for all parameters, avoiding in this way the computational issues. An advantage of this approach is that it allows researchers to give answers to questions beyond those of localization and also the parameters of the model can interpreted in terms of physiology of hemodynamic response. In 2004 Woolrich et al. proposed a model that not only models the hemodynamic response but also introduces a spatiotemporal noise component. The advantages of this approach is that allows for model comparison and the formulation of the HRF is not restricted by the experimental design. A different perspective on the Bayesian analysis is presented in Hartvig (2002), where marked point processes are used to describe the spatial activation pattern. Although, Bayesian framework is widely applied in fMRI analysis the potential of this framework is not fully

exploited. A comparison of classical and Bayesian framework is given in (Friston and Penny, 2002).

4.3 Multivariate analysis

In this section we give a short description of multivariate or model free approaches such as component, correlation and clustering analysis of fMRI data. Component analysis includes principal and independent component analysis while correlation analysis includes canonical and maximum correlation analysis. Clustering include methods such as k-means or fuzzy k-means. In contrast to the methods described in previous sections which were voxel based, the techniques which are presented aim to finding or characterizing the multivariate nature of the data, looking in subspaces or higher dimensional directions of common behavior. These directions may be in space, time or both depending on how the analysis is performed.

4.3.1 Component analysis

A classical multivariate statistical analysis technique is the Principal Component Analysis (PCA). The goal of PCA is to explain the variance-covariance structure of the data through linear combinations of the original data. It aims in: a) data reduction and b) interpretation. Although, the original dataset contains p variables, often much of the variability can be accounted for by a smaller number, m, of principal components. Hence, data reduction is necessary. A PCA can show relationships that were not previously suspected, and it allows interpretations that would not ordinarily result. PCA of fMRI data is often performed through a Singular Value Decomposition (SVD) technique after centering the dataset. The SVD simply decomposes the dataset into mutually orthogonal spatio-temporal components. On the contrary, Independent Component Analysis (ICA) aims to derive statistically independent components either in the spatial or in the temporal domain but not in both. This is justified since the independence of the random variables is a much more constrained problem than their correlation. The ICA uses information available in higher moments; hence it does not assume normality. Application of ICA involves two main preprocessing steps, data reduction and whitening. PCA is often used for the data reduction step. It is used in such a way that the majority of the variability in the data is captured. The innovative characteristic is that even if the number of required components is large, it will still be smaller than either the number of time points or the number of voxels in a typical fMRI study. PCA is also used to prewhiten the data. Whitening transforms the search space to an orthogonal one. A variety of algorithms, which constrain the results to be correlated and take advantage of the higher order features of the data are available to actually perform the ICA.

Comparison of PCA and ICA reveals the following differences. First, the frame of reference into which one projects the multivariate data with ICA is no more inevitably orthogonal. Second, the direction of the axes in ICA is not only computed from the second order statistics like in PCA but also from higher orders statistics. A third difference is the ordering of the components. More specifically, in PCA, the first principal component accounts for as much of the variability in the data as possible, and each successive orthogonal component accounts for as much of the residual variability as possible. The PCA can be used to decrease the dimension of the problem by considering only the first components which explain most of the variance in the data. With ICA, the number of sources to be computed must be selected first. By changing the dimensions of the unmixing matrix to be estimated, the number of independent sources is computed by the algorithm. The obtained independent sources depend on the postulated number of sources, which is not the case in PCA (Lazar, 2008, Bugli & Lambert, 2007).

4.3.2 Extensions of PCA and ICA

An extension of PCA is its nonlinear version (Friston et al., 1999, Friston et al., 2000b). The motivation for this extension is the observation that the conventional analysis imposes biologically implausible constraints on the solutions. These constraints are: a) the components are orthogonal and account successively for the greatest amount of remaining variance, b) the decomposition is into linearly separable components. The last constraint precludes the possibility of interactions among brain systems. However, neuroscientists believe that brain systems interact with each other in a complex way.

Another form of PCA is functional PCA (Viviani et al., 2005). The data delivered by the functional magnetic resonance imaging (fMRI) scans are considered as continuous functions of time sampled at the inter scan interval and subject to observational noise. These functions may be estimated by fitting a set of basis functions to each voxel time series. Collectively, the functions replace the voxels of a series of images with a single "functional image." In functional PCA, the eigenanalysis is carried out directly on these functions. It requires two steps: a) smoothing time series and b) application of PCA on the estimated functions. As an explorative tool, functional PCA can be used as an alternative to other multivariate methods. This is justified in (Viviani et al., 2005).

Kernel PCA is a modification of the original PCA using techniques of kernel methods (Thirion & Faugeras, 2003). It does not assume that underlying structures of interest are uncorrelated spatially and temporally. The reason for this modification is that the assumption reported previously does not always hold for fMRI data. Kernel PCA is a two step procedure. In the first step each voxel time series is analyzed univariately, resulting in a temporal characterization of that voxel's behavior. Then, the voxel based models are subjected to a multivariate analysis. The aim of the kernel PCA is to preserve temporal patterns extracted in the first modeling step, something that is not attainable with ordinary PCA because of the assumption that components are uncorrelated.

As far as it concerns modification of the basic ICA approach these are spatial ICA, temporal ICA, spatiotemporal ICA, skew ICA and combination of spatiotemporal and skew ICA (Biswal & Ulmer, 1999, Calhoun et al., 2001, Calhoun et al., 2003a, McKeown et al., 1998, Calhoun et al., 2003b, Stone et al., 2002). Spatial ICA seeks a set of mutuall independnent source images, temporal seeks a set of independent source time courses, while spatiotemporal ICA decomposes an image sequence into a set of spatial images and a corresponding set of time courses such that signals in both sets are maximally independent. It is based on the observation that the underlying source images and time courses associated with brain tissue tend towards statistical independence, but neither source images nor time courses are independent in such cases. These approaches are based on the assumption that the probability density function (PDF) of the independent sources is highly kyrtotic and symmetric. Skew ICA is based on the assumption that images are characterized by the skewness (rather than the kurtosis) of their PDF's. This assumption is consistent with spatially localized regions of activity. Spatiotemporal skew ICA combines the ideas of spatiotemporal ICA and skew ICA and produces better results both spatially and temporally.

4.3.3 Correlation analysis

Correlation analysis includes canonical and maximum correlation analysis methods. Canonical Correlation Analysis (CCA) (Friman et al., 2001, Nandy & Cordes, 2003, Lazar, 2008) is a way of quantifying the correlation between sets of variables. More specifically, it is a mean to detect the subcomponents of two multivariate datasets that are maximally correlated. It has been proposed as a way of investigating fMRI datasets with two possible applications: a) the derivation of temporal components that are maximally correlated and b) the derivation of the most spatially smooth maps of the dataset. An advantage of this approach is that the transformation of the original variables into the new scale reveals the correlation structure between the sets. This would not always be apparent if the simple pairwise correlations between components of the two sets were calculated instead.
Maximum correlation analysis of maximum correlation modeling (MCM) (Friman et al., 2002a, Friman et al., 2002b, Lazar, 2008) is a technique related to CCA. It works as follows: it considers the eight neighbors around each voxel. From this neighborhood five new time series are created. These are: a) time series of the center voxel, b) the average of the voxels to the immediate left and right of the center, c) the average of the voxels above and below the center, d) the average of the voxels in the upper left and low corners, and e) the average of the voxels in the upper right and lower left corners. The five new time series are combined linearly via weights ($w1$, $w2$, $w3$, $w4$, $w5$) which are positive numbers and sum to one. Also the weight applied to the center voxel is greater than the others. The correlation of this spatially smoothed time courses with the convolution of the stimulus and the hemodynamic response function is calculated. The aim is to find the values of the weights and the parameters of the model such that the correlation is maximized.

4.3.4 Clustering

Clustering is another exploratory method based on the following statistical viewpoint. The dataset X is a set of N features (the temporal time series) that belong to a given signal manifold or feature space F. The literature on fMRI data clustering deals with the following problems: a) the method for constructing the final clusters, b) the definition of the feature space F, c) the assessment of the quality of clustering results, and d) the determination of the number of clusters. Clustering algorithms also try to isolate patterns of no interest since the lack of prior knowledge. Flandin et al. (2003) suggest that introducing anatomical and functional information improves the generality and the precision of the method. Unlike PCA and ICA they do not decompose the data into components, and thus, do not benefit from the associated denoising effect.

4.4 Wavelets and fMRI

Wavelet analysis of fMRI data has gained the attraction of researchers due to the numerous advantages of wavelet basis functions. These advantages are: a) wavelets are multi-resolutional, b) they are adaptive to nonstationary or local features, c) wavelet transform has a whitening effect and this may be statistically convenient for modeling purposes, d) the wavelet transform is useful for data compression and denoising, e) the discrete wavelet transform is very fast computationally, even compared to the fast Fourier transform, and f) the brain has a fractal nature, and wavelets are an effective way of modeling such processes. Thus, wavelet analysis has three main uses: a) creation of activation maps (Fadili & Bullmore, 2004), b) modeling, and c) resampling. The most traditional application of wavelets is the last one.

Wavelet resampling has been proposed to assess the presence of activation with colored noise. It was introduced by Bullmore et al. (2001) and it is remarkably simple. First, the discrete wavelet transform of fMRI time series is applied. It is adjusted to have zero mean. Second, the coefficients are resampled at each level of detail. Finally, the inverse wavelet transform of the permuted coefficients is applied to obtain a reconstructed time series that has the same variance and covariance as the original. Breakspear et al. (2004) proposed a two step procedure that aims to preserve both spatial and temporal second-order structure which is presented in the original data. Also, issues such as which is the best way to resample coefficients in each direction at each level are addressed. As far as it concerns the choice of wavelet family, the order of the wavelet, the number of vanishing moments, the way of resampling in multiple directions (jointly or independently), the management of edge effects are discussed in (Bullmore et al., 2001, Breakspear et al., 2004). Resampling can also be achieved in the frequency domain. At each frequency the components are approximately independent and so the same rationale, as for wavelet resampling, holds. A comparison of these two methods is given in (Laird et al., 2004), while a detailed comparison of prewhitening with an autoregressive mode, wavelet and Fourier resampling is presented in (Friman and Westin, 2005).

As already mentioned above, wavelet has also been used in fMRI analysis for data compression and modeling. The latter is of specific interest because attempts are presented to directly use prior anatomical information, and hence, to derive a set of functions that have intrinsic physiological meaning and interpretation. Fadili & Bullmore, (2002) propose a wavelet generalized least squares algorithm. The advantage of transforming the data into the wavelet domain is that the variance-covariance matrix of the error is approximately diagonal, which facilitates inference. The novel characteristic of this procedure is that the parameters of the long-range dependency process are estimated simultaneously with the parameters of the linear model.

5. Connectivity analysis

So far only the estimation of sites of activation and their relationship to stimulation or cognitive activity were discussed. No special reference to the relationships between different sites in the brain has been made. Connectivity analysis attempts to estimate such networks, in order to build up a more shopisticated picture of the functioning of the brain. Connectivity analysis is carried out on the basis of either similarities in time seires or relationships between final activation levels. There are two types of connectivity, functional and effective connectivity. Functional connectivity is defined as the temporal correlations between spatially remote neurophysiological events (Friston et al., 1993b). This definition provides a simple characterization of functional interactions, and it does not comment on how these interactions are mediated. Effective connectivity is the influence one neuronal system exerts over another (Friston et al., 1993c). Effective connectivity depends on two models: a mathematical model describing how are connected and a neuroanatomical model describing which areas are connected. From the definitions given above it is understood that functional and effective connectivity differ fundamentally at a practical level. This is because the time scale and the nature of neurophysiological measurements are very different.

Functional connectivity is a statistical concept since it can be defined as the extent of correlation in brain activity measured across a number of spatially distinct brain regions. Studies regarding the presence or the absence of functional connectivity between a set of brain regions depend on: a) the type of measurement (e.g. EEG, fMRI, MEG), b) the type of the analysis, and c) the state of the subject during the recording of brain activity (e.g. rest, stimulation or cognitive task). However, the majority of the studies have employed only two approaches: a) coherence of EEG signals, and b) inter-regional correlation in fMRI time series. Studies of patterns of functional connectivity (based on coherence or correlation) among cortical regions have demonstrated that functional brain networks exhibit small-world attributes possibly reflecting the underlying structural organization of anatomical connections. More detailed graph theoretical analysis of functional brain connectivity helped to identify functional hubs, which are highly connected and central to information flow and integration. It should be noted that functional connectivity does not make any explicit reference to specific directional effects or to an underlying structural model (Friston, 2003, David et al., 2004, Achard et al., 2006).

The methods for measuring functional connectivity can be categorized according to the mathematical domain in which they are implemented (time, frequency). Functional connectivity is highly time-dependent. Statistical patterns between neuronal elements fluctuate on multiple time scales, some as short as tens or hundreds of milliseconds. While the majority of the methods have been developed in the time domain, considerable fewer methods have been developed in Fourier or wavelet domain. The motivation is that associations between brain regions may not be equally subtended by all frequencies. Some frequency bands may be of special importance in mediating functional connectivity. Functional connectivity studies in the frequency domain have provided evidence for a fractal organization of functional brain networks (Friston, 2003, David et al., 2004, Achard et al., 2006).

As far as it concerns effective connectivity its computation is more challenging than the computation of functional connectivity. More specifically, there are linear and nonlinear models for effective connectivity such as multiple linear regression, covariance structural equation modeling and variable parameter regression. Multiple linear regressions (Friston et al. 1995b, Buchel & Friston, 2001) demonstrated that nonlinear interactions can be characterized using simple extensions of the linear models. Structural equation modeling (Penny et al., 2004, Buchel & Friston, 2001, Buchel & Friston, 1997a, McIntosh & Gonzalez-Lima, 1994) was introduced as a technique that allows combining observed changes in cortical activity and anatomical models. Variable parameters regerssion (Buchel & Friston, 2001, Buchel & Friston, 1998) was introduced as a flexible regression technique, allowing the regression coefficients to smoothly vary over time. Multiple linear regression models are sufficient to analyze effective connectivity to one region at a time. Structural equation modeling allows for more complicated models compromising many regions and demonstrates how nonlinear interaction are dealt withing this context. The basic idea behind this approach differs from the usual statistical approach of modeling individual observations. In muliple linear regression models the regression coefficients derive from the minimisation of the sum of squared differences of the predicted and observed dependent variable. Structural equation modeling approaches the data from a different perspective. The emphasis lies on the variance-covariance structure. Thus, the models are solved by minimizing the difference between the observed variance-covariance structure and the one implied by a structural or path model. An important issue in structural equation modeling is the determination of the participating regions and the underlying anatomical model. Several approaches can be adopted. Those include categorical comparisons between different conditions, statistical images highlighting structures of functional connectivity and non-human electrophysiological and anatomical studies. Due to the fact that the goal of some experiments is not to compute effective connectivity but to demonstrate changes in effective connectivity, variational parameter regression is proposed. Variational parameter regression allows the characterization of the variance of regression coefficients by using the framework of state space models and the Kalman filter (Buchel & Friston, 1997b).

6. Applications of fMRI

Functional neuroimaging has revolutionized the way that cognitive neuroscientists investigate the relationship between brain and behavior. Functional MRI is contributing to that revolution by providing a widely available, non-invasive technique which combines high spatial resolution with critical information about the temporal dynamics of the cortical and sub-cortical signal changes observed. It is widely accepted as a tool for identifying brain regions that are associated with certain perceptual, cognitive, emotional, and behavioral functions, such as visual, sensorimotor, language, and memory. It is suitable for accessing many aspects of human cognition and plays an important role in assisting presurgical planning in neurosurgery and in providing additional diagnostic information in the clinical management of patients who have functional disorders due to neurological diseases and mental illness. Some other fundamental application of fMRI is the management of pain, the improved assessment of risk, and the improved seizure localization.

The ability of fMRI to depict brain activity *in vivo* makes it a promising tool for the diagnosis, interpretation, and treatment evaluation of clinical disorders involving brain function. Presurgical planning is an area of clinical importance where fMRI plays an active role. When surgeons are going to remove a part of a patient's brain, it is critical to know exactly where various motor and sensory functions are mapped in that individual's brain. Functional MRI is a non-surgical technique for obtaining critical information before any surgical intervention starts.

Other areas of obvious clinical potential, such as psychopharmacology, neurology, stroke treatment and recovery, drug addiction, and psychiatric disorders, are under research. As already mentioned in previous sections fMRI allows for the creation of maps of brain activity corresponding to the performance of a specific task. A way to exploit these maps is to identify areas of the brain which are functionally important and therefore should be carefully avoided during neurosurgery. An important characteristic of these maps is that they are specific to the individual patient and they do not based on averages across many subjects.

Pharmacology is another area where fMRI has great potential. Although, fMRI is not recommended for the identification of the binding sites of a drug, due to its good spatial and temporal resolution, it can be utilized for the indication of brain areas that a drug influences.

A better understanding of the anatomy and physiology of addiction may eventually lead to more effective treatment.
As far as it concerns the application of fMRI to neurological and psychiatric disorders is still under development. Also fMRI has great potential in the area of medical diagnosis, since the analysis of this modality reveals a great variety of differences between healthy and diseased subjects. Many such studies have been conducted already concerning various diseases. In the future the fusion of fMRI with other medical image modalities will offer a significant amount of valuable information for the better understanding of human brain anatomy and function (Owen et al., 2001, Thulborn & Gisbet, 2001, Faro & Mohamed, 2006).

7. References

Achard, S.; Salvador, R., Whitcher, B., Suckling, J. & Bullmore, E. (2006). A resilient, low-frequency, small-world human brain functional network with highly connected association cortical hubs. Journal of Neuroscience, Vol. 26, 2006, 63–72

Balslev, D.; Nielsen, F., Frutiger, S., Sidtis, J., Christiansen, T., Svarer, C., Strother, S., Rottenberg, D., Hansen, L., Paulson, O. & Law, I. (2002). Cluster analysis of activity-time series in motor learning. Human Brain Mapping, Vol. 15, 2002, 135–145

Baumgartner, R.; Windischberger, C. & Moser, E. (1998). Quantification in functional magnetic resonance imaging: Fuzzy clustering vs. correlation analysis. Magnetic Resonance Imaging, Vol. 16, 1998, 115–125

Benjamini, Y. & Hochberg, Y. (1995). Controlling the false discovery rate: A practical and powerful approach to multiple testing. Journal of the Royal Statistical Society, Series B, Vol. 57, 1995, 289–300

Biswal, B. & Ulmer, J. (1999). Blind source separation of multiple signal sources of fMRI data sets using independent component analysis. Journal of Computer Assisted Tomography, Vol. 23, 1999, 265–271.

Bowman, F. & Patel, R. (2004). Identifying spatial relationships in neural processing using a multiple classification approach. NeuroImage, Vol. 23, 2004, 260–268

Breakspear, M.; Brammer, M., Bullmore, E., Das, P. & Williams, L. (2004). Spatiotemporal wavelet resampling for functional neuroimaging data. Human Brain Mapping, Vol. 23, 2004, 1–25

Buchel, C. & Friston, K. (1997b). Functional connectivity. In: Human Brain Function, R.S.J. Frackowiak (Ed.), K.J. Friston (Ed.), C. Frith (Ed.), R. Dolan (Ed.), K.J. Friston (Ed.), C.J. Price (Ed.), S. Zeki (Ed.), J. Ashburner (Ed.), & W.D. Penny (Ed.), Academic Press, 1st edition, 1997

Buchel, C. & Friston, K. (1998). Dynamic Changes in Effective Connectivity Characterized by Variable Parameter Regression and Kalman Filtering. Human Brain Mapping, Vol. 6, 1998, 403-408

Buchel, C. & Friston, K. (2001). Extracting Brain Connectivity. In: Functional MRI: An Introduction to Methods, Peter Jezzard (Ed.), Paul Matthews (Ed.), Stephen Smith (Ed.), 295-308, Oxford University Press, Oxford New York

Büchel, C. & Friston, K. (1997a). Modulation of connectivity in visual pathways by attention: Cortical interactions evaluated with structural equation modelling and fMRI. Cerebral Cortex, Vol. 7, 1997, 768–78

Bugli, C. & Lambert, P. (2007). Comparison between Principal Component Analysis and Independent Component Analysis in Electroencephalograms Modelling, Biometrical Journal, Vol. 2, 2007, 312-327

Bullmore, E.; Long, C., Suckling, J., Fadili, J., Calvert, G., Zelaya, F., Carpenter, T. & Brammer, M. (2001). Colored noise and computational inference in neurophysiological (fMRI) time series analysis: Resampling methods in time and wavelet domains. Human Brain Mapping, Vol. 12, 2001, 61–78

Burock, M. & Dale, A. M. (2000). Estimation and detection of event related fMRI signals with temporally correlated noise: A statistically efficient and unbiased approach. Human Brain Mapping, Vol. 11, No. 4, 2000, 249–269.

Calhoun, V. D., Adali, T., Pearlson, G. D., and Pekar, J. J. (2001). Spatial and temporal independent component analysis of functional MRI data containing a pair of task-related waveforms. Human Brain Mapping, Vol. 13, 2001, 43–53

Calhoun, V.; Adali, T., Hansen, L., Larsen, J. & Pekar, J. (2003a). ICA of functional MRI data: An overview. 4th International Symposium on Independent Component Analysis and Blind Signal Separation, 2003, 281–288

Calhoun, V.; Adali, T., Pekar, J. & Pearlson, G. (2003b). Latency (in)sensitive ICA: Group independent component analysis of fMRI data in the temporal frequency domain. NeuroImage, Vol. 20, 2003, 1661–1669

David, O.; Cosmelli, D. & Friston, K. (2004). Evaluation of different measures of functional connectivity using a neural mass model. NeuroImage, Vol. 21, 2004, 659-673

Descombes, X.; Kruggel, F. & von Cramon D. (1998). fMRI signal restoration using and edge preserving spatio-temporal Markov Random Field. NeuroImage, Vol. 8, 1998, 340-349

Fadili, M. & Bullmore, E. (2002). Wavelet-generalized least squares: A new BLU estimator of linear regression models with 1/f errors. NeuroImage, Vol. 15, 2002, 217–232

Fadili, M. & Bullmore, E. (2004). A comparative evaluation of wavelet-basedmethods for hypothesis testing of brain activation maps. NeuroImage, Vol. 23, 2004, 1112–1128

Fadili, M.; Ruan, S., Bloyet, D. & Mazoyer, B. (2000). A multistep unsupervised fuzzy clustering analysis of fMRI time series. Human Brain Mapping, Vol. 10, 2000, 160–178

Faro, S. & Mohamed, F. (2006). Clinical Overview and Future fMRI Applications. In: Functional MRI

Basic Principles and Clinical Applications, S. Faro (Ed.), & F. Mohamed, (Ed.), 496-502, Springer New York

Filzmoser, P.; Baumgartner, R. & Moser, E. (1999). A hierarchical clustering method for analyzing functional MR images. Magnetic Resonance Imaging, Vol. 17, 1999, 817-826

Flandin, G.; Penny, W., Pennec, X., Ayache, N. & Poline J. (2003). A multisubject anatomo-functional parcellation of the brain. NeuroImage (HBM'03), New York, USA, 2003

Friman, O. & Westin, C. (2005). Resampling fMRI time series. NeuroImage, Vol. 25, 2005, 859–867

Friman, O.; Borga, M., Lundberg, P. & Knutsson, H. (2002a). Detection of neural activity in fMRI using maximum correlation modeling. NeuroImage, Vol. 15, 2002, 386–395

Friman, O.; Borga, M., Lundberg, P. & Knutsson, H. (2002b). Exploratory fMRI analysis by autocorrelation maximization. NeuroImage, Vol. 16, 454–464

Friman, O.; Cedefamn, J., Lundberg, P., Borga, M. & Knutsson, H. (2001). Detection of neural activity in functional MRI using canonical correlation analysis. Magnetic Resonance in Medicine, Vol. 45, 2001, 323–330

Friston, K. (2003). Functional connectivity. In: Human Brain Function, R.S.J. Frackowiak (Ed.), K.J. Friston (Ed.), C. Frith (Ed.), R. Dolan (Ed.), K.J. Friston (Ed.), C.J. Price (Ed.), S. Zeki (Ed.), J. Ashburner (Ed.), & W.D. Penny (Ed.), Academic Press, 2nd edition, 2003

Friston, K., Jacquie, P., Chawal, D. & Bucher, C. (1999). Revealing interactions among brain systems with nonlinear PCA. Human Brain Mapping, Vol. 8, 1999, 92-97

Friston, K., Jacquie, P., Chawal, D. & Bucher, C. (2000b). Nonlinear PCA: Characterizing interactions between modes of brain activity. Philosophical Transactions The Royal Society of Biological Sciences, Vol. 355, 2000, 135-146

Friston, K.; Frith, C., and Frackowiak, R. (1993b) Timedependent changes in effective connectivity measured with PET. Human Brain Mapping, Vol. 1, 1993, 69–80

Friston, K.; Frith, C., Liddle, P., and Frackowiak, R. (1993c). Funcational connectivity: The principal and component analysis of large (PET) data sets. Journal of Cerebral Blood Flow in Metabolism, Vol. 13, 1993, 5–14

Friston, K.; Holmes, A., Poline, J., Grasby, P., Williams, S., Frackowiak, R. & Turner, R. (1995a). Analysis of fMRI time series revisited. NeuroImage, Vol. 2, No. 1, 1995, 45-53

Friston, K.; Josephs, O., Zarahn, E., Holmes, A., Rouquette, S. & Poline, J., (2000a). To smooth or not to smooth. NeuroImage, Vol. 12, No. 2, 2008, 196-208

Friston, K.; Penny, W., Phillips, C., Kiebel, S., Hinton, G. & Ashburner, J. (2002). Classical and Bayesian inference in neuroimaging:Theory. Neuroimage, Vol. 16, 2002, 465-483

Friston, K.; Ungerleider, L., Jezzard, P. & Turner, R. (1995b). Characterizing modulatory interactions between V1 and V2 in human cortex with fMRI. Human Brain Mapping, Vol. 2, 1995, 211–24

Friston, K.; Worsley, K., Frackowiak, R., Mazziotta, J. & Evans, A. (1993a). Assessing the significance of focal activations using their spatial extent. Human Brain Mapping, Vol. 1, No. 3, 1993, 210-220

Genovese, C. (2000). A Bayesian time-course model for functional magnetic resonance imaging (with discussion). Journal of the American Statistical Association, Vol. 95, 2000, 691–719.

Genovese, C.; Lazar, N. & Nichols, T. (2002). Thresholding of statistical maps in functional neuroimaging using the false discovery rate. NeuroImage, Vol. 15, 2002, 870–878

Goutte, C.; Toft, P., Rostrup, E., Nielsen, F. A. & Hansen, L. K. (1999). On clustering fMRI time series. NeuroImage, Vol. 9, 1999, 298–310

Hartvig, N. & Jensen, J. (2000). Spatial mixture modeling of fMRI data. Human Brain Mapping, Vol. 11, 2000, 233–248

Hartvig, N. (2002). A stochastic geometry model for functional magnetic resonance images. Scandinavian Journal of Statistics, Vol. 29, 333–353.

Hoge, R. & Pike, B. (2001). Quantitative measurement using fMRI. In: Functional MRI: An Introduction to Methods, Peter Jezzard (Ed.), Paul Matthews (Ed.), Stephen Smith (Ed.), 159-174, Oxford University Press, Oxford New York.

Jezzard, P. & Clare, S. (2001). Principles of nuclear magnetic resonance and MRI. In: Functional MRI: An Introduction to Methods, Peter Jezzard (Ed.), Paul Matthews (Ed.), Stephen Smith (Ed.), 67-92, Oxford University Press, Oxford New York.

Jezzard, P. ; Matthews, P. & Smith, S. (2001). Functional MRI: An introduction to methods, Oxford University Press, Oxford New York

Katanoda, K.; Matsuda, Y. & Sugishita, M. (2002). A spatio-temporal regression model for the analysis of functional MRI data. NeuroImage, Vol. 17, 1415–1428

Kershaw, J., Ardekani, B., & Kanno, I. (1999). Application of Bayesian inference to fMRI data analysis. IEEE Transactions on Medical Imaging, Vol. 18, No. 12, 1999, 1138–1153

Kruggel, F.; von Cramon, D. & Descombes, X. (1999). Comparison of filtering methods of fMRI datasets. NeuroImage, Vol. 10, No. 5, 1999, 530-543

Laird, A.; Rogers, B. & Meyerand, M. (2004). Comparison of Fourier and wavelet resampling methods. Magnetic Resonance in Medicine, Vol. 51, 2004, 418–422

Lazar, N. (2008). The Statistical Analysis of Functional MRI Data, Springer Science+Business Media, LLC, ISBN 978-0-387-78190-7, USA

Long, C.; Brown, E., Manoach, D. & Solo, V. (2004). Spatiotemporal wavelet ananlysis for functional MRI. NeuroImage, Vol. 23, No. 2, 2004, 500-516

Lowe, M. & Sorenson, J. (1997). Spatially filtering functional magnetic resonance imaging data. Magnetic Resonance in Medicine, Vol. 37, No. 5, 1997, 723-729

Marchini, J. & Presanis, A. (2004). Comparing methods of analyzing fMRI statistical parametric maps. NeuroImage, Vol. 22, 2004, 1203-1213

Marchini, J. & Ripley, B. (2000). A new statistical approach to detecting significant activation in functional MRI. NeuroImage, Vol. 12, No.4, 2000, 366–380

McIntosh, A. & Gonzalez-Lima, F. (1994). Structural equation modelling and its application to network analysis in functional brain imaging. Human Brain Mapping, Vol. 2, 1994, 2–22

McKeown, M.; Makeig, S., Brown, G., Jung, T., Kindermann, S., Bell, A., & Sejnowski, T. (1998). Analysis of fMRI data by blind separation into independent spatial components. Human Brain Mapping, Vol. 6, 1998, 160–188

Menon, R. & Goodyear, B. (2001). Spatial and temporal resolution in fMRI. In: Functional MRI: An Introduction to Methods, Peter Jezzard (Ed.), Paul Matthews (Ed.), Stephen Smith (Ed.), 145-158, Oxford University Press, Oxford New York.

Nandy, R. & Cordes, D. (2004). Improving the spatial specificity of canonical correlation analysis in fMRI. Magnetic Resonance in Medicine, Vol. 52, No. 4, 2004, 947-952

Nandy, R. and Cordes, D. (2003). Novel nonparametric approach to canonical correlation analysis with applications to low CNR functional MRI data. Magnetic Resonance in Medicine, Vol. 50, 2003, 354–365

Owen, A.; Epstein, R. & Johnsrude, I. (2001). fMRI applications to cognitive neuroscience. In: Functional MRI: An Introduction to Methods, Peter Jezzard (Ed.), Paul Matthews (Ed.), Stephen Smith (Ed.), 311-327, Oxford University Press, Oxford New York

Parrish, T.; Gitelman, D., LaBar, K. & Mesulam, M. (2000). Impact of signal-to-noise on functional MRI. Magnetic Resonance in Medicine, Vol. 44, No. 6, 2000, 925-932

Penny W.; Stephan, K., Mechelli, A. & Friston, K. (2004). Modelling Functional Integration: A Comparison of Structural Equation and Dynamic Causal and Models. NeuroImage, Vol. 23, 2004, 264-274

Poline, J. & Mazoyer, B. (1995). Enhanced detection in brain activation maps using a multifiltering approach. Journal of Cerebral Blood Flow Metabolism, Vol. 14, No. 4, 1994, 639-642

Purdon, P. & Weisskoff, R. (1998). Effect of temporal autocorrelation due to physiological noise and stimulus paradigm on voxel-level false positive rates in fMRI. Human Brain Mapping, Vol. 6, 1998, 239-249

Purdon, P.; Solo, V., Weisskoff, R. & Brown. E. (2001). Locally regularized spatiotemporal modeling and model comparison of functional MRI. NeuroImage, Vol. 14, No. 4, 2001, 912-923

Skudlarski, P.; Constable, P. & Core J. (1999). ROC analysis of statistical methods used in functional MRI: Individual subjects. NeuroImage, Vol. 9, No. 3, 1999, 311-329

Smith, M. & Fahrmeir, L. (2007). Spatial Bayesian variable selection with application to functional magnetic resonance imaging. Journal of the American Statistical Association, Vol. 102, 417–431

Smith, M.; Putz, B., Auer, D. & Fahrmeir, L. (2003). Assessing brain activity through spatial Bayesian variable selection. NeuroImage, Vol. 20, 802–815

Smith, S. (2001). Preparing fMRI data for statistical analysis. In: Functional MRI: An Introduction to Methods, Peter Jezzard (Ed.), Paul Matthews (Ed.), Stephen Smith (Ed.), 229-242, Oxford University Press, Oxford New York.

Sole, A.; Ngan S., Sapiro, G., Hu. X. & Lopez, A. (2001). Anisotropic 2-D and 3-D averaging of fMRI signals. IEEE Transactions on Medical Imaging, Vol. 20, No. 2, 2001, 86-93

Solo, V.; Purdon, P., Weisskoff, R. & Brown E. (2001). A signal estimation approach to functional MRI. IEEE Transactions on Medical Imaging, Vol. 20, 2001, 26-35

Stone, J.; Porrill, J., Porter, N. & Wilkinson, I. (2002). Spatiotemporal Independent Component Analysis of Event-Related fMRI Data Using Skewed Probability Density Functions. NeuroImage, Vol. 15, 2002, 407–421

Strother, S. (2006). Evaluating fMRI preprocessing pipelines. IEEE Engineering in Medicine and Biology, Vol. 25, No. 2, March/April 2006, 27-41.

Strother, S.; La Conte, S., Kai Hansen, L., Anderson, J., Zhang, J., Pulapura, J. & Rottenberg, D. (2004). Optimizing the fMRI data-processing pipeline using prediction and reproducibility performance metrics: I. A preliminary group analysis. NeuroImage, Vol. 23, Suppl. I, 2004, S196-S207

Thirion, B. & Faugeras, O. (2003). Dynamical components analysis of fMRI data through kernel PCA. NeuroImage, Vol. 20, 34–49

Thulborn, K. & Gisbert, A. (2001). Clinical applications of mapping neurocognitive processes in the human brain with functional MRI. In: Functional MRI: An Introduction to Methods, Peter Jezzard (Ed.), Paul Matthews (Ed.), Stephen Smith (Ed.), 329-349, Oxford University Press, Oxford New York.

Viviani, R.; Gron, G. & Spitzer, M. (2005). Functional principal component analysis of fMRI data. Human Brain Mapping, Vol. 24, 2005, 109–129

Wink, A. & Roerdink, J. (2004). Denoising functional MR images: A comparison of wavelet denoisng and Gaussian smoothing. IEEE Transaction on Medical Imaging, Vol. 23, No. 3, 2004, 374-387

Woolrich, M.; Jenkinson, M., Brady, J. & Smith, S. (2004). Fully Bayesian spatio-temporal modeling of FMRI data. IEEE Transactions on Medical Imaging, Vol. 23, 213–231.

Worsley, K. (2000). Comment on "A Bayesian time-course model for functional magnetic resonance imaging data". Journal of the American Statistical Association, Vol. 95, 711-716.

Worsley, K.; Liao, C., Aston, J., Petre, V., Duncan, G., Morales, F. & Evans, A. (2002). A general statistical approach for fMRI data. NeuroImage, Vol. 15, 2002, 1-15

Worsley, K.; Marrett, S., Neelin, P. & Evans, A. (1996). Searching scale space for activation in PET images. Human Brain Mapping, Vol. 4, No. 1, 1996, 74-90

Carbon Nanotubes in Bone Tissue Engineering

Kaveh PourAkbar Saffar[1,2] , Nima JamilPour[3] and Gholamreza Rouhi[4]
[1]Department of Biomedical Engineering, Amirkabir University of Technology, Tehran, Iran
[2]Department of Mechanical and Manufacturing Engineering, University of Calgary, Calgary, Alberta, Canada
[3]School of Mechanical Engineering, Semnan University, Semnan, Iran
[4]Department of Mechanical Engineering and School of Human Kinetics, University of Ottawa, Ontario, Canada

1. Introduction

Exceptional properties of carbon nanotubes (CNTs) such as electrical, mechanical, chemical and thermal, attract growing attention and interest among different disciplines toward their usage in modern technologies. A more recent implementation of the concept is encountered within the field of bioengineering where researchers are focusing on the bioactivity and biocompatibility of CNTs. Carbon is the main component of biomolecules, and this makes CNT to be considered as a biocompatible material. Several studies report increase in the activity of living cells adjacent to CNTs. Electrical response of CNTs to mechanical loading makes them piezoelectric biosensors. Having the highest strength known so far, CNTs are believed to be an ideal reinforcement for composites. Use of such versatile functions of carbon nanotubes, as composite matrix reinforcements, may have the potential to apply this unique nano-structured material to tissue engineering issues such as replacement, healing, and growth (Abarrategi et al., 2008). At the same time, cell adhesion, viability, and accelerated growth support the idea of using CNTs as substrates for tissue regeneration (Lobo et al., 2008). These potentials and many others point at the suitability of CNTs for bone tissue engineering applications (Usui et al., 2008). For example, CNTs can be viewed as reinforcement to orthopedic materials such as bone cement (Marrs et al., 2006; 2007). It has also the ability to act as a biosensor to report bone growth adjacent to an implant (Sirivisoot & Webster, 2008). Having a density similar to graphite and much lower than that of other metallic bone scaffold materials, CNTs have been viewed as excellent stimulant scaffolds for growth and proliferation of osteoblasts, the bone forming cells (Zanello et al., 2006). Therefore, bone regeneration on CNT reinforced scaffolds is increasingly favored. This suggests making a mechanically enhanced nano-bio-composite for applications in both curative and preventative approaches in bone tissue engineering.

In this chapter, first, a brief explanation about the bone structure as a biocomposite at different hierarchical levels and a quick review on bone mechanics and remodeling process will be provided. Next, the most important approaches to CNT applications in bone tissue engineering will be reviewed and a new area of applicable researches will be introduced.

This includes investigation on the idea of bone mineral phase formation on CNTs as a replacement for collagen fibers in the infrastructure of bone. The initial steps of such a study should include modeling and simulation of the phenomenon, since it is dealing with a living tissue and many difficulties come along with experimental studies. Therefore, modeling issues will be addressed and discussed based on the recent experimental findings on the potentials of CNT as a biocompatible reinforcement and scaffold for bone tissue growth. Some results of modeling will be presented and also some predictions of our theoretical model will be provided and discussed based on both mechanical and biological functions of bone tissue.

2. Bone Structure, Mechanics and Remodeling Process

Bone is the main constituent of the skeletal system and differs from the connective tissues in rigidity and hardness. The rigidity and hardness of bone enable the skeleton to maintain the shape of the body; to protect the vital organs; to supply the framework for the bone marrow; and also to transmit the force of muscular contraction from one part to another during movement (Cowin, 2001). It is made basically of the fibrous protein collagen, impregnated with a mineral closely resembling calcium phosphate (Currey, 2002). The mineral content of bone acts as a reservoir for ions, particularly calcium (almost 99% of the calcium of our body is stored in bone), and it also contributes to the regulation of extracellular fluid composition (Cowin, 2001). It also contains water, which is very important mechanically, some not well-understood proteins and polysaccharides, living cells and blood vessels. The organic matrix of bone consists of 90% collagen, the most abundant protein in the body, and about 10% of various noncollagenous proteins (Behari, 1991). The protein part, mainly collagen type I, forms a model for the subsequent deposition of hyroxyapatite, the mineral phase of bone which provides rigidity to the structure. From mechanical point of view, bone is a non-homogeneous and anisotropic material. Spongy and cortical bones can be considered as an orthotropic (with 9 independent material constants) and transversely isotropic materials (with 5 independent material constants), respectively. In the physiological range of loading, bone can be assumed as a linear elastic material, with negligible viscoelastic effects (Rouhi, 2006a). Bone is stronger in compression than in tension, and much greater young's moduli of elasticity than shear modulus (Bartel et al., 2006).
The term composite is usually employed for those materials in which two or more distinct phases are separated on a scale larger than the atomic, and in which their material properties such as stiffness and strength are changed compared with those of a homogeneous material. On the basis of the definition of a composite and also by considering bone structure, it is evident that bone is a composite material. Bone, as a biocomposite, shows hierarchical structures at different scales (Lakes, 1996). For example, in cortical bone, on the microstructural level, there are osteon (or havesian systems), which are large hollow fibers (200 to 250 μm outer diameter) composed of concentric lamellae and of pores. The lamellae are made up of fibers, and the fibers contain fibrils. At the nanosclae, the fibers are a composite of mineral hydroxyapatite and the protein collagen. These well organized structural features have been associated with various unique structural properties. For instance, the stiffness of bone is related to the composite structure of mineral microcrystals and collagen (mostly type I) fibers (Lakes & Saha, 1979); and the cement lines as weak interfaces convey a degree of toughness to bone (Piekarski, 1970).

Bone is produced inside the body and is usually covered with cells throughout life. Because of its nonexpendable nature, all bone resorption and formation occurs at the bone surfaces, as opposed to soft biological tissues which can have both interstitial and appositional growth. Bone is a porous structure with different values of porosity depending on its macrostructure. At the macroscopic level, there are basically two types of bone structures: cortical (compact or Haversian) and cancellous (spongy, or trabecular) bone. Cortical bone is a dense, solid mass with only microscopic channels, and with a maximal density of about 1.8 gr/cm^3. Approximately 80% of the skeletal mass in the adult human is cortical bone, which forms the outer wall of all bones and is largely responsible for the supportive and protective function of the skeleton. The main structural unit of the cortical bone is called osteon. A typical osteon is a hollow cylinder with the outer and inner diameteres of about 200 (or 250) and 50 μm, respectively. An osteon is made up of 20 to 30 concentric lamellae, and surrounding the outer border of each osteon there is a cement line, a 1-2 μm thick layer of mineralized matrix deficient in collagen fibers, which it is believed they act as crack stoppers when cracks are present. On the other hand, cancellous (spongy or trabecular) bone is a lattice of narrow rods and plates (70 to 200 μm in thickness) of calcified bone tissue called trabeculae, with an average thickness of of 100-150 μm (Van der Meulen & Prendergast, 2000). The trabeculae are surrounded by bone marrow that is vascular and provides nutrients and waste disposal for the bone cells. The symmetry of structure in cancellous bone depends upon the direction of applied loads. If the stress pattern in spongy bone is complex, then the structure of the network of trabeculae is also complex and highly asymmetric. Comparison of micrograph structures with the density maps show that low density, open cell, rod like structure develops in regions of low stress while greater density, closed cell, plate like structures occur in regions of higher density in cancellous bone (Gibson, 1985). There are no blood vessels within the trabeculae, but there are vessels immediately adjacent to the tissue. Trabecualr bone is less mineralized than cortical bone, and experimental evidence and data suggest that spongy bone is much more active in remodeling than in cortical bone (Guo & Goldstein, 1997). The major cellular elements of bone include osteoclasts (bone resorbing cells), osteoblasts (bone making cells), osteocytes (it is believed that they act as mechano-sensors), (Burger & Klein-Nulend, 1999) and bone-lining cells (inactive cells on the resting surfaces of bone). While osteoblasts and osteoclasts have opposite functions and have different developmental origins, they exhibit several parallel features, particularly with respect to their life cycles. Osteoblasts and osteoclasts are both temporary cells with relatively short life spans (Parfitt, 1995).

Skeletal development begins as mesenchymal condensations that appear early in the fetal period. These condensations ossify to form membrane bones through intramembranous ossification and cartilaginous bones through endochondral ossification. In both types of ossifications, bone formation is similar, beginning with an increase in the number of cells and fibers. The cells differentiate into osteoblasts, which lay down an unmineralized matrix, and the osteoid that mineralizes almost immediately. During growth, bone is formed in the necessary places and resorbed as needed to attain the final shape, in a process called modeling. Modeling involves resorption drifts and formation drifts that remove *or* add bone over wide regions of bone surfaces. Thus, in modeling bone resorbing and making cells act independently and at different spots. Modeling controls the growth, shape, size, strength, and anatomy of bones and joints. Collectively, modeling leads to increasing the outside cortex and marrow cavity diameters, shaping the ends of long bones. Modeling allows not only the development of normal architecture during growth, but also the modulation of this architecture and mass when the mechanical condition changes. When bone trains exceed a modeling threshold window, the minimum effective strain, modeling in the formation mode is turned on to increase bone mass and strength, and lower its strains toward the bottom of the window. When strains remain below the modeling threshold, mechanically controlled formation drifts stay inactive. As the forces on bone increases 20 times in size between birth and maturity, modeling in the formation mode keeps making bones strong enough to keep their strains from exceeding the modeling threshold, and therefore from reaching the microdamage threshold (Jee, 2001). In the adult age, the localized and independent activities of cells in modeling, are replaced by a distributed and coordinated work of the cells, resulting in a dynamic state called remodeling process. The actual remodeling occurs in two steps: the osteoclasts attach to the bone surface, dissolve the mineral, and later the organic phase of the bone, opening a hole that is subsequently filled by a number of osteoblasts, which produce the collagen matrix and secrete a protein which stimulates the calcium phosphate deposition. This state can be shifted in favour of bone formation or resorption by mechanical stimulation, hormonal effects, nutrition, or diseases among other factors (Rouhi, 2006a). There are several reasons for the necessity of remodeling process, for examples: immature bone formed at the metaphyses is structurally inferior to mature bone; or the quality of adult bone deteriorates with time; or microcracks produced in bone by daily activity should be removed to attain a desired strength in bone; and/or ions concentration (e.g. calcium) should be adjusted to lie in an acceptable range; and, most likely, other factors that will be known in the future (Rouhi, 2006a). Assuming normal rates of adult bone remodeling, cortical bone has a mean age of 20 years and cancellous bone 1 to 4 years (Parfitt, 1983). Many diseases are related to global shift in the remodeling balance, for example: Osteoporosis, which is caused by increased osteoclast activity; Ostetrosis, which is an abnormal increase in bone density by reduced osteoclast activity, Osteopenia, which is the bone loss by decreased osteoblast activity. The treatment of these diseases is based on drugs that intend to restore the remodeling equilibrium. Most of the work on osteoporosis, probably the most important of these diseases, seems to be currently in the osteoclast inhibition side (Rodan & Martin, 2000; Teitelbaum, 2000; Rouhi et al., 2007).

An early hypothesis about the dependence of the structure and form of bones on their mechanical function was proposed by Galileo in 1638 (Ascenzi, 1993). The nature of this dependence was first described in a semi-quantitative manner by Wolff (Wolff, 1886), who stated that remodeling of bone occurs in response to physical stresses or to the lack of them - in that bone is deposited in sites subjected to stress and is resorbed from sites where there is not enough stress. Several mechanisms have been proposed to relate changes in mechanical loads to the adaptive responses in bone, including (among many others): piezoelectric and streaming potentials (Gjelsvik, 1973a,b; Pollack et al., 1984); mechanical fatigue microdamage (Frost,1960; Carter & Hayes, 1977; Carter & Cayler, 1983; 1985; Martin, 1992; 1995; Prendergast & Taylor, 1994); and extra- cellular fluid pressure gradient effects on bone cells (Cowin et al., 1991; 1995). Experimental evidence can be found in support of each of the above-mentioned mechanisms. In 1964, Frost subgrouped bone remodeling into surface and internal remodeling (Frost, 1964). Surface remodeling refers to the remodeling of bone on the external surfaces, i.e. on endosteal and periosteal surfaces. The phenomenological model for surface remodeling postulates a causal relationship between the rate of surface deposition or resorption and the strain in the surface of the bone (Cowin, 2003). On the basis of the fact that all bone resorption and formation occurs on bone free surfaces, a newly defined quantity so-called free surface density, was used instead of commonly used volume fraction in the adaptive elasticity theory (Cowin & Hegedus, 1976) and surface remodeling equations are resulted (Rouhi et al., 2004). Interestingly, in the newly developed model of surface remodeling, one can see a strong dependency between the rate of surface bone remodeling and the geometry of bone mass distribution. It is also well accepted that bone microdamages can initiate and also accelerate bone remodeling process (Taylor et al., 2007). Introducing a microcracks factor besides bone specific surface into adaptive elasticity theory, a much more complex form of bone remodeling equation will be resulted (Rouhi et al., 2006b), in which not only the mechanical stimuli, but also their rate and history play a role in the rate of bone remodeling process.

A preliminary review on the bone structure, bone mechanics, and bone remodeling process, helps in better understanding of the bone tissue engineering problems. As the main subject of this chapter, the following section deals with most important applications of carbon nanotubes in bone tissue engineering.

3. Quick Review on CNT Applications in Bone Tissue Engineering

Polymer matrix composites have recently been the focus of attention in many researches and a considerable number of such studies are dealing with the application of biopolymers. Acrylic bone cement, namely poly methyl-methacrylate (PMMA), is an example of a common biopolymer. This is a biomaterial widely used in orthopedic surgeries as a bone filling cement, though is extremely weak in comparison with natural bone tissue regarding mechanical properties. This becomes meaningful when the stresses applied to a load-bearing bone in human daily activities are considered. Experimental and theoretical studies show that there is an increase in Young's modulus and fracture toughness of PMMA when reinforced with CNTs (Marrs et al., 2006). The resulting composite also exhibits improved fatigue and fracture resistance by bridging and arresting cracks and also absorbing energy (Marrs et al., 2007). Embedding functionalized CNTs into PMMA matrix thus improves the clinical functions of bone cement, mechanically, while chemical functional groups on CNT surface and tips can induce cross-links to the surrounding matrix material and contribute in load transfer from PMMA matrix to CNT. This leads to further enhancement of the mechanical properties of the bone cement.

Ninety-five percent of bone organic phase contains collagen (Judex et al., 1999). Collagen is a fibrous protein which exists in both soft and hard tissues, and plays a critical role in providing them with mechanical tensile strength. Although many researchers studying carbon nanotubes in collagen matrices are focusing on CNTs as scaffolds for muscle tissue engineering, the approach is most likely applicable in the area that is dealing with bone tissue. Scanning electron microscopy (SEM) observation shows physical interactions between CNT and collagen matrix, after mixing solubilized Type I collagen with the solution of carboxyl functionalized CNTs at different concentrations (MacDonald et al., 2005). Type I collagen is an interesting biomolecule that has self-assembly properties and thus may be useful in inducing assembly and alignment of CNTs. Through applying mechanical strains, the mechanism of self-assembly and alignment offers possible production of ordered and anisotropic CNT composite materials (Voge et al., 2008). This, beside proven cell viability on such a scaffold, offers utilities of the composite for various medical applications.

Bone, itself, in many studies is considered as a fiber reinforced ceramic matrix composite material for modeling purposes (Raeisi Najafi et al., 2007a,b; 2009). The complicated

structure of bone should provide high strength, for body support, and go through the remodeling process in response to applied stresses caused by everyday normal and/or strenuous physical activity. Bone should also be porous so that oxygen and other nutrients can be available for internal cells, while, at the same time, this porosity must not reduce its resistance to fracture. Bone is also a main reservoir of minerals in the body. It is a composite of minerals, organics, and water. The fundamental nano-structure of bone is mineralized collagen. Type I collagen fibril (organic phase) in bone is made up of three polypeptide chains of amino acids in a triple helix. Such a triple-helical molecule can be viewed as a fiber with 1.5 nm in diameter and 300 nm in length. This stiff protein provides tensile strength of bone and is the main component of the matrix in which the mineral phase forms. Mineral component of bone is dahllite, or carbonated apatite $(Ca_{10}(PO_4, CO_3)_6(OH)_2)$, in the form of plate-shaped crystals of 50×25 nm, and a third dimension of about 1.5 to 4 nm. Long axis of the plate is generally parallel to bone axis, maximizing its compressive strength (Weiner & Wagner, 1999; Meyers et al., 2008).
Hydroxyapatite (HAp), with a chemical formula of $(Ca_{10}(PO_4)_6(OH)_2)$ is a bioceramic material, often used for clinical bone grafting and implantation. HAp has the ability to bond chemically with living bone tissue because of its chemical, compositional, biological, and crystal structure similarities to native apatite, bone mineral phase, in the human skeleton. Furthermore, the bioactivity and biocompatibility of HAp inspire osteoblast adhesion and proliferation (Rabiei et al., 2007). However, brittle HAp is fragile in tension and offers low fracture toughness in comparison with natural bone, and thus is unsuitable for main load bearing sites. On the other hand, excellent mechanical and biological characteristics of CNTs suggest the chance of strengthening and toughening HAp, while keeping its bioactivity (White et al., 2007). Measurements on HAp-CNT composite coatings fabricated by laser surface alloying show increase in elastic modulus and hardness of HAp due to adding CNT (Chen et al., 2006). Scratching tests also indicate enhanced wear resistance and lower friction coefficient as a result of raising the amount of CNTs in the composite (Chen et al., 2007). Therefore, HAp-CNT composite is introduced as a favorable coating material for load-bearing metallic implants. Bending strength and fracture toughness of sintered HAp-CNT composite is reported to improve compared to pure HAp (Li et al., 2007). Scattered CNTs in HAp coating by plasma spraying method, result in promotion of fracture toughness and crystallinity of the composite. Higher crystallinity leads to enhanced precipitation of apatite over the CNT surface, observed by SEM. Moreover, unlimited growth of cultivated human osteoblast cells is also detected near the CNT surface (Balani et al., 2007).
CNTs, on the other hand, can be considered as the mineralization site for HAp. Carboxyl functionalized CNTs (CNT-COOH) are used to chemically synthesize HAp, as an effective template. This is due to the capability of carboxylate ions (COO^-) to absorb calcium ions (Ca^{2+}) and contribute in HAp crystallization as a result of exposure to phosphate ions (PO_4^{3-}) (Aryal et al., 2006a). The method is also examined using simulated body fluid to provide physiological conditions. These synthesized composites are found to chemically resemble natural bone. Initiation of HAp nucleation is shown (by physico-chemical characterization of the composites) to take place within carboxyl group (Aryal et al., 2006b).
Other chemically functionalized CNTs are shown to be capable of conducting the scaffold role for artificial bone material growth, as well. Nucleation and crystallization of HAp is observed on functionalized CNTs with phosphonates and poly amino-benzene sulfonic acid

in the solution phase. Mineral ions attracted to these functional groups on CNTs can lead to enhanced HAp self-assembly compared to carboxylated CNTs (Zhao et al., 2005).

CNTs are close in size to the triple helical collagen fibrils which can act as templates for nano-sized HAp crystallization when functionalized and are also capable of providing structural tensile strength to the HAp-matrix composite material. However, due to the differences in mechanical behavior of CNTs and collagen fibers under loading, there is a serious necessity to look into the mechanical response of such an artificial bone nano-composite to physiological loading for possible future applications. It is consequently essential to prepare a mechanical model of CNT reinforced HAp. The model can be utilized to obtain a preliminary evaluation of the suitability of such an artificial bone tissue under physiological loading conditions.

In the following section, therefore, a model for the HAp-CNT composite is provided by incorporating cross-links which represent the bonds between CNT (reinforcement) and HAp (matrix) through functionalized sites. The cross-links are taken to be responsible for load transfer between the two phases of the composite. This model is to provide preliminary predictions for effective Young's modulus of HAp-CNT composite. The model can also be developed to predict tensile axial strength and consequently the energy absorbed prior to fracture (fracture toughness) of the CNT reinforced bone tissue.

4. Establishment of the Model

In the presented model, carboxylated CNT is considered as the substratum on which the bone mineral phase, i.e. HAp, forms. To explore the model, first, a brief description of the mechanism of HAp formation on this scaffold is required. The carbon atom of the carboxyl group (-COOH) is attached to a carbon atom on the CNT which already has three sp^2 covalent bonds with three adjacent carbon atoms on the CNT surface. This happens while the hybridization of the carbon atom on the CNT bonded to the carbon atom on functional group changes to sp^3 (Odegard et al., 2005). Therefore, carboxyl group attaches to the CNT through a sp^3 carbon-carbon (C-C) bond (see Fig. 1).

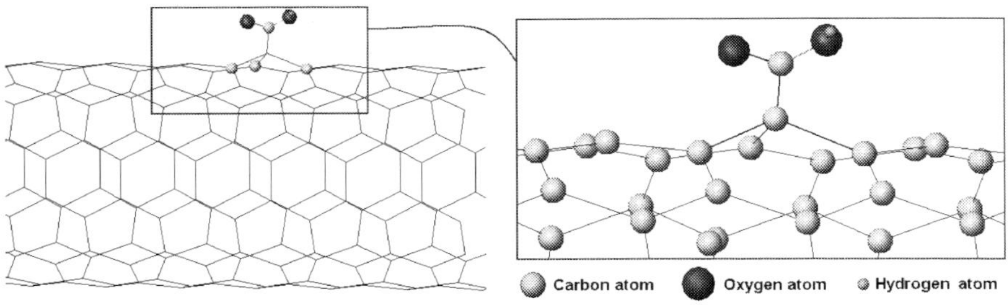

Fig. 1. Illustration of a -COOH functional group on CNT surface (PourAkbar Saffar et al., 2009a)

Carboxyl group loses hydrogen and obtains a negative electrical charge. The negative charge is evenly distributed on the two remaining oxygen atoms, causing an unstable configuration. This negative charge is tending to attract positively charged calcium ions. After that, by exposing this unstable assemblage to phosphate and hydroxide ions, it is anticipated to form a similar type of calcium phosphate to what is called HAp on the CNT surface through the carboxyl functionalized site. This mechanism is believed to be responsible for the initiation of HAp precipitation on CNT surface (Aryal et al., 2006a,b). The calcium phosphate-like material induces ionic interaction with -COO's head due to oppositely charged ions at the contact sites. Further supply of mineral ions can lead to growth of the HAp in different directions. Other probable functional sites on the CNT may also contribute simultaneously in local HAp deposition on the CNT and this, in turn, will result in the formation of a homogeneous and continuous mineral material surrounding the CNT (see Fig. 2).

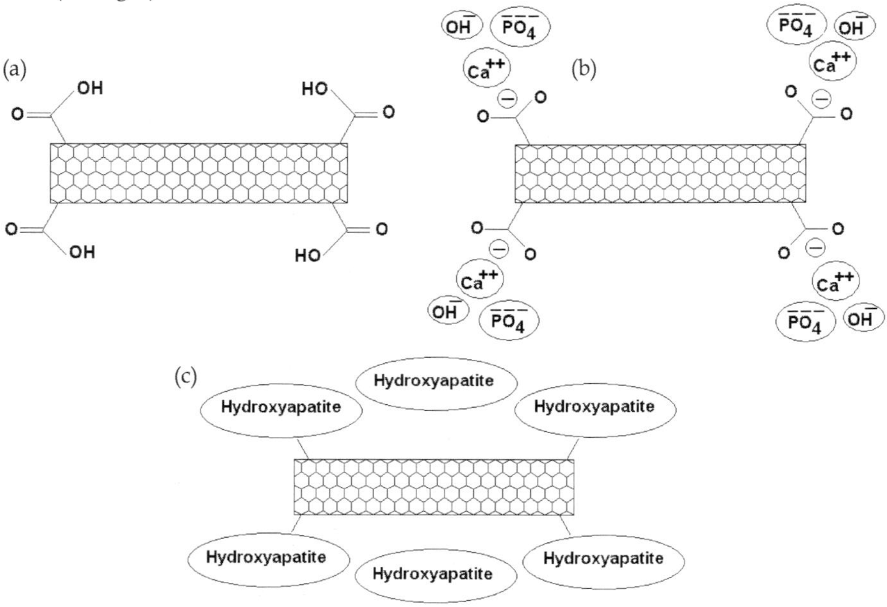

Fig. 2. (a) -COOH functionalized CNT; (b) Attraction of calcium, phosphate, and hydroxide ions; and (c) HAp formation around CNT (PourAkbar Saffar et al., 2009a)

To derive the model, a representative volume element (RVE) of the CNT-HAp composite is considered. For building the RVE, a tip-functionalized (carboxylated) armchair (8,8) single walled carbon nanotube (SWCNT) with a length of 2L is assumed onto which the HAp matrix is assembled. The CNT is considered as an elastic cylindrical beam element with a diameter of 1.08 nm for (8,8) SWCNT, at the center of the RVE. Two C-C covalent bonds are assumed at the two tips of the RVE, inducing bonding between CNT and HAp matrix. They are presented as elastic beam elements, referred to as cross-links, using a structural mechanics approach introduced by (Li & Chou, 2003). Each cross-link has total strain energy equal to the C-C bonding energy in sp^3 hybridization. Since electrostatic interactions within an ionic solid are strong enough, the ionic bonding area between carboxylate ion and HAp phase is taken as a continuous region in the model. HAp matrix in the RVE is, thus, assumed as a homogeneous, continuous hollow cylindrical beam element, and concentric with the CNT. The C-C bond length is taken to be 0.1522 nm (Cornell et al., 1995) (Fig. 2).

Outer diameter of this element is determined according to the CNT volume fraction in the RVE.

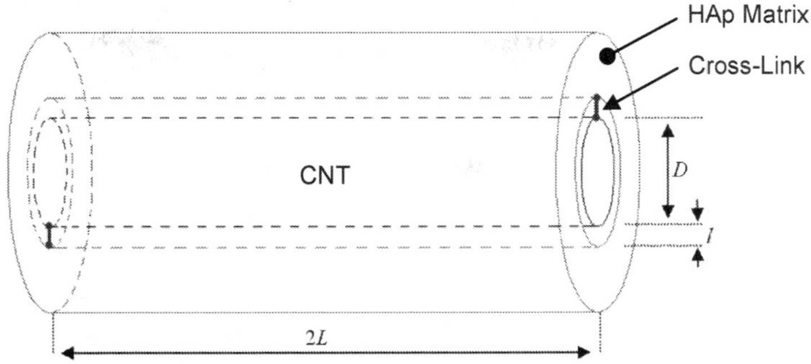

Fig. 3. RVE of HAp formed on tip-functionalized CNT

The cross-link is responsible for stress transfer from HAp matrix to the CNT, and thus, takes part in the reinforcing mechanism in the composite when subjected to an axial load. Elastic constants for CNT and HAp are indicated in Table 1.

	Young's Modulus (GPa)	Poisson's Ratio
SWCNT	1010	0.28
HAp Matrix	130	0.3

Table 1. Elastic constants of SWCNT and HAp matrix

For evaluating the characteristics of cross-link beam element, a connection between molecular and structural continuum mechanics is used. The method has been previously applied for simulating SWCNTs as space-frame structural elements, where covalent bonds are treated as beam elements. In this approach, the total atomic bonding energy in the C-C covalent bond is set equal to total strain energy of a uniform beam with length l and circular cross-sectional area A (Tserpes & Papanikos, 2005). If relatively negligible electrostatic forces and non-bonding interactions are discarded, the total bonding energy can be expressed as:

$$U_{total} = \sum U_r + \sum U_\theta + \sum U_\tau \tag{1}$$

U_r, U_θ, and U_τ are the energies due to stretch, bending, and sum of dihedral angle and out-of-plane torsion interactions, respectively. If the bond stretching increment, the bond angle variation, and the angle variation of bond twisting are represented by Δr, $\Delta\theta$, and $\Delta\phi$, respectively, then each energy can be expressed as:

$$U_r = \frac{1}{2}k_r(\Delta r)^2, \qquad U_\theta = \frac{1}{2}k_\theta(\Delta\theta)^2, \qquad U_\tau = \frac{1}{2}k_\tau(\Delta\phi)^2 \tag{2}$$

where in molecular mechanics, k_r, k_θ, and k_τ represent the resistance force constants for the bond stretching, bending, and torsion, respectively. So, direct relationships between molecular and structural mechanics parameters can be determined as:

$$\frac{EA}{l}=k_r,\qquad \frac{EI}{l}=k_\theta,\qquad \frac{GJ}{l}=k_\tau \tag{3}$$

Here, E and G are the Young's modulus and shear modulus of elasticity for the beam element. Cross-sectional area, moment of inertia, and polar moment of inertia, for a cylindrical beam with a diameter of d can be obtained as $A=\pi d^2/4$, $I=\pi d^4/64$, and $J=\pi d^4/32$, respectively. The values of molecular mechanics parameters for a C-C covalent bond in sp^3 hybridization are found to be $k_r = 4.39\times10^{-7}$ N/nm, $k_\theta = 8.76\times10^{-10}$ N.nm/rad^2, and $k_\tau = 2.78\times10^{-10}$ N.nm/rad^2 (Cornell et al., 1995; Jorgensen & Severance, 1990). Therefore, the values for d, E, and G are obtained as 0.179 nm, 2.67 TPa, and 0.42 TPa, respectively.

Once the RVE model is built as a combination of elastic elements in series and parallel orders, the problem can be tackled for axial loading condition to determine the mechanical response of the RVE in the form of elastic deformation (PourAkbar Saffar et al., 2008). This, thus, can give the effective axial Young's modulus of the RVE. Uniform axial loading causes deformation in the RVE elements. Clearly, larger deformation occurs in the element representing HAp due to its lower Young's modulus in comparison with the CNT, although this deformation is significantly smaller than non-reinforced HAp under similar loading condition. The difference in HAp and CNT deformation causes stretching in the cross-link. Therefore, cross-link participates in the reinforcing mechanism by transferring stresses from the HAp matrix to the CNT.

A criterion can be assumed for the determination of the axial tensile strength of the RVE. In this approach, the axial tensile stress applied on the RVE cross-section leads to a combination of stresses within each element, since the linking beam element transfers stresses from the matrix to the reinforcement. The resulting stresses in either HAp matrix or the C-C bond representing element may exceed the ultimate value, i.e., defined tensile strength for that element, and cause failure. Therefore, the value of axial tensile stress which causes failure in either HAp or C-C bond can be calculated as the tensile strength of the RVE (PourAkbar Saffar et al. 2009b). Here, failure of the RVE is supposed to occur without any non-linear deformations.

The effective Young's modulus defines the slope of the stress-strain curve, when neglecting the non-linear response of the chemical bonding and assuming overall linear elastic behavior for the RVE. On the other hand, the same assumption leads to the determination of the fracture strain at the point in which fracture strength is known. As a result, the area under the stress-strain curve, up to the fracture point, can be obtained as fracture toughness. This is a critical parameter which describes the energy dissipated prior to fracture.

5. Modeling Results

The head cross-linked model illustrated in Fig. 3 predicts different values of the RVE effective axial Young's modulus for various CNT volume fractions and RVE lengths (CNT aspect ratio = 2L/D). Fig. 4 illustrates plots of the Young's modulus versus CNT volume fraction for different RVE lengths. Results of current model, as seen in Fig. 4, can be compared to that of classical micromechanics models for composite materials. For the sake of comparison, Rule-of-Mixtures predictions (Voigt, 1889; Reuss, 1929), Hashin-Shtrikman upper and lower bounds (Hashin & Shtrikman, 1961a,b; 1962a,b; 1963), and Mori-Tanaka model results (Mori & Tanaka, 1973) for the composite consisting of CNT and HAp are also provided in Fig. 4.

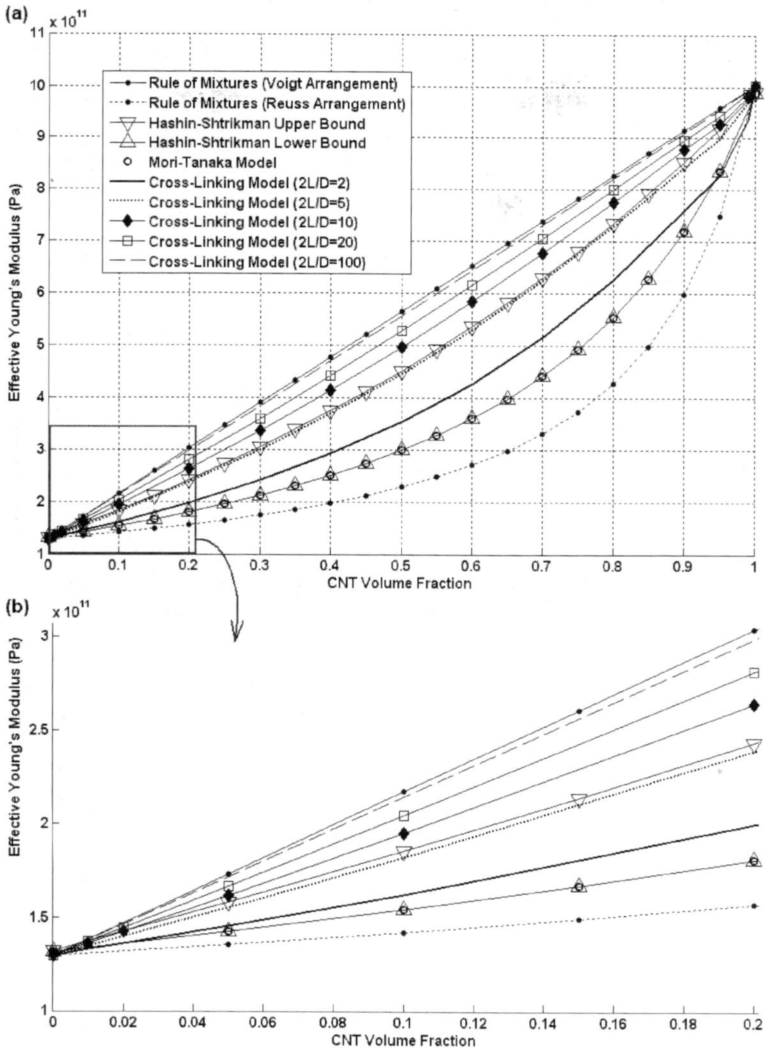

Fig. 4. RVE effective axial Young's modulus predicted by some classical models and the cross-linking model with respect to CNT volume fraction

Although primary configuration presumes head cross-linked RVEs, in an alternative configuration, this can be in the shape of additional C-C bonds with the matrix on the CNT surface, since functionalization is practically feasible on both CNT heads and sidewalls. A simple case is considered here for a RVE of a length of 10 nm, with 4 equidistance cross-links evenly distributed throughout the length. Results of the simulation for this case and also Rule-of-Mixtures (Voigt) results for different values of CNT volume fraction (from 1 to 10%) are illustrated in Fig. 5.

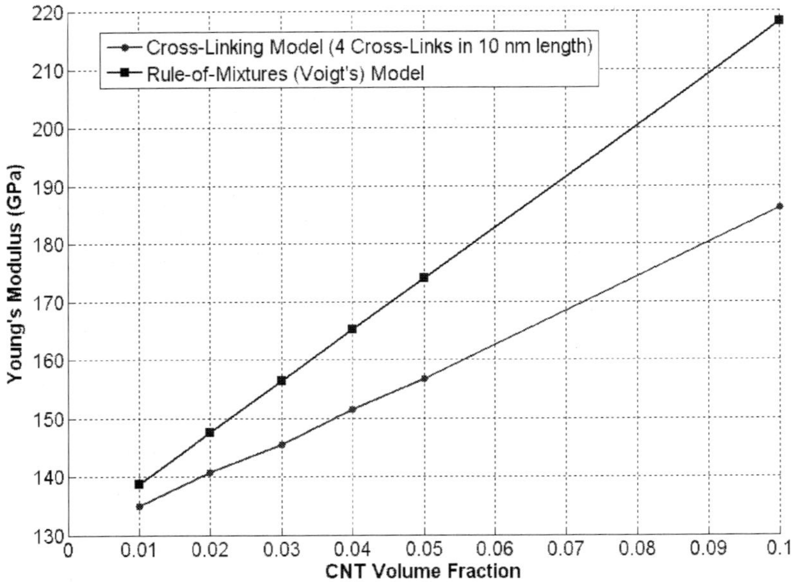

Fig. 5. Young's modulus versus CNT volume fraction predicted by Rule-of-Mixtures and the current model having 4 equidistance cross-links in 10 nm RVE length

Fig. 6 illustrates the case that cross-links are distributed in the RVE length holding equal distances of 4 nm from each other. This means that each 4 nm increase in the RVE length adds a cross-link to the RVE. This configuration is regarded for a CNT volume fraction of 10%.

Fig. 7 presents Young's moduli for two types of RVEs. The first is associated with RVEs of different length, each having only two end cross-links. The second is for the RVEs of similar lengths, having one cross-link per each 4 nm of their length. CNT volume fraction is 10% for both.

The predicted tensile strength of the RVE is shown in Fig. 8 for different CNT aspect ratios versus CNT volume fraction. This figure indicates that reinforcing mechanism acts more effectively to increase the tensile strength, when there is an increase in CNT volume fraction and/or aspect ratio.

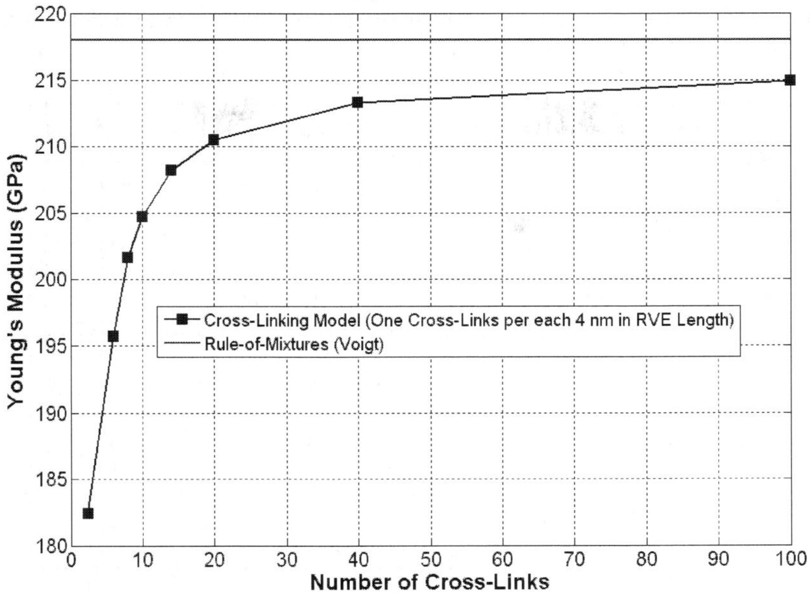

Fig. 6. Young's modulus versus number of evenly distributed cross-links in different RVE lengths (CNT volume fraction=10%)

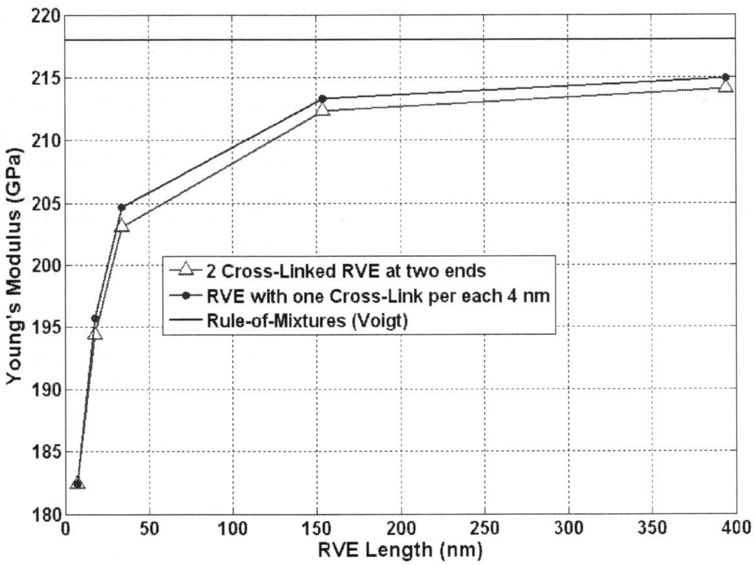

Fig. 7. Young's modulus versus RVE length (CNT volume fraction=%10)

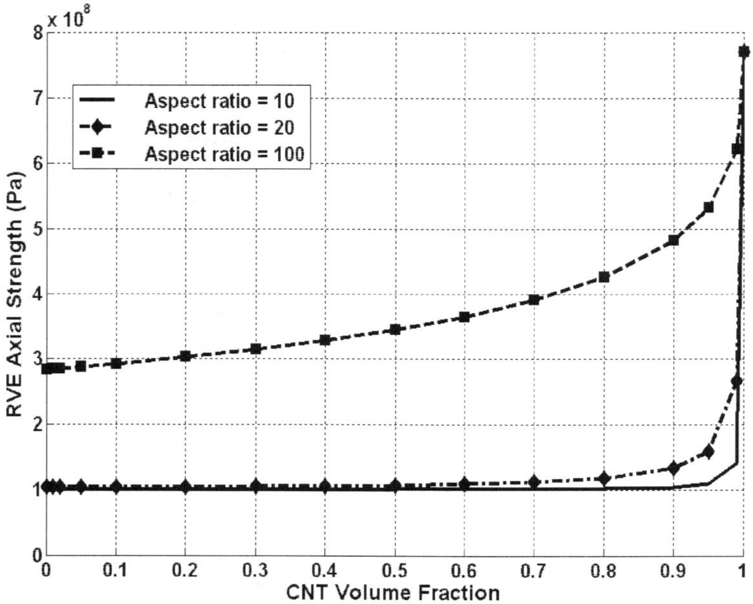

Fig. 8. Axial tensile strength versus CNT volume fraction

6. Discussions on the Model Predictions

Ordinary outputs of developed models for predicting mechanical properties of fiber-reinforced composites include consideration of microstructural Young's, shear, and/or bulk moduli with respect to volume fraction of reinforcement phase. Rule-of-Mixtures gives two general cases of isostrain and isostress arrangements of material constituents proposed by (Voigt, 1889) and (Reuss, 1929), respectively. Voigt suggests the upper limit of a range of elastic constants, while the lower limit of this range is given by Reuss's model. Results of other classical models lie between Rule-of-Mixtures estimated limits. So-called Hashin-Shtrikman upper and lower bounds (Hashin & Shtrikman, 1961a,b; 1962a,b; 1963) for the composite material behavior are the most adopted bounds for the overall properties of composites. Mori and Tanaka proposed their well-known method (Mori & Tanaka, 1973), matching Hashin-Shtrikman's lower bound for the composite behavior in certain conditions. The key point in different approaches is the pre-assumed interaction between composite phases. Voigt's model, assuming perfect bonding between matrix and reinforcement, considers isostrain condition in which deformations of the elements are equal at every contact point between the two phases. Perfect bonding assumption in such a situation, provides the uppermost limit of effective properties of the composite. However, the cross-linking model presented here, represents the inter-phase interaction only at cross-links sites which results in a significant deviation from Voigt's prediction. When interface contact is less perfect, as is the case for our cross-linking model compared to isostrain model, it is expected to see a weaker reinforcing mechanism and so a smaller value for the Young's modulus of the composite.

According to Fig. 4, the Young's modulus of the RVE of CNT-HAp predicted by the cross-linking model, lies under Voigt's model result and adjacent to Hashin-Shtrkman bounds. For a CNT aspect ratio of 5, with RVE at the same length as CNT, the cross-linking model adapts interestingly near the Hashin-Shtrikman's upper bound. It is apparent that by increasing aspect ratio, the results obtained by the current model approach those of Voigt. When the aspect ratio is approaching 100 or higher, this model's results match roughly the Voigt's prediction illustrated as a straight line in Fig. 4. This is in agreement with the general concept that increasing the CNT volume fraction and/or length leads to an improved reinforcement (Thostenson et al., 2005; Haque & Ramasetty, 2005).

The Young's modulus predicted by the present model, even for a very small aspect ratio, e.g. for a CNT aspect ratio of 2, lies above the Hashin-Shtrikman's lower bound which is also far above Reuss's prediction. This is caused by the cross-linking, and it is contrary to the isostress situation which is based on Reuss's assumption that both matrix and fibers carry the same amount of load. In the current model, however, the cross-link carries just part of the load which is caused by a combination of parallel and series elements. The phenomenon can be explained by considering the apparent difference between the Young's moduli of CNT and the matrix.

When increasing dilute volume fractions (see Figs. 4b and 5), model deviation from Voigt's prediction increases. This difference is directly related to the perfect bonding assumption in Voigt's model which results in overestimating the Young's modulus. In the cross-linking model, however, it is assumed that the only interaction between matrix and CNT is through cross-links, unlike the assumption made by Voigt, i.e., at every point throughout the contact surface there is a perfect bond between fibers and the matrix. Interesting to note that Young's moduli predicted by various models here, get closer for high CNT volume fractions; and approach a unique value when the volume fraction is 1. However, this is not of immediate interest, since empirical studies tend to concentrate on lower volume fractions of CNTs in such nano-composites (Thostenson et al., 2005; Haque & Ramasetty, 2005).

Voigt, Hashin-Shtrikman, and Mori-Tanaka models tend to predict similar curves for the Young's modulus versus volume fraction, independent of RVE lengths. The presented model, however, indicates that the longer the CNT, the more efficient the reinforcement becomes. In addition, longer CNTs have the potential to support a greater number of cross-links. The cross-linking model shows that an increase in the number of cross-links will increase the Young's modulus and in its limit will approach the value predicted by the Voigt formulation. If the number of cross-links distributed uniformly along the RVE goes to infinity, the interaction can be considered as perfect bonding. So, for such a critical condition, similar results are expected from both Voigt and the cross-linking models.

According to Fig. 6, the greater the number of cross-links, the stronger is the interaction between composite phases. The effect of increasing the CNT length, however, is much more apparent than the effect of increasing the number of cross-links in constant RVE length, as can be seen in Fig. 7. This could raise the issue of comparing the reinforcement efficiency of tip and side wall functionalized CNTs. The important point here is that adding more functional groups to the CNT surface alters the regular cylindrical shape of the CNT as a result of changes in hybridization of carbon atoms on its surface. Although the current model fails to describe this phenomenon, but on the basis of experimental observation and theoretical predictions, such modification can adversely affect nanotube properties due to induced structural defects (Balasubramanian & Burghard, 2005).

Results show a significant increase in both axial Young's modulus and tensile strength of the HAp when reinforced with CNT. A simple comparison leads to the understanding that fracture toughness of the synthesized HAp-CNT is several times higher than that of the natural bone which is structurally composed of HAp and collagen fibers (PourAkbar Saffar et al. 2009b) (see Fig. 9 as an example). Fracture toughness as a measure and indicator of the capacity of a material to resist failure, is an important parameter that can be used to determine to which category of materials, a material belongs. It is well known that pure HAp is a brittle material, while bone tissue behaves in a quasi-brittle manner (Raeisi Najafi et al., 2009), and this is due to the collagen inclusion as a flexible phase which can increase bone toughness. The enhanced elastic properties of CNTs in the HAp matrix, however, introduce the doubt on change of the material behavior as to ductile. Microcracking is a common toughening mechanism in bone, as a quasi-brittle material, which occurs near the main crack tip to resist the crack growth (Raeisi Najafi et al., 2007a,b; 2009). Moreover, it is well accepted that microcracks and microdamages in bone can initiate and accelerate bone remodeling process in which there will be a break for the crack propagation and can encourage making new bony material at the deteriorated sites (Rouhi et al., 2006; Vahdati & Rouhi, 2009). It seems reasonable, by considering the differences between the mechanical properties of the natural and artificial bone (HAp-CNTs), to assume that the rate of bone remodeling process will be altered, and possibly disturbed when CNTs replace the collagen fibers in natural bone tissue.
Assuming that CNT reinforcement increases bone fracture toughness, and decreases possibility of microcracks generation, another aspect of future researches should also be addressing whether the HAp-CNT composite is more suitable than collagen I-HAp from bone remodeling point of view or this can be seen as a drawback for the artificial bone.

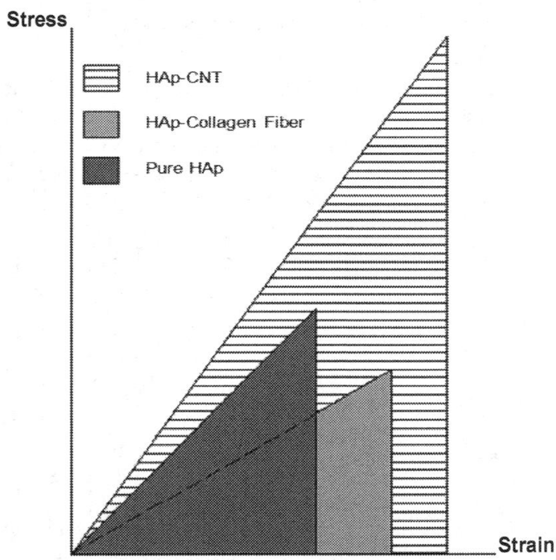

Fig. 9. Schematic stress-strain curves for HAp-CNT, HAp-collagn fiber, and pure Hap

Although promising results are shown in initial steps toward the bioapplications of CNTs as scaffolds for bone growth, more investigations need to be done to address the question of: "Is replacing collagen fibers by CNTs beneficial for bone from the bone adaptation point of view or can be seen as a disturbing factor in the remodeling process?" This study is therefore aimed at exploring the mechanical characteristics of the HAp-CNT composite in order to lay emphasize on the importance of the evaluation of the biological related effects of CNT reinforcement in such an artificial bone tissue.

7. Summary

The idea of HAp precipitation on functionalized CNTs suggests a new avenue in bone tissue engineering. For instance, implanting functionalized CNTs as solutions or substratum in the bone injury site may result in generation of the composite material. This could exemplify an appropriate application of the concept, to bone tissue therapy. A critical investigation of the applicability of CNTs as a reinforcement to a living tissue could thus find tangible potentials in preventative or post traumatic measures. This approach, however, necessitates a multidisciplinary research encompassing such subjects as Mechanical and Biomedical Engineering. The interaction between the mechanical behavior of the living tissue and the biological functions in the organism is almost totally accepted. This work is therefore aiming to evaluate such applications by exploring the mechanical properties of the HAp-CNT composite.

As the very first step in evaluating the mechanical response of the composite, a model has been presented here to obtain the effective axial Young's modulus of a RVE of HAp formed on functionalized CNT. This study predicts close behavior of the material to those suggested by classical micromechanical models. This model predicts higher Young's moduli and tensile strengths for RVEs with higher CNT contents and/or aspect ratios, as it is expected based on current knowledge of fiber composite materials. When CNT length increases, possibly, there may exist more cross-links distributed on the CNT surface in addition to those on the CNT tips, resulting in a stronger interfacial force and so bigger Young's modulus and tensile strength, as our model predicts in this study. Although initial results are promising, further careful studies are necessary to find out whether they support or cast doubt on the proposed suggestion of CNT application as bone tissue engineering scaffold.

8. Acknowledgement

Dr. A.R. Arshi from Amirkabir University of Technology, Dr. A. Raeisi Najafi from University of Illinois at Urbana-Champaign, and Dr. L. Sudak from University of Calgary are also acknowledged for collaborative supports.

9. References

Abarrategi, A.; Gutiérrez, M.C.; Moreno-Vicente, C.; Hortigüela, M.H.; Ramos, V.; López-Lacomba; J.L.; Ferrer, M.L. & del Monte, F. (2008). Multiwall carbon nanotube scaffolds for tissue engineering purposes, *Biomaterials*, Vol. 29, pp. 94-102.

Aryal, S.; Bahadur, K.C.R.; Dharmaraj, N.; Kim, K-W. & Kim, H.Y. (2006). Synthesis and characterization of hydroxyapatite using carbon nanotubes as a nano-matrix, *Scripta Materialia*, Vol. 54, pp. 131-135.

Aryal, S.; Bhattarai, S.R.; Bahadur, K.C.R; Khil, M.S.; Lee, D-R. & Kim, H.Y. (2007). Carbon nanotubes assisted biomimetic synthesis of hydroxyapatite from simulated body fluid, *Materials Science & Engineering A*, Vol. 426pp. 202-207.

Ascenzi, A. (1993). Biomechanics and Galileo Galilei, *Journal of Biomechanics*, Vol. 26, pp. 95-100.

Balani, K.; Anderson, R.; Laha, T.; Andara, M.; Tercero, J.; Crumpler, E. & Agarwal, A. (2007). Plasma-sprayed carbon nanotube reinforced hydroxyapatite coatings and their interaction with human osteoblasts in vitro, *Biomaterials*, Vol. 28, pp. 618-624.

Balasubramanian, K. & Burghard, M. (2005). Chemically functionalized carbon nanotubes. *Small*, Vol. 1, pp. 180-192.

Bartel, L.B.; Dwight T.D. & Keaveny T.M. (2006). *Orthopaedic Biomechanics Mechanics and Design in Musculoskeletal Systems*, Chap. 3, Pearson Prentice Hall.

Behari, J. (1991). Solid state bone behaviour, *Progress in Biophysics & Molecular Biology*, Vol. 56, pp. 1-41.

Burger, E.H. & Klein-Nulend, J. (1999). Mechanotransduction in bone-role of the lacuno-canalicular network, *FASEB Journal*. Vol. 13, pp. S101-S112.

Carter, D.R. & Hayes, W.C. (1977). Compact bone fatigue damage-I. Residual strength and stiffness, *Journal of Biomechanics*, Vol. 10, pp. 325-337

Carter, D.R. & Cayler, W.E. (1983). Cycle dependent and time dependent bone fracture with repeated loading, *Journal of Biomechanical Engineering*, Vol. 105, pp. 166-170.

Carter, D.R. & Cayler, W.E. (1985). A cumulative damage model for bone fracture, *Journal of Orthopedic Research*, Vol. 3, pp. 84-90.

Chen, Y.; Zhang, Y.Q.; Zhang, T.H.; Gan, C.H.; Zheng, C.Y. & Yu, G. (2006). Carbon nanotube reinforced hydroxyapatite composite coatings produced through laser surface alloying, *Carbon*, Vol. 44, pp. 37-45.

Chen, Y.; Zhang, T.H.; Gan, C.H.; & Yu, G. (2007). Wear studies of hydroxyapatite composite coating reinforced by carbon nanotubes, *Carbon*, Vol. 45, pp. 998-1004.

Cornell, W.D.; Cieplak, P.; Bayly, C.I.; Gould, I.R.; Merz, Jr. K.M.; Ferguson, D.M.; Spellmeyer, D.C.; Fox, T.; Caldwell, J.W. & Kollman, P.A. (1995). A second generation force field for the simulation of proteins, nucleic acids, and organic molecules. *Journal of American Chemical Society*, Vol. 117, pp. 5179-5197.

Cowin, S.C. & Hegedus, D.M. (1976). Bone Remodeling I: A theory of adaptive elasticity, *Journal of Elasticity*, Vol. 6, pp. 313-325.

Cowin, S.C.; Moss Salentijn, L.; & Moss, M.L. (1991). Candidates for the mechanosensory system in bone, *Journal of Biomechanical Engineering*, Vol. 113, pp. 191-197.

Cowin, S.C.; Weinbaum, S.; & Zeng, Y. (1995). A case for bone canaliculi as the anatomical site of strain generated potentials, *Journal of Biomechanics*, Vol. 28, pp. 1281-1297.

Cowin, S.C. (2001). *Bone Mechanics Handbook*, 2nd edition, CRC Press, Boca Raton, FL, USA.

Cowin, S.C. (2003). Adaptive elasticity: a review and critique of a bone tissue adaptation model, *Engineering Transactions, Polish Academy of Science*, Vol. 51 (2-3), pp. 113-193.

Currey, J.D. (2002). *Bone Structure and Mechanics*, Princeton University Press.

Frost, H.M. (1960). Presence of microscopic cracks in vivo in bone, *Bulletin of Henry Ford Hospital*, Vol. 8, pp. 25-35.

Frost, H.M. (1964). *The laws of bone Structure*; Charles C. Thomas, Springfield, IL, USA.

Gibson, L.J. (1985). The mechanical behaviour of cancellous bone, *Journal of Biomechanics*, Vol. 18, pp. 317-328.
Gjelsvik, A. (1973a). Bone remodeling and piezoelectricity-I, *Journal of Biomechanics*, Vol. 6, pp. 69-77.
Gjelsvik, A. (1943b). Bone remodeling and piezoelectricity-II. *Journal of Biomechanics*, Vol. 6, pp. 187-193.
Guo, X.E. & Goldstein, S.A. (1997). Is trabecular bone tissue different from cortical bone?, *Forma*, Vol. 12, pp. 3-4.
Haque, A. & Ramasetty, A. (2005). Theoretical study of stress transfer in carbon nanotube reinforced polymer matrix composites, *Composite Structures*, Vol. 71, pp. 68-77.
Hashin, Z. & Shtrickman, S. (1961a). Note on a variational approach to the theory of composite elastic materials, *Journal of the Franklin Institute*, Vol. 271, pp. 336-341.
Hashin, Z. & Shtrickman, S. (1961b). Note on the effective constants of composite materials, *Journal of the Franklin Institute*, Vol. 271, pp. 423-426.
Hashin, Z. & Shtrikman, S. (1962a). On some variational principles in anisotropic and nonhomogeneous elasticity, *Journal of the Mechanics & Physics of Solids*, Vol. 10, pp. 335-342.
Hashin, Z. & Shtrikman, S. (1962b). A variational approach to the theory of the elastic behavior of polycrystals, *Journal of the Mechanics & Physics of Solids*, Vol. 10, pp. 343-352.
Hashin, Z. & Shtrikman, S. (1963). A variational approach to the theory of the elastic behavior of multiphase materials, *Journal of the Mechanics & Physics of Solids*, Vol. 11, pp. 127-140.
Jee, W.S.S. (2001). Integrated bone tissue physiology: anatomy and physiology, in *Bone Mechanics Handbook* (Ed. Cowin, S.C.), Chap.1.
Jorgensen, W.L. & Severance, D.L. (1990) .Aromatic-aromatic interactions-free energy profiles for the benzene dimmer in water chloroform and liquid benzene, *Journal of American Chemical Society*, Vol. 112, pp. 4768-4774.
Judex, S.; Whiting, W. & Zernicke, R. (1999). Bone Biomechanics and Fracture, In: *Biomechanics in Ergonomics*, Kumar, S., (Ed.), Taylor & Francis, ISBN, London.
Lakes, R.S. & Saha, S. (1979). Cement line motion in bone, *Science*, Vol. 204, pp. 501-503.
Lakes, R. (1993). Materials With Structural Hierarchy, *Nature*, Vol. 361, pp. 511-515.
Li, A.; Sun, K.; Dong, W. & Zhao, D. (2007). Mechanical properties, microstructure and histocompatibility of MWCNTs/HAp biocomposites, *Materials Letters*, Vol. 61, pp. 1839-1844.
Li, C.Y. & Chou, T-W. (2005). A structural mechanics approach for the analysis of carbon nanotubes, *International Journal of Solids & Structures*, Vol. 40, pp. 2487-2499.
Lobo, A.O.; Antunes, E.F.; Machado, A.H.A; Pacheco-Soares, C.; Trava-Airoldi, V.J. & Corat, E.J. (2008). Cell viability and adhesion on as grown multi-wall carbon nanotube films, *Materials Science & Engineering C*, Vol. 28, pp. 264-269.
MacDonald, R.A.; Laurenzi, B.F.; Viswanathan, G.; Ajayan, P.M. & Stegemann, J.P. (2005). Collagen-carbon nanotube composite materials as scaffolds in tissue engineering, *Journal of Biomedical Materials Research*, Vol. 74A, pp. 489-496.
Marrs, B.; Andrews, R.; Rantell., T. & Pienkowski, D. (2006). Augmentation of acrylic bone cement with multiwall carbon nanotubes, *Journal of Biomedical Materials Research*, Vol. 77A, pp. 269-276.

Marrs, B.; Andrews, R. & Pienkowski, D. (2007). Multiwall carbon nanotubes enhance the fatigue performance of physiologically maintained methyl methacrylate-styrene copolymer, *Carbon,* Vol. 45, pp. 2098-2104.

Martin, R.B. (1992). A theory of fatigue damage accumulation and repair in cortical bone. *Journal of Orthopedic Research,* Vol. 10, pp. 818-825.

Martin, R.B. (1995). Mathematical model for repair of fatigue damage and stress fracture in osteonal bone, *Journal of Orthopedic Research,* Vol. 13, pp. 309-316.

Meyers, M.A.; Chen, P-Y.; Lin, A. & Seki, Y. (2008). Biological materials: Structure and mechanical properties, *Progress in Materials Science,* Vol. 53, pp. 1-206.

Mori, T. & Tanaka, K. (1973). Average stress in matrix and average elastic energy of materials with misfitting inclusions, *Acta Metallurgica et Materiala,* Vol. 21, pp. 571-574.

Odegard, G.M.; Frankland, S.J.V. & Gates, T.S. (2005). Effect of chemical functionalization on mechanical properties of nanotube/polymer composites, *AIAA Journal,* Vol. 43, No. 8, pp. 1828-1835.

Parfitt, A.M. (1983). The physiologic and clinical significance of bone histomorphometric data, in *Bone Histomorphometry: Techniques and Interpretation,* (Ed. Recker, R.R.), CRC Press, Boca Raton, FL, pp. 143-223.

Parfitt, A.M. (1995). Problems in the application of *in vitro* systems to the study of human bone remodeling, *Calcified Tissue International,* Vol. 56 (Suppl. 1), pp. S5-S7.

Piekarski, K.J. (1970). Fracture of bone, *Journal of Applied Physics,* Vol. 41, pp. 215-223.

Pollack, S.R.; Salzstein, R. & Pienkowski, D. (1984). The electric double layer in bone and its influence on stress-generated potentials, *Calcified Tissue International,* Vol. 36 (Suppl. 1), pp. S77-S81.

PourAkbar Saffar, K.; JamilPour, N.; Raeisi Najafi, A.; Rouhi, G.; Arshi, A.R. & Fereidoon, A. (2008). A finite element model for estimating Young's modulus of carbon nanotube reinforced composites incorporating elastic cross-links, *International Journal of Mechanical Systems Science and Engineering,* Vol. 2, No. 3, pp. 172-175.

PourAkbar Saffar, K.; Arshi, A.R.; JamilPour, N.; Raeisi Najafi, A.; Rouhi, G. & Sudak, L. (2009a). A cross-linking model for estimating Young's modulus of artificial bone tissue grown on carbon nanotube scaffold, *Journal of Biomedical Materials Research A (Submitted)*

PourAkbar Saffar, K.; JamilPour, N.; Rouhi, G.; Raeisi Najafi, A.; Arshi, A.R. & Sudak, L. (2009b). Fracture toughness of carbon nanotube reinforced artificial bone tissue, *12th International Conference on Fracture (ICF12),* July 2009, Ottawa, Canada.

Prendergast, P.J. & Taylor, D. (1994). Prediction of bone adaptation using damage accumulation, *Journal of Biomechanics,* Vol. 27, pp. 1067-1076.

Rabiei, A.; Blalock, T.; Thomas, B.; Cuomo, J.; Yang, Y. & Ong, J. (2007). Microstructure, mechanical properties, and biological response to functionally graded HA coatings, *Materials Science & Engineering C,* Vol. 27, pp. 529–533.

Raeisi Najafi, A.; Arshi, A.R.; PourAkbar Saffar, K.; Eslami, M.R.; Fariborz, S. & Moeinzadeh, M.H. (2009). A fiber-ceramic matrix composite material model for osteonal cortical bone fracture micromechanics: Solution of arbitrary microcracks interaction, *Journal of the Mechanical Behavior of Biomedical Materials,* Vol. 2, pp. 217-223.

Raeisi Najafi, A.; Arshi, A.R.; Eslami, M.R.; Fariborz, S. & Moeinzadeh, M. (2007a). Haversian cortical bone model with many radial microcracks: An elastic analytic solution, *Medical Engineering and Physics,* Vol. 29, pp. 708-717.

Raeisi Najafi, A.; Arshi, A.R.; Eslami, M.R.; Fariborz, S. & Moeinzadeh, M.H. (2007b). Micromechanics fracture in osteonal cortical bone: A study of the interactions between microcrack propagation, microstructure and the material properties. *Journal of Biomechanics*, Vol. 40, pp. 2788-2795.

Reuss, A. (1929). Berechnung der Fliessgrenze von Mischkristallen auf Grund der Plästizitatsbedingung für Einkristalle, *Zietschrift für Angewandte Mathematik und Mechanik (Journal of Applied Mathematics and Mechanics)*, Vol. 9, pp. 49-58.

Rodan, G.A. & Martin, T.J. (2000). Therapeutic approaches to bone diseases, *Science*, Vol. 289, pp. 1508-1514.

Rouhi, G. (2006a). Theoretical aspects of bone remodeling and resorption process, *PhD Dissertation*, University of Calgary, AB, Canada.

Rouhi, G.; Firoozbakhsh, K.; Epstein, M.; Herzog, W. & Sudak, L. (2004). Free surface density instead of volume fraction in the bone remodeling equation: theoretical considerations. *Forma*, Vol. 19, Issue 3, pp. 165-182.

Rouhi, G.; Epstein, M.; Sudak, L. & Herzog, W. (2006b). Free surface density and microdamage in the bone remodeling equation: Theoretical considerations, *International Journal of Engineering Science*, Vol. 44, pp. 456-469.

Rouhi, G.; Epstein, M.; Sudak, L. & Herzog, W. (2007). Modeling bone resorption using mixture theory with chemical reactions. *Journal of Mechanics of Materials and Structures*, Vol. 2, Issue 6, pp. 1141-1156.

Sirivisoot, S. & Webster, T.J. (2008). Multiwalled carbon nanotubes enhance electrochemical properties of titanium to determine in situ bone formation, *Nanotechnology*, Vol. 19, p. 295101(12pp).

Taylor, D.; Hazenberg, J.G. & Lee, T.C. (2007). Living with cracks: Damage and repair in human bone, *Nature*, Vol. 6, pp. 263-268.

Teitelbaum, S.L. (2000). Bone resorption by osteoclasts, *Science*, Vol. 289, pp. 1504-1508.

Thostenson, E.T.; Li, C., & Chou, T-W. (2005). Nanocomposites in context, *Composites Science & Technology*, Vol. 65, pp. 491-516.

Tserpes, K.I. & Papanikos, P. (2005). Finite element modeling of single-walled carbon nanotubes, *Composites Part B*, Vol. 36, pp. 468-477.

Usui, Y.; Aoki, K.; Narita, N.; Murakami, N.; Nakamura, I.; Nakamura, K.; Ishigaki, N.; Yamazaki, H.; Horiuchi, H.; Kato, H.; Taruta, S.; Kim, Y.A.; Endo, M. & Saito, N. (2008). Carbon nanotubes with high bone-tissue compatibility and bone-formation acceleration effects, *Small*, Vol. 4, No. 2, pp. 240-246.

Vahdati, A. & Rouhi, G. (2009a). A model for mechanical adaptation of trabecular bone incorporating cellular accommodation and effects of microdamage and disuse, *Mechanics Research Communications*, Vol. 36, Issue 3, pp. 284-293.

Vahdati A.; Rouhi G.; Ghalichi, F. & Tahani, M. (2009b). Mechanically induced trabecular bone remodeling including cellular accommodation effect: A computer simulation, *Transactions of the Canadian Society for Mechanical Engineering*, Vol. 32, Issues 3-4, pp. 371-382.

Van der Meulen, M.C.H. & Prendergast, P.J. (2000). Mechanics in skeletal development, adaptation and disease, *Philosophical Transactions for the Royal Society of London A*, Vol. 358, pp. 565-578.

Voge, C.M.; Kariolis, M.; MacDonald, R.A. & Stegemann, J.P. (2008). Directional conductivity in SWNT-collagen-fibrin composite biomaterials through strain-induced matrix alignment, *Journal of Biomedical Materials Research,* Vol. 86A, pp. 269-277.

Voigt, W. (1889). Über die Beziehung zwischen den beiden Elastizitätskonstanten isotroper Körper, *Wiedmanns Annalen der Physik und Chemie,* Vol. 38, pp. 573-587.

Weiner, S. & Wagner, H.D. (1998). The material bone: structure-mechanical function relations, *Annual Reviews in Materials Science,* Vol. 28, pp. 271–298.

White, A.A.; Best, S.M. & Kinloch, I.A. (2007). Hydroxyapatite-carbon nanotube composites for biomedical applications: A review, *International Journal of Applied Ceramic Technology,* Vol. 4, pp. 1-13.

Wolff, J.L. (1886). *The law of bone remodeling,* Springer, Berlin.

Zanello, L.P; Zhao, B.; Hu, H. & Haddon, R.C. (2006). Bone cell proliferation on carbon nanotubes, *Nano Letters,* Vol. 6, pp. 562-567.

Zhao, B.; Hu, H.; Mandal, S.K. & Haddon, R.C. (2005). A bone mimic based on the self-assembly of hydroxyapatite on chemically functionalized single-walled carbon nanotubes, *Chemical Materials,* Vol. 17, No. 12, pp. 3235 -3241.

Traditional and Dynamic Action Potential Clamp Experiments with HCN4 Pacemaker Current: Biomedical Engineering in Cardiac Cellular Electrophysiology

Arie O. Verkerk and Ronald Wilders
Heart Failure Research Center, Academic Medical Center, University of Amsterdam
The Netherlands

1. Introduction

The sinoatrial (SA) node is the normal pacemaker of the mammalian heart and generates the electrical impulse for the regular, rhythmic contraction of the heart. Pacemaker activity—or spontaneous electrical activity—of SA nodal cells is based on the presence of a special phase of the action potential, the diastolic depolarization, in which cells depolarize spontaneously towards the action potential threshold. This diastolic depolarization phase is due to a very small net inward current across the cell membrane, which is the result of a complex interaction of multiple inwardly and outwardly directed ion currents (see reviews by Boyett et al. (2000), Dobrzynski et al. (2007), and Mangoni & Nargeot (2008)). Among these currents, the hyperpolarization-activated 'funny' current (I_f) is of particular importance and is traditionally also named 'pacemaker current'. The ion channels carrying I_f are encoded by the hyperpolarization-activated cyclic nucleotide-modulated (HCN) gene family, with HCN4 as the dominant HCN isoform in the SA node (Moosmang et al., 2001; Dobrzynski et al., 2007). Despite a large body of experimental data from voltage clamp experiments, the contribution of I_f to pacemaker activity in the adult SAN is still controversial and not fully established (see Verkerk et al. (2009a) and primary references cited therein).

In this chapter, we demonstrate how the 'action potential clamp' technique, as an alternative to traditional voltage clamp, can provide insights into the role of I_f in SA nodal pacemaker activity. We have used the action potential clamp technique to study the behaviour of HCN4 channels expressed—by transfection with the ion channel gene cDNA—in cells from the HEK-293 human embryonic kidney cell line, which express little or no endogenous HCN channels (Varghese et al., 2006). The current in response to a voltage clamp command potential with the shape of an SA nodal action potential then reflects the behaviour of the expressed HCN4 channels during that action potential. We also show how this technique can be turned into a dynamic technique with continuous feedback between the SA nodal action potential and the HEK-293 cell current. With this 'dynamic action potential clamp' technique, the voltage clamp command potential is not a predefined action potential, but is the free-running membrane potential of an SA nodal cell that is simulated in real time, with the measured HEK-293 cell current contributing to its net membrane current. In this approach, it is immediately clear how the HCN4 channels affect the SA nodal action potential.

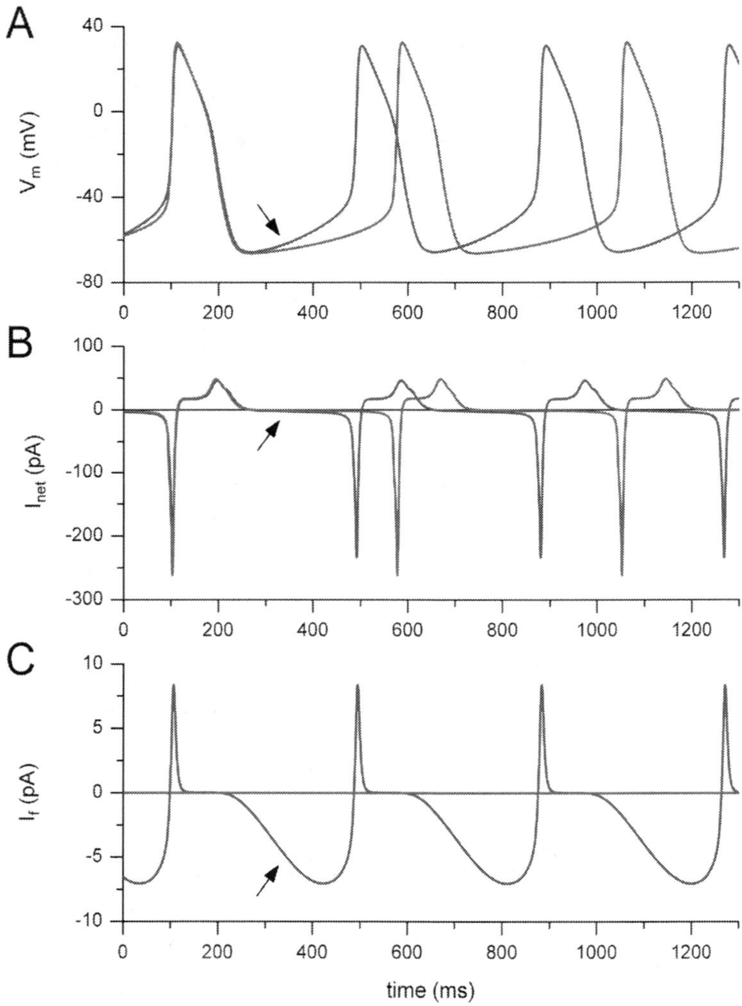

Fig. 1. Pacemaker activity a single pacemaker cell isolated from the rabbit sinoatrial node. Computer simulation using the Wilders et al. (1991) model under control conditions (blue traces) and with the hyperpolarization-activated 'pacemaker current' I_f set to zero (red traces). (A) Spontaneous action potentials. (B) Underlying net membrane current (I_{net}). (C) Hyperpolarization-activated current (I_f). Note difference in ordinate scales between panels B and C.

2. Pacemaker activity of the sinoatrial node

Figure 1 illustrates the intrinsic pacemaker activity of the cells that constitute the SA node. Figure 1A (blue trace) shows spontaneous action potentials of a rabbit SA nodal cell, according to the mathematical model of such cell by Wilders et al. (1991). The arrow indicates the diastolic depolarization phase of the action potential, during which the cell undergoes a spontaneous depolarization towards the action potential threshold. Figure 1B (blue trace) shows the net current across the cell membrane (I_{net}) that charges and discharges the membrane capacitance and underlies the spontaneous electrical activity. By convention, a net inward inflow of cations, which depolarizes the cell, is shown as a negative current. During diastolic depolarization, I_{net} is a tiny net inward current (arrow), which results from a complex interaction of several inwardly and outwardly directed cation currents. On a different ordinate scale, Figure 1C (blue trace) shows the 'pacemaker current' I_f, which makes an important contribution to this net inward current (arrow). Note that I_f turns into an outward current during the subsequent upstroke of the action potential, reflecting the I_f reversal potential of −24 mV. Although I_f is an important current, it is not a prerequisite for pacemaker activity. This is illustrated by the red traces in Fig. 1, which were obtained with the same action potential model, but with I_f set to zero. The main effect of 'blocking' I_f is a significant slowing of diastolic depolarization and an increase in the cycle length of the spontaneous electrical activity from 388 tot 474 ms (Fig. 1A).

3. Patch clamp

3.1 Recording from single cells

In today's cardiac cellular electrophysiology, 'patch clamp' is the common technique to

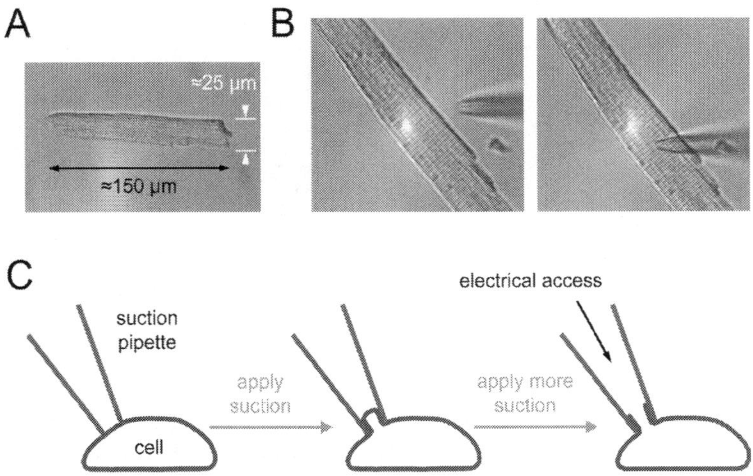

Fig. 2. Recording electrical activity of single cardiac myocytes. (A) Enzymatically isolated single ventricular myocyte. (B) Approaching the myocyte with a recording pipette. (C) Applying suction to obtain electrical access to the cell interior.

record the electrical activity of single cardiac cells, e.g. SA nodal cells. Cardiac myocytes are isolated from (pieces of) the hearts of laboratory animals by dedicated enzymatic isolation techniques. Cell suspensions are then put into a recording chamber on the stage of an inverted microscope and continuously superfused with Tyrode's solution, i.e. a salt solution with a composition in accordance with the interstitial fluid of the intact heart. Apparently healthy spindle or elongated spindle-like SA nodal cells or rod-shaped working myocardial cells with clear cross-striations (Fig. 2A) are selected for electrophysiological measurements. If not stimulated, pacemaker cells isolated from SA nodal tissue show regular rhythmic contractions, whereas cells isolated from atrial or ventricular tissue are quiescent.
For electrophysiological recording, pipettes are pulled from small borosilicate glass capillaries and heat polished. A pipette is filled with a salt solution mimicking the intracellular fluid. When filled with this 'pipette solution', the pipette typically has a 2–3 MΩ resistance, contributing to an unwanted 'series resistance', which can be electronically compensated by the 'patch clamp amplifier'. With the use of a micromanipulator that holds the pipette, the myocyte is approached with the recording pipette (Fig. 2B). When the pipette tip is in close vicinity of the myocyte (Fig. 2C, left), a little suction is applied and an omega-shaped seal is obtained (Fig. 2C, middle). If some more suction is applied, the seal is broken and electrical access to the cell interior is obtained (Fig. 2C, right). The thus obtained recording configuration is known as the 'whole-cell patch clamp configuration'.

3.2 Current clamp and voltage clamp

The 'whole-cell patch clamp configuration' of Fig. 2C (right) can be used in different recording modes. The main recording modes are 'current clamp' (Fig. 3A) and 'voltage clamp' (Fig. 3B). In either case, the bath solution is grounded to earth, as indicated by '$V = 0$' in Fig. 3A. In current clamp mode, the free-running membrane potential of the myocyte (V_m) is recorded. When recording from SA nodal myocytes, spontaneous action potentials, as in Fig. 1A, can be acquired. When recording from intrinsically quiescent cells, like atrial or ventricular myocytes, a brief current pulse can be injected into the myocyte through the

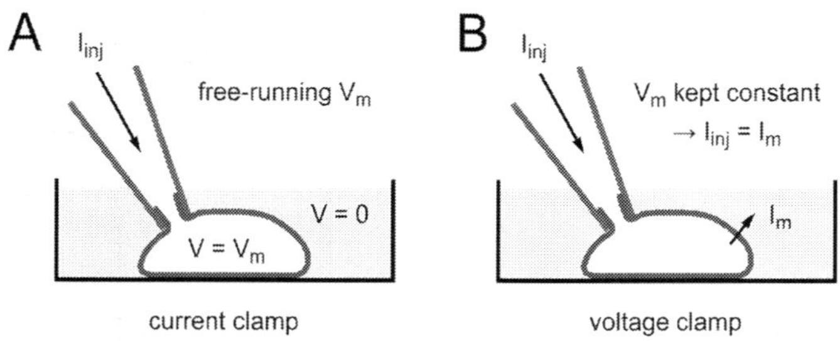

Fig. 3. Different recording modes of the whole-cell patch clamp configuration. (A) Current clamp mode. A current (I_{inj}) can be injected into the myocyte through the recording pipette, e.g. as a stimulus to elicit an action potential in a normally quiescent cell, and the free-running membrane potential of the myocyte (V_m) is recorded. (B) Voltage clamp mode. The membrane potential of the myocyte is held at a set level through a feedback circuit in the patch clamp amplifier. Consequently, the current that enters the cell through the recording pipette (I_{inj}) matches the current that leaves the cell through its membrane (I_m).

recording pipette as a stimulus to elicit an action potential (I_{inj}). In the voltage clamp mode, the membrane potential of the myocyte is held at a set level through a feedback circuit in the patch clamp amplifier. Consequently, there is no (dis)charging of the cell membrane capacitance and the current that enters the cell through the recording pipette (I_{inj}) matches the current that leaves the cell through its membrane (I_m). This way, ion currents can be studied under carefully controlled conditions, applying dedicated 'voltage clamp protocols' (cf. Section 4).

4. Voltage clamp recordings of HCN4 current

Figure 4 shows data obtained from voltage clamp experiments carried out on HEK-293 cells expressing HCN4 channels. The HCN4 gene was bicistronically expressed with green fluorescent protein (GFP) as a reporter of successful transfection with HCN4. Cell suspensions were put into a recording chamber on the stage of an inverted microscope, and superfused with Tyrode's solution (36±0.2°C) containing (in mmol/L): NaCl 140, KCl 5.4, $CaCl_2$ 1.8, $MgCl_2$ 1.0, glucose 5.5, and HEPES 5.0; pH was set to 7.4 with NaOH. Single HEK-293 cells exhibiting green fluorescence, indicating presence of HCN4 channels, were selected for electrophysiological measurements. The HCN4 current was recorded by the whole-cell patch clamp technique using an Axopatch 200B amplifier (Molecular Devices, Sunnyvale, CA, USA). The recording pipette was filled with a solution containing (in mmol/L): K-gluconate 125, KCl 20, NaCl 10, and HEPES 10; pH was set to 7.2 using KOH. Signals were low-pass filtered (cut-off frequency: 5 kHz) and digitized at 5 kHz. Series resistance was compensated by ≥80%, and potentials were corrected for the estimated 15 mV 'liquid junction potential'. Voltage control, data acquisition, and data analysis were accomplished using custom software.

Figure 4A shows representative HCN4 current recordings. The HCN4 current was measured during 6-s hyperpolarizing steps (range −30 to −120 mV) from a holding potential of −30 mV. Next, a 6-s step to −120 mV was applied to record 'tail current' followed by a 1-s pulse to 10 mV to ensure full deactivation (see Fig. 4A, top, for protocol; cycle length of protocol: 18 s). We observed large, time-dependent inward currents in response to the hyperpolarizing voltage steps (Fig. 4A, bottom). Typical for HCN4, the current amplitude and activation rate increased with more hyperpolarized potentials. The activation properties of the HCN4 current were measured during the 6-s hyperpolarizing steps. The average current voltage (I-V) relationship of the fully-activated HCN4 current at the end of the 6-s hyperpolarizing steps is shown in Fig. 4B. To correct for differences in current amplitude due to differences in cell size—larger cells have more channels in their membrane—currents were normalized to the cell membrane capacitance (in pF), which is a reliable measure of the cell membrane surface area.

The amplitude of the tail current immediately following the 6-s hyperpolarizing step reflects the amount of channels that activated during the preceding hyperpolarizing step. To characterize the voltage dependence of activation of the HCN4 current, we therefore plotted the normalized tail current amplitude (I/I_{max}) against the preceding hyperpolarizing potential. Average data are shown in Fig. 4C. The solid line is a Boltzmann fit to the data, for which we used the equation

$$I/I_{max} = A/\{1.0 + \exp[(V_m - V_{1/2})/k]\} \tag{1}$$

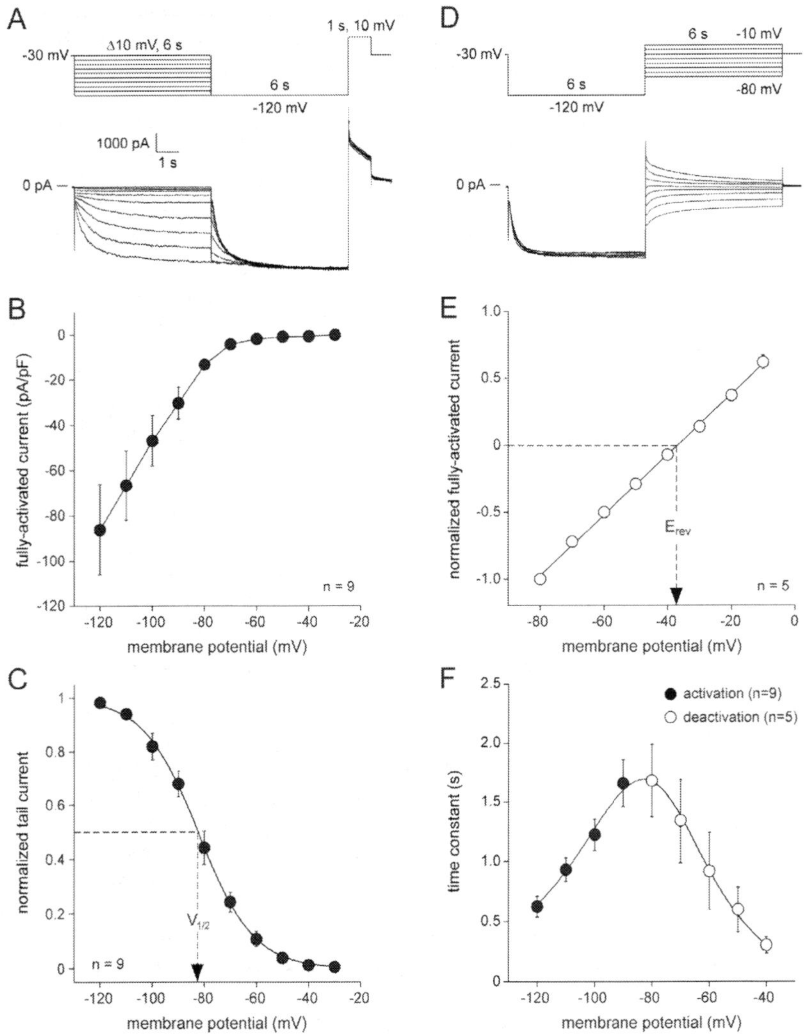

Fig. 4. Voltage clamp recordings of HCN4 current expressed in human embryonic kidney cells (HEK-293 cells). (A) Voltage pulse protocol to measure activation properties (top) and typical HCN4 current traces in response to this protocol (bottom). (B) Average current-voltage (I-V) relationship of the fully-activated HCN4 current at the end of the hyperpolarizing steps. (C) Voltage dependence of HCN4 current activation. Solid line is the Boltzmann fit to the experimental data. (D) Voltage pulse protocol to measure deactivation properties (top) and typical HCN4 current traces in response to this protocol (bottom). (E) I-V relationship of the fully-activated HCN4 current at the beginning of the depolarizing steps. Solid line is the linear fit to the experimental data. (F) Time constant of (de)activation.

In this equation, V_m denotes membrane potential and the fitting parameters $V_{1/2}$ and k are half-maximum activation voltage and slope factor, respectively. For the data of Fig. 4C, $V_{1/2}$ and k amounted to −87.7 ± 2.4 and 11.5 ± 2.4 mV (n=9), respectively.

Deactivation kinetics and reversal potential (E_{rev}) were measured during depolarizing steps (range −80 to −10 mV, duration 6 s) after a 6-s prepulse to −120 mV to ensure full activation (see Fig. 4D, top, for protocol and Fig. 4D, bottom, for a typical example of associated current recordings; cycle length of protocol: 15 s). E-4031 (5 μM) was added to the Tyrode's solution to block the delayed rectifier like endogenous current of HEK-293 cells (Yu & Kerchner, 1998; Jiang et al., 2002). The voltage dependence of the fully−activated current was evaluated over the entire range of depolarizing test potentials, i.e. −80 to −10 mV, by measuring the amplitude of the tail currents immediately following the 6-s hyperpolarizing step to −120 mV. Figure 4E shows the thus obtained average I-V relationship of the fully-activated HCN4 current normalized to its value measured at −120 mV. The average reversal potential was −36.8 ± 1.0 mV (n=5).

Activation of the HCN4 current during the hyperpolarizing steps of Fig. 4A was characterized by a monoexponential fit to each of the normalized current traces, using the equation

$$I/I_{max} = A \times [\,1 - \exp(-t/\tau)\,] \tag{2}$$

In this equation, t denotes time and the fitting parameter τ is the time constant of activation. Similarly, deactivation of the HCN4 current during the depolarizing steps of Fig. 4D was characterized by a monoexponential fit to each of the normalized current traces, using the equation

$$I/I_{max} = A \times \exp(-t/\tau) \tag{3}$$

In this equation, t again denotes time and the fitting parameter τ now is the time constant of deactivation. In the above Eqs. 2 and 3, the variable initial delay in HCN4 current (de)activation is ignored (van Ginneken & Giles, 1991; Verkerk et al., 2009a). Figure 4F shows the average activation and deactivation time constants of the HCN4 current. The activation time constant (closed symbols) ranged from ≈625 ms at −120 mV to ≈1.6 s at −90 mV, and the deactivation time constant (open symbols) from ≈1.7 s at −80 mV to ≈305 ms at −40 mV. The bell-shaped curve in Fig. 4F was obtained by fitting the data to the equation

$$\tau = 1 \,/\, [\, A_1 \times \exp(-V_m/B_1) + A_2 \times \exp(V_m/B_2)\,] \tag{4}$$

In this equation, τ is the activation or deactivation time constant, V_m is membrane potential, and A_1, A_2, B_1, and B_2 are fitting parameters (Qu et al., 2004).

5. Action potential clamp

In this section, we first explain the traditional 'action potential clamp' technique and then the 'dynamic action potential clamp'. The techniques are presented by means of examples of recent applications aimed at investigating differences in kinetics of wild-type (WT) and mutant ion channels encoded by the human ether-à-go-go-related gene (HERG), i.e. the gene encoding the pore-forming α-subunit of the channels underlying the cardiac rapid delayed rectifier current (I_{Kr}). This outward potassium current is one of the ion currents underlying the repolarization phase of the action potential of ventricular cells (and also of SA nodal pacemaker cells).

5.1 Traditional action potential clamp

Essentially, action potential clamp is a particular refinement of the voltage clamp technique. Instead of the traditional step protocols (cf. Fig. 4, A and D), a prerecorded action potential waveform is used as voltage clamp command potential. Figure 5 shows a recent application

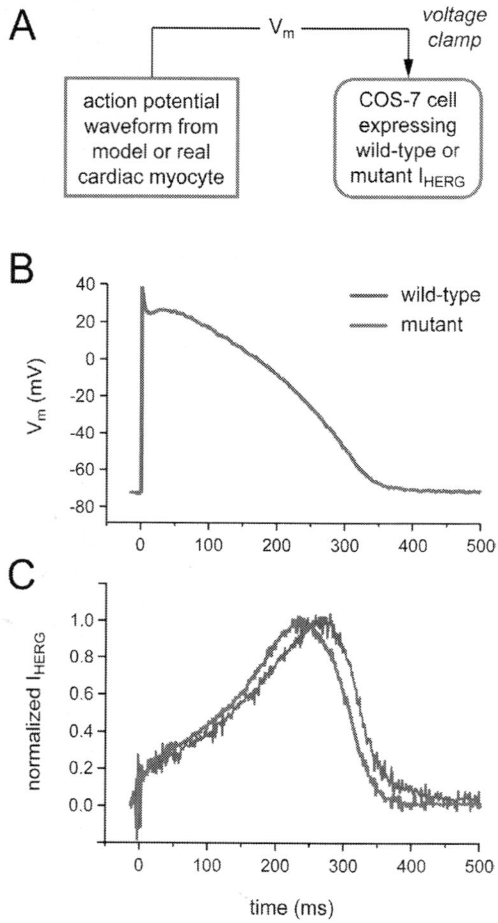

Fig. 5. Traditional action potential clamp experiment, exploring the effect of the A561P mutation in HERG. African green monkey kidney cells (COS-7 cells) were either transfected with human wild-type (WT) HERG cDNA or co-transfected with WT and A561P mutant HERG cDNA. (A) Experimental configuration. (B) Action potential recorded from a human ventricular myocyte, paced at 1 Hz, used as command voltage to clamp HERG-transfected COS-7 cells. Note that this command voltage is identical for WT ('wild-type', blue trace) and WT + A561P mutant ('mutant', red trace). (C) Normalized HERG current in response to the command voltage of B. Data from Bellocq et al. (2004).

of traditional action potential clamp by Bellocq et al. (2004) to investigate differences in kinetics of wild-type (WT) and A561P mutant HERG current. To this end, both WT + A561P mutant HERG channels, representing heterozygous carriers of the long-QT syndrome associated A561P mutation, and WT HERG channels, representing non-carriers, are expressed in the COS-7 cell line. Like HEK-293 cells, cells of this African green monkey cell line express little or no endogenous membrane current. As diagrammed in Fig. 5A, a previously recorded human ventricular action potential (Fig. 5B) is used as voltage clamp command potential and applied to HERG channel expressing COS-7 cells at a rate of 1 Hz. The associated normalized HERG current is shown in Fig. 5C. The current traces demonstrate a more rapid activation of WT + A561P current (red trace) compared to WT (blue trace), which would decrease action potential duration, but also a more rapid deactivation, which would increase action potential duration. From these data, it is difficult to predict the net effect of these changes in kinetics on the action potential. This is where dynamic action potential clamp can provide a direct and unambiguous answer.

5.2 Dynamic action potential clamp

'Dynamic clamp', which is widely used in neurophysiology but has its roots in cardiac electrophysiology (Wilders, 2005), has been used to introduce artificial conductances into real excitable cells by injecting a real-time computed current into a current-clamped cell, thus simulating, e.g., synaptic input in an isolated neuron or the presence of an additional membrane ionic current in an isolated cardiac cell (see reviews by Goaillard and Marder (2006) and Wilders (2006)). As a novel application of 'dynamic clamp', we recently developed the 'dynamic action potential clamp' (dAPC) technique, which was used to study the effects of ion channel mutations by effectively replacing a native ionic current of a cardiac myocyte with wild-type or mutant current expressed in HEK-293 cells (Berecki et al., 2005; Berecki et al., 2006; Berecki & van Ginneken, 2006; Berecki et al., 2007). Dynamic action potential clamp differs from traditional 'dynamic clamp' and 'action potential clamp' in that it combines current clamp, as used in dynamic clamp, and voltage clamp, as used in action potential clamp.

The diagram of Fig. 6A illustrates the concept of dynamic action potential clamp. Like in the study of Fig. 5, WT or mutant HERG channels are expressed in cells of a mammalian cell line, in this case HEK-293 instead of COS-7 cells, and subjected to voltage clamp to investigate differences in kinetic properties of these channels. This time, however, the voltage clamp command potential is not a prerecorded action potential, but the free-running membrane potential of a freshly isolated, patch-clamped ventricular cell (or cell model) with its native HERG-encoded current, i.e. I_{Kr}, blocked by a pharmacological agent (or set to zero in case of a model cell). The measured HERG current is injected into the ventricular myocyte in real time. Thus, there is continuous feedback between action potential and HERG current. The WT or mutant HERG channels are allowed to follow the natural time course of the ventricular action potential (through the voltage clamp), upon being simultaneously allowed to contribute current for the generation of this action potential as if they were incorporated into the membrane of the myocyte (through injection of the HERG current into the current-clamped myocyte).

The experiment of Fig. 6 directly demonstrates that the long-QT syndrome associated R56Q mutation results in significant action potential prolongation (Fig. 6B) and provides insights in the underlying mechanism (Fig. 6C). Notably, this action potential prolongation occurs despite the larger initial HERG current in the mutant case. This demonstrates that the change in action potential profile is not only the result of changes in HERG current but also of changes in other membrane currents through their dependence on membrane potential.

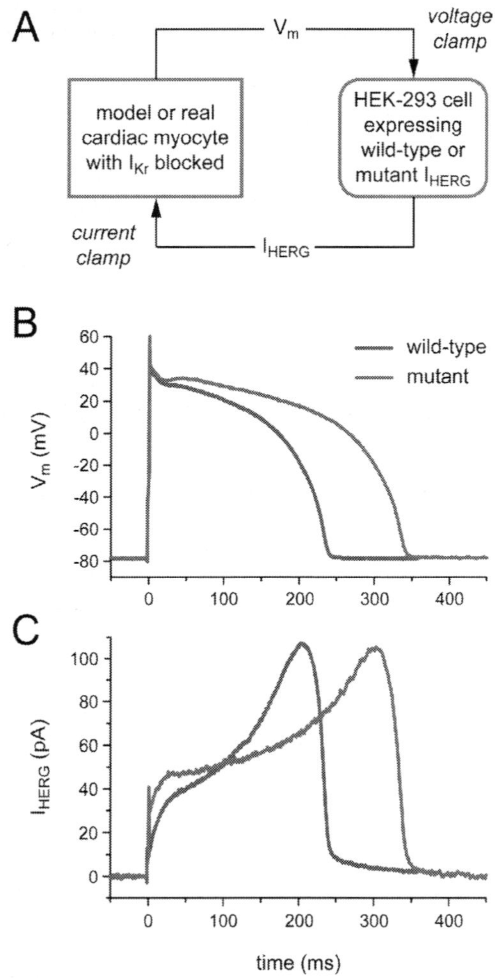

Fig. 6. Dynamic action potential clamp experiment, exploring the effect of the R56Q mutation in HERG. A single isolated rabbit ventricular myocyte was successively coupled to a HEK-293 cell expressing wild-type HERG current ('wild-type', blue traces) and a HEK-293 cell expressing R56Q mutant HERG current ('mutant', red traces). The myocyte had its native rapid delayed rectifier current (I_{Kr}) blocked by E-4031 and was paced at 1 Hz. (A) Experimental configuration. (B) Superimposed action potentials of the myocyte. (C) Associated HERG current. Data from Berecki et al. (2005).

The latter changes can be assessed using the recorded action potentials as voltage waveforms in traditional action potential clamp experiments or computer simulations. In the experiment of Fig. 6, WT and mutant HERG current were both scaled down to produce a HERG current density comparable to the native I_{Kr} density of the real isolated myocyte, as estimated using the I_{Kr} blocker E-4031. This scaling procedure seemed appropriate because the R56Q mutation is associated with altered gating properties rather than impaired trafficking of the HERG channel protein from the endoplasmic reticulum to the cell membrane.

5.3 Technical considerations

The experimental setup for the experiment of Fig. 6 is detailed in Fig. 7. The central desktop PC running the Real-Time Linux (RT-Linux) operating system (Barabanov & Yodaiken, 1997) is connected to two patch-clamp amplifiers, one in current clamp mode (amplifier 1) and the other in voltage clamp mode (amplifier 2). Through the command potential $V_{cmd,2}$ the central PC tells amplifier 2 to make the HEK-293 cell follow the free-running membrane potential of the myocyte. At the same time, through the command potential $V_{cmd,1}$, it tells amplifier 1 to inject the HERG current recorded from the HEK-293 cell into the myocyte. This is typically done with an update rate of 20 kHz, i.e. with the time step Δt set to 50 µs. Given the relatively high expression level of HERG channels in HEK-293 cells, the HERG current is scaled down to achieve an appropriate current amplitude. Any endogenous current included in the current recorded from the HEK-293 cell (Yu & Kerchner, 1998; Jiang et al., 2002) is then also scaled down, so that this endogenous current becomes negligible. However, if the expressed current needs to be scaled up, precautions should be made to avoid distortion by endogenous current, e.g. through a subtraction procedure as used in the study on sodium current by Berecki et al. (2006). The real isolated cardiac myocyte may be replaced by a real-time simulation of such cell, computed in the central PC. The differential equations of the mathematical model of the myocyte are then integrated with the above time step Δt.

As long as real-time simulations are not required, dAPC experiments can also be carried out using analogue circuitry, but if ease of use and high flexibility are important, the use of custom software running on an RT-Linux PC, or another operating system suitable for time-critical applications, equipped with a multifunction data acquisition board is the best option. Dynamic clamp software is not commercially available, but several research groups have made their custom software, mainly developed for use in neurophysiology, publicly available (Wilders, 2006). Our 'DynaClamp' dAPC software is available for download from our institutional website (URL: http://www.amc.nl/index.cfm?pid=4922).

As illustrated in Fig. 7, dAPC software should be able to continuously sample two analogue signals, carry out computations based on the acquired data, and send out two analogue signals based on the outcome of these computations. This implies that, in contrast with traditional data acquisition software, data buffering is not useful because individual samples are processed immediately after they are acquired. With today's computer processor speed the limiting factor for the overall speed (update rate) of the dAPC system is the rate of signal input and output operations, even if complex mathematical models are used in the computations of the current to be injected. With proper selection of hardware and software, an update rate of 10–50 kHz, corresponding with a cycle time of 20–100 µs, can be achieved. Considerations on this matter have been published elsewhere (see Wilders

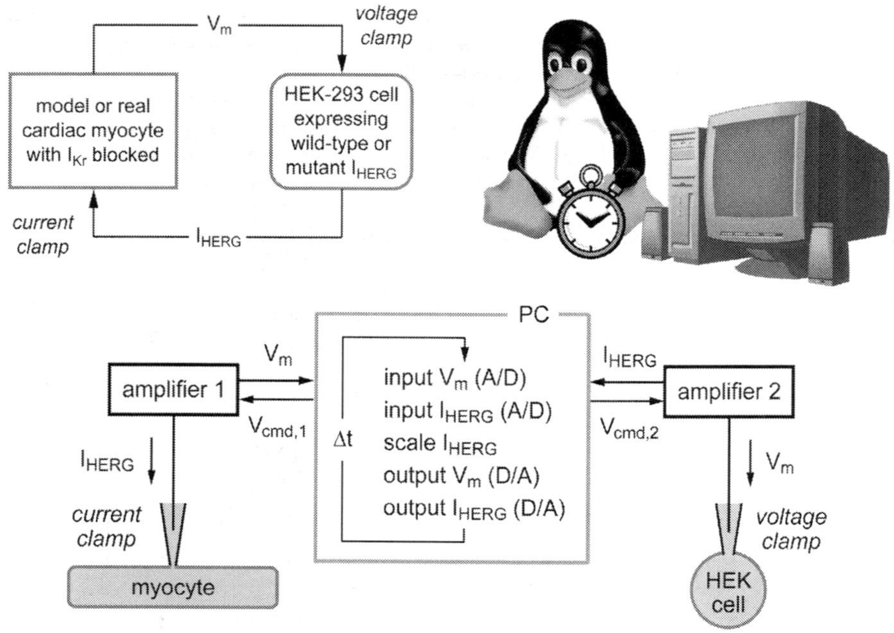

Fig. 7. Dynamic action potential clamp (dAPC) technique, when used to effectively replace the native HERG-encoded cardiac delayed rectifier potassium current (I_{Kr}) of a ventricular cell (or cell model) with the HERG current (I_{HERG}) recorded from a HEK-293 cell transfected with wild-type or mutant HERG cDNA. In a continuous cycle (with cycle time Δt), controlled through a PC running the Real-Time Linux (RT-Linux) operating system, I_{HERG} is recorded from the voltage-clamped HEK-293 cell, appropriately scaled, and then applied as external current to the ventricular myocyte, which is in current clamp mode and has its native I_{Kr} blocked pharmacologically (or set to zero in case of a model cell). The free-running action potential of the myocyte, co-shaped by the input I_{HERG}, is applied as voltage clamp command potential to the HEK-293 cell, thus establishing dAPC.

(2006) and primary references cited therein). In general, one should realize that carrying out dAPC experiments is not straightforward and that there are numerous distorting factors that should be taken care of (Bettencourt et al., 2008; Preyer & Butera, 2009).

6. Action potential clamp recordings of HCN4 current

With the availability of HEK-293 cells expressing HCN4 channels (Fig. 4), it is possible to record the HCN4 current that would flow during a prerecorded SA nodal action potential. We have carried out such traditional action potential clamp experiment, with the same electrophysiological recording conditions as for Fig. 4. We used the Wilders et al. (1991) rabbit SA nodal cell model with I_f set to zero to generate an action potential waveform and, in a 10-s run, continuously applied the resulting action potential waveform to the HEK-293 cell as voltage clamp command potential (Fig. 8A; cf. Fig. 1A, red trace). Figure 8B shows the associated HCN4 current recorded from the HEK-293 cell.

There are several differences between the recorded HCN4 current (Fig. 8B) and the I_f 'pacemaker current' of the SA nodal cell model (Fig. 1C), which is computed from the second-order Hodgkin & Huxley type kinetic scheme put forward by van Ginneken & Giles (1991), based on their voltage clamp data on I_f obtained from rabbit SA nodal cells. Most strikingly, the HCN4 current has a large outward component, partly due to the more negative reversal potential of the HCN4 current (−43 mV in this particular cell, compared to −24 mV for the model I_f), and is available early during diastolic depolarization. Interestingly, the more pronounced outward component and early availability during

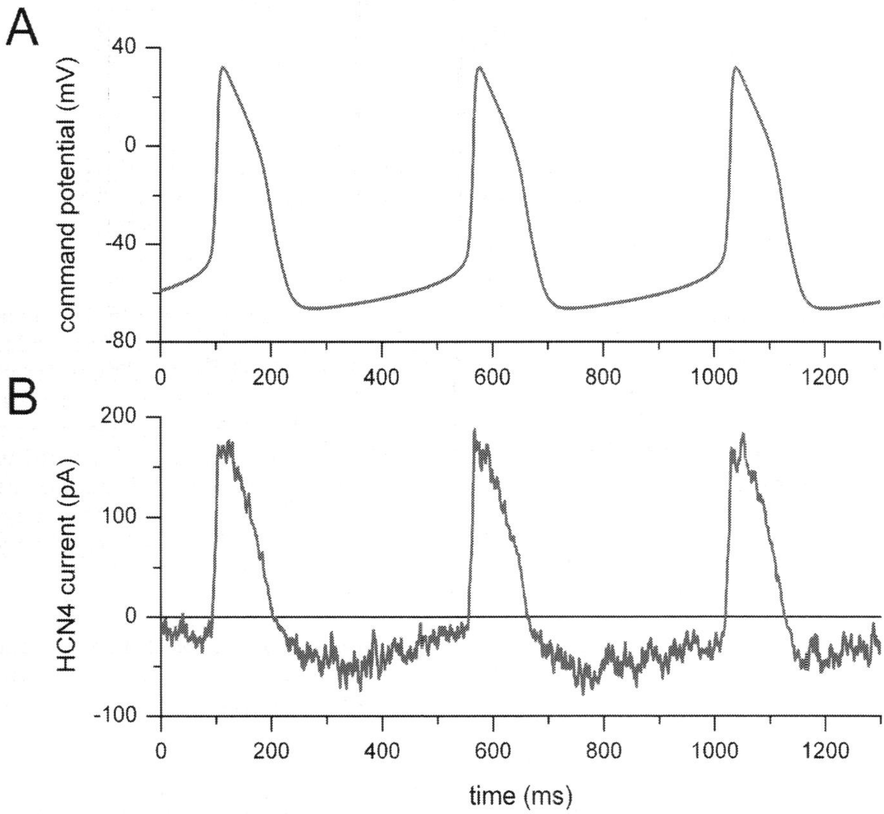

Fig. 8. Traditional action potential clamp experiment with a HEK-293 cell expressing HCN4 channels. (A) Sinoatrial (SA) nodal action potential waveform (Wilders et al. (1991) SA nodal cell model with I_f set to zero, cf. Fig. 1A) applied to the HEK-293 cell as voltage clamp command potential. (B) HCN4 current recorded from the HEK-293 cell.

diastole are in agreement with action potential clamp data from rabbit SA nodal cells by Zaza et al. (1997), who studied I_f as the current sensitive to 2 mmol/L Cs^+, and our recent numerical reconstructions, based on a first-order Hodgkin & Huxley type kinetic scheme, of I_f in human SA nodal cells (Verkerk et al., 2008; Verkerk et al., 2009a). The experiment of Fig. 8 underscores the importance of carrying out action potential clamp experiments in addition to traditional voltage clamp experiments and computer simulations.

7. Dynamic action potential clamp experiments with HCN4 current

The action potential clamp experiment of Fig. 8 reveals the HCN4 current that would flow during the prerecorded SA nodal action potential of Fig. 8A. However, it does not show how this current modulates the SA nodal action potential. Therefore, we also carried out a dynamic action potential clamp experiment with an HCN4-transfected HEK-293 cell in combination with the Wilders et al. (1991) model of a rabbit SA nodal pacemaker cell with its native I_f set to zero, as illustrated here in Fig. 9 and published elsewhere in the light of engineering a gene-based biological pacemaker (Verkerk et al., 2008; Verkerk et al., 2009c). A time step of 50 μs was used in the dAPC setup (cf. Fig. 7) and in the Euler type integration scheme that we used to solve the differential equations of the cell model.

In the Wilders et al. (1991) model, as in other (rabbit) SA nodal cell models (Wilders, 2007), the cycle length increases significantly upon blockade of I_f, mainly due to a decrease in the rate of diastolic depolarization (Fig. 1). As diagrammed in Fig. 9A, we used the action potential of the model cell—with its I_f set to zero—to voltage-clamp the HEK-293 cell and fed the recorded HCN4 current back into the current-clamped model cell, thus establishing the dAPC configuration. Given the large HCN4 currents expressed in HEK-293 cells (Fig. 4), we applied scaling factors of 0.0–1.0% to the recorded HCN4 current before adding it to the model. With the scaling factor set to zero (Fig. 9B, red trace labeled '0.0'), the resulting action potential is identical to that of the model cell with its I_f set to zero (Fig. 1A, red trace). With a scaling factor of 1.0% (Fig. 9B, blue trace labeled '1.0'), the cycle length shortens and becomes almost identical to that of the original model with its default I_f (Fig. 1A, blue trace). Intermediate shortening occurs with intermediate values for the scaling factor (Fig. 9B, traces labeled '0.5', '0.7' and '0.9').

The data of Fig. 9 suggest that the HCN4 current can functionally, in terms of modulating pacemaker frequency, replace the native I_f. However, unlike I_f, increasing the HCN4 current not only increases the rate of diastolic depolarization, but also clearly depolarizes the maximum diastolic potential to less negative values. This emphasizes that the kinetics of HCN4 channels need not be identical to those of native I_f channels (Qu et al., 2002) and that HCN4 channels should not simply be regarded as a replacement of I_f 'pacemaker channels' in gene therapy strategies. In addition, it stresses that the behaviour of HCN4 channels is more complex than reflected in the description of I_f in currently available SA nodal cell models (Wilders, 2007). A caveat that should be put in place here is that the depolarization of the maximum diastolic potential may, at least to some extent, be due to inward 'leakage current' of the HEK-293 cell, although the scaling factor of 0.01 or less also applies to this current. Ideally, the experiment of Fig. 9, and also that of Fig. 8, should have been carried with a human SA nodal cell model instead a rabbit model, but such model is not available due to a paucity of data from human SA nodal cells (Verkerk et al., 2007; Verkerk et al., 2009a; Verkerk et al., 2009b).

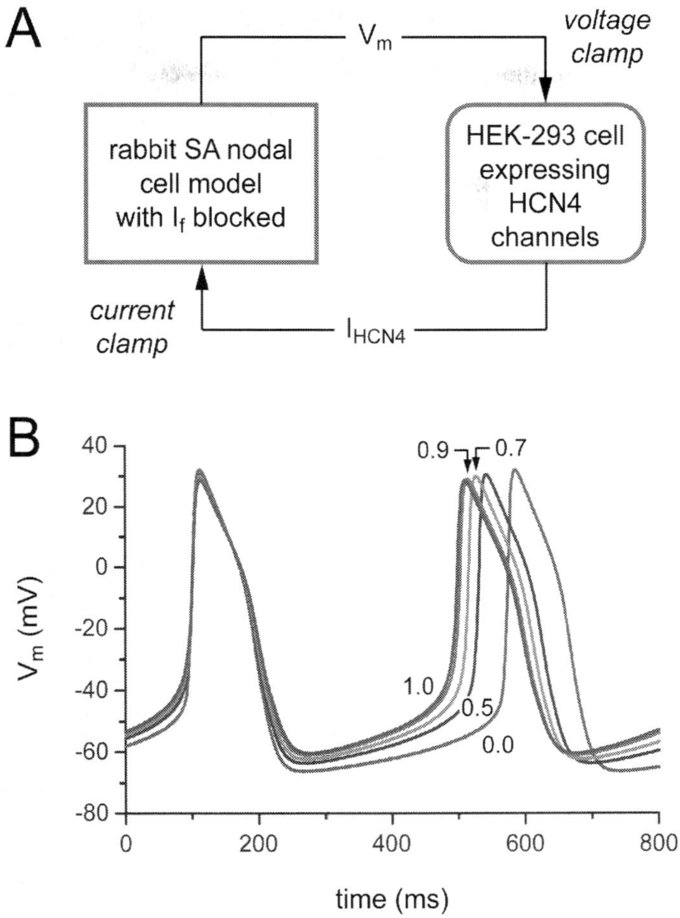

Fig. 9. Dynamic action potential clamp (dAPC) experiment with a real-time simulation of a sinoatrial (SA) nodal pacemaker cell and a HEK-293 cell expressing HCN4 channels. (A) Experimental configuration. An SA nodal pacemaker cell is simulated in real time using the Wilders et al. (1991) model of a rabbit SA nodal myocyte. The HCN-encoded hyperpolarization-activated current I_f, also known as 'pacemaker current' or 'funny current', of the model cell is set to zero and replaced with HCN4 current recorded from the HEK-293 cell (I_{HCN4}). (B) Effect of adding increasing amounts of HCN4 current to the SA nodal cell with its native I_f set to zero. A scaling factor of 0.0, 0.5, 0.7, 0.9, or 1.0%, as indicated by numbers near traces, was applied to the HCN4 current recorded from the HEK-293 cell.

8. Conclusion

In this chapter we have shown how our dynamic action potential clamp technique can provide important insights into the ionic mechanisms underlying intrinsic pacemaker activity of SA nodal cells. This underscores the important role that biomedical engineering can play in the field of cardiac cellular electrophysiology.

9. References

Barabanov, M. & Yodaiken, V. (1997). Introducing real-time Linux. *Linux Journal,* 34, February 1997, 19–23, ISSN: 1075-3583

Bellocq, C.; Wilders, R.; Schott, J.-J.; Louérat-Oriou, B.; Boisseau, P.; Le Marec, H.; Escande, D. & Baró, I. (2004). A common antitussive drug, clobutinol, precipitates the long QT syndrome 2. *Molecular Pharmacology,* 66, 5, 1093–1102, ISSN: 0026-895X

Berecki, G.; Zegers, J.G.; Verkerk, A.O.; Bhuiyan, Z.A.; de Jonge, B.; Veldkamp, M.W.; Wilders, R. & van Ginneken, A.C.G. (2005). HERG channel (dys) function revealed by dynamic action potential clamp technique. *Biophysical Journal,* 88, 1, 566–578, ISSN: 0006-3495

Berecki, G. & van Ginneken, A.C.G. (2006). Cardiac channelopathies studied with the dynamic action potential clamp technique. *Physiology News,* 63, Summer 2006, 28–29, ISSN: 1476-7996

Berecki, G.; Zegers, J.G.; Bhuiyan, Z.A.; Verkerk, A.O.; Wilders, R. & van Ginneken, A.C.G. (2006). Long-QT syndrome-related sodium channel mutations probed by the dynamic action potential clamp technique. *The Journal of Physiology,* 570, Pt. 2, 237–250, ISSN: 0022-3751

Berecki, G.; Zegers, J.G.; Wilders, R. & van Ginneken, A.C.G. (2007). Cardiac channelopathies studied with the dynamic action potential-clamp technique, In: *Patch-Clamp Methods and Protocols,* Molnar, P. & Hickman, J.J. (Eds.), 233–250, Humana Press, ISBN: 978-1-58829-698-6, Totowa, NJ, USA

Bettencourt, J.C.; Lillis, K.P.; Stupin, L.R. & White, J.A. (2008). Effects of imperfect dynamic clamp: computational and experimental results. *Journal of Neuroscience Methods,* 169, 2, 282–289, ISSN: 0165-0270

Boyett, M.R.; Honjo, H. & Kodama I. (2000). The sinoatrial node, a heterogeneous pacemaker structure. *Cardiovascular Research,* 47, 4, 658–687, ISSN: 0008-6363

Dobrzynski, H.; Boyett, M.R. & Anderson, R.H. (2007). New insights into pacemaker activity: promoting understanding of sick sinus syndrome. *Circulation,* 115, 14, 1921–1932, ISSN: 0009-7322

Goaillard, J.-M. & Marder, E. (2006). Dynamic clamp analyses of cardiac, endocrine, and neural function. *Physiology,* 21, 3, 197–207, ISSN: 1548-9213

Jiang, B.; Sun, X.; Cao, K. & Wang, R. (2002). Endogenous K_V channels in human embryonic kidney (HEK-293) cells. *Molecular and Cellular Biochemistry,* 238, 1-2, 69–79, ISSN: 0300-8177

Mangoni, M.E. & Nargeot, J. (2008). Genesis and regulation of the heart automaticity. *Physiological Reviews,* 88, 3, 919–982, ISSN: 0031-9333

Moosmang, S.; Stieber, J.; Zong, X.; Biel, M.; Hofmann, F. & Ludwig, A. (2001). Cellular expression and functional characterization of four hyperpolarization-activated pacemaker channels in cardiac and neuronal tissues. *European Journal of Biochemistry*, 268, 6, 1646–1652, ISSN: 0014-2956

Preyer, A.J. & Butera, R.J. (2009). Causes of transient instabilities in the dynamic clamp. *IEEE Transactions on Neural Systems and Rehabilitation Engineering*, 17, 2, 190–198, ISSN: 1534-4320

Qu, J.; Altomare, C.; Bucchi, A.; DiFrancesco, D. & Robinson, R.B. (2002). Functional comparison of HCN isoforms expressed in ventricular and HEK 293 cells. *Pflügers Archiv - European Journal of Physiology*, 444, 5, 597–601, ISSN: 0031-6768

Qu, J.; Kryukova, Y.; Potapova, I.A.; Doronin, S.V.; Larsen, M.; Krishnamurthy, G.; Cohen, I.S. & Robinson, R.B. (2004). MiRP1 modulates HCN2 channel expression and gating in cardiac myocytes. *The Journal of Biological Chemistry*, 279, 42, 43497–43502, ISSN: 0021-9258

van Ginneken, A.C.G. & Giles, W. (1991). Voltage clamp measurements of the hyper-polarization-activated inward current I_f in single cells from rabbit sino-atrial node. *The Journal of Physiology*, 434, Pt. 1, 57–83, ISSN: 0022-3751

Varghese, A.; TenBroek, E.M.; Coles, J. Jr. & Sigg, D.C. (2006). Endogenous channels in HEK cells and potential roles in HCN ionic current measurements. *Progress in Biophysics and Molecular Biology*, 90, 1–3, 26–37, ISSN: : 0079-6107

Verkerk, A.O.; Wilders, R.; van Borren, M.M.G.J.; Peters, R.J.G.; Broekhuis, E.; Lam, K.Y.; Coronel, R.; de Bakker, J.M.T. & Tan, H.L. (2007). Pacemaker current (I_f) in the human sinoatrial node. *European Heart Journal*, 28, 20, 2472–2478, ISSN: 0195-688X

Verkerk, A.O., Zegers, J.G., van Ginneken, A.C.G. & Wilders, R. (2008). Dynamic action potential clamp as a powerful tool in the development of a gene-based bio-pacemaker. *Conference Proceedings of the IEEE Engineering in Medicine and Biology Society*, 2008, 1, 133–136, ISSN: 1557-170X

Verkerk, A.O., van Ginneken, A.C.G. & Wilders, R. (2009a). Pacemaker activity of the human sinoatrial node: role of the hyperpolarization-activated current, I_f. *International Journal of Cardiology*, 132, 3, 318–336, ISSN: 0167-5273

Verkerk, A.O.; Wilders, R.; van Borren, M.M.G.J. & Tan, H.L. (2009b). Is sodium current present in human sinoatrial node cells? *International Journal of Biological Sciences*, 5, 2, 201–204, ISSN: 1449-2288

Verkerk, A.O., Zegers, J.G., van Ginneken, A.C.G. & Wilders, R. (2009c). Development of a genetically engineered cardiac pacemaker: insights from dynamic action potential clamp experiments, In: *Dynamic-Clamp: From Principles to Applications*, Destexhe, A. & Bal, T. (Eds.), 399–415, Springer, ISBN: 978-0-387-89278-8, New York, NY, USA

Wilders, R.; Jongsma, H.J. & van Ginneken, A.C.G. (1991). Pacemaker activity of the rabbit sinoatrial node: a comparison of mathematical models. *Biophysical Journal*, 60, 5, 1202–1216, ISSN: 0006-3495

Wilders, R. (2005). 'Dynamic clamp' in cardiac electrophysiology. *The Journal of Physiology*, 566, Pt. 2, 641, ISSN: 0022-3751

Wilders, R. (2006). Dynamic clamp: a powerful tool in cardiac electrophysiology. *The Journal of Physiology*, 576, Pt. 2, 349–359, ISSN: 0022-3751

Wilders, R. (2007). Computer modelling of the sinoatrial node. *Medical & Biological Engineering & Computing*, 45, 2, 189–207, ISSN: 0140-0118

Yu, S.P. & Kerchner, G.A. (1998). Endogenous voltage-gated potassium channels in human embryonic kidney (HEK293) cells. *Journal of Neuroscience Research,* 52, 5, 612–617, ISSN: 0360-4012

Zaza, A.; Micheletti, M.; Brioschi, A. & Rocchetti, M. (1997). Ionic currents during sustained pacemaker activity in rabbit sino-atrial myocytes. *The Journal of Physiology,* 505, Pt. 3, 677–688, ISSN: 0022-3751

Medical Remote Monitoring using sound environment analysis and wearable sensors

Dan Istrate[1], Jérôme Boudy[2], Hamid Medjahed[1,2] and Jean Louis Baldinger[2]
[1]*ESIGETEL-LRIT, 1 Rue du Port de Valvins, 77210 Avon France*
[2]*Telecom&Management SudParis, 9 Rue Charles Fourier, 91011 Evry France*

1. Introduction

The developments of technological progress allow the generalization of digital technology in the medicine area, not only the transmission of images, audio streams, but also the information that accompany them. Many medical specialties can take advantage of the opportunity offered by these new communication tools which allow the information share between medical staff. The practice of medicine takes a new meaning by the development and diffusion of Information and Communication Technologies (ICT). In the health field, unlike other economic sectors, the technical progress is not necessarily generating productivity gains but generate more safety and comfort for patients.

Another fact is that the population age increases in all societies throughout the world. In Europe, for example, the life expectancy for men is about 71 years and for women about 79 years. For North America the life expectancy, currently is about 75 for men and 81 for women[i]. Moreover, the elderly prefer to preserve their independence, autonomy and way of life living at home the longest time possible. The number of medical specialists decreases with respect to the increasing number of elderly fact that allowed the development of technological systems to assure the safety (telemedicine applications).

The elderly living at home are in most of the cases (concerning Western and Central Europe and North America) living alone and with an increased risk of accidents. In France, about 4.5 % of men and 8.9% of women aged of 65+ years has an everyday life accident[ii]. Between these everyday life accidents, the most important part is represented by the domestic accidents; about 61% (same source) and 54% of them take place inside the house. In France, annually, 2 millions of elderly falls take place, which represent the source of 10 000 deaths[iii]. Between 30% and 55% of falls cause bruises and only 3% to 13% of falls are the causes of serious injuries such as fractures, dislocation of a joint, or wounds. Apart from physical injury and hospitalization, a fall can cause a shock (especially if the person cannot recover only after the fall). This condition can seriously affect the senior psychology, he might looses the confidence in his abilities and can result in a limitation of daily activities and, consequently, in a decrease of the life quality.

In order to improve the quality of life of elderly several applications has been developed: home telemonitoring in order to detect distress situations and audio-video transmission in order to allow specialists to diagnose patient at distance.

This chapter describe a medical remote monitoring solution allowing the elderly people to live at home in safety.

2. Telemedecine applications

The term "telemedicine" appears in a dictionary of the French language for the first time in the early 1980's, the prefix "tele" denoting "far away". Thus, telemedicine literally means remote medicine and is described as "part of medicine, which uses telecommunication transmission of medical information (images, reports, records, etc.) in order to obtain remote diagnosis, a specialist opinion, continuous monitoring of a patient, a therapeutic decision." Using a misnomer, one readily associates the telemedicine to the generic term "health telematics". This term has been defined by the World Health Organization in 1997 and "refers to the activities, services and systems related to health, performed remotely using information technology and communication needs for global promotion of health, care and control of epidemics, management and research for health."

The interest of telemedicine is far from being proved and is not without stimulating reflection, particularly in the areas ethical, legal and economic. The main telemedicine applications are:

- **Telediagnostic** = The application which allow a medical specialist to analyze a patient at distance and to have access to different medical analysis concerning the patient. A specific case can be if a specialist is at the same place with the patient but need a second opinion from another one.
- **Telesurgery** = technical system allowing a surgery at distance for spatial or military applications. Also in this category we can have the distant operation of a complex system like an echograph or the augmented reality in order to help the medicine in the framework of a surgery.
- **Telemonitoring** = an automatic system which survey some physiological parameters in order to monitor a disease evolution and/or to detect a distress situation.
- **Tele-learning** = teleconferencing systems allowing medical staff to exchange on medical information.

Among the main telemedicine applications, telediagnostic and telemonitoring are more investigated solutions. The telediagnostic allows medical specialist to consult the elderly through audio video link in order to avoid unnecessary travel for both patient and medical staff. Several systems were currently developed between hospital and nursing home, or between medical staff and a mobile unit. The main challenges are the audio-video quality, the possibility to transmit also other medical data (ECG, medical records) and data security. In order to guarantee a good audio-video quality a high bandwidth network is needed.

The medical remote monitoring or telemonitoring can prevent or reduce the consequences of accidents at home for elderly people or chronic disease persons. The increase of aging population in Europe involves more people living alone at home with an increased risk of home accidents or falls. The remote monitoring aims to detect automatically a distress situation (fall or faintness) in order to provide safety living to elderly people.

The medical remote monitoring consists in establishing a remote monitoring system of one or more patients by one or more health professionals (physician, nursing...). This monitoring is mainly based on the use of telecommunication technology (ie the continuous analysis of patient medical parameters of any kind: respiratory, cardiac, and so on...). This technique is used in the development of hospitalizations at home, ie where the patient is medically monitored at home, especially in cases of elderly people. In addition, this method avoids unnecessary hospitalizations, increasing thus the patient comfort and security. The main aim of remote monitoring systems is to detect or to prevent a distress situation using different types of sensors.

In order to improve the quality of life of elderly several research teams have developed a number of systems for medical remote monitoring. These systems are based on the deployment of several sensors in the elderly home in order to detect critical situations. However, there are few reliable systems capable of detecting automatically distress situations using more or less non intrusive sensors. Monitoring the activities of elderly people at home with position sensors allows the detection of a distress situation through the circadian rhythms (Bellego et al., 2006). However, this method involves important data bases and an adaptation to the monitored person (Binh et al., 2008). Other studies monitor the person activity through the use of different household appliances (like oven or refrigerator) (Moncrieff et al., 2005). More and more applications use embedded systems, like smart mobile phones, to process data and to send it trough 3G networks (Bairacharya et al., 2008). In order to detect falls, several wearable sensors was developed using accelerometers (Marschollek et al., 2008), magnetic sensors (Fleury et al., 2007) or data fusion with smart home sensors (Bang et al., 2008).

There are many projects which develop medical remote monitoring system for elderly people or for chronic disease patient like TelePat project[iv] which was aimed at the realization of a service of remote support in residence for people suffering of cardiac pathologies (Lacombe et al., 2004). Other National projects like RESIDE-HIS and DESDHIS[v] have developed different modality to monitor like infra-red sensor, wearable accelerometer sensor and sound analysis. At European level (FP6) several projects has investigated the domain of combination of smart home technologies with remote monitoring like SOPRANO project which aims at the design of a system for the assistance of the old people in the everyday life for a better comfort and safety (Wolf et al., 2008).

Consequently, devices of the ambient intelligence are connected continuously to a center of external services as in the project EMERGE[vi]. This last aims by the behavior observation through holistic approach at detecting anomalies, an alarm is sent in the case of fall, faintness or another emergency.

Three institutions (TELECOM & Management SudParis, INSERM U558 and ESIGETEL) have already developed a medical remote monitoring modality in order to detect falls or faintness. The TELECOM & Management SudParis has developed a mobile device which detects the falls, measures the person pulse, movement and position and is equipped with panic button (Baldinger et al., 2004). The ESIGETEL has developed a system which can recognize abnormal sounds (screams, object falls, glass breaking, etc.) or distress expressions (Help!, A doctor please! etc.) (Istrate et al., 2008).

Each remote monitoring modality, individually, present cases of missed detections and/or false alarms but the fusion of several modalities can increase the system reliability and allow a fault tolerant system (Virone et al., 2003). These two modalities and others are combined in the framework of CompanionAble project.

3. CompanionAble Project

A larger telemedicine application which includes sound environment analysis and wearable sensor is initiated in the framework of a European project. CompanionAble[1] project (Integrated Cognitive Assistive & Domotic Companion Robotic Systems for Ability & Security) provides the synergy of Robotics and Ambient Intelligence technologies and their semantic integration to provide for a care-giver's assistive environment. CompanionAble project aims at helping the elderly people living semi or independently at home for as long as possible. In fact the CompanionAble project combines a telemonitoring system in order to detect a distress situation, with a cognitive program for MCI patient and with domotic facilities. The telemonitoring system is based on non intrusive sensor like: microphones, infra-red sensors, door contacts, video camera, pills dispenser, water flow sensor; a wearable sensor which can detect a fall and measure the pulse and a robot equipped with video camera, audio sensors and obstacles detectors.

4. Proposed telemonitoring system

Two modalities sound and wearable sensors are presented by following. A multimodal data fusion method is proposed in the next section.

4.1 ANASON

The information from the everyday life sound flow is more and more used in telemedical applications in order to detect falls, to detect daily life activities or to characterize physical status. The use of sound like an information vector has the advantage of simple and cheapest sensors, is not intrusive and can be fixed in the room. Otherwise, the sound signal has important redundancy and need specific methods in order to extract information. The definition of signal and noise is specific for each application; e.g. for speech recognition, all sounds are considered noise. Between numerous sound information extraction applications

[1] *www.companionable.net*

we have the characterization of cardiac sounds (Lima & Barbarosa, 2008) in order to detect cardiac diseases or the snoring sounds (Ng & Koh, 2008) for the sleep apnea identification. Using sound for the fall detection has the advantage that the patient not need to carry a wearable device but less robust in the noise presence and depend from acoustic conditions (Popescu et al., 2008), (Litvak et al., 2008). The combination of several modalities in order to detect distress situation is more robust using the information redundancy.

The sound environment analysis system for remote monitoring capable to identify everyday life normal or abnormal and distress expressions is in continuous evolution in order to increase the reliability in the noise presence. Currently in the framework of the CompanionAble project a coupled smart sensor system with a robot for mild cognitive impairment patients is being developed. The sound modality is used like a simplified patient-system interface and for the distress situation identification. The sound system will participate to the context awareness identification, to the domotic vocal commands and to the distress expressions/sounds recognition. This system can use a classical sound card allowing only one channel monitor or an USB acquisition card allowing a real time multichannel (8 channels) monitoring covering thus all the rooms of an apartment.

Current systems use mainly the speech information from sound environment in order to generate speech command or to analyze the audio scene. Few studies investigate the sound information. The (Moncrieff et al., 2005) uses the sound level coupled with the use of household appliances in order to detect a threshold on patient anxiety. In (Stagera et al., 2007) some household appliances sounds are recognized on an embedded microcontroller using a vectorial quantization. This method was used to analyze the patient activities, a distress situation being possible to be detected through a long time analysis. In (Cowling & Sitte, 2002) a statistical sound recognition system is proposed but the system was tested only on few sound files.

The proposed smart sound sensor (ANASON) analyzes in real time the sound environment using a first module of detection and extraction of useful sound or speech based on the Wavelet Transform (Istrate et al., 2006). The module composition of the smart sound sensor can be observed in the Fig.1. This module is applied on all audio channels simultaneously, in real time. Only extracted sound signals are processed by the next modules. The second module classifies extracted sound event between sound and speech. This module, like the sound identification engine, is based on a GMM (Gaussian Mixture Model) algorithm. If a sound was detected the signal is processed by a sound identification engine and if a speech was detected a speech recognition engine is launched. The speech recognition engine is a classical one aiming at detecting distress expressions like "Help!" or "A doctor, please!".

Signal event detection and extraction. This first module listen continuously the sound environment in order to detect and extract useful sounds or speech. Useful sounds are: glass breaking, box falls, door slap, etc. and sounds like water flow, electric shaver, vacuum cleaner, etc. are considered noise. The sound flow is analyzed through a wavelet based algorithm aiming at sound event detection. This algorithm must be robust to noise like neighbourhood environmental noise, water flow noise, ventilator or electric shaver. Therefore an algorithm based on energy of wavelet coefficients was proposed and evaluated. This algorithm detects precisely the signal beginning and its end, using properties of wavelet transform even at signal to noise ratio (SNR) of 0 dB. The signals extracted by this module are recorded in a safe communication queue in order to be processed by the second parallel task.

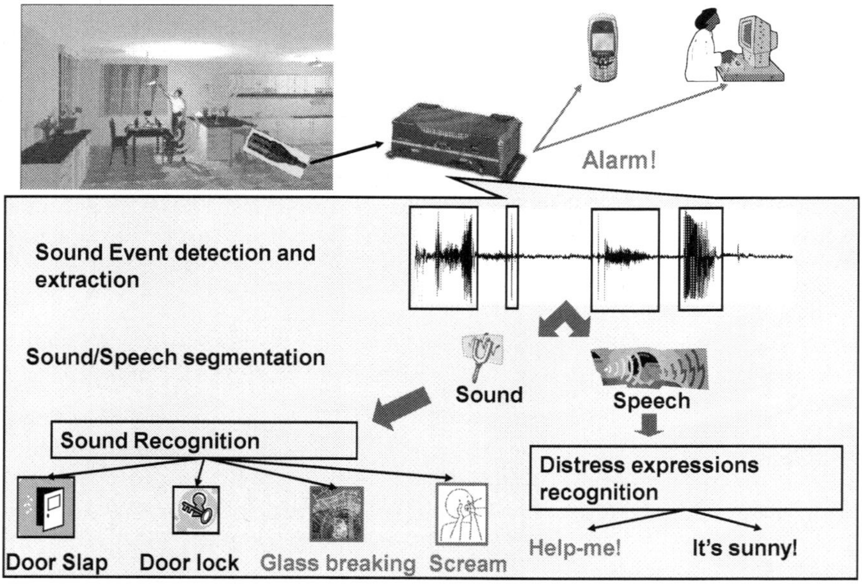

Fig. 1. Sound environment analysis system (ANASON)

Sound/speech segmentation. The second module is a low-stage classification one. It processes the extracted sounds in order to separate the speech signals from the sound ones. The method used by this module is based on Gaussian Mixture Model (GMM). There are other possibilities for signal classification: Hidden Markov Model (HMM), Bayesian method, etc. Even if similar results have been obtained with other methods, their high complexity and high time consumption prevent from real-time implementation.

A preliminary step before signal classification is the extraction of acoustic parameters: LFCC (Linear Frequency Cepstral Coefficients) - 24 filters. The choice of this type of parameters relies on their properties: bank of filters with constant bandwidth, which leads to equal resolution at high frequencies often encountered in life sounds. Other types of acoustical parameters like zero crossing rate, roll-off point, centroid or wavelet transform based was tested with good results.

Sound recognition. This module composes with the previous one the second parallel task and classifies the signal between several predefined sound classes. This module is based, also, on a GMM algorithm. The 16 MFCC (Mel Frequency Cepstral Coefficients) acoustical parameters have been used coupled with ZCR (Zero crossing rate), Roll-off Point and Centroid. The MFCC parameters are computed from 24 filters. A log-likelihood is computed for the unknown signal according to each predefined sound classes; the sound class with the biggest log likelihood constitute the output of this module.

In the current version, the number of Gaussians is optimized according to data base size which allows having different number of Gaussians for each sound class. Taking into account that for some sounds, especially for abnormal ones, is difficult to record an important number, we have chosen to allow a variation between 4 and 60 Gaussians for the sound models.

Distress expressions recognition. In order to detect distress expressions two possibilities can be considered: the use of a classical speech recognition engine followed by a textual detection of distress expressions or a word spotting system. The first solution has tested with good results through a vocabulary optimization with specific words.

If an alarm situation is identified (the sound or the sentence is classified into an alarm class) this information and the sound signal are sent to the data fusion system. In the case of a typical everyday life sound, only the extracted information (and not the sound) is sending to the data fusion system.

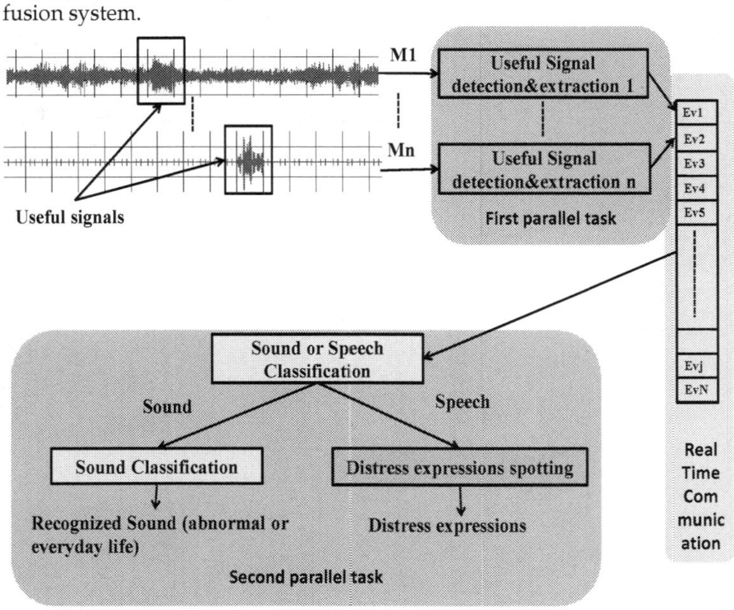

Fig. 2. ANASON real time implementation

ANASON system has been implemented in real time on PC or embedded PC using three parallel tasks (Fig. 2.):

1. Sound Acquisition + Sound Event Detection & Extraction

2. Hierarchical Sound Classification
3. Graphical User Interface and Alarm management

ANASON modality carries out also localization information concerning the microphone which has been used to recognize the abnormal sound or speech and a confidence measure in the output (SNR value).

The speech monitoring allows the system to detect a distress request coming from the patient, if the patient in the distress situation is conscious (the same role that panic button of RFPAT).

Globally, ANASON software has no false alarms and 20 % of missed detections for signals with SNR between 5 and 20 dB (real test conditions). The Useful signal detection and extraction module and the Sound or Speech Classification module work correctly even for signals with a SNR about 10 dB but the sound or speech recognition modules need at least a SNR of 20 dB. We work currently to ameliorate these performances by adding specific filtering and noise adaptation modules.

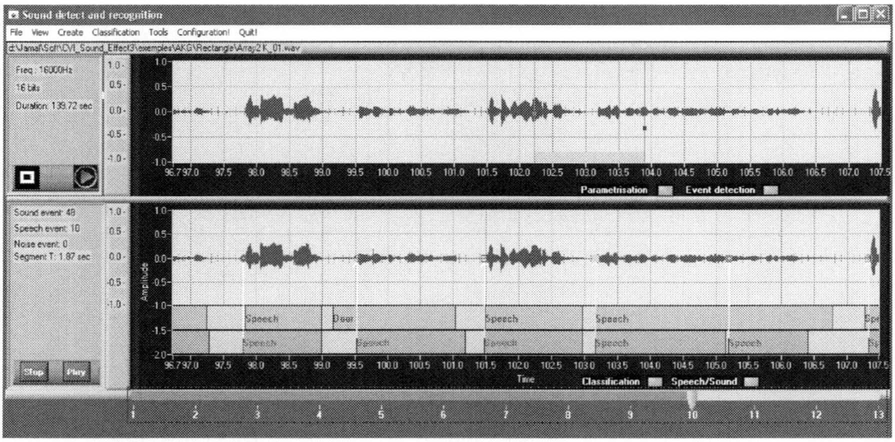

Fig. 3. Example of sound/speech detection and recognition

Fig.3. shown the ANASON algorithm application on a signal recorded in our laboratory. In the second window the blue rectangle represent the automatic output of ANASON and the gray ones the reference labels (manually labels). We can observe some reduced errors on the start/stop time of each event. All detected events were correctly classified.

4.2 RFPAT

The remote monitoring modality RFPAT consists in two fundamental modules (Fig. 2.):

- A mobile terminal (a waist wearable device that the patient or the elderly clips to his belt, for instance, all the time he is at home; it measures the person's vital data and sends it to a reception base station)

- A fixed reception base station (a receiver connected to a personal computer (PC) through a RS232 interface; it receives vital signals from the patient's mobile terminal, analyzes and records them).

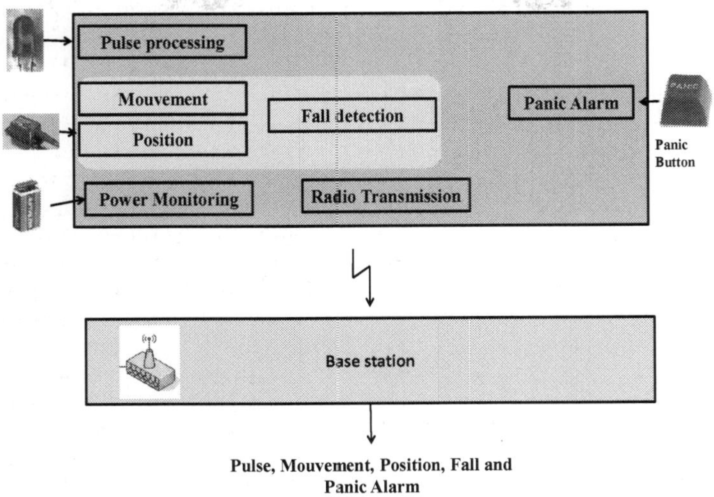

Fig. 4. Wearable device (RFPAT)

All the data gathered from the different RFPAT sensors are processed within the wireless wearable device. To ensure an optimal autonomy for the latter, it was designed using low consumption electronic components. Namely, the circuit architecture is based on different micro-controllers devoted to acquisition, signal processing and emission. Hence, the mobile wearable terminal (Fig. 4.) encapsulates several signal acquisition and processing modules:

- to records pulse rate, actimetric signals (posture, movement) and panic button
- to pre-process the signals in order to reduce the impact of environmental noise or user motion noise.

This latter point is an important issue for in-home healthcare monitoring. In fact, monitoring a person in ambulatory mode is a difficult task to achieve. For the RFPAT system, the noise is filtered in the acquisition stage inside the wearable device using digital noise reduction filters and algorithms. These filters and algorithms were applied respectively to all acquired signals: movement data, posture data and namely the pulse signal (heart rate).

Movement data describes the movement of the monitored person. It gives us information like: "immobile", "normal life movements", "stressed person", etc. Movement data consists also in the percentage of movement, it computes the total duration of the movements of the monitored person for each time slot of 30 seconds (0 to 100% during 30 seconds).

The posture data is information about the person posture: standing up/laying down. The posture data is a quite interesting measurement which gives us useful information about the person's activity.

Thanks to an actimetric system embedded in the portable device, we can detect the situations where the person is approaching the ground very quickly. This information is interpreted as a "fall" when the acceleration goes through a certain threshold in a given situation.

The pulse signal is delivered by a photoplethysmographic sensor connected to the wearable device. After pre-conditioning and algorithmic de-noising it gives us information about the heart rate every 30 seconds.

In the ambulatory mode, the challenging process consists in noise reduction (Baldinger et al., 2004). We afford to reduce the variations of pulse measurement lower than 5% for one minute averaging, which remains in conformity with the recommendations of medical professionals.

Data gathered from the different sensors are transmitted, via an electronic signal conditioner, to low power microcontroller based computing unit, embedded in the mobile terminal.

Currently, a fall-impact detector is added to this system in order to make the detection of falls more specific.

5. EMUTEM platform

A data synchronization and fusion platform, EMUTEM (Multimodal environment for medical remote monitoring), was developed (Medjahed et al., 2009).

In order to maximize correct recognition of the various activities daily live (ADL) like sleeping, cleaning, bathing etc..., and distress situation recognition, data fusion over the different sensors types is studied. The area of data fusion has generated great interest among researchers in several science disciplines and engineering domains. We have identified two major classes of fusion techniques:

- Those that are based on probabilistic models (such as Bayesian reasoning (Cowel et al., 1999) and the geometric decision reasoning like Mahanalobis distance), but their performances are limited when the data are heteregeneous and insufficient for the correct statistical modeling of classes, therefore the model is uncontrollable.
- Those based on connectionist models (such as neural networks MLP (Dreyfus et al., 2002) and SVM (Bourges, 1998)) which are very powerful because they can model the strong nonlinearity of data but with complex architecture, thus lack of intelligibility.

Based on those facts and considering the complexity of the data to process (audio, physiologic and multisensory measurements) plus the lack of training sets that reflect activities of daily living, fuzzy logic has been found useful to be the decision module of the multimodal ADLs recognition system. Fuzzy logic can gather performance and intelligibility and it deals with imprecision and uncertainty. It has a background application history to clinical problems including use in automated diagnosis (Adlassnig, 1986), control systems (Mason et al., 1997), image processing (Lalande et al., 1997) and pattern recognition (Zahlmann et al., 1997). For medical experts is easier to map their knowledge onto fuzzy relationships than to manipulate complex probabilistic tools.

Everyday life activities in the home split into two categories. Some activities show the motion of the human body and its structure. Examples are walking, running, standing up, setting down, laying and exercising. These activities may be most easily recognized using sensors that are placed on the body (e.g. (Makikawa & Iizumi, 1995)(Himberg et al., 2001)(Lee and Mase, 2002)). A second class of activities is recognized by identifying or looking for patterns in how people move things. In this work we focus on some activities identification belong to these both categories by using fuzzy logic. The use of fuzzy logic is motivated by two main raisons from a global point of view:

- Firstly the characteristic of data to merge which are measurements obtained from different sensors, thus they could be imprecise and imperfect.
- Secondly, the history of fuzzy logic proves that it is used in many cases which are necessary for pattern recognition applications.

5.1 Fuzzy Logic

Fuzzy logic is a powerful framework for performing automated reasoning. It reflects human reasoning based on inaccurate or incomplete data. It uses the concept of partial membership, each element belongs partially or gradually to fuzzy sets that have been already defined. In contrast to classical logic where the membership function $m(x)$ of an element x belonging to a set S could take only two values: $m_S(x) = 1$ if $x \in S$ or $m_S(x) = 0$ if $x \notin S$, Fuzzy logic introduces the concept of membership degree of an element x to a set S and $m_S(x) \in [0, 1]$, here we speak about truth value.

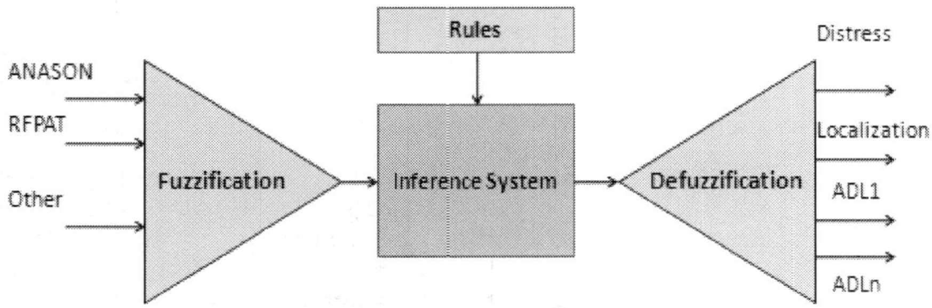

Fig. 5. Fuzzy Logic data fusion

The Fig. 5. shows the main fuzzy inference system steps:

- **Fuzzification**: First step in fuzzy logic is to convert the measured data into a set of fuzzy variables. It is done by giving value (these will be our variables) to each of a membership functions set. Membership functions take different shape: triangular, trapezoidal, Gaussian, generalized Bell, sigmoidally shaped function, single function etc. The choice of the function shape is iteratively determinate, according to type of data and taking into account the experimental results.

- **Fuzzy rules and inference system**: The fuzzy inference system uses fuzzy equivalents of logical AND, OR and NOT operations to build up fuzzy logic rules. An inference engine operates on rules that are structured in an IF-THEN format. The IF part of the rule is called the antecedent, while the THEN part of the rule is called the consequent. Rules are constructed from linguistic variables. These variables take on the fuzzy values or fuzzy terms that are represented as words and modelled as fuzzy subsets of an appropriate domain. There are several types of fuzzy rules, we mention only the two mains used in our system:
    - Mamdani rules (Jang et al., 1997) which is of the form: If x_1 is S_1 and x_2 is S_2 and...and x_p is S_p Then y_1 is T_1 and y_2 is T_2 and...and y_p is T_p. Where S_i and T_i are fuzzy sets that define the partition space. The conclusion of a Mamdani rule is a fuzzy set. It uses the algebraic product and the maximum as Tnorm and S-norm respectively, but there are many variations by using other operators.
    - Takagi/Sugeno rules (Jang et al., 1997): If x_1 is S_1 and x_2 is S_2 and...and x_p is S_p Then $y = b_0 + b_1x_1 + b_2x_2 + \ldots + b_px_p$. In the Sugeno model the conclusion is numerical. The rules aggregation is in fact the weighted sum of rules outputs.
- **DeFuzzification:** The last step of a fuzzy logic system consists in turning the fuzzy variables generated by the fuzzy logic rules into real value again which can then be used to perform some action. There are different defuzzification methods; in our platform decision module we could use Centroid of area (COA), Bisector of area (BOA), Mean of Maximum (MOM), Smallest of Maximum (SOM) and Largest of Maximum (LOM).

5.2 Fuzzy Logic for medical telemonitoring

The first step for developing this approach is the fuzzification of system outputs and inputs obtained from each sensor and subsystem.

From ANASON subsystem three inputs are built. The first one is the sound environment classification; all sound class and expressions detected are labelled on a numerical scale according to their source. Nine membership functions are set up in this numerical scale according to sound sources as it is in Table 1. N other inputs are associated to each SNR calculated on each microphone (N microphones are used in the current application), and these inputs are split into three fuzzy levels: low, medium and high.

RFPAT produce five inputs: heart rate for which three fuzzy levels are specified normal, low and high; activity which has four fuzzy sets: immobile, rest, normal and agitation; posture is represented by two membership functions standing up/setting down and lying; fall and call have also two fuzzy levels: Fall/Call and No Fall/Call. The defined area of each membership function associated to heart rate or activity is adapted to each monitored elderly person.

The time input has five membership functions morning, noon, afternoon, evening and night which are also adapted to patient habits.

Membership Function	Composition
Human Sound	snoring, yawn, sneezing, cough, cry, scream, laught
Speech	key words and expressions
Multimedia Sounds	TV, radio, computer, music
Door sounds	door claping, door knob, key ring
Water sounds	water flushing, water in washbasin, coffee filter
Ring tone	telephone ring, bell door, alarm, alarm clock
Object sound	chair, table, tear-turn paper, step foot
Machine sounds	coffee machine, dishwasher, electrical shaver, microwave, vaccum cleaner, washing machine, air conditioner
Dishwasher	glass vs glass, glass wood, plastic vs plastic, plastic vs wood, spoon vs table

Table 1. Fuzzy sets defined for the ANASON classification input

The output of the fuzzy logic ADL recognition contains some activities and distress situation identification. They are sleeping, getting up, toileting, bathing, washing hands, washing dishes, doing laundry, cleaning, going out of home, enter home, walking, standing up, setting down, laying, resting, watching TV and talking on telephone. These membership functions are ordered, firstly according to the area where they maybe occur and secondly according to the degree of similarity between them.

The next step of the fuzzy logic approach is the fuzzy inference engine which is formulated by a set of fuzzy IF-THEN rules. This second stage uses domain expert knowledge regarding activities to produce a confidence in the occurrence of an activity. Rules allow the recognition of common performances of an activity, as well as the ability to model special cases. A confidence factor is accorded to each rule and in order to aggregate these rules we have the choice between Mamdani or Sugeno approaches available under the fuzzy logic component. After rules aggregation the defuzzification is performed by the centroid of area for the ADL output.

The proposed method was experimentally achieved on a simulated data in order to demonstrate its effectiveness. The first study was devoted to the evaluation of the system by taking into account rules used in this fuzzy inference system. The used strategy consisted in realizing several tests with different combination rules, and based on obtained results one rule is added to the selected set of rules in order to get the missed detection. With this strategy good results are reached for the ADL output (about 97% of good ADL detection).

6. Conclusions

This chapter has presented the usage of the sound environment information in order to detect a distress situation and the data fusion using Fuzzy Logic between sound extracted information and a wearable sensor. All presented system is the basis of the development of a complex companion system (CompanionAble project). The telemonitoring systems using redundant sensors in order to detect distress situation but also to prevent trough a long time analysis represents a solution to the lack of medical staff. These systems do not replace the care givers but represent only a help for them.

7. References

Adlassnig K. P. (1986). Fuzzy set theory in medical diagnosis. *IEEE Transactions On System, Man and Cybernetics*, Vol. 16, No. 2, pp. 260–265.

Bairacharya A.; Gale T.J.; Stack C.R. & Turner P. (2008). 3.5G Based Mobile Remote Monitoring System, *Proceedings of EMBC 2008,* pp. 783-786, doi: 10.1109/IEMBS.2008.4649269, Vancouver, Canada, August 2008

Baldinger J.L.; Boudy J.; Dorizzi B.; Levrey J.; Andreao R.; Perpre C.; Devault F.; Rocaries F. & Lacombe A. (2004). Telesurveillance system for patient at home: The medeville system, *Proceedings of ICCHP 2004,* pp. 400-407, Paris, France, July 2004

Bang S.; Kim M.; Song S.K. & Park S.J. (2008). Toward real time detection of the basic living activity in home using a wearable sensor and smart home sensors, *Proceedings of EMBC 2008,* pp. 5200-5203, doi: 10.1109/IEMBS.2008.4650386, Vancouver, Canada, August 2008

Bellego G. L.; Noury N.; Virone G.; Mousseau M. & Demongeot J. (2006). Measurement and model of the activity of a patient in his hospital suite. *IEEE Transactions on TITB,* Vol. 10, No. 1, pp. 92–99

Binh X.L.; Mascolo M.; Gouin A. & Noury N. (2008). Health Smart Home for elders - A tool for automatic recognition of activities of daily living, *Proceedings of EMBC 2008,* pp 3316-3319, doi: 10.1109/IEMBS.2008.4649914, Vancouver, Canada, August 2008

Burges C. J. C. (1998). A tutorial on SVM for Pattern Recognition. *Data Mining and Knowledge Discovery,* Vol. 2, No. 2, pp. 121–167.

Cowell R.; Dawid A.; Lauritzen S. & Spiegelhalter D. (1999). *Probabilistic Networks and Expert Systems,* Springer, ISBN: 0-387-98767-3, New York.

Cowling M. & Sitte R. (2002). Analysis of speech recognition techniques for use in a non-speech sound recognition system. *Digital Signal Processing for Communication Systems,* Vol. 703, No. 1, pp. 31-46

Dreyfus G.; Martinez J.M.; Samuelides M.; Gordon M.; Badran F.; Thiria S. & Hrault L. (2002). *Réseaux de neurones. Méthodologie et applications,* Eyrolles, ISBN 2-212-11019-7, France.

Fleury A.; Noury N. & Vuillerme N. (2007). A Fast Algorithm to Track Changes of Direction of a Person Using Magnetometers, *Proceedings of IEEE EMBS 2007,* pp. 2311-2314, doi: 10.1109/IEMBS.2007.4352788, Lyon, France, August 2007

Himberg J.; Mantyjarvi J. & Seppanen T. (2001). Recognizing human motion with multiple acceleration sensors, *IEEE Transactions on Systems, Man, and Cybernetics,* Vol. 2, No. 2, pp. 747-52

Istrate D.; Castelli E.; Vacher M.; Besacier L. & Serignat J.F. (2006). Information extraction from sound for medical telemonitoring. *IEEE Transactions on TITB*, Vol. 10, No. 4, pp. 264–274

Istrate D.; Binet M. & Cheng C. (2008). Real Time Sound Analysis for Medical Remote Monitoring, *Proceedings of EMBC 2008*, pp. 4640-4643, doi: 10.1109/IEMBS.2008.4650247, Vancouver, Canada, August 2008

Jang J.-S. R.; Sun C. T. & Mizutani E. (1997). *Neuro-Fuzzy and Soft Computing: A Computational Approach to Learning and Machine Intelligence*, Prentice Hall, ISBN 0132610663, USA

Lacombe A.; Baldinger J.L.; Boudy J.; Dorizzi B.; Levrey J.P.; Andreao R.; Perpere C.; Delavault F.; Rocaries F. & Dietrich C. (2004). Tele-surveillance System for Patient at Home: the MEDIVILLE system, *Lecture Notes in Computer Science*, Springer-Verlag GmbH, Vol. 3118, pp 400-407, June 2004

Lalande A.; Legrand L.; Walker P. M.; Jaulent M. C.; Guy F.; Cottin Y. & Brunotte F. (1997). Automatic detection of cardiac contours on MR images using fuzzy logic and dynamic programming, Proceedings of AMIA'97, pp. 474–478, ISBN 978-3-540-62709-8, Lecture Notes in Artificial Intelligence 1211, Springer-Verlag, Berlin

Lee S.W. & Mase K. (2002). Activity and location recognition using wearable sensors. *IEEE Pervasive Computing*, Vol. 1, No. 3, pp. 24-32

Lima C. S. & Barbosa D. (2008). Automatic segmentation of the second cardiac sound by using wavelets and hidden markov models, *Proceedings of IEEE EMBC 20008*, pp. 334–337, Vancouver, Canada, August 2008

Litvak D.; Zigel Y. & Gannot I. (2008). Fall detection of elderly through floor vibrations and sound, *Proceedings of IEEE EMBC 2008*, pp. 4632–4635, Vancouver, Canada, August 2008

Makikawa M. & Iizumi H. (1995). Development of an ambulatory physical activity monitoring device and its application for categorization of actions in daily life. MEDINFO, pp. 747-750

Marschollek M.; Wolf K.H.; Gietzelt M.; Nemitz G.; Meyer zu Schwabedissen H. & Haux R. (2008). Assessing elderly persons' fall risk using spectral analysis on accelerometric data - a clinical evaluation study, *Proceedings of the EMBC 2008*, pp. 3682-3685, doi: 10.1109/IEMBS.2008.4650008, Vancouver, Canada, August 2008

Mason D.;Linkens D. & Edwards N. (1997). Self-learning fuzzy logic control in medicine, *Proceedings of AIME'97*, pp. 300–303, ISBN 978-3-540-62709-8, Lecture Notes in Artificial Intelligence 1211, Springer-Verlag, Berlin

Medjahed H.; Istrate D.; Boudy J. & Dorizzi B. (2009). A Fuzzy Logic System for Home Elderly People Monitoring (EMUTEM), *Proceedings of Fuzzy Systems 2009*, pp. 69-75, ISBN 978-960-474-066-6, Prague, Czech Republic, Mars 2009

Moncrieff S.; Venkatesh S.; West G. & Greenhill S. (2005). Incorporating contextual audio for an actively anxious smart home, *Proceedings of the Intelligent Sensors, Sensor Networks and Information Processing Conference*, pp. 373-378, ISBN: 0-7803-9399-6, Melbourne, Australia, December 2005

Ng A.K. & Koh T.S. (2008). Using psychoacoustics of snoring sounds to screen for obstructive apnea, *Proceedings of IEEE EMBC 2008*, pp. 1647–1650, Vancouver, Canada, August 2008

Popescu M.; Li Y.; Skubic M. & Rantz M. (2008). An acoustic fall detector system that uses sound height information to reduce the false alarm rate, *Proceedings of IEEE EMBC 2008*, pp. 4628–4631, Vancouver, Canada, August 2008

Stagera M.; Lukowiczb P. & Trostera G. (2007). Power and accuracy tradeoffs in sound-based context recognition systems. *Pervasive and Mobile Computing*, Vol. 3, No. 3, pp. 300–327, ISSN:1574-1192

Virone G.; Istrate D.; Vacher M.; Serignat J.F.; Noury N. & Demongeot J. (2003). First Steps in Data Fusion between a Multichannel Audio Acquisition and an Information System for Home Healthcare, *Proceedings of IEEE Engineering In Medicine And Biology Society Conference*, pp. 1364-1367, doi: 10.1109/IEMBS.2003.1279557, Cancun, Mexique, September 2003

Wolf P.; Schmidt A. & Klein M. (2008). SOPRANO - An extensible, open AAL platform for elderly people based on semantical contracts, Proceedings of 3rd Workshop on Artificial Intelligence Techniques for Ambient Intelligence 2008 (AITAmI'08), pp. 225-228, Patras, Greece

Zahlmann G.; Scherf M. & Wegner A. (1997). A neurofuzzy classifier for a knowledge-based glaucoma monitor, *Proceedings of AIME'97*, pp. 273–284, ISBN 978-3-540-62709-8, Lecture Notes in Artificial Intelligence 1211, Springer-Verlag, Berlin

8. ACKNOWLEDGMENTS

The authors gratefully acknowledge the contribution of European Community's Seventh Framework Program (FP7/2007-2011), CompanionAble Project (grant agreement n. 216487).

---

[i] INSEE. Espérance de vie, taux de mortalité et taux de mortalité infantile dans le monde; Population Reference Bureau of INSEE; 2007; www.insee.fr/fr/themes/tableau.asp?reg_id=98&ref_id=CMPTEF02216; retrieved in November 2008

[ii] C. Duval, M.-L. Bouvet and J. Yacoubovitch. Accidents de la vie courante - Données statistiques. Health Ministry France; 2000; http://www.sante.gouv.fr/htm/pointsur/acc_dom/donnees03.htm#22; retrieved on November 2008

[iii] Le Figaro, Accidents domestiques : les personnes âgées très exposées; October 14, 2007; http://www.lefigaro.fr/france/20070604.FIG000000130_accidents_domestiques_les_personnes_agees_tres_exposees.html; retrieved on November 2008

[iv] TelePat project RNTS 2003-2006, http://www.esiee.fr/~research/documents/Index/Projets/Telepat.html; retrieved on November 2008

[v]DESDHIS, ACI Technologies for health 2002/2004

[vi] http://www.emerge-project.eu/; retrieved on November 2008:

Standard model, file formats and methods in Brain-Computer Interface research: why?

Lucia Rita Quitadamo[1,2], Donatella Mattia[2], Febo Cincotti[2], Fabio Babiloni[3], Gian Carlo Cardarilli[4], Maria Grazia Marciani[1,2] and Luigi Bianchi[1,2,5]
[1]*University of Tor Vergata, Department of Neuroscience*
[2]*Fondazione Santa Lucia, IRCCS, Neuroelectrical Imaging and BCI Laboratory*
[3]*University of La Sapienza, Department of Physiology and Pharmacology*
[4]*University of Tor Vergata, Department of Electronic Engineering*
[5]*University of Tor Vergata, Centro di Biomedicina Spaziale*
[1,2,3,4,5]*Rome, Italy*

1. Introduction

Assistive Technologies (AT) include all the assistive, adaptive and rehabilitation devices that help people with disabilities to interact with the external environment without or with minimal need of care assistant. They have become very wide spread in the last decades as they promote independence for those people that are unable to perform a task, by providing them methods of interacting with the technology needed to accomplish such tasks.
Brain-Computer Interface (BCI) represents a subset of the more general AT; its main purpose is to help disables to communicate by creating a direct channel of interaction between brain and external environment, without the need of muscles or nerves (Wolpaw et al., 2002; Kübler & Neumann, 2005): in fact, people who lost the control on their muscles, after strokes, spinal cord injuries, cerebral palsy, traumas or degenerative diseases (see Amyotrophic Lateral Sclerosis), may lie in the so-called "locked-in" state, that is, they are confined into a body which does not meet their intents and desires anymore, while their cognitive activity is still intact; these people can keep on communicating their thoughts by means of a BCI, which translates their brain signals into output controls that can be commands to select characters on a speller or to pilot a wheelchair or a robotic arm, as well as commands to control a cursor on a screen or a domotic environment and so on.
It is evident that the BCI field is a very complex one, as it deals either with human beings feelings and technology aspects; in fact BCI must involve different research areas such as engineering, informatics, computer science, neurology, neurophysiology, psychology, rehabilitation, that must interact to implement an efficient and user-centric BCI system.
It follows that one of the greatest problem that can be found in BCI research is a difficulty in the communication among the people who are involved in it: in fact, a lot of research labs are interested in BCI all around the world, each of them focusing on some particular aspects of these systems (enhancing the acquisition quality of the signals, improving the communication rate, finding the best algorithms to classify data, choosing the best

peripheral according to the user requirements) and maybe most of them have dealt with the same problems and found different solutions to them, so that a multitude of BCI systems has been implemented to date, which are very different and almost incompatible among each other (Cincotti et al., 2006).

Hence a question arises: is it possible to define a common language for BCI systems that allows all the researches to talk the same language and so to share their knowledge?

This question comes from the necessity of defining **standards** in BCI, that mean a common language for BCI systems and that are fundamental to promote some progresses, such as:

- **Easy data sharing** among different research labs. Today many different file formats are used for storing physiological and BCI data, such as BCI2000 (Schalk et al., 2000), Ascii, GDF (Schlögl, 2006), EDF and EDF+ (Kemp & Olivan, 2003), Matlab, etc, and each of them has its own features. This prevents a practical circulation of data among the different scientific communities and hinders the sharing of knowledge.
- **Unique BCI model.** Different structures and protocols for BCI systems have been implemented to date and, due to the lack of a standard model to describe them, there is often a disagreement even on the names of the basic components which constitute them (for example, *trial, run, session*). This adds some difficulties when different modules of a system have to be exchanged or different systems have to be compared.
- **Reliable comparison among different systems.** Today many different metrics are used to evaluate the performances of a BCI system (bit-rate, Mutual Information, Entropy, characters per second, error rate) and each of them focuses on a different problem (e.g. classifier performance, spelling speed, etc…). This leads to a misunderstanding of the effective behavior of a system and makes it difficult to identify the best one for a specific application.
- **Easy module substitution (SW and HW) without compatibility issues.** Actually each lab has its own systems as regarding recording devices, analysis and optimizing tools, classifiers, etc., which are not compatible each other. This, again, hinders the sharing of tools and results among labs.

In the following paragraphs, some solutions to the problems previously mentioned will be provided; a unique model for BCI systems, a new file format, a metric for evaluating their performances and tools for optimizing them will be illustrated. All these features together contribute to the creation of a standard language for talking about BCI, that is necessary for the dissemination of knowledge, for the sharing of data and results and finally for the standardization and unification of BCI systems.

2. Open file formats in BCI: a XML-based proposal

The problem of data sharing has always been very compelling in the neuroscience research field, and mainly in the BCI one, as exchanging data among different researchers and laboratories can lead to the sharing of results and to the dissemination of resources. Unfortunately, the actual situation is that each lab uses its own file format and still needs to convert other labs' files in its own format if wants to use them, with waste of resources and time.

The solution to this problem could be reached by means of a common file format that is flexible, easily accessible and comprehensible by everyone and suitable for storing information about all possible kinds of physiological signals and BCI-related components.

This would be a great achievement in the BCI field as it would allow to overcome all the obstacles due to the fact that each laboratory has its own file format to save data.
For this reason, open standard file formats have been recently proposed (Bianchi et al., 2007b), which can be accessible and modified by everyone, by adding or removing information, without breaking the backward compatibility. This file format is based on the XML (eXensible Markup Language) technology and then called NeuroPhysiological data in XML (NPX). XML has some important features, such as, *extensibility,* that is, data can be added by everyone without altering the overall structure of the document and without breaking the backward compatibility; *portability,* that is, the user can define new tags and attributes for the objects, without special libraries for reading them; *platform-independence,* that is, the technology can be used with different operating systems without any problem; *data-independence,* that is, the content of a file is kept separate from its presentation, so that one can store the content in an XML file only once and then extract and visualize it in the desired format. All these features have made XML the standard technology for the communication world.
The NPX format was successfully used for the storage of electroencephalography (EEG), magnetoencephalography (MEG), electromyography (EMG), electrocardiography (EKG) and event-related potentials (ERP) data; it supports a virtually unlimited number of sensors, events and montages; data can also be stored in various ways with respect to the accuracy (8, 16, 32, 64 bits) and the internal representation (integer, floating point). Sometimes, if a faster access to data is needed, an XML file can be linked to a binary file: for example, if the amount of sampled data is huge (e.g. an EEG recording) they can be stored in an additional distinct binary file, otherwise (e.g. ERP, spectral data) they can be stored in the XML file itself. In both cases the XML file will contain a complete description of the sensors (dynamics, number of bits, gain, coordinates, etc...), events (type, occurrence, etc...), processing, etc....
The XML technology has been also adopted for the storage of BCI experiments parameters, such as feedback rules for sensory motor protocols, virtual keyboard layout for spellers, classifiers performances, etc. (Quitadamo et al., 2007).
All these features show that an XML-based file format can be a valuable solution for BCI data storage and handling; the necessity of a common file format is compelling if a unification of BCI resources is the ultimate goal that standardization can achieve.

3. A unique functional model: structural and temporal characterization

A further step that is necessary for the standardization of BCI systems is to outline a set of common definitions for all the BCI components, which are embedded in a functional model. A wide-accepted functional model has been fully described in the literature (Mason & Birch, 2003; Bianchi et al., 2007a; Quitadamo et al., 2008) and is depicted in Fig. 1.
In this model the two most important functional blocks are the Transducer and the Control Interface. The Transducer is the only module that deals with physiological signals; it includes, in fact, different sub-modules for the acquisition and processing of brain signals:

- **The Collector,** that is the module which deals with the acquisition of brain signals and is usually constituted by sensors. Different signals have been used to implement a BCI, some of them being recorded with a non-invasive modality such

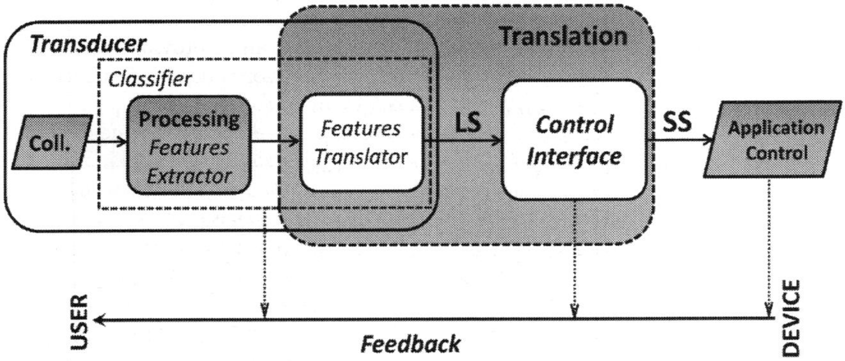

Fig. 1. Functional Model of a BCI system

as, EEG, MEG (Mellinger & al., 2007), functional Magnetic Resonance Imaging (fMRI, Weiskopf et al., 2004; Yoo et al., 2004) and near-infrared spectroscopy (NIRS, Coyle et al., 2007) signals, and some others in an invasive modality, such as electrocorticography (ECoG, Schalk et al. 2008) and intra-electrocortigraphy signals.

For example, in the case of EEG-based BCIs, which are the most diffused ones, scalp signals are recorded by means of a set of electrodes, whose number spans from 2 to 128, according to the application.

- **The Classifier**, that is the module which is devoted to the processing of bioelectrical signals and is formed by the Features Extractor and the Features Translator. The Features Extractor deals with the extraction of some features of interest from brain signals; these features can be manifold, such as P300 (Donchin et al., 2000; Sellers at al., 2006), μ-rhythm (Wolpaw & McFarland, 2004), Slow Cortical Potentials (Kübler et al., 2001), Steady-State Visual Evoked Potentials (Trejo et al., 2006), etc., and lead to the implementation of different BCI protocols. Then these features are linearly or non-linearly combined, by means of the Features Translator, into some Logical Symbols, LSs, which belong to a Logical Alphabet (LA); a LS corresponds to the actual mental task performed by the subject and is usually the result of a classification process. For example, in the fMRI-based protocol implemented by Yoo (Yoo et al., 2004), the subject learnt to control the movement of a cursor through a maze by exploiting four mental tasks: right and left hand motor imagery, mental calculation and mental speech generation. These four tasks have to be recognized by the system, and this corresponds to the generation of a LS (for example, one among the α, β, γ, δ symbols), which has actually no semantic meaning but is useful for the successive translation phase.

The LSs, in fact, are then inputted to the Control Interface which deals with the second stage of translation: in fact, it contains encoders which allow the translation of LSs into Semantic Symbols, SSs, which belong to a Semantic Alphabet (SA) and are meaningful for the Control Interface itself. Some example of SSs are the English Alphabet for a speller application, the items selected into a menu, the directions of the movements of a robotic arm, etc.

SSs are finally mapped into physical controls toward the output application, that can be the movement of a cursor on a screen, a prosthesis, a wheelchair, a speller, and so on.
During the whole duration of a BCI session, some feedback can be provided to the user of the system, that can be a feedback on the classification performances, a feedback on the translation of LSs into SSs or, finally, a feedback from the output peripherals.
As previously mentioned, a lot of different protocols have been implemented in BCI research, according to the features extracted by the brain signals, and different BCI systems have been designed to date, everyone being characterized by different structures and components. However, it has been demonstrated in a recent work (Quitadamo et al., 2008) that a unique standard model is able to describe different BCI systems both from the static point of view and from the dynamic one; in particular, the temporal characterization of different BCI protocols under a unique dynamic scheme is very innovative and meaningful, as it demonstrates that a common basic description can be possible for all them, leading to a standardization of BCI systems.
This is very important for such a complex field as the BCI one, because a unique model avoids that each BCI lab has its own terminology and structures to refer to BCI components, and helps in the process of unification and dissemination of tools and resources among researchers.
The model that has been recently proposed, has been implemented with the Unified Modelling Language (UML) which is a well established visual language for model-driven technologies, which include system development, engineering and architecture. It allows a universal representation of common concepts like classes, components, generalization, aggregation, and behaviors. Also it is very simple to understand, as it makes use of diagrams that even a non-programmer is able to design, modify and reuse. The two most important UML diagrams types that have been used in this model are **class diagrams** and **sequence diagrams.** Class diagrams represent structural correlations among the objects of a system, by means of classes, that are the components of a system, characterized by attributes and methods, that are the operations the class performs. In UML notation classes are represented by means of rectangles divided into compartments, where the name of the class, its attributes and its operations are listed, and connections among classes are represented by means of relationships. Sequence diagrams, instead, describe the temporal relationships occurring between the objects of the system by means of messages running from the sending class to the receiving one.
In this model a clear description of the timing of a trial has been furnished so that the system is characterized not only from the static point of view but from the dynamic one too, that is, the temporal relationships occurring between the objects of the system have been identified. In the following paragraphs some general aspects on the static and dynamic characterizations of the implemented model will be furnished.

3.1 Structure of a trial

The Trial is the main entity of a BCI session, as it leads to the classification of a symbol that can be logical or semantic. For example, in a P300 protocol (Sellers et al., 2006; Krusienski, 2008) a semantic trial leads to the classification of one semantic symbol in a 2D matrix (formed by the English alphabet characters plus the space one and the numbers from 1 to 9); in a μ-rhythm protocol (Wolpaw & McFarland, 2004) a logical trial leads to the selection of a target among those shown on a PC screen. A trial is constituted by a set of processing

quanta (PQs) that are the operations iterated for the update of the internal state of the classifier.
Then four main phases have been identified in a trial, that lead to the classification of a symbol: Preparation, Target Request, Brain Performance and Performance Notification. These four phases are slightly different if the system runs in asking or operating mode; in fact, in asking mode the user of the system is asked to perform a mental task in order to train and test the classifier to recognize his mental states while in operating mode the user communicates what he wants and the system is supposed to be already well-adapted to correctly classify the user intents.
Therefore, in the Preparation phase the system is set to a rest state until the subject is ready to start a BCI experimental session. Then, in the Target Request phase, only possible if the system runs in asking mode, the subject is requested to perform a mental task.
In the Brain Performance phase the subject generates a symbol as a consequence of a specific mental task; his mental states are then classified in order to generate a LS or a SS and he can be provided with a feedback for the adjustments on the performances. The result of the classification is finally communicated to the subject in the Performance Notification phase. At the end of the last phase a rest period can occur.
In Fig. 2 a schematic representation of a trial in a μ-rhythm protocol is reported: in asking mode, after the warning message at the end of the preparation phase, the subject is notified with the request of the mental task. In this example he has to select the middle target among those represented on the monitor; the reaching of the desired target on the screen corresponds to the generation of a LS. In the Brain Performance phase he does his mental task to reach the target and, at the end of each PQ, the classifier updates its internal state. A symbol is generated at the end of this phase and the result is notified to the subject in the Performance Notification. In operating mode, during which there is not a Target Request phase, after the warning, the subject performs mental tasks to select the bottom target among those available.

3.2 Actors of the system

Four main actors have been defined which attend to the correct execution of a trial and that in the UML notation are identified by classes: the Session Manager, the Transducer, the Control Interface and the Feedback Manager.
The Session Manager is active for the whole duration of the BCI experimental session and, in particular, it manages the trial execution by invoking methods on all the other actors.
The Transducer is constituted by the collector and the classifier (Features Extractor and Features Translator) so it acquires the physiological signals and attends to their translation into LSs.
The Control Interface encodes sequences of LSs into SSs and stores the classification performances history. It would be noteworthy to avoid direct dependence relationship between the transducer and the control interface in order to realize a better software modularization.
The Feedback Manager handles both the feedback in the Brain Performance phase (for example, after getting the results of the analysis performed by the Transducer on the physiological signals, it updates the position of a cursor on the screen) and the feedback to the system's user, by notifying special signals and events, and in general manages all the features regarding the direct interface with the subject.

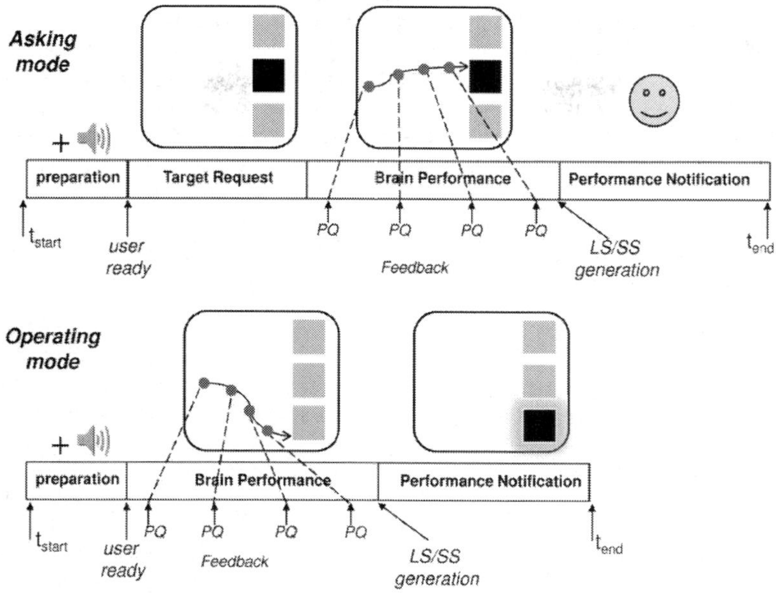

Fig. 2. Structure of a trial

In Fig. 3 a class diagram of the four actors is reported. Dotted arrows denote dependency relationships between actors; black diamonds are for composition relationships, as for the transducer class which is composed by the classifier and the collector module.

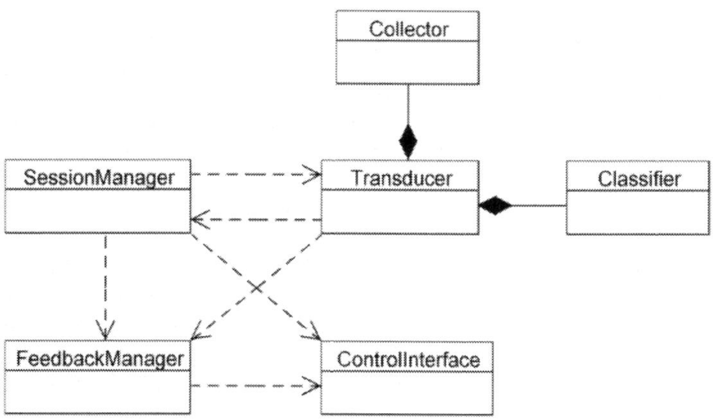

Fig. 3. Class diagram of the actors

3.3 Timing of a trial

Up to now static features of the model have been described. However a static characterization of BCI systems is not sufficient if, for example, an easy substitution of hardware and software modules is desirable; in fact, the temporal sequence of operations tells when and in which manner two different objects of the system communicate each other and if this communication is not standardized, how can different modules be interchanged?
For this reasons, the timing of a trial is the most important novelty that the model proposed in (Quitadamo et al., 2008) can add to those already presented in the literature: the identification of the flux of operations that characterize a typical BCI trial is fundamental for the demonstration that a unique model is able to describe different protocols.
Also, by means of this model, it is possible to define unique interfaces that allow to freely substitute a module with another one: Lab 1 could use Lab 2's classifier without any effort, or an EEG manufacture could simply provide a driver so that the system can freely be changed according to the specific requirements.
Note that here it will be illustrated a simplified version of the whole model that has been fully described in (Quitadamo et al., 2008): so the reader can refer to the cited article for a more detailed description of the model and for having an idea on how it can be easily used to explain five BCI protocols (P300, SCP, μ-rhythms, SSVEP, fMRI).
The timing of the trial has been UML-modeled by means of a sequence diagram (Fig. 4) in which the four actors previously mentioned communicate by means of messages. From the diagram it is possible to follow the temporal evolution of the different phases of the trial and the way each actor acts during them.
The Session Manager resets the internal clock of the system after receiving a message from the outside which invokes the starting of a trial (*StartTrial()*). In asking mode (*opt,* optional operations), the Session Manager notifies the asked symbol (the logical mental task to perform, the SS to select) to the Control Interface, which manages the encoding strategies, and to the Feedback Manager (*setAskedSymbol()*), which is responsible of the communication of the symbol to the subject. Then it communicates the starting of the trial to all the other actors which eventually get ready (*onTrialBegin()*). The Feedback Manager notifies to the subject that the active phase is going to start (for example by means of a sound, a fixation cross, etc.) and which task he is asked to perform (*onRequestNotify()*). Then the processing phase begins (*onProcessingBegin()*), with a loop of operations in which the Session Manager scans the starts of the PQs to the Transducer (*onPQBegin()*), which on its turn communicates the starts and the ends of the PQs to the Feedback Manager (*onPQBegin(), onPQEnd()*); the Feedback Manager gets the analysis results (*getAnalysisResult()*) and updates the feedback if necessary (for example, it updates the position of a cursor on a screen).
When the classification of a symbol is reached, that is the Classifier is able to give a result (*alt* fragment indicates an alternative), or the time established for it has elapsed (the internal clock of the system interrupts the classification and the Classifier abstains from giving a result), the trial ends (*EndTrial()*); the Transducer communicates the classification result to the Session Manager which communicates it to all the remaining actors (*onClassificationReached()*). Finally the Feedback Manager notifies the overall performance to the subject (*onPerformanceNotify()*) and the trial definitively ends.
It is important to underline that all the protocols previously mentioned have successfully been described with this unique temporal structure and this can be considered a preliminary step towards the unification of BCI systems.

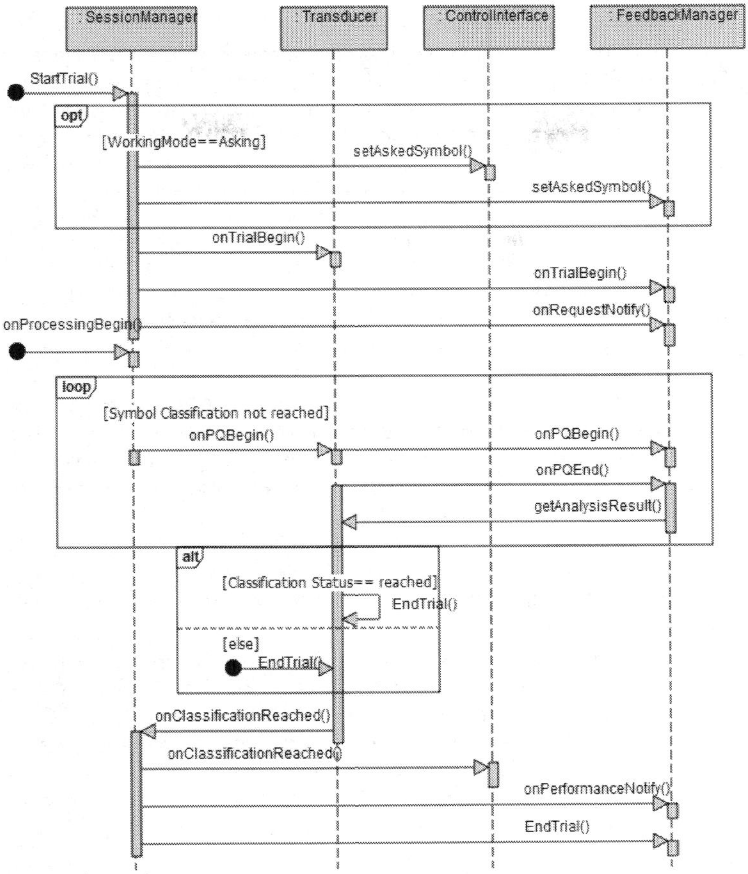

Fig. 4. Timing of a trial

4. A new performance indicator: the Efficiency

The evaluation of the performances of BCI systems is a capital item in BCI research. Different metrics have been proposed to date, such as Bit-Rate, Error-Rate and Mutual Information (Schlögl et al., 2003; Wolpaw, 2002), but all of them are somehow incomplete in characterizing a real-world application, as they do not take into account, for example, errors consequences and strategies to correct them. In particular, errors consequences strictly depend upon the final application that the BCI is intended to pilot: if the subject is communicating by means of a P300 speller, an error into communication is something that involves simply the selection of an UNDO command and a new mental task to reselect the desired character; in these cases errors do not affect severely system performances. However, if the BCI is piloting a wheelchair, an error in the detection of the exact intents of the subject can lead to situations that could be dangerous for the subject himself. These last

are particular cases in which errors weight a lot in the evaluation of the system performances and it is preferable that the classifier abstains from classification unless the certainty on it is maximal.
For all these reasons, a new metric has been proposed which evaluates the performances of a system as a function of the performances of both the Transducer and the Control Interface (Bianchi et al., 2007). This metric is strictly correlated to the functional model described in the previous section and gives some costs to the errors in the communication, so that a more reliable evaluation of systems is achievable.

4.1 Describing the Transducer performances: the Extended Confusion Matrix

The Extended Confusion Matrix (ECM) evaluates the performances of a transducer, that is, it stores the results of the classifications of the mental tasks performed by the subject. In facts it represents on the rows the LSs to be classified and on the columns the LSs actually classified; the last column of the matrix represents the cases in which the classifier was not able to classify and so abstained from decisions (*abstaining classifiers*). Abstentions are really important in such kinds of application which must be as much safe as possible. Then the elements of the principal diagonal are the correct classifications, while the remaining non-diagonal elements constitute the wrong ones.
As an example, suppose that the mental tasks that the subject is required to perform are associated to a logical alphabet of four logical symbols, α, β, γ, δ.
An example of ECM is now reported:

$$ECM = \begin{array}{c|c|c|c|c|c} & \alpha & \beta & \gamma & \delta & abst \\ \hline \alpha & 84 & 8 & 0 & 8 & 0 \\ \hline \beta & 4 & 96 & 0 & 0 & 0 \\ \hline \gamma & 12 & 0 & 80 & 8 & 0 \\ \hline \delta & 12 & 4 & 12 & 72 & 0 \end{array} \quad (1)$$

As it can be seen from (1), most of the classification errors are associated to the generation of the fourth symbol δ; this is of great importance in the choice of the encoding strategy to implement, as selecting an encoding which minimizes the occurrence of the δ symbol will result in the minimization of the errors and this can represent an optimization strategy.
From an ECM, a Misclassification Probability Matrix (MPM) can be defined in the following way (N_{LA} is the length of the logical alphabet) (eq. 2-5):

$$MPM[i,j] = \frac{ECM[i,j]}{n_i}, i \neq j \quad (2)$$

$$MPM[i,j] = 0, i = j \quad (3)$$

$$n_i = \sum_{j=1}^{N_{LA}+1} ECM[i,j] \tag{4}$$

$$MPM = \begin{array}{c|c|c|c|c|c} & \alpha & \beta & \gamma & \delta & abst \\ \hline \alpha & 0 & 0.08 & 0 & 0.08 & 0 \\ \hline \beta & 0.04 & 0 & 0 & 0 & 0 \\ \hline \gamma & 0.12 & 0 & 0 & 0.08 & 0 \\ \hline \delta & 0.12 & 0.04 & 0.12 & 0 & 0 \end{array} \tag{5}$$

and an Extended Overtime Matrix (EOM) is defined as in (6):

$$EOM = \begin{array}{c|c|c|c|c|c} & \alpha & \beta & \gamma & \delta & abst \\ \hline \alpha & 0 & 2 & 2 & 2 & 1 \\ \hline \beta & 2 & 0 & 2 & 2 & 1 \\ \hline \gamma & 2 & 2 & 0 & 2 & 1 \\ \hline \delta & 2 & 2 & 2 & 0 & 1 \end{array} \tag{6}$$

The MPM represents the probabilities concerning incorrect classifications and EOM represents the "costs" associated to errors and indeterminateness cases and which depend on the Control Interface error correction strategy. In the example in (6), a cost of "0" means that no error was done during the selection of the LS; a cost of "1" is associated to indeterminate cases and means that, when a classifier abstains from a decision, only a reselection of the correct LS is needed; finally a cost of "2" means that, after an error, one has to perform two additional steps to correct the error, that is, one to delete the wrong LS and one to reselect the right one. However, different correction strategies can be implemented, which can be somehow smart; for example they can take into account some thresholds for the decision of the correct symbol to be classified so reducing the cost associated to some errors. The strategies therefore are characteristic of the Control Interface and can be manifold according to the requirements of the system itself.

4.2 Measuring error consequences: Super Tax Vector

When a misclassification or an abstention occur the loss of information can be quantified with the Super Tax Vector, whose i-*th* element is given by:

$$ST(i) = \sum_{j=1}^{N_{LA}+1} MPM[i,j] \cdot EOM[i,j] \tag{7}$$

$$ST = \begin{bmatrix} 0.32 \\ 0.08 \\ 0.40 \\ 0.56 \end{bmatrix} \qquad (8)$$

where each element of ST represents the fraction of additional selections that are necessary to correct a mistake. In (8), the (7) has been applied to our example.

One can easily see that the generation of the fourth symbol appears to be the most difficult, as already pointed out. In fact, the ST value associated to it is the highest one.

The elements of the ST vector (ST(i)) represent the additional selections that must be done to recover an error; however, these additional selections are not error-free, as they imply a classification too, and the classification process implies misclassifications on its turn. Misclassifications lead to the same ST(i) elements, so that $ST(i)^2$ new selections are needed, that are on their turn subject to misclassification.

The geometric series can be recognized in (9):

$$\sum_k ST(i)^k = 1 + ST(i) + ST(i)^2 + ST(i)^3 + \dots \qquad (9)$$

which converges to (10):

$$\sum_k ST(i)^k = \frac{1}{1 - ST(i)}, \text{ if } |ST(i)| < 1 \qquad (10)$$

Finally, the Expected mean Selection Cost (ESC), that is the number of classifications required to generate a correct LS, is defined as in (11):

$$\overline{ESC} = \sum_{j=1}^{N_{LA}} \frac{p_{occ}(i)}{1 - ST(i)} \qquad (11)$$

where $p_{occ}(i)$ is the probability of the ith LS to occur.

If N_{SA} is the length of the SA, $p_{SS}(n)$ is the probability of the nth SS to occur and $l(n)$ is the number of LSs used for the encoding, then the mean codeword length can be defined as in (12):

$$\overline{L_{CW}} = \sum_{j=1}^{N_{LA}} p_{ss}(n) \cdot l(n) \qquad (12)$$

An example of an encoding map between LA and SA (the English Alphabet plus the space character) is given in Table 1. Note that the symbol δ is used as an UNDO key. Choosing different encodings (e.g. variable length encodings), L_{CW} can be reduced, leading to a compression of the message.

CHAR	E	CHAR	E	CHAR	E
A	ααα	J	βαα	S	γαα
B	ααβ	K	βαβ	T	γαβ
C	ααγ	L	βαγ	U	γαγ
D	αβα	M	ββα	V	γβα
E	αββ	N	βββ	W	γββ
F	αβγ	O	ββγ	X	γβγ
G	αγα	P	βγα	Y	γγα
H	αγβ	Q	βγβ	Z	γγβ
I	αγγ	R	βγγ	Sp	γγγ

Table 1. Example of an encoding map between SA and LA.

Finally the Efficiency (*Eff*) of a system is defined as in (13):

$$Eff = \frac{1}{\overline{L_{CW}} \cdot \overline{ESC}} \tag{13}$$

It is easy to see that the *Eff* of a system depends on both the Transducer (L_{CW}, ECM and MPM) and the Control Interface (EOM) even if they have been separately implemented; so the choice of the best BCI system to adapt to the user requirements can be performed only after the evaluation of the best Transducer-Control Interface combination.
It has been demonstrated in (Bianchi et al., 2007) that Efficiency is a better indicator of the performances of a BCI system than Mutual Information in a copy-spelling task.

5. Optimizing BCI systems: BF++Toys

The metric and the file format defined in the previous paragraphs allowed the implementation of a set of tools dedicated to the simulation of BCI systems and to the prediction of the their performances (Quitadamo, 2007). They were called BF++Toys because they are included in the Body Language Framework (Bianchi et al., 2003) and have been developed in C++. Their main feature is the open-source nature that makes it possible for everyone to modify and adjust them according to the need of his system. They can be downloaded at www.brainterface.com.
BF++ Toys deal with logical and semantic alphabets, encoders, confusion matrices, errors correction strategies and are actually formed by four main applications:

- the ECM generator, which can simulate different transducers with different errors and abstentions distributions and finally create new ECMs;
- the Encoding Generator, which can create new encoders by using a LA and a SA;
- the Simulator, which, given an ECM and an encoding, can generate realistic sequences of LSs in copy spelling task;

- the Optimizers, which can find the best combination of Transducers and Control Interfaces on the basis of the metric described in the previous paragraphs.

The most important thing that has to be underlined here, is that BF++ Toys were a direct derivation of the XML file format and the BCI definitions previously illustrated; this means that they can be used to optimize whatever BCI system independently from the protocol to be implemented (P300, μ-rhythms, etc.) or from the final application, as they entirely respect the described standards.

Finally, the possibility to simulate different BCI systems and to find the solution with the highest efficiency is very valuable as it can help in the choice of the system that best fits to the users' requirements.

6. Conclusions

The necessity of standards in the research is effective as they can enhance the dissemination of data and information among all the groups that are interested in it or want to cooperate. The main goal of standards is to harmonize the resources available in a particular research field and create a common language for defining its components, that anyone can refer to, by avoiding confusion or misunderstandings due to different semantics.

This necessity is compelling mostly in the BCI research field, where a lot of systems, protocols, frameworks, file formats, have been established to date, lacking a concrete collaboration among different groups and so leading to a concrete difficulty when data have to be exchanged, different systems have to be evaluated and compared, different hardware and software modules have to be substituted, etc.

Standards in BCI can be defined on three different main levels: file formats, functional model and methods. These three levels are strictly interconnected and functional to each other: in fact, while a common file format is essential for an easy storage and exchange of all the data related to BCI, a functional model with standard definitions allow to use a common language to talk about BCI and so makes the dissemination of BCI-related resources much easier. Finally, common methods for evaluating the performances of systems allow the comparison of different systems and so the choice of the most suitable system for the final application.

In conclusion all the three levels together lead to common shared tools whose ultimate aim is to build systems that definitively fit to the patients' residual skills and requirements and from which they can derive real benefits to improve the quality of their lives.

7. Acknowledgments

This work is partially supported by the European ICT Programme Project FP7-224631 and by the DCMC Project of the Italian Space Agency. This paper only reflects the authors' views and funding agencies are not liable for any use that may be made of the information contained herein.

8. References

Bianchi, L.; Babiloni, F.; Cincotti, F.; Salinari, S. & Marciani, M. G. (2003). Introducing BF++: A C++ Framework for Cognitive Bio-Feedback Systems Design. *Methods of Information in Medicine,* Vol. 42, No. 1, (July 2003) 104-110, 0026-1270.

Bianchi, L.; Quitadamo, L. R.; Garreffa, G.; Cardarilli, G. C. & Marciani, M. G. (2007a). Performances evaluation and optimization of brain computer interface systems in a copy spelling task. *IEEE Transactions on Neural Systems and Rehabilitation Engineering,* Vol. 15, No. 2, (June 2007) 207-16, 1534-4320.

Bianchi, L.; Quitadamo, L. R.; Marciani, M. G.; Maraviglia, B.; Abbafati, M. & Garreffa, G. (2007b). How the NPX data format handles EEG data acquired simultaneously with fMRI. *Magnetic Resonance Imaging,* Vol. 25, No. 6, (July 2007) 1011-4, 0730-725X.

Cincotti, F.; Bianchi, L.; Birch, G.; Guger, C.; Mellinger, J.; Scherer, R.; Schmidt, R. N.; Yáñez Suárez, O. & Schalk, G. (2006). BCI meeting 2005--workshop on technology: hardware and software. *IEEE Transactions on Neural Systems and Rehabilitation Engineering,* Vol. 14, No. 2 (June 2006) 128-31, 1534-4320.

Coyle, S. M.; Ward, T. E. & Markham, C. M. (2007). Brain-computer interface using a simplified functional near-infrared spectroscopy system. *Journal of Neural Engineering,* Vol. 4, No. 3, (September 2007) 219-26, 1741-2560.

Donchin, E.; Spencer, K. M. & Wijesinghe, R. (2000). The Mental Prosthesis: Assessing the Speed of a P300-Based Brain-Computer Interface. *IEEE Transactions on Rehabilitation Engineering,* Vol. 8, No. 2, (June 2000) 174-179, 1063-6528.

Kemp, B. & Olivan, J. (2003). European data format 'plus' (EDF+), an EDF alike standard format for the exchange of physiological data. *Clinical Neurophysiology,* Vol. 114, No. 9, (September 2003) 1755-1761, 1388-2457.

Krusienski, D. J.; Sellers, E. W.; McFarland, D. J.; Vaughan, T. M. & Wolpaw, J. R. (2008). Toward enhanced P300 speller performance. *Journal of Neuroscience Methods,* Vol. 167, No. 1, (January 2008) 15-21, 0165-0270.

Kübler, A. & Neumann, N. (2005). Brain-computer interfaces-the key for the conscious brain locked into a paralyzed body. *Progress in Brain Research,* Vol. 150, (2005) 513-25, 0079-6123.

Mason, S. G. & Birch, G. E. (2003). A general framework for brain-computer interface design. *IEEE Transactions on Neural Systems and Rehabilitation Engineering,* Vol. 11, No. 1, (March 2003) 70-85, 1534-4320.

Mellinger, J.; Schalk, G.; Braun, C.; Preissl, H.; Rosenstiel, W.; Birbaumer, N. & Kübler, A. (2007). An MEG-based brain-computer interface (BCI). *NeuroImage,* Vol. 36, No. 3, (July 2007) 581-93, 1053-8119.

Quitadamo, L. R.; Marciani, M. G.; Cardarilli, G. C. & Bianchi, L. (2008). Describing different brain computer interface systems through a unique model: a UML implementation. *Neuroinformatics,* Vol. 6, No. 2, (June 2008) 81-96, 1559-0089.

Quitadamo, L. R; Marciani, M. G & Bianchi, L. (2007). Optimization of Brain Computer Interface systems by means of XML and BF++ Toys. *International Journal of Bioelectromagnetism,* Vol. 9, No. 3, (December 2007) 172-184.

Schalk, G.; McFarland, D. J.; Hinterberger, T.; Birbaumer, N. and Wolpaw, J. R. (2000) BCI2000: a general-purpose brain-computer interface (BCI) system. *IEEE Transactions on Biomedical Engineering,* Vol. 51, No. 6, (June 2000) 1034-43, 0018-9294.

Schalk, G.; Miller, K. J.; Anderson, N. R.; Wilson, J. A.; Smyth, M. D.; Ojemann, J. G.; Moran, D. W.; Wolpaw, J. R. & Leuthardt, E. C. (2008). Two-dimensional movement control using electrocorticographic signals in humans. *Journal of Neural Engineering,* Vol. 5, No. 1, (March 2008) 75-84, 1741-2560.

Schlögl, A. (2006) GDF - A general dataformat for BIOSIGNALS. *cs/0608052* (Aug 2006), available at http://arxiv.org/abs/cs/0608052.

Schlögl, A.; Keinrath, C.; Scherer, R. & Pfurtscheller G. (2003). Information transfer of an EEG-based brain computer interface, *Proceedings of the 1st International IEEE EMBS Conference on Neural Engineering,* pp. 641-644, Capri Island, Italy, March 20-22, 2003.

Sellers, E. W.; Krusienski, D. J.; McFarland, D. J.; Vaughan, T. M. & Wolpaw, J. R. (2006). A P300 event-related potential brain-computer interface (BCI): the effects of matrix size and inter stimulus interval on performance. *Biological Psychology,* Vol. 73, No. 3, (October 2006) 242-52, 0301-0511.

Weiskopf, N.; Mathiak, K.; Bock, S. W.; Scharnowski, F.; Veit, R.; Grodd, W.; Goebel, R. & Birbaumer, N. (2004). Principles of a brain-computer interface (BCI) based on real-time functional magnetic resonance imaging (fMRI). *IEEE Transactions on Bio-Medical Engineering,* Vol. 51, No. 6, (June 2004) 966-70, 0018-9294.

Wolpaw, J. R. & McFarland, D. (2004). Control of a two-dimensional movement signal by a non invasive brain-computer interface in humans. *Proc. Natl. Acad. Sci,* Vol. 101, No. 51, (December 2004) 17849-17854, 0027-8424.

Wolpaw, J. R.; Birbaumer, N.; McFarland, D. J.; Pfurtscheller, G. & Vaughan, T. M. (2002). Brain-computer interfaces for communication and control. *Clinical Neurophysiology,* Vol. 113, No. 6, (June 2002) 767-91, 1388-2457.

Yoo, S. S; Fairneny, T.; Chen, N. K; Choo, S. E.; Panych, L. P.; Park, H.; Lee, S. Y. & Jolesz, F. A. (2004). Brain-computer interface using fMRI: spatial navigation by thoughts. *Neuroreport,* Vol. 15, No. 10, (July 2004) 1591-5, 0959-4965.

30

Tonometric Vascular Function Assessment

Jeon Lee[1] and Ki Chang Nam[2]
[1]*Daegu Haany University*
[2]*Korea Electrotechnology Research Institute*
South Korea

1. Introduction

Recently, the number of patients suffered from cardiovascular disease has increased world-widely. Thus, the importance on vascular function assessment has been emphasized and many researchers have tried to develop some non-invasive but effective method for vascular function assessment. If the assessment methods are divided into two, theses are methods based on blood pressure and based on arterial stiffness respectively.

As well known, the cardiovascular risk found to be related to the levels of mean blood pressure (MBP), systolic blood pressure (SBP) and diastolic blood pressure (DBP). And, these three blood pressures were found to be strong determinants of the risks to the brain, heart and kidney. Additionally, in a cross-sectional analysis, the pulse pressure (PP) was shown to be independently related to the degree of cardiac hypertrophy and to be a good predictor of myocardial infarction (MI) (Darne et al., 1989). In the last few years, these parameters of central blood pressure have been verified to more strongly relate to cardiovascular disease than those of brachial blood pressure (Roman et al., 2007).

Meanwhile, arteries store part of the stroke volume during systolic period and drain it during diastolic period. This so called "Windkessel function" thus transforms the pulsatile flow of central arteries into the steady flow required in the peripheral tissues. Under normal condition, approximately 40% of stroke volume is forwarded directly to peripheral tissues during systole and the remainder (60%) is stored in the capacitive arteries. In diastole, the stored blood is squeezed forward into the peripheral circulation (Gerard & Alain, 1999). Increased arterial stiffness causes dysfunction of this function, increasing the incidence of fracture, rupture, and aneurysm formation in arteries and, potentially, the development of atherosclerosis. So, in recent years, great emphasis has been placed on the role of arterial stiffness in the development of cardiovascular diseases.

Even there have been several methods for the assessment of arterial stiffness, two non-invasive methods with PWV (pulse wave velocity) and with AIx (augmentation index) are most widely studied these days. The former is based on the fact that, between two local positions, the pulse wave travels faster for increased arterial stiffness and the latter based on the fact that the reflected pulse wave comes back earlier so to cause the augmentation of systolic pressure. Both PWV and AIx can be calculated by analyzing pulse wave measured with tonometric sensors but, through AIx, the estimation of arterial stiffness has more controversial and challenging issues.

So, in this chapter, the assessment of arterial function with AIx computed from pulse wave measured by tonometric sensors will be dealt. This chapter is composed of brief introduction, outline of arterial tonometry with operation principle, mathematical model and reliable measurement procedure, explanation on arterial stiffness estimation method, introduction of emerging issues arising in this field and conclusion. While we deal with contents mentioned above, we want to share our recent works in between.

2. Arterial tonometry

In the early 1960, applanation tonometry was first implemented by Pressman and Newgard and was shown to be able to measure the pulse wave of a superficial artery non-invasively, so called as 'arterial tonometry' (Pressman & Newgard, 1963). While the sphygmomanometer measures only systolic and diastolic pressure, it provides continuous pulse waveform with pressure sensor placed over a superficial artery. In this section, the operation principle and mathematical model of arterial tonometry are explained to increase the understanding of tonometric measurement.

2.1 Operation principle

The operation principles of arterial tonometry are similar to those of ocular tonometry. But, in arterial tonometry, a rigid structure as like bone is required to support the arterial vessel unlike ocular tonometry. Therefore, the method has been applied mainly to the radial arteries. In Fig. 1, a simplified arterial tonometry principle is shown.

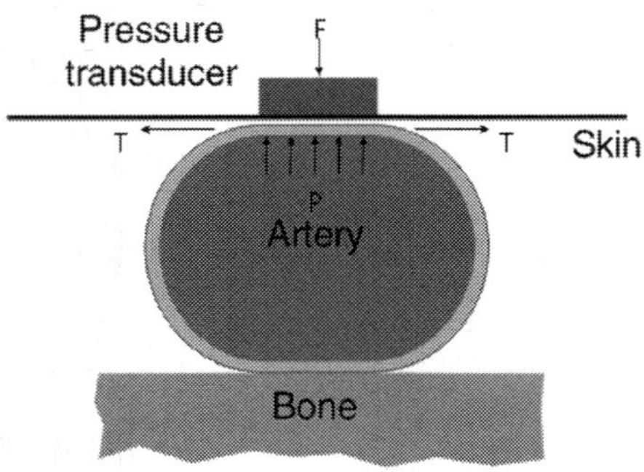

Fig. 1. Arterial tonometry principle

P represents the blood pressure in superficial artery and *F* is the force measured by tonometer transducer. When a pressure transducer is placed over the artery and appropriate pressure is applied so as to partially flatten the artery, the tension vector, *T*, is perpendicular to the pressure vector. Therefore the force, *F*, is independent of *T* and the sensor receives only internal arterial pressure. In practice, to obtain an accurate measurement, several conditions should be satisfied (Eckerle, 2006):

- The artery is supported by rigid structure as like radius.
- The hold-down force flattens a portion of the artery wall, but does not occlude the artery.

- The thickness of the skin over the artery is insignificant, compared to the artery diameter.
- The artery wall behaves essentially like an ideal membrane.
- The artery rider, a force transmission structure to a transducer, is smaller than the flattened area of the artery, and it is centered over the flattened area.
- The spring constant of the force transducer is larger than the effective spring constant of the artery.

2.2 Mathematical model

Deeper insights of arertial tonometry principle can be given by a realistic mathematical model. The first reasonable but simple model for an arterial tonometer was developed by Pressman and Newgard, and consisted of lumped linear elastic elements which represented those the artery, the adjacent tissue, the skin, the tonometer sensor element, and sensor's mounting (Pressman & Newgard, 1963). Although this model provided the relationships among inter-arterial pressure, displacement of sensor frame, and sensor system positioning force, this lumped model was not suitable to analyze remaining problems.

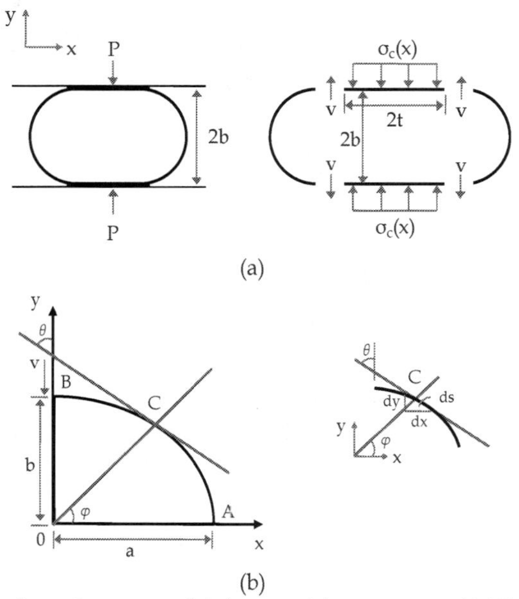

Fig. 2. Cross-sectional continuous model for arterial tonometry. (a) The deflection shape such that the vessel wall consist of free and surface constrained sections. (b) A quadrant of the original cross-section deflected by shear force v=1/2P (Drzewiecki et al., 1983)

So, a mathematical model, which treats the artery and tonometer as solid mechanical structures, was developed and it dealt with the bending and shear deformation neglected in the lumped model (Drzewiecki et al., 1983). In this model shown in Fig. 2, the artery was regarded as a thin cylindrial shell positioned between two rigid and parallel planes; that is, tonometer and underlying bone. The undeformed radius of the artery is r and the distance between the planes is $2b$.

While hold-down pressure increases, arterial wall is deformed and the distance of planes decreases. And, the total external force and the length of contact can be formulated as a function of the distance b. The solution for the end shear force, V, and half length of flattened section, t, can be written as a function of planes separation, b,

$$V(b) = (0.7157/b^2)EI \tag{1}$$

$$t(b) = \frac{\pi}{2}(r - \frac{b}{0.7185}) \tag{2}$$

where E and I represent the Young's modulus and the moment of inertia of the artery, respectively.

If the dimensions and forces acting on the ends of the flattened wall segment are known, the contact stress σ_c can be calculated. When the segment of artery has changed shape from cicular to straight, the flexure equation can ben written as a difference in curvature as equation (3).

$$\frac{1}{r_1} - \frac{1}{r} = \frac{-M}{EI} + \frac{\alpha}{AG}\frac{dV}{dx} \tag{3}$$

where r = initial radius; r_1 = radius after distortion; M = applied bending moment; I = moment of inertia for flattened wall cross-section; α = a geometric constant, 1.5; A= cross-sectional area of flattened wall; G = shear modulus of arterial wall, $E/2(1+\upsilon)$; υ = Poisson's ratio.

Then, considering the balance of shear forces and bending moments in a radial plane of the vessel wall, $dM/dx-V=0$ is given and let $\beta^2=AG/\alpha EI$, equation (3) can be modified as

$$\frac{d^2M}{dx^2} - \beta^2 M = -\frac{\beta^2 EI}{r} \tag{4}$$

Then, $M(x)$'s general solution can be expressed,

$$M(x) = C_1 e^{\beta x} + C_2 e^{-\beta x} + \frac{EI}{r} \tag{5}$$

As $V(x)$ can be obtained by the differential of $M(x)$, the constants C_1 and C_2 are dtermined from the shear foce relations,

$$V(x) = C_1 \beta e^{\beta x} - C_2 e^{-\beta x} \tag{6}$$

Considering the contact force per unit length $q(x)$ and substitition $q(x)=dV/dx=0$ with contact stress defined as $\sigma_c(x)=-q(x)/\Delta L$, then, the relationship between contact stress and deformed distance is given,

$$\sigma_c = V(b)\beta \frac{\cosh \beta x}{\sinh \beta t} \tag{7}$$

In Fig. 3, the computed contact stress distribution along the flattened vessel wall is plotted. In this computation, the radial artery is supposed to be isotropic and geometric and material values are summarized below (Westerhof et al., 1969):

$E = 8 * 10^6$ dynes/cm^2
$G = 2.67 * 10^6$ dynes/cm^2
$\upsilon = 0.5$
$r = 0.172$ cm
$h = 0.043$ cm.

The computed contact stress, $\sigma_c(x)$ is plotted as function of x and x=0 corresponds to a point directly over the axis of the vessel. Each percentile number of curves represents a ratio of given deflection, y to initial radius, r. From the results, we can gain much insights of the relationships between the degree of deflection and contact stress distribution. In detail, as the degree of deflection increases, the contact length between pressure transducer system and arterial wall increases so to be almost 0.10cm (-0.05~0.05cm) at the deflection of 70%. And, we can also know that, at 30% deflection, the larger deformational stress are needed than that at the other degrees of deflection shown in Fig. 3 and the minimum contact stress under a contact section is in inverse proportion to the degree of deflection.
Consequently, with this mathematical model, not only the operation principle can be explained thoroughly but also it is expected to help set up a proper measuring process and design a reliable sensor system.

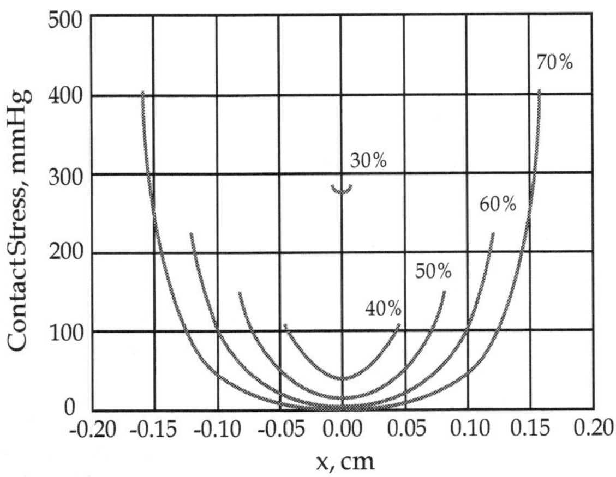

Fig. 3. Computed contact stress distribution for given deflection in the y direction (Drzewiecki et al., 1983)

2.3 Reliable measurement

The arterial tonometry is easy and useful non-invasive measurement technique but is susceptible to wrong measurement. To deal with this problem, the subject's variation caused by physiological and psychological variations, movements, and so on during the measurement should be minimized first and, then, the several conditions mentioned in section 2.1 should be satisfied. An overriding factor, the subject's variation, can be suppressed by following the standardized measurement conditions as listed in Table 1 (Van Bortel et al., 2002). For example, some radial and aortic pulse parameters, such as time to 1st and 2nd peak at radial artery, ejection duration, augmentation index, heart rate etc., were significantly different between upright position and supine position (Nam, 2009).

Confounding factor	In practice
Room temperature	Controlled environment kept at 22±1°C
Rest	At least 10 min in recumbent position
Time of the day	Similar time of the day for repeated measurements
Smoking, eating	Subjects have to refrain, for at least 3h before measurements, particularly from drinking beverages containing caffeine
Alcohol	Refrain from drinking alcohol 10h before measurements
Speaking, sleeping	Subjects may neither speak nor sleep during measurements
Positions	Supine position is preferred. Position (supine, sitting) should be mentioned
White coat effect	Influence on blood pressure and pressure dependent stiffness
Cardiac arrhythmia	Be aware of possible disturbance

Table 1. Recommendations for standardization of subject conditions

A major practical problem is how to make the sensor centered on the artery. Actually, reliable measurements can be obtained only after painstaking adjustment of the sensor location (Kelly et al., 1989). To solve this problem, multi-element sensors, which consist of multi-force transducers and arterial riders at the end of each transducer, have been developed (Terry et al., 1990). The array needs to be positioned with enough precision so that one or more elements of the array are centered over the artery and they can be identified by comparing the measured pressure values at each element. The first step to identify the center positioned element is to examine the measured pulse amplitudes, that is, differences between the maximum and the minimum of a pulse waveform. If an element is precisely centered over the artery, this element will get the largest amplitude. However, it is not sufficient to determine the centered element so that second step is followed. In the second step, the pressure distribution of sensor at a diastolic period is examined.

In Fig. 4, a multi-element tonometer sensor and an underlying and partially compressed artery at the instant of diastole are illustrated. Assuming that the diastolic pressure is 80mmHg, elements 4-6 lying over the flattened artery wall measure the intra-arterial pressure, 80mmHg. However, the pressures of elements 2, 3, 7, and 8 are all significantly greater because the artery wall under these elements is bent to a very small radius and, at the both ends, large bending moments (or contact stresses) are transmitted by the artery wall as shown in Fig. 3 in section 2.2. So, the sensor element corresponding to the local minimum should be determined as the centered element (Drzewiecki et al., 1983).

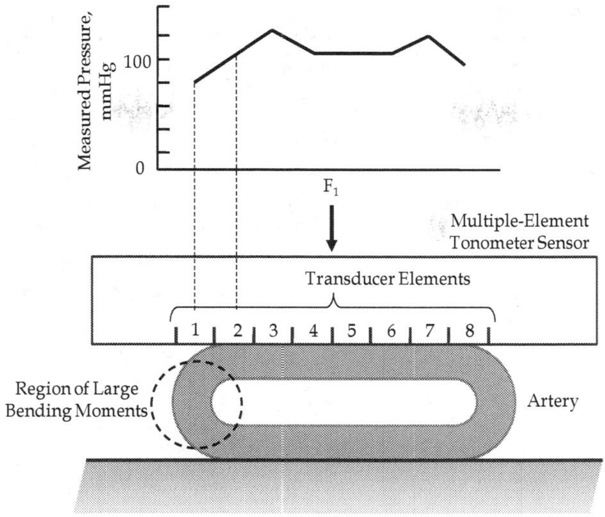

Fig. 4. Bending effect on pressure distribution (Eckerle, 1981)

Determining the centered sensor element is not enough for reliable measurement; the degree of arterial flattening is also important. Arterial flattening depends on the interaction of anatomical factors with the hold-down force, F_1 in Fig. 4. The appropriate hold-down force, which minimizes the contact stress of arterial wall and maximizes the amplitude of pulse pressure, must be determined for each subject before reliable tonometric measurement can be made. An algorithm for automatic identification of the appropriate hold-down pressure was developed (Eckerle et al., 1989). Briefly, the algorithm fits a third order polynomial to the signal recorded while increasing or decreasing hold-down pressure and then determines the timing of the appropriate hold-down pressure from polynomial coefficients.

To determine this hold-down pressure more exactly, we have developed a step motor controlled robot arm including a multi-array sensor on its tip and a laser displacement sensor (LK-G30, Keyence Co., Japan) embedding an algorithm for the elimination of diffused reflection effects which happens on skin inevitably. We lowered the robot arm by increasing the number of motor steps so that the tip of robot arm approaches the skin closely and, then, indented the skin over the radial artery gradually. Therefore we could record the displacement of the robot arm which is roughly related to the degrees of arterial deflection in section 2.2, as well as hold-down pressure and radial pulse waveforms simultaneously. The displacement and approximated degrees of deflection can be used to check whether the determined appropriate hold-down pressure corresponds to the reasonable range of deflection degrees (60%-70%); Assuming the thickness of skin and tissue layer as 3.0 mm, the diameter of radial artery as 3.0 mm and the maximum decrement of skin/tissue layer thickness as 0.5 mm or less, the appropriate hold-down pressure will correspond to 2.3-.2.6 mm displacement from skin contact level approximately. In Fig. 5, an example of robot arm displacement values and corresponding radial pulse waveforms depicted as dimensionless are shown. Since the skin contact seems to occur at around 3.5 mm in y-axis and the pulse pressure can be found to be biggest at near 1 mm in y-axis, the decreased diameter is presumed to be about 2.5 mm and it falls within the reasonable range of deflection degrees well.

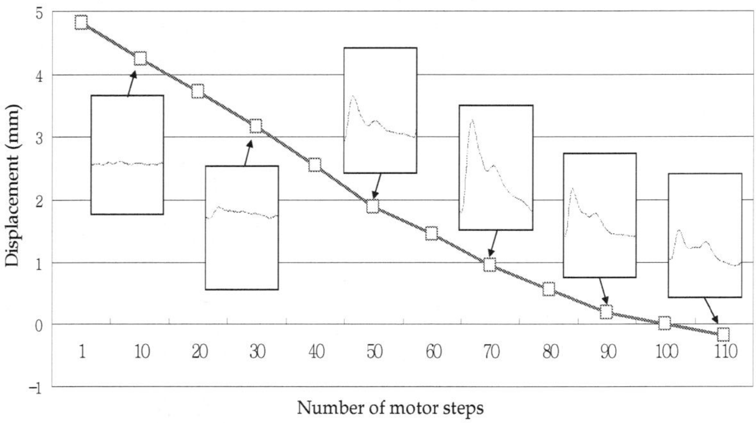

Fig. 5. Displacements of the robot arm and corresponding radial pulse waveforms

Consequently, despite the easiness to be performed, the reliable measurement needs to pay much attention to keep the subject's variation minimized and to have sophisticated strategies to determinate the centered sensor element and the appropriate hold-down pressure.

3. Arterial stiffness estimation

Increased arterial stiffness accelerates the speed at which the left ventricular ejection pressure wave travels through the arteries, and leads to an earlier return of the reflected pressure wave back to the left ventricle. As a result, the reflected pressure wave arrived during systole causes the augmentation of the late systolic pressure (afterload) on the left ventricle. So, the degrees of augmentation can be used as one of the arterial stiffness estimators.

3.1 Augmentation index

The arterial pressure waveform is a composite of the forward pressure wave generated ventricular contraction and a reflected wave. Waves are reflected from the periphery, mainly at branch points or sites of impedance mismatch. In elastic vessels, because PWV is low, reflected wave arrives back at the central arteries earlier, adding to the forward wave and augmenting the systolic pressure. This phenomenon can be quantified through the augmentation index (AIx) - defined as the ratio of the difference between the second and first systolic peaks (P2-P1) to the pulse pressure as shown in Fig. 6. The augmentation index is dimensionless and usually expressed in percentage, but it does not depend on the absolute pressure. While pacing the heartbeat rhythm, AIx was shown to be significantly and inversely related to heart rate ($r= -0.70$, $p <.001$) due to an alteration in the relative timing of the reflected pressure wave (Wilkinson et al., 2002). So, using the relationship between AIx and heart rate, corrected AIx at 75 bpm (AIx@75) has been commonly used. Even though peak systolic pressures are similar, different augmentation indexes explain that different loading effects arise on the left ventricle. Increased AIx due to arterial stiffening may occur with aging or in disorders such as hypertension, diabetes or hypercholesterolemia. And, because the augmentation means the increase of afterload in systolic period and the eduction of coronary artery perfusion pressure and leads to greater risk of angina, heart attack, stroke and heart failure, it is quite useful clinically.

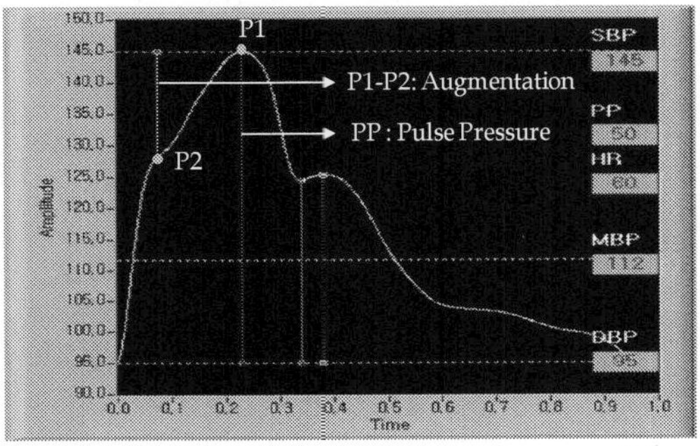

Fig. 6. An example of aortic pulse pressure waveform and augmented pressure

3.2 Transfer function

Aortic pressure waveform for AIx calculation can be estimated either from the radial artery waveform, using a transfer function, or from the common carotid waveform.

And, a transfer function between aortic pressure radial pressure signals can be derived by the linear ARX model. The ARX linear model describes the properties of a system on the basis of its immediate past input and output data as

$$T(t)=-a_1T(t-1)-a_2T(t-2)-...-a_m(t-m) \\ +b_1P(t-1)+...+b_nP(t-n) \quad (8)$$

where T(t) and T(t-i) [i=1, 2, ..., m] are present and previous output (radial tonometer), respectively, and P(t-i) are previous input (aortic pressure). The a's and b's are the parameters of the model, and m and n represent the order of the model, that is, the number of previous input-output values used to describe the present output. This methodology yields more statistically stable and thus reliable spectral estimates from limited data compared with nonparametric approaches, for example, a Fourier transform.

The transfer function is estimated with the aortic pressure used as input and the radial tonometer signal as output. An inverse TF derived from TF can be used to reconstruct the aortic pressure from the radial pulse as follows:

$$P(t-1)=-b_2/b_1P(t-2)-...-b_n/b_1P(t-n) \\ +1/b_1T(t)+a_1/b_1T(t-1)+...+a_m/b_1T(t-m) \quad (9)$$

In general, the model order for TF estimate is selected as 10, that is, 10 'a' coefficients and 10 'b' coefficients are used. Meanwhile, a critical problem lies on this approach. The low gain of the TF in the frequency range above 8 to 10 Hz brings out the high gains of the inverse TF so that it amplifies high-frequency noise and distorts the reconstructed aortic pressure waveform. This problem can be solved by convolving the inverse TF with a low-pass filter having a cut-off frequency at which the magnitude of the TF gain function declines below 1. While the mean TF of an individual at several steady-states is called as an individual transfer function (ITF), a global transfer function (GTF) are obtained by averaging the ITF from all participated patients. Chen et al. have reported that TFs varied among patients; coefficient of variation was 24.9% for peak amplitude and was 16.9% for frequency at peak amplitude, respectively. Despite this, the GTF estimated central arterial pressure to ≤0.2±3.8mmHg error, arterial compliance to 6±7% accuracy, and augmentation index to within -7% points (30±45%) (Chen et al., 1997). In addition, because the radial blood pressure is higher than the brachial blood pressure, brachial artery pressure is used as surrogate of radial artery pressure for the calibration of central pressure.

3.3 Augmentation point detection algorithm

As an augmentation pressure is a determinate factor in AIx calculation, a reliable AIx estimation depends on accurate detection of augmentation point mostly. Even if one can indicate the timing of the augmentation point easily such a local minimum in the first derivative that was in the range from 0 to 50 msec of the peak flow (Chen et al., 1996), it is hard to detect an exact augmentation point. In late 80's, utilizing a non-invasively measured flow velocity signal, an earnest algorithm which could detect an augmentation point of ascending aortic pressure was developed (Kelly et al., 1989). Kelly et al. showed that the first zero-crossing of the fourth derivative corresponded to the beginning of the pressure wave upstroke and the second zero crossing in the same direction corresponded to the shoulder, that is, the augmentation points. And, they also found a good correlation between the time to the second zero crossing of the fourth derivative (x) and the timing of the peak of flow (y), which was the time-delayed sign to arrival of reflected wave; y=0.91+1.31x, R=0.75. So, it was suggested that an augmentation points could be determined as the second zero crossing of the fourth derivative as shown in Fig. 7. Recently, a detection method with only carotid pulse pressure was proposed (Gatzka et al., 2001). In this study, the augmentation point was defined as the first zero crossing from positive to negative of the fourth derivative and occurs 55 msec after the onset of systole pressure.

However, these mentioned studies do not fit well to all types of aortic pressure waveform; the aortic pressure waveform can be divided into three broad categories generally (Murgo et al., 1980). Particularly, a subject-sensitive searching interval for the detection of augmentation point should be fixed empirically so to lack in flexibility.

So, our colleague suggested a syntactic algorithm in which they tried first to indicate an augmentation point on the first derivative with a searching condition, if failed, then, on the second derivative with another searching condition, if failed again, lastly on the third derivative with the other searching condition within a first searching range from the first peak to second negative slope zero crossing of the first derivative (Im & Jeon, 2008). Nevertheless, if no augmentation point were detected, they considered the augmentation point located after the systolic peak of aortic pulse not before the systolic peak. Then, within a second searching range from the first negative slope zero crossing to the second positive slope zero crossing of the first derivative, they tried to detect an augmentation point with similar strategy mentioned above. Finally, they reported that the percentage error in AIx was 4.82± 16.9, smaller than 39.5± 39.4 reported by Fetics et al. (Fetics et al., 1999) and smaller than 27± 22 reported by Chen et al. (Chen et al., 1997).

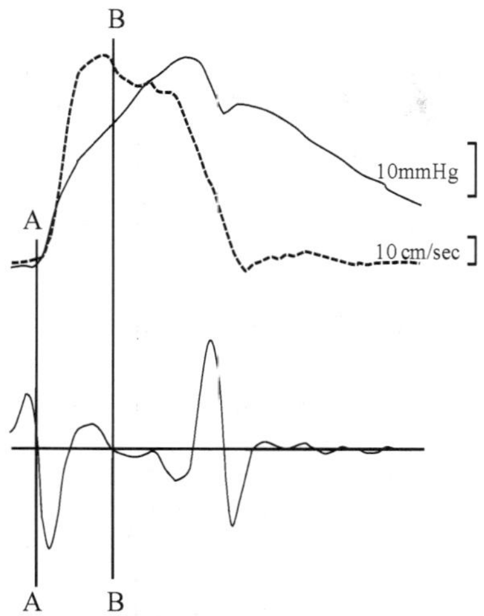

Fig. 7. An example of ascending aortic pressure form(solid line above), blood flow (dashed line above) and corresponding fourth derivative of pressure waveform(solid line below) (Kelly et al., 1989)

4. Emerging issues

Although the radial areterial tonometry has been widely used to estimate the arterial function, there remains many research issues to be studied. For examples, the geometric and hemodynamic characteristics of radial artery and the effects of measuring position selection on AIx have not be studied thoroughly. One the other hand, there is criticism for the use of transfer function. So, in the following sections, we want to deal with the radial artery characteristics and the importance of measuring position. And, we will introduce the latest attempts to estimate the arterial stiffness with radial pulse waveform itself and to apply the radial tonometry to the oriental pulse diagnosis.

4.1 Geometric and hemodynamic characteristics of radial artery

In oriental medicine, before at least about 2,000 years, it has been asserted that the pulse pressures, the optimal hold-down pressures for pulse diagnosis and even the pulse images are different among adjacent three diagnosis positions over the radial artery. So, we performed an experiment of ultrasonography on radial artery to examine the geometrical and hemodynamic characteristics in 2007. The six measuring positions on each hand were selected as shown in Fig. 8. The distal three positions were the well-known oriental pulse diagnosis positions and the other proximal three positions were non-pulse diagnosis positions which were located at regular intervals. The intervals between adjacent positions ranged from 1.20cm to 1.45cm and it was determined as to be proportional to the length of elbow individually by a skillful oriental medical doctor.

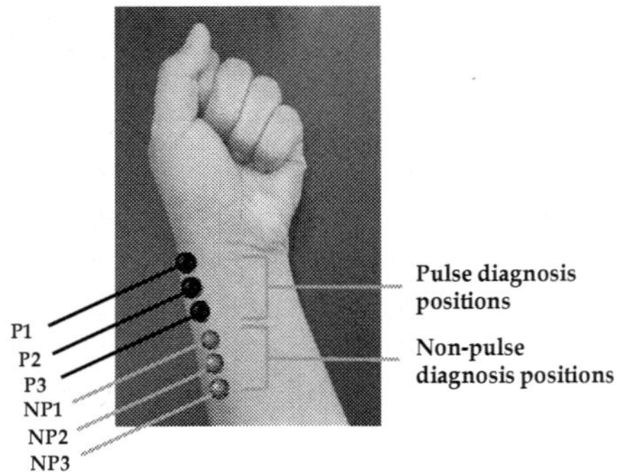

Fig. 8. An example of selected measuring positions composed of three pulse diagnosis positions and three non-pulse diagnosis positions

Under the approval of the Institutional Review Board of the Oriental Medicine Hospital at Daejeon University, South Korea, 44 healthy male and female in their 20s were participated as subjects. The geomtrical parameters, the depth and diameter of radial artery, and the hemodynamic parameters, the maximum and average blood velocities, were measured three times in random order at 12 positions, that is, each 6 positions in left and right sides. These positions are marked with tiny metal wires so to be recognized in an ultrasound image. In this experiment, a medical ultrasonography equipment (Volusion 730 Pro, GE Medical, USA) was utilized to measure the geometrical parameter values in B-Mode and the hemodynamic parameter values in PW Doppler mode. In the geometrical measurement, because the geometrical parameters varied dynamically during a heartbeat, the geometrical parameters were obtained only from the B mode images frozen at diastolic periods. The timing of diastolic period was determined with simultaneously measured photo-plethysmogram (PPG) from the index finger of each subject.
The measured values of parameters at 12 positions are summarized in Table 2 and reported as mean±SD. And, the variation tendency of all parameters from P1 to NP3 is also shown with mean values in Fig. 9. One-way ANOVA was conducted to examine whether the depths, the diameters and the blood flow velocities among 6 positions were different for each hand. A p-value<0.05 was considered statistically significant. As a result, the vessel depths($p < .001$), vessels diameter ($p < .001$) and average flow velocities($p < .001$) among 6 positions, that is, P1, P2, P3, NP1, NP2 and NP3 were showed to be significantly different in each hand. And, when those parameters of left and right hand were compared, the vessel depths of P1, NP2 and NP3, the vessel diameter of P3 and the average flow velocity of all 6 positions were found to be also different signifcantly between left and right hand. In details, as for the vessel depths, those among P1, P2 and P3 differed significantly (left: $p = 0.001$; right: $p < .0001$), but no significant differences were observed among non-pulse dianosing positions. Contrarily, when the vessel diameter was evaluated, no significant differences

were observed among P1, P2 and P3. However, there was a statistically significant difference among NP1, NP2, and NP3 (left: $p = 0.0002$; right: $p = 0.0032$).
Consequently, in further studies on radial pulse wave, 1) the geometrical difference between the pulse diagnosis positions and the non pulse diagnosis positions, and even among P1, P2 and P3 and 2) the hemodynamic radical change near the periphery must be considered.

	Parameters	P1	P2	P3	NP1	NP2	NP3
Left	Vessel depth (mm)	3.26± (0.71)	2.74 ± (0.66)	3.32 ± (0.85)	3.79 ± (1.09)	3.90± (1.11)	4.17 ± (1.26)
	Vessel diameter (mm)	2.52 ± (0.36)	2.42 ± (0.35)	2.52 ± (0.30)	2.54 ± (0.32)	2.51 ± (0.31)	2.51 ± (0.31)
	Maximum blood flow velocity (cm/sec)	41.68 ± (12.39)	55.34 ± (14.70)	56.26 ± (11.82)	54.98 ± (12.23)	56.36± (12.21)	57.66 ± (13.57)
	Average blood flow velocity (cm/sec)	5.75± (3.25)	9.24 ± (4.86)	9.51 ± (4.44)	9.81 ± (5.24)	9.66 ± (4.51)	10.14 ± (5.04)
Right	Vessel depth (mm)	3.60± (0.82)	2.74 ± (0.72)	3.36± (1.14)	3.95± (1.36)	4.32 ± (1.42)	4.64 ± (1.41)
	Vessel diameter (mm)	2.47 ± (0.39)	2.37 ± (0.32)	2.46 ± (0.33)	2.53 ± (0.41)	2.55 ± (0.34)	2.55 ± (0.33)
	Maximum blood flow velocity (cm/sec)	35.50± (4.64)	49.28 ± (11.95)	50.91 ± (11.55)	51.43± (12.53)	52.85± (13.15)	53.94 ± (12.13)
	Average blood flow velocity (cm/sec)	4.64 ± (2.99)	7.46 ± (4.24)	7.98± (4.41)	8.26± (4.44)	8.45 ± (5.12)	8.39 ± (4.43)

Table 2. Summarized measurement results: the depth, the diameter of radial artery, and the blood blow velocity at 12 positions

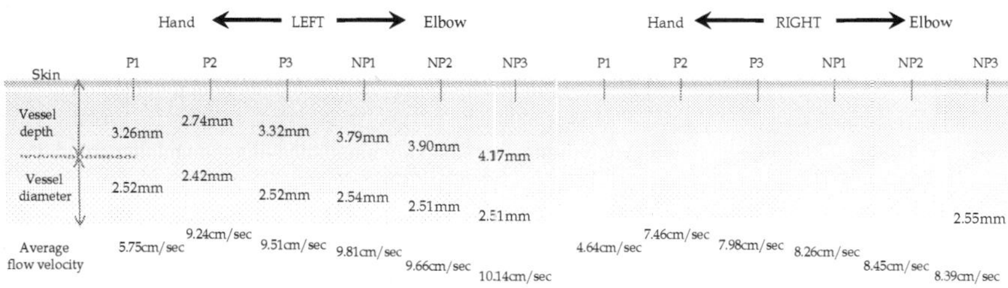

Fig. 9. The variation of parameters along the 6 positions composed of three pulse diagnosis positions and three non-pulse diagnosis positions in both hands

4.2 Measuring position effects on AIx

As referred in section 4.1, the geometric and hemodynamic characteristics are different among pulse diagnosis positions. So, we examined the measuring position effects on AIx.
In this study, 20 young male persons were involved, who had no cardiovascular disease history and were in twenties, normotensive and within the normal range (18.5~24.9 kg/m^2) of the body mass index (BMI). And, using the SphygmoCor apparatus (AtCor Medical, Australia), we measured twice the baseline and the signal strength, which correspond to the hold-down pressure and the measured pulse pressure, respectively, and the AIx@75 at the

P1, P2, and P3 of left hand. To avoid any bias in data collection, we randomized the order of measuring positions for each subject. Especially, to obtain the noise minimized and high intensity signals, the signal strength, which represents the difference between the maximum and the minimum of the pulse waveform, were kept over 360 and the variation of signal strength and baseline were monitored to be within ±100, ±200, respectively. If these were not contented, the measurement of radial pulse waveform was designed to be performed again. Furthermore, the signals, of which the OI (operator index) provided by the SphygmoCor software were over 90 and the sub-parameters of OI, that is, average pulse height, pulse height variation, diastolic variation, shape deviation, and maximum dP/dT fell in agreeable green range, were only selected for the statistical analysis. First, we tested the repeatability of measurement with two-way repeated measures ANOVA, by which the differences in the average of baseline, pulse strength, and AIx@75 between first and second measurement for each position were examined.
As a result, we could not find any difference at 5% of statistical significance level so that the measurement process was showed to be well-controlled. In detail, the mean and the standard error (mean±SEM) of the differences between AIx@75s of the two repeated measures were estimated respectively as -0.45±0.63, 0.05±0.72, and -0.15±0.68 at P1, P2, and P3. Then, we tested the differences of baseline, pulse strength, and AIx@75 among P1, P2 and P3 with two-way repeated measures ANOVA analysis. In Table 3, the measured values (mean±SD) of three parameters at each positions and p-values calculated by the two-way repeated measures ANOVA are summarized. Finally, in all parameters including AIx@75, significant differences among P1, P2 and P3 were found. From this, we could conclude that careless selection of measuring position might bring out different or wrong estimation of augmentation index. Interestingly, no significant difference was found in the radial waveform parameters including radial AIxs among P1, P2 and P3.

	P1	P2	P3	*p*-value
Baseline	1108.8±273.6	962.5±170.9	1033.8±246.4	4.625E-4
Signal strength	511.5±78.0	543.1±82.6	472.6±69.5	2.354E-8
AIx@75	-0.23±5.56	-1.83±5.97	-2.28±5.73	0.004

Table 3. Differences of baseline, signal strength and AIx@75 among P1, P2 an dP3

We also analyzed the difference of AIx among P1, P2 and P3 using a well-known multiple comparison analysis, Duncan test, and the results are shown in Table 4. It probably seemed to be correlated with the fact that the blood flow velocity at P1 was quite different from that of P2 and P3 as described in section 4.1. Consequently, we want to suggest that it is necessary to establish a more detailed guideline for the selection of measuring positions so to minimize the mistakes in treatment based on the AIx.

	P1	P2	P3
Mean	-0.225	-1.825	-2.275
SD	5.558	5.597	5.729
F		5.867	
p-value		0.004	
Group	A	B	B

Table 4. Multiple comparisons on AIx@75

4.3 Stiffness estimation without a transfer function

The transfer function has been widely used to reconstruct the aortic pressure waveform from the measured radial waveform. However, the reliability of this is still controversial. Although the use of a general transfer function has been well established and has demonstrated its reliability for calculating central PP (Williams et al., 2006), the accuracy of this method for the calculation of aortic AIx has been disputed (Millasseau et al., 2003). Indeed, even though the general transfer function has been reported to provide accurate estimates of central PP, compliance, and other low-frequency component features of the central waveform, it has been urged to be less accurate and to induce greater between-subject variability at high frequency components which contributes to determine the augmentation index (Segers et al., 2005). So, an alternative and direct approach without a transfer function has been needed. In a recent study, the reliability of carotid AIx estimation from nontransformed radial AIx has been shown (Melenovsky et al., 2007). The major results can be summarized are below:

- Carotid AIx significantly correlated with radial AIx independent of age, mean BP, gender and body mass index. This correlation was significant under baseline conditions, during a cold-pressor test, and after sublingual administration of nitro-glycerine.
- The changes in radial AIx and carotid AIx caused by provocative maneuver were also significantly correlated.
- The non-linear correlation between radial (or carotid) AIx and late systolic pressure-time integral, defined as afterload was found.

If more cases of radial AIx's or a third index's compatibility to the aortic AIx in the treatment of hypertension are accumulated, the AIx estimation method with a transfer function might be disused spontaneously.

4.4 Applications in the oriental medicine

In oriental medicine, the radial arterial pulse has been widely believed as a reflection of health condition for over at least two thousand years. However, the pulse diagnosis, which is similar to the radial artery tonometry but more complex, has been criticized as having some ambiguities and a susceptibility to being subjectified because almost procedure have been quite dependent on the subjective and not-exchangeable feeling of oriental medical doctors (OMDs).

A patient's pulse diagnosis has been determined with one or more of the 28 types of so-called pulse image defined as pulsation pressure distributions on the 3 pulse diagnosis positions while varying hold-down pressure. All verbal descriptions related with the 28 types of pulse image could be divided into the readily measurable physical components, that is, the depth, the frequency, the strength, the width, and the length of pulsation, and the others (Ryu et al., 2007). With these 5 components, 10 types of pulse images are able to diagnosed: that is, floating and sinking pulses, slow pulse and fast pulses, forceful and deficient pulses, large and fine pulses, and long and short pulses. To measure these quantities reliably, our colleagues in KIOM (Korea Institute of Oriental Medicine) have tried to develop a few types of pulse diagnosis devices based on 3 or 5 degrees of freedom robot arms embedding a multi-array pressure sensor on its tip since 2006 (Lee, 2007). The multi-

array sensor can measure the hold-down pressure and the pulsation pressure distribution simultaneously at 10 different hold-down pressures ranged from 0 to 500g·f. From these obtained signals, we can extract some useful information for the pulse diagnosis such as the profile of pulse pressure vs. hold-down pressure, the maximum pulse pressure at a certain hold-down pressure defined as an optimal hold-down pressure, the pulsation frequency, the pressure distribution under the array sensor at the optimal hold-down pressure etc.
On the other hand, we have obtained over 4,000 volunteer's data with one of these systems and have also collected their clinical information including blood pressures, body temperatures, health questionnaires, and quantitative pulse diagnosis records by 3 OMDs. In these pulse diagnosis records by OMD, the membership degrees to 10 pulse images each have been included. With this database, we are examining the normal and abnormal range of each quantity and the interactions between each quantity, and each quantity's contributions to diagnosis into 10 types of pulse images and we are developing some pulse diagnosis discriminant functions (Lee et al., 2007).
For now, the floating and sinking pulses might be correlated to the blood pressure - systolic pressure($r=0.405$, $p<0.005$) and diastolic pressure($r=0.398$, $p<0.005$). And, between the pulse waveforms of the forceful and deficient pulses, significant differences has been shown in the maximum pulse pressure ($p=0.000$) and the systolic pulse width ($p=0.000$). No doubt, the slow and fast pulses are highly correlated to the heart rate. The wide and fine pulse are inferred to be related to the contact length described in section 2.2 so that they should be examined on its correlation with the blood vessel's diameter directly, the elasticity of blood vessel, or E involved in equation (7) as a factor of β. Lastly, the long and short pulses are guessed to be related with the effective systolic time and systolic volume.
In further studies, we hope to reveal the underlying physiological factors of these pulse images and to examine the relationship between these pulse images and clinical symptoms mentioned in oriental medicine literatures. In that case, with radial arterial tonometry, we can provide unheard of healthcare contents originated from the oriental medicine.

5. Conclusion

In this chapter, we presented the one of most attractive arterial stiffness estimation method with AIx calculated from radial pulse waveform measured by radial arterial tonometry.
In the first part, we tried to enhance the understanding of arterial tonometry by explaining the operation principle and continuous mathematical model of the relationship between arterial wall deformation and contact stress. We also dealt with three causes of measurement errors; subject's variation, uncertainty of sensor location and non-appropriate hold-down pressure. Concerning these, we summarized factors affect subject's variation and introduced some algorithms of searching the centered sensor element and of determining the optimal hold-down pressure for reliable measurement.
In the middle part, the estimation method of arterial stiffness with AIx was elucidated. In details, the clinical importance of AIx was explained and some ways to generate an aortic pressure waveform with transfer function and to detect an augmentation point for calculating AIx were surveyed.
In the latter part, some emerging issues on radial tonometry were provided. First two were about the geometric and hemodynamic characteristics of radial artery and the effect of measuring position on AIx ignored comparatively heretofore. Next one was about recent

attempts to estimate arterial stiffness with radial AIx extracted from radial pulse waveform itself. In last, we exclusively reported the development of robot arm adopting the radial tonometry for oriental pulse diagnosis in Korea, and the possibility of offering new healthcare contents with this system.

Though further studies, we expect, all underlying principles are revealed and all conditions for reliable measurement are established and made controllable. And, we hope that more concrete clinical evidences are accumulated and potential applications are established so that arterial tonometry would be used usefully and frequently as much as electrocardiography does.

6. References

Chen, C. H.; Ting, C. T.; Nussbacher, A.; Nevo, E.; Kass, D. A.; Pak, P.; Wang, S. P.; Chang, M. S. & Yin, F. C. P. (1996). Validation of carotid artery tonometry as a means of estimating augmentation index of ascending aortic pressure. *Hypertension*, Vol. 27, pp. 168-175

Chen, C.; Nevo, E.; Fetics, B.; Pak, P. H.; Yin, F. C. P.; Maughan, W. L. & Kass. D. A. (1997). Estimation of central aortic pressure waveform by mathematical transformation of radial tonometry pressure. *Circulation*, Vol. 95, pp. 1827-1836

Darne, B.; Girerd, X.; Safar, M.; Cambien, F. & Guise, L. (1989). Pulsatile versus steady component of blood pressure : a cross-sectional analysis and a prospective analysis on cardiovascular mortality. *Hypertension,* Vol. 13, pp. 392-400

Drzewieki, G. M.; Melbin, J. & Noordergraff, A. (1983). Arterial tonometry : Review and anlysis. *J. Biomechanics,* Vol. 16, No. 2, pp. 141-152

Eckerle, J. S. (1981). Noninvasive blood pressure monitoring transducer. *US Patent* 4,269,193

Eckerle, J. S. (1989). Blood pressure monitoring method and apparatus. *US Patent* 4,799,491

Eckerle, J. S. (2006). Tonometry, Arterial, In: *Encyclopedia of Medical Devices and Instrumentation,* Webster, J. G., 2nd Edition, 402-409, Wiley, ISBN: 978-0-471-26358-6

Fetics, B.; Nevo, E.; Chen, C. H. & Kass, D. A. (1999). Parametric model derivation of transfer function for noninvasive estimation of aortic pressure by radial tonometry. *IEEE Transcations on Biomdeical Engineering*, Vol. 46, pp. 698-706

Gatzka, C. D.; Cameron, J. D.; Dart, A. M.; Berry, K. L.; Kingwell, B. A.; Dewar, E. M.; Reid, C. M. & Jennings, G. L. R. (2001). Correction of carotid augmentation index for heart rate in elderly essential hypertensives. *Am J Hypertens*, Vol. 14, pp. 573–577

Gerard, M. & Alain, P. G. (1999). Influence of arterial pulse and reflective waves on blood pressure and cardiac function. *American Heart Journal,* Vol. 138, No. 3, pp. S220-S224

Im, J. J. & Jeon, Y. J. (2008). Estimation of the central aortic pulse using transfer function and improvement of an augmentation point detection algorithm, *Korean Journal of Electronics Engineering*, Vol. 45, No. 3, pp. 68-79 (*in Korean*)

Kelly, R.; Hayward, C.; Avolio, A. & O'Rourke, M. (1989). Noninvasive determination of age-related changes in the human arterial pulse. *Circulation*, Vol. 80, pp. 1652-1659

Lee, J. (2007). Traditional Medicine Instrument in Korea - Development States of Pulse Analyzer, *7th Annual Meeting for Japanese Society of Integrative Medicine,* pp. 50, Ichinobo hotel, Dec. 2007, Matsushima, Japan

Lee, Y. J.; Lee, J.; Jang, E. S.; Choi, E. J.; Lee, H. J. & Kim, J. Y. (2007). A study of floating and sink pulse diagnosis : analysing of pulse wave parameter and typical pulse pattern, *ICMART2007*, pp. 14-17, ISBN, Hotel Fira Palace, Jun. 2007, Barcelona, Spain

Melenovsky, V.; Borlaug, B. A.; Fetics, B.; Kesseler, K.; Shively, L. & Hass, D. A. (2007). Estimation of central pressure augmentation using automated radial artery tonometry. *J Hypertens*, Vol. 25, pp. 1403-1409

Millasseau, S. C.; Patel, S. J.; Redwood, S. R.; Ritter, J. M. & Chowienczyk, P. J. (2003). Pressure wave reflection assessed for the peripheral pulse. Is a transfer function necessary? *Hypertension*, Vol. 41, pp. 1016-1020

Murgo, J. P.; Westerhof, N.; Giolma, J. P. & Altobelli, S. A. (1980). Aortic input impedance in normal man: relationship to pressure wave forms. *Circulation*, Vol. 62, No. 1, pp. 105-116

Nam, K.C.; Kim E.G.; Heo, H.; Huh, Y. (2009). Effect of Subject Posture on Pulse Wave Measurement, *The 24th International Technical Conference on Circuits/Systems, Computers and Communications (ITC-CSCC 2009)*, pp. 499-501, Jeju KAL Hotel, Jul. 2009, Jeju, Korea

Pressman, G. & Newgard, P. (1963). A transducer for the continuous external measurement of arterial blood pressure. *IEEE Trans. Bio-Med. Electron.*, Vol. BME-10, pp. 73-80

Roman, M. J.; Devereux, R. B.; Kizer, J. R.; Lee, E. T.; Galloway, J. M.; Ali, T.; Umans, J. G. & Howard, B. V. (2007). Central pressure more strongly relates to vascular disease and outcome than does brachial pressure. *Hypertension*, Vol. 50, pp. 197-203

Ryu, H. H.; Lee, S. W.; Lee, J.; Lee, Y. J. & Kim, J. Y. (2007). The Literary Study on the Physical Quantification of Pulse Types. *Korean J. Oriental Physiology & Pathology*, Vol. 21, No. 6, pp. 1381-1387 (*in Korean*)

Segers, P.; Rietzschel, E.; Heireman, S.; Du Buyzere, M.; Gilbert, T.; Verdonk, P. & Van Bortel, L. (2005). Carotid tonometry versus synthesized aorta pressure waves for the estimation of central systolic blood pressure and augmentation index. *Am J Hypertens*, Vol. 18, pp. 1168-1173

Terry, S.; Eckerle, J. S.; Kornbluh, R. D.; Low, T. & Ablow, C. M. (1990). Silicon pressure transducer arrays for blood-pressure measurement. *Sensors and Actuators*, Vol. A21-A23, pp. 1070-1079

Van Bortel, L. M; Duprez, D.; Starmans-Kool, M. J.; Safar, M. E.; Giannattasio, C.; Cockfroft, J.; Kaiser, D. R. & Thuillez, C. (2002). Applications of arterial stiffness, Task Force III: recommendations for user procedures. *Am J Hypertens*, Vol. 15, pp. 445-452

Wilkinson, I. B.; Mohammad, N. H.; Tyrrell, S.; Hall, I. R.; Webb, D. J.; Paul, V. E.; Levy, T. & Cockcroft, J. R. (2002). Heart rate dependency of pulse pressure amplification and arterial stiffness. *Am J Hypertens*, Vol. 15, No. 1, pp. 24-30

Williams, B.; Lacy, P. S.; Thom, S. M.; Cruickshank, K.; Stanton, A. & Collier, D. (2006). Differential impact of blood pressure-lowering drugs on central aortic pressure and clinical outcomes: principal results of the Conduit Artery Function Evaluation (CAFE) study. *Circulation*, Vol. 113, pp. 1213-1225

31

New Methods for Atrial Activity Extraction in Atrial Tachyarrhythmias

Raúl Llinares and Jorge Igual
Universidad Politécnica de Valencia
Spain

1. Introduction

Atrial fibrillation (AF) is the most common human arrhythmia. The analysis of the associated atrial activity (AA) provides features of clinical relevance. In particular, the fibrillatory rate has primary importance in AF spontaneous behavior (Asano et al., 1992), response to therapy (Stambler et al., 1997) or cadioversion (Manios et al., 2000). Previously, the atrial signal must be obtained. Hence, the identification of the AA is necessary. AA is embedded into the surface electrocardiogram (ECG), including the rest of the signals, such as the ventricular rhythm, breathing or noise. The cancellation of the ventricular signal can be done in different ways: from template matching subtraction to source separation approaches. One of these AA extraction methods is implemented on a commercially ECG system available on the market. It features ECG recording and signal processing for non-invasive assessment of atrial fibrillatory activity (Grubitzsch et al., 2008).

This chapter presents further developed algorithms to extract the AA in the frequency domain. The methods presented are extensions of classical ICA methods based on second and higher order statistics. The algorithms exploit the prior assumption about the sources in order to obtain the source extraction algorithms that are focused on the extraction of the atrial component.

The chapter is organized as follows. Section 2 describes the AF. Section 3 reviews the methods of AA extraction existent in the literature. Section 4 outlines the new methods in detail. In Section 5, the quality parameters of AA extraction are discussed. Numerical simulations and comparisons are provided in Section 6. Finally, concluding remarks are given in Section 7.

2. Atrial Fibrillation

The importance of atrial tachyarrhythmias in humans, such as atrial fibrillation (AF) or atrial flutter (AFL), is revealed by statistics: AF affects 0.4% of the general population, but the probability of developing it rises with age, less than 1% for people under 60 years of age and greater than 6% in those over 80 years (Fuster et al., 2001).

During AF, the atria beat chaotically and irregularly, out of coordination with the ventricles, increasing the risk of stroke and death. There is no unique theory about the mechanisms of

AF, but some characteristics of AF in the ECG are well established: the atrial activity is irregular in timing and shape; there is a substitution of the P-waves by an oscillating baseline that consists of low amplitude fibrillatory F-waves (Petrutiu et al., 2006). The shape, amplitude and frequency of the F-waves depend obviously on the patient, being more regular in the AFL case. Atrial rates are usually in the range 240-540 waves per minute in AF and 240-320 in the case of AFL (Stridh et al., 2006). In addition, the ventricular response during AF episodes becomes irregular, with higher average rate (shorter RR intervals). Figure 1 shows an episode of AF (a) and a normal sinus rhythm (b). Note the fibrillatory waves between the R peaks, the absence of the P waves and the irregular ventricular rhythm in (a). The normal sinus rhythm (b) contains the P waves and it is more regular.

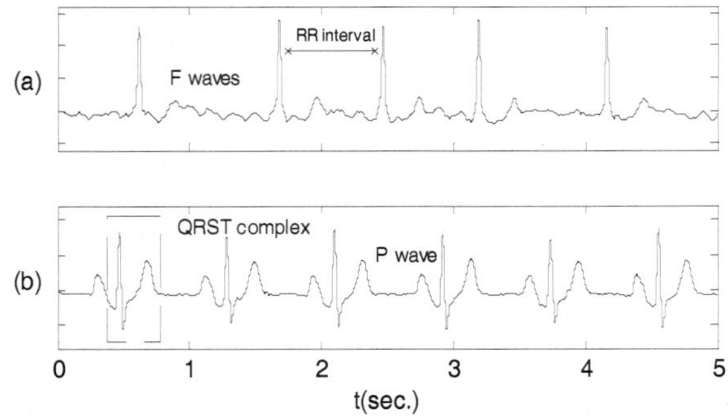

Fig. 1. Comparison between Atrial Fibrillation (a) and Normal Sinus Rhythm (b)

From the signal processing point of view, AA shows a power spectral density concentrated around a main peak in a frequency band (narrowband signal), with slight variations depending on the authors; for example, 4-9 Hz. (Petrutiu et al. 2006, Stridh et al. 2006), 5-10 Hz. (Langley et al. 2000) or 3.5-9 Hz. (Castells et al., 2005a). This spectrum is a key feature to distinguish between AF and other non fibrillatory rhythms. Figure 2 represents two examples of atrial activity: AF in (a) and AFL in (c); (b) and (d) plot their spectra and the corresponding peak frequencies.

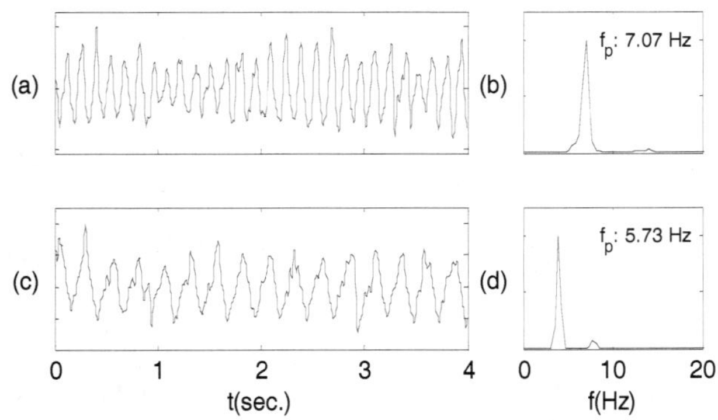

Fig. 2. Two examples of AA, their spectra and the corresponding peak frequencies

Analyzing the AA from a statistical point of view, the AA shows a Gaussian or subgaussian distribution (zero or negative kurtosis value, depending on the patient and the stage of the disease). From a time series point of view, it can be modeled as a sawtooth signal consisting of a sinusoid with several harmonics (Stridh & Sornmo 2001). In this case, the kurtosis values are close to zero. In Figure 3 the histograms of the atrial activities of Figure 2 are represented together with their associated kurtosis values. The continuous solid lines on the plots represent the closest Gaussian approximations to the observed distributions.

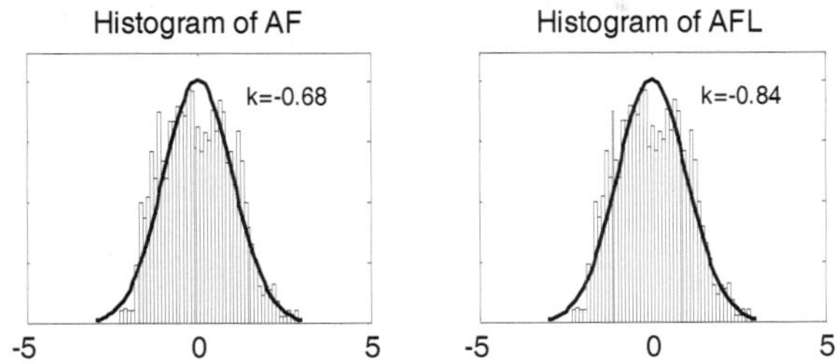

Fig. 3. Histogram of the atrial activities in Fig. 2

3. Methods of Atrial Activity Extraction in the Time Domain

3.1 Strategies

Two main approaches are used to extract the AA: techniques based on exploiting the spatial diversity of multi-lead ECG recordings and single-lead techniques. The first group includes algorithms based on averaged beat subtraction (ABS) and algorithms based on source separation performing an independent component analysis (ICA) or a principal component analysis (PCA) of the recorded ECG. Similar results were obtained when these algorithms were compared (Langley et al., 2006). The single-lead methods to extract the AA are mainly based on averaged beat subtraction. Single-lead algorithms are not benefited by the information present in all the leads. However, single-lead algorithms permit the analysis of early stages of AF with Holter systems where there is no more than two or three available leads, that are not sufficient to exploit the spatial diversity.

3.2 Averaged Beat Subtraction

ABS methods are the most widespread techiques of atrial signal extraction. These methods are based on QRST cancellation in the time domain. They assume two premises: (i) the atrial and ventricular activity are decoupled during AF episodes, and (ii), each individual beat can be represented approximately by an average (template) beat. Once the template is created, it is used to subtract the ventricular activity (VA) from each individual beat, obtaining a remainder or residual ECG containing only the F-waves.

ABS methods can be applied directly to single leads (Slocum et al., 1992, Shkurovich et al., 1998). They differ in the clustering of the different beat morphologies and the estimation of the template. One key point in ABS methods is the time alignment of the average beat and the QRST complex before the subtraction. The alignment can be carried out directly from the R wave timings or maximizing the cross-correlation between the template and the processed beat for different time shifts.

Other ABS methods work in a multi-lead ECG environment. Spatiotemporal QRST cancellation (Stridh & Sornmo, 2001) takes advantage of the spatial diversity to compensate for variations in the electrical axis, variations in the tissue conductivity and heart position. In this case, the ventricular activity is modeled by:

$$\mathbf{X} = \mathbf{J}_\tau \bar{\mathbf{X}} \mathbf{D} \mathbf{Q} \tag{1}$$

where $\mathbf{J}_\tau = \left[\mathbf{0}_{Nx(\Delta+\tau)} \quad \mathbf{I}_{NxN} \quad \mathbf{0}_{Nx(\Delta-\tau)} \right]$ is the shift matrix used for time alignment (with τ an integer time shift and $\pm\Delta$ the maximum corrected alignment error), $\bar{\mathbf{X}}$ is the average beat, $\mathbf{D}$ is a diagonal amplitude scaling matrix and $\mathbf{Q}$ is a rotation matrix.
The optimization of the parameters $\mathbf{D}$, $\mathbf{Q}$ and $\mathbf{J}_\tau$ is solved by means of a minimization problem:

$$\varepsilon_{\min}^2 = \min_{\mathbf{D},\mathbf{Q},\tau} \left\| \mathbf{Y} - \mathbf{J}_\tau \bar{\mathbf{X}} \mathbf{D} \mathbf{Q} \right\|_F^2 \tag{2}$$

where $\mathbf{Y} = \mathbf{X} - \tilde{\mathbf{X}}_A$ perfoms the AF reduction step with $\mathbf{X}$ the beat being processed and $\tilde{\mathbf{X}}_A$ the TQ-based fibrillation signal (Stridh & Sornmo, 2001). Note that when $\mathbf{Y} = \mathbf{X}$ (no AF reduction step) and $\mathbf{DQ} = \mathbf{I}$, the algorithm corresponds to a traditional ABS algorithm applied to a single-lead.
Lemay et al. (2007) propose a method that processes the QRS complexes separated from the T waves basing on the different nature of the repolarization and depolarization waves.
The main problem of these methods is the reduction of the performance when a high quality QRST cancellation template is difficult to obtain. This is the case of clinical practice where there is only available no more than 10 seconds (Lemay et al. 2007). Other limitations are their high sensitiveness to variations in QRST morphology or the difficulty of finding the optimal selection of the complexes to generate the template (Alcaraz & Rieta, 2008).

3.3 Independent Component Analysis

ICA is a signal processing tool for estimating individual source components from mixtures of them recorded at sensors. The estimation is carried out only with the statistical independence of the sources as assumption. The most basic formulation of ICA is the linear noiseless instantaneous mixture model for real-valued sources and mixtures:

$$\mathbf{x} = \mathbf{A}\mathbf{s} \tag{3}$$

where $\mathbf{x}$ $(Mx1)$ is the observed vector that is a linear transformation (mixing matrix $\mathbf{A}$ (MxK)) of a source vector $\mathbf{s}$ $(Kx1)$ whose components are statistically independent, i.e., the joint probability is the product of the marginal densities $p(\mathbf{s}) = \prod_i p(s_i)$.

The source distributions are not available, so the independence condition cannot be enforced and a measure of the independence is required. ICA algorithms differ in the way that they approximate the independence condition (Hyvarinen et al., 2001).

ICA based on higher order statistics (HOS) has been applied to AA extraction problem (Rieta et al., 2004). The approach satisfies the basic conditions of ICA: independence of the sources, non-gaussianity and generation of observations by instantaneous linear mixing of the sources. The identification of the AA among the set of separated sources was carried out using a kurtosis-based reordering of the separated signals followed by spectral analysis of the subgaussian sources.

Taking advantage of the time structure of the ECG recordings, ICA based on second order statistics (SOS) has also been applied successfully to this problem (Llinares et al., 2006). The sources in the ECG have different spectra allowing the application of SOS-based algorithms. In this case, the identification of the atrial activity was carried out using spectral analysis and kurtosis values.

Castells et al. (2005) proposed a two-step solution based on HOS-ICA (first stage) and SOS-ICA (second stage) to extract the AA. The identification of the atrial activity was done in frequency domain searching for the source with a peak in the range of 3-10 Hz.

Regarding the approach, ICA is a multi-lead technique that suffers a decrement of the quality of the extraction as the number of leads is reduced. Recent studies focus on the optimization of the location of the leads to apply blind source separation (BSS) techniques with a reduced number of leads (Igual et al., 2006). Starting from 64-leads recordings (body surface potential mapping), the AA was extracted using only two leads and an ICA technique.

The methods based on source separation waste computational load in the separation of non interesting sources. In addition, they need an additional step to choose the atrial signal among the recovered sources.

3.4 Principal Components Analysis

PCA is a statistical technique that applies a linear transformation $\mathbf{V}$ (MxK) to the observation data $\mathbf{x}$ $(Mx1)$ obtaining a vector of uncorrelated variables $\mathbf{z}$ $(Kx1)$:

$$\mathbf{z} = \mathbf{V}\mathbf{x} \tag{4}$$

where the elements of $\mathbf{z}$ are called the principal components. The first principal components will retain most of the variation present in all of the original variables.

PCA has been applied to multi-lead ECG for extracting the AA (Raine et al., 2004). The first components are related to ventricular activity and its variability since this activity presents the largest energy. Among the rest of principal components, the AA is identified in the frequency domain since it exhibits a narrowband spectrum. PCA applied to multi-lead ECG provides the optimal solution for orthogonal mixtures. However, the mixing matrix may have an arbitrary structure, obtaining non-satisfactory results. In addition, if the signals are Gaussian, decorrelation means independence, so in this case PCA and ICA are the same transformation.

PCA has also been applied to single-lead ECG for extracting the AA successfully exploiting the interbeat redundancy. When PCA is applied to several consecutive beats from the same lead, it outputs the principal components and their projections on each beat. The first principal component is related to the main QRST waveform, several components are related to AA and the rest of the components correspond to noise. In the case of several QRST morphologies in the lead or non-regular QRST waveforms, other principal components will appear representing the different patterns or the dynamics of the QRST waveforms. Castells et al. (2005) estimate the AA reconstructing the atrial subspace from the projections of the non-ventricular components:

$$\mathbf{s}_{AA} = \mathbf{V}_{AA}\mathbf{z} \tag{5}$$

Other application of PCA to extract the AA in single-lead ECGs is presented by Alcaraz & Rieta (2008). They calculate the singular value decomposition of a matrix containing N QRST complexes of the analyzed lead with L samples each one. They use the first non-normalized principal component as a QRST template to cancel out VA with a previous amplitude adaptation between each QRST complex and the template. The method also avoids sudden transitions at the beginning or the end of each QRST segment provoked by the subtraction of the template to each individual complex.

4. Atrial Fibrillation Extraction in the Frequency Domain

Considering the aforementioned approaches to extract the atrial activity, the specific characteristics of the target signal, i.e., the F-waves, are not included in the separation process. In fact, the spectrum of the F-waves that characterizes this signal is a key feature to distinguish between AF and other non fibrillatory rhythms. Llinares & Igual (2009) presented two algorithms that exploits this discriminative frequency information of the atrial rhythm, focusing only on the extraction of the atrial component in a more effective and simpler manner.
The blind source extraction of the atrial component $y_A(t)$ is:

$$y_A(t) = \mathbf{b}^T\mathbf{x}(t) \tag{6}$$

The recorded signals are first whitened by PCA in order to reduce the dimensions of the problem, to exhaust the use of the second order statistics and to assure that all the sources have the same variance: $\mathbf{z}(t) = \mathbf{V}\mathbf{x}(t)$, where $\mathbf{V}$ is the NxM whitening matrix, so $E\{\mathbf{z}(t)\mathbf{z}(t)^T\} = \mathbf{I}$. The new problem reads:

$$y_A(t) = \mathbf{w}^T\mathbf{z}(t) \tag{7}$$

with the restriction $\mathbf{w}^T\mathbf{w} = 1$ (to assure unit power signals). The aim is to estimate $y_A(t)$, i.e., the recovering unit norm vector $\mathbf{w}$, maximizing the independence using HOS-based or SOS-based ICA algorithms and at the same time looking for a signal that is as close as possible to the known spectral properties of the atrial signal. This implies the addition to the independence criterion (HOS or SOS) of a new term that models prior information. The new combined cost function to be maximized can be expressed as $J(\mathbf{w}) = J_1(\mathbf{w}) + \lambda J_2(\mathbf{w})$. The first term, $J_1(\mathbf{w})$, is the ICA only contrast function; it is maximum when a (independent) source is extracted. The second term, $J_2(\mathbf{w})$, models the prior information about the spectral content of the atrial signal. It is maximum when the extracted signal corresponds to the F-

waves that define the atrial signal. The tradeoff between the ICA term and the prior is controlled by the parameter λ that is experimentally adjusted.
The mathematical formulation of the power spectral density information about the atrial waveform corresponds to the integral of the power spectrum in the proper range of frequencies:

$$J_2(\mathbf{w}) = \int_{f_1}^{f_2} \phi_y(f)df \quad (8)$$

where $\phi_y(f)$ is the power spectrum of the recovered signal $y(t)$. It is maximum for the atrial activity $y_A(t)$; the interval of integration $[f_1, f_2]$ depends on prior information about the patient and the criterion to fix the bandwidth. This interval is calculated from a central frequency f_c (maximum of the power spectral density function) and a bandwidth $2B$: $f_1 = f_c - B$ and $f_2 = f_c + B$.
The estimation of the central frequency must be first addressed. Llinares & Igual (2009) propose a simple procedure for the estimation of the peak frequency. First, starting from leads V1 or II (they have the largest ratio of atrial to ventricular signal amplitude (Petrutiu et al., 2006)), the time intervals where there is no QRST complex are extracted, i.e., the signal corresponding only to the T-Q intervals is obtained; second, these T-Q segments are joined smoothly; third, the spectrum of the new signal composed of only T-Q fragments is calculated; fourth, the peak frequency is obtained as the maximum of the FFT in the interval of frequencies 3-9 Hz. Another option for estimating the initial peak frequency is to follow the procedure described by Sassi et al. (2007). From leads V1 or II, the time intervals of the QRST complex (QT intervals) are eliminated and a spectral analysis of the rest of the signal (T-Q interval) is made with a method appropriate for unevenly sampled data, the Lomb-Scargle periodogram (Flannery et al., 1988). Although the automated measurement of the QT interval in atrial fibrillation episodes is complex (Pai & Rawles, 1989), satisfactory results were obtained applying a simple rule based on Bazzet formula (Bazzet, 1997) and fixing $QT_c = 550$ ms (Sassi et al. 2007).

4.1 Atrial Activity Extraction based on HOS

The HOS-ICA cost function $J_1(\mathbf{w})$ chosen is the approximation of the negentropy given by Hyvarinen (1999):

$$J_{HOS}(u) \,\alpha\, \left(E[g(u)] - E[g(u_G)]\right)^2 \quad (9)$$

where E is the expectation operator, u is a random variable, u_G is a Gaussian with the same variance of u and g is the non linear function $g(u) = \frac{1}{a_1}\log\cosh(a_1 u)$ with $1 \le a_1 \le 2$.

This non-linear function is a good general-purpose contrast function that avoids possible problems of outliers associated with the kurtosis based contrast function. The final formulation of the optimization problem is:

$$\arg\max_{\mathbf{w}}\left(\left(E[g(y)]-E[g(y_G)]\right)^2+\lambda\int_{f_1}^{f_2}\phi_y(f)df\right)\quad \textit{subject to } \mathbf{w}^T\mathbf{w}=1 \tag{10}$$

where the spectrum $\phi_y(f)$ is estimated by means of the periodogram.

The final updating rule consists of two terms. The first one corresponds to the independence criterion, i.e., the negentropy term (Hyvarinen, 1999). The second one implements the optimization of the cost function corresponding to the prior information. See (Llinares & Igual, 2009) for details in the optimization process:

$$\begin{aligned}&\mathbf{w}\leftarrow E\left[\mathbf{z}\tanh\left(a_1\mathbf{w}^T\mathbf{z}\right)\right]-E\left[a_1\left(1-\tanh^2\left(a_1\mathbf{w}^T\mathbf{z}\right)\right)\right]\mathbf{w}+\lambda(\mathbf{C}\mathbf{w}+\mathbf{C}^T\mathbf{w}),\quad \mathrm{C}=\frac{1}{N}\sum_{i=I_1}^{I_2}\mathbf{Z}\boldsymbol{\omega}_i\boldsymbol{\omega}_i^{*T}\mathbf{Z}^T\\&\mathbf{w}\leftarrow\mathbf{w}/\|\mathbf{w}\|\end{aligned} \tag{11}$$

where $[I_1,I_2]$ is the interval of digital frequencies corresponding to $[f_1,f_2]$ and $\mathbf{Z}=[\mathbf{z}(0),\mathbf{z}(1),\ldots,\mathbf{z}(N-1)]$ is the matrix of whitened observations. The second step of the algorithm enforces that $\mathbf{w}$ is a unit norm vector, a necessary condition in order to maintain the unit variance of the recovered source.

4.2 Atrial Activity Extraction based on SOS

The SOS-ICA cost function $J_1(\mathbf{w})$ chosen consists in a "sequential diagonalization" of the autocovariance matrices (Li et al., 2007). The cost function to be maximized is:

$$J_{SOS}\left(\mathbf{w},\mathbf{t},d_0,d_1,\ldots,d_Q\right)=-\sum_{\tau=0}^{Q}\left\|\mathbf{R}_\tau\mathbf{w}-d_\tau\mathbf{t}\right\|^2 \tag{12}$$

where $R_\tau=E\left[\mathbf{z}(t)\mathbf{z}^T(t-\tau)\right],\tau=0,1,\ldots,Q$ are $Q+1$ autocorrelation matrices of the whitened mixtures, $d_0,d_1,\ldots,d_Q$ are $Q+1$ unknown scalars, and $\|\cdot\|$ denotes the Euclidean length of vectors. In order to avoid the trivial solution, the constraints $\|\mathbf{t}\|=1$ and $\left\|\left[d_0,d_1,\ldots,d_Q\right]\right\|=1$ are imposed. One source is perfectly extracted when $\mathbf{R}_\tau\mathbf{w}=d_\tau\mathbf{t}$, since $\mathbf{t}$ is collinear with one column vector in $\mathbf{A}$, and $\mathbf{w}$ is orthogonal to the other $K-1$ column vectors in $\mathbf{A}$. The final formulation of the optimization problem is:

$$\arg\max_{\mathbf{w}}\left(-\sum_{\tau=0}^{Q}\left\|\mathbf{R}_\tau\mathbf{w}-d_\tau\mathbf{t}\right\|^2+\lambda\int_{f_1}^{f_2}\phi_y(f)df\right),\quad \text{subject to } \mathbf{w}^T\mathbf{w}=1 \tag{13}$$

The final updating rule consists of three steps. The first one adjusts the independence criterion together with the implementation of the prior information. The second one adjusts the value of $\mathbf{d}$ and the third one adjusts the value of $\mathbf{t}$. The final algorithm reads (see (Llinares & Igual, 2009) for details in the optimization process):

$$
\begin{aligned}
&(i)\quad \mathbf{w} \leftarrow \mathbf{T}\left(\sum_{\tau=0}^{Q} d_\tau \mathbf{R}_\tau\right)\mathbf{t} + \lambda\left(\mathbf{C}\mathbf{w} + \mathbf{C}^T\mathbf{w}\right), \quad \mathbf{T} = \left[\sum_{\tau=0}^{Q} \mathbf{R}_\tau^2\right]^{-1}; \ \mathbf{C} = \frac{1}{N}\sum_{i=I_1}^{I_2} \mathbf{Z}\boldsymbol{\omega}_i \boldsymbol{\omega}_i^{*T}\mathbf{Z}^T \\
&\qquad \mathbf{w} \leftarrow \mathbf{w} / \|\mathbf{w}\| \\
&(ii)\quad \mathbf{d} = \left[(\mathbf{R}_0\mathbf{w})^T\mathbf{t}, (\mathbf{R}_1\mathbf{w})^T\mathbf{t}, \ldots, (\mathbf{R}_Q\mathbf{w})^T\mathbf{t}\right]^T \qquad (14) \\
&\qquad \left[d_0, d_1, \ldots, d_Q\right] \leftarrow \mathbf{d} / \|\mathbf{d}\| \\
&(iii)\quad \mathbf{v} = \sum_{\tau=0}^{Q} d_\tau \mathbf{R}_\tau \mathbf{w} \\
&\qquad \mathbf{t} \leftarrow \mathbf{v} / \|\mathbf{v}\|
\end{aligned}
$$

5. Quality Parameters in Atrial Activity Extraction

To quantify the quality of the extraction with real ECG recordings is not a simple task. In fact, the problem is unsolvable: the true atrial signal is an unobserved random process that is only measured mixed with not only the QRST complexes, but other biologic and non biologic signals, such as 60 (50) Hz powerline interference, instrumentation noise, baseline drift and wander or electromyogram. It makes impossible to compare the residual ECG with the real one, so it is not possible to obtain the typical measures of error in signal processing such as the mean squared error (MSE) or correlation coefficients. As a consequence, the quality of the extraction (bad-good) cannot be quantified with a distance measure from the real solution. This section reviews some of the most extended measures found in the literature and proposes two new quality indexes.

5.1 Parameters Defined in the Frequency Domain

Two parameters in the AA extraction are defined in the frequency domain: the peak frequency and the spectral concentration around the peak frequency.
The peak frequency is defined as the frequency at which the power spectral density is the highest in the 3 - 10 Hz band. It is not really a quality measurement by itself, but a parameter to characterize the AA. The dispersion of its value when we apply the different algorithms can be used to assure the goodness of the extraction.
The Spectral Concentration (SC) is defined as (Castells et al., 2005a):

$$
SC = \frac{\int_{0.82 f_p}^{1.17 f_p} P_A(f)df}{\int_0^\infty P_A(f)df} \qquad (15)
$$

where $P_A(f)$ is the power spectrum of the extracted atrial signal and f_p the main peak frequency. SC is a measure of the relative power contained in the narrow band around the peak frequency. This means that when we compare different algorithms applied to the same patient, a higher SC value indicates a better extraction of the atrial F-waves.
We propose another index that explains the kind of noise present in the estimated signal. For every patient, the true atrial signal has an unknown peak frequency and SC value. This

is equivalent to say that, assuming the bandwidth of the atrial signal from 3 to 10 Hz, every patient has a centroid frequency, defined such as:

$$f_c = \frac{\int_3^{10} f \cdot S_{y_A}(f)df}{\int_3^{10} S_{y_A}(f)df} \tag{16}$$

The centroid frequency measures the form of the distribution of the spectrum over the bandwidth of the atrial signal. If the SC is very large, it should be close to the peak frequency. If not, the centroid frequency will move in the frequency direction where there is more power. Remember that the spectrum of the ventricular activity includes frequencies above the 10 Hz and below 3 Hz. With respect to other non atrial signals, their spectrum is also known in advance, e.g., the high frequency powerline interference or the low frequency breathing. We propose an index that measures the centroid frequency displacement when we calculate the centroid frequency of the estimated atrial rhythm considering the atrial bandwidth or the full range of frequencies. It will give us an idea about the kind of noise remaining:

$$\hat{I}_l = \frac{\int_3^{10} f \cdot S_{y_A}(f)df}{\int_0^{10} f \cdot S_{y_A}(f)df} \tag{17}$$

$$\hat{I}_h = \frac{\int_3^{10} f \cdot S_{y_A}(f)df}{\int_3^{\infty} f \cdot S_{y_A}(f)df} \tag{18}$$

In the case of perfect atrial estimation, both indexes equals to one. If not, the indexes are lower than one. A value close to one means a better estimation. In addition, it gives us information about the kind of noise. For example, $\hat{I}_h$ will be large for an algorithm that does not cancel the powerline interference.

5.2 Parameters Defined in the Time Domain

Four parameters in the AA extraction are defined in the time domain: the ventricular residue, the ventricular depolarization reduction, the percentage of significant QRS residua detected and the relations between amplitudes of the AA and the different segments of a reference lead in QT and TQ intervals.

The ventricular residue (VR) proposed by Alcaraz & Rieta (2008) permits to estimate ventricular residua in the extracted AA. VR is defined as:

$$VR_i = \frac{1}{\frac{1}{Q}\sum_{n=1}^{Q} y_A^2(n)} \sqrt{\frac{1}{2H+1}\sum_{k=r_i-H}^{r_i+H} y_A^2(k)} \cdot \max_{k=r_i-H \cdots k=r_i+H}\left(\left|y_A(k)\right|\right) \tag{19}$$

where $2H+1$ is the duration of the QRS interval in samples for a value of H corresponding to 50 ms. In this case, high values of VR indicate greater QRS residua, i.e., a poor AA extraction.

The ventricular depolarization reduction (VDR) measures the reduction of the R-peak amplitude achieved by the algorithm under evaluation (Rieta & Hornero, 2007). VDR is defined as:

$$VDR(dB) = 10\log\left(R_{RL} / R_{VR}\right) \tag{20}$$

where R_{RL} is the R-peak amplitude of a reference lead and R_{VR} is the R-peak amplitude of the recovered AA. High values of VDR indicate good performance of the algorithm.

Other parameter used to evaluate the quality of the atrial activity is the percentage of significant QRS residua detected (Lemay et al., 2007). The method identifies the significant ventricular residua comparing the absolute values of the QRS intervals with a threshold $\varsigma = m + 2\sigma$ where m is the median of the amplitude distribution of $y_A(t)$ and $\sigma = qr / 0.6745$ is the standard deviation estimated from the interquartile range qr of the amplitude distribution of $y_A(t)$. Those QRS complexes with absolute values above the threshold are considered as significant. Finally, the parameter is presented showing the percentage of significant QRS residua (PSQRS).

Langley et al. (2006) compared the amplitudes of the extracted atrial signal with a reference lead, V1, in QRST segments. In addition, they defined a reference atrial signal as the segments of V1 containing no ventricular activity and compared this reference atrial signal with noQRST and QRST segments of the extracted AA. The amplitude of each segment was the peak-to-peak amplitude.

The above parameters (VR, VDR and PSQRS) are designed for ABS methods. They only take into account the recovered atrial signal in QRST segments, ignoring the form of the signal in noQRST segments. Respect to the comparison of amplitudes, it can be carried out only with methods that do not modify the amplitude of the original signal. ICA and PCA returns signals with unit power, distorting the results when comparing the amplitudes of the signals.

We propose the kurtosis as quality measure of the atrial signal extraction. It considers the whole signal (QRST and noQRST segments) and it is valid for signals with unit power. The kurtosis of a subgaussian (supergaussian) random variable is negative (positive), allowing distinguish between atrial and ventricular activities. In the cases where the kurtosis of the atrial activity is marginally positive, it will be always lower than the ventricular activity. This property can also be extended to measure the quality of the atrial activity extraction. Since the atrial activity is near the Gaussian distribution, a high absolute value of the kurtosis means a poor extraction.

6. Results

In this section, we demonstrate the use of the new algorithms in the AA extraction and the accuracy of the proposed quality parameters compared with other quality parameters found in the literature.

We have used two different databases for a total amount of 50 patients. Ten belong to the "PTB Diagnostic ECG Database" from the MIT database Physionet (Goldberger et al., 2000). Each record includes 15 simultaneously measured signals: the conventional 12 leads together with the 3 Frank lead ECG. The other forty belong to a clinical database recorded at the Clinical University Hospital, Valencia, Spain, and were taken with a commercial recording system with 12 leads (Prucka Engineering Cardiolab system). For both databases, the signals are digitized at 1000 samples per second with a resolution of 16 bits.

In our experiments, we have used all the available leads for a period of 10 s for every patient. The signals were preprocessed in order to reduce the baseline wander, high frequency noise and power line interference for the later signal processing. The recordings were filtered with an 8 coefficients highpass Chebyshev filter and with a 3 coefficients lowpass Butterworth filter to select the bandwidth of interest: 0.5 – 40 Hz. In order to reduce the computational load, the data were downsampled to 200 samples per second with no significant changes in the quality of the results.

The detection of the R peak wave event is carried out by means of a parabolic fitting algorithm (Illanes Manriquez & Zhang, 2007). The power spectrum is obtained with the modified periodogram using the Welch-WOSA method with a Hamming window of 4096 points length, a 50% overlapping between adjacent windowed sections, and an 8192-point fast Fourier transform (FFT).

We use the following acronyms for the algorithms: cFastICA (constrained FastICA) corresponding to Eq. (11) and cSAD (constrained Sequential Approximate Diagonalization) to Eq. (14). The parameter λ is 4 for cFastICA and 2 for cSAD and the bandwidth used in both cases is ±0.85 Hz.

In Table 1 the results of the quality indexes in the frequency domain are shown. Note the agreement between the SC values and the centroid frequency indexes: cSAD obtains slightly better results in SC and I_l and I_h.

	cFastICA	*cSAD*
f_p (Hz)	5.543 ± 1.233	5.556 ± 1.247
SC	0.541 ± 0.149	0.555 ± 0.145
f_c (Hz)	5.604 ± 0.855	5.622 ± 0.885
I_l	0.945 ± 0.040	0.950 ± 0.045
I_h	0.565 ± 0.132	0.581 ± 0.125

Table 1. Quality indexes in the frequency domain

Figure 4 shows two examples of AA recovered from different patients by cFastICA (a) and cSAD (b) and their respective spectra (c) and (d) with the associated value of the peak frequency of each AA.

Figure 5 represents one example of AA with low value of I_l (a) and another one with low value of I_h (b) and their respective spectra (c) and (d) together with the values of the indexes. The first case presents low frequency content and the second case shows high frequency content.

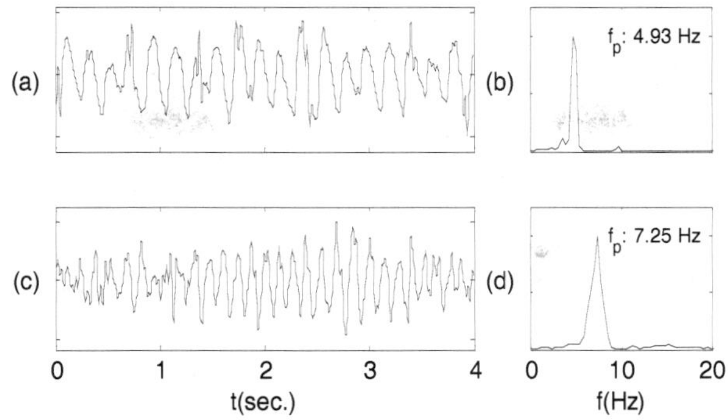

Fig. 4. Two examples of AA recovered by cFastICA (a) and cSAD (c), their spectra and the corresponding peak frequencies (b) and (d)

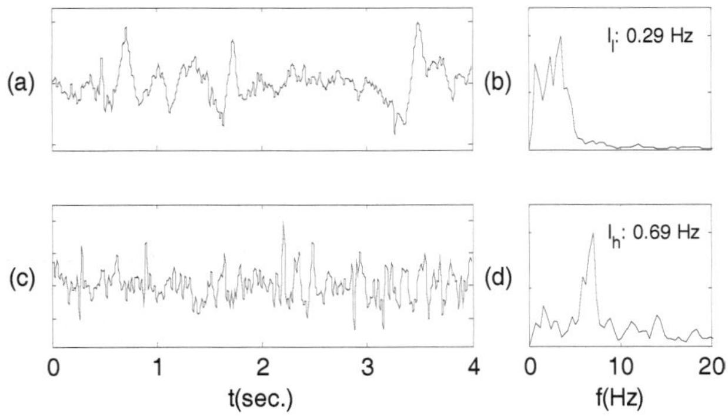

Fig. 5. (a) Atrial signal with low I_l value and its spectrum (b); (c) atrial signal with low I_h value and its spectrum (d)

Finally, we show a scatter plot of SC values and the indexes I_l (a) and I_h (b) for both methods in the Figure 6. Clearly, there exists a positive correlation between these parameters, i.e., both parameters increase together.

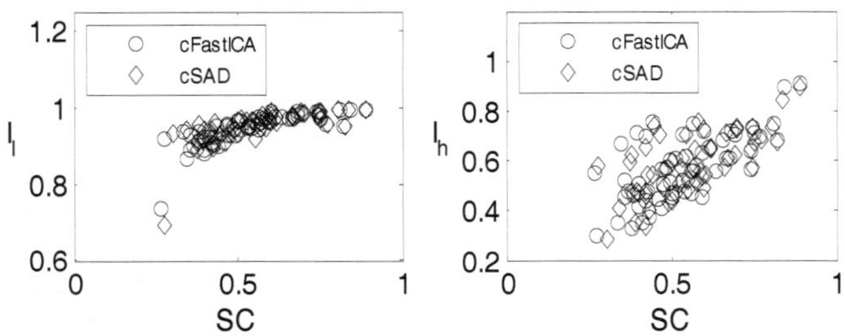

Fig. 6. Scatter plot between SC and the indexes I_l (left) and I_h (right) values

In the case of time domain quality indexes, for the sake of simplicity, we only use the parameter VR and the kurtosis. Table 2 summarizes the results obtained. Note the agreement between the VR values and the kurtosis: low values of kurtosis imply low values of VR.

	cFastICA	*cSAD*
VR	2.893 ± 1.051	3.129 ± 1.169
Kurtosis	-0.030 ± 0.648	0.219 ± 0.794

Table 2. Quality indexes in the time domain

In Figure 7 we analyze the effect of an extraction where the kurtosis of the estimated atrial signal is high (3.80), due to the presence of QRST residua near 0.6 seconds, 2 seconds and 3.5 seconds.

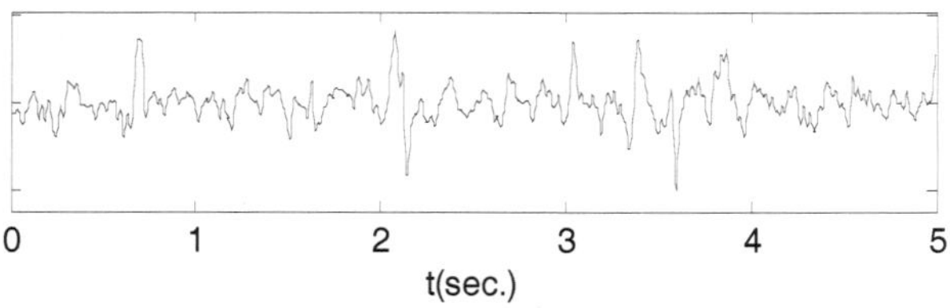

Fig. 7. Example of AA with high kurtosis value

Finally, Figure 8 represents the scatter plot between VR and kurtosis for both methods. The figure confirms the relation between the correct cancellation of the QRST complexes and the low values of the associated kurtosis.

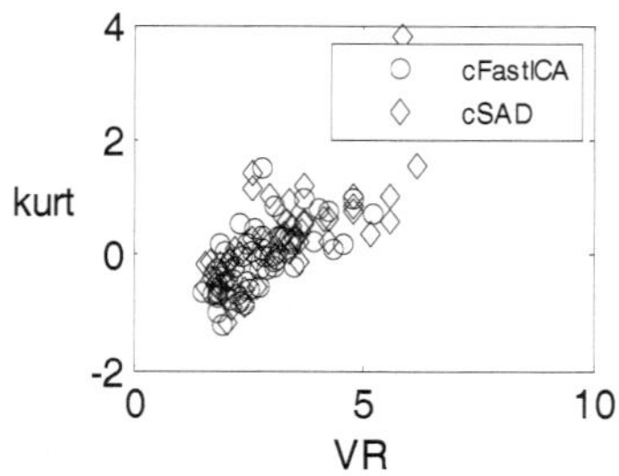

Fig. 8. Scatter plot between VR and kurtosis values

7. Conclusion

The extraction of the atrial signal in atrial fibrillation has attracted the attention of many researchers in the last years. We have reviewed the statement of the problem and the different approaches to solve it. We have shown how the traditional multilead solutions can be adapted considering the characteristics of the signals involved in the problem. In addition, we have paid attention to the difficult goal of how to measure the quality of the extraction since the solution (the true atrial rhythm) is unknown. We have presented some indexes that can help in order to analyze the goodness of the extraction.

8. Acknowledgments

The authors would like to thank Francisco Castells and Jose Millet for sharing the real AF database provided by the cardiologists Ricardo Ruiz and Roberto Garcia-Civera during the project TIC2002-00957.

9. References

Alcaraz, R. & Rieta, J. (2008). Adaptive singular value cancelation of ventricular activity in single-lead atrial fibrillation electrocardiograms. *Physiological Measurement*, Vol. 29, No. 12, 1351–1369, ISSN 0967-3334

Asano, Y.; Saito, J.; Matsumoto, K.; Kaneko, K.; Yamamoto, T. & Uchida, M. (1992). On the mechanism of termination and perpetuation of atrial fibrillation. *Am J Cardiol*, Vol. 69, No. 12, 1033–1038, ISSN 0002-9149

Bazzet, H. (1997). An analysis of the time-relations of electrocardiograms. *Annals of Noninvasive Electrocardiology*, Vol. 2, 177–194, ISSN 1082-720X

Castells, F.; Mora, C.; Rieta, J.; Moratal-Perez, D. & Millet, J. (2005). Estimation of atrial fibrillatory wave from single-lead atrial fibrillation electrocardiograms using principal component analysis concepts. *Medical and Biological Engineering and Computing*, Vol. 43, No. 5, 557– 560, ISSN 0140-0118

Castells, F.; Rieta, J.; Millet, J. & Zarzoso, V. (2005a). Spatiotemporal blind source separation approach to atrial activity estimation in atrial tachyarrhythmias. *IEEE Transactions on Biomedical Engineering*, Vol. 52, No. 2, 258– 267, ISSN 0018-9294

Flannery, B.; Press, W.; Teukolsky, S. & Vetterling, W. (1988). Numerical Recipes in C: The Art of Scientific Computing, *Cambridge University Press*, ISBN 0-521-43108-5

Fuster, V.; Ryden, L.E.; Asinger, R.W.; Cannom, D.S.; Crijns, H.J.; Frye, R.L.; et al (2001). ACC/AHA/ESC guidelines for the management of patients with atrial fibrillation: executive summary, *Circulation*, Vol. 104, 2118-2150, ISSN 0009-7322

Goldberger, A.L.; Amaral, L.A.N.; Glass, L, Hausdorff, J.M.; Ivanov, P.Ch.; Mark, R.G. et al. (2000). PhysioBank, PhysioToolkit, and PhysioNet: components of a new research resource for complex physiologic signals, *Circulation*, Vol. 101, 215-220, ISSN 0009-7322

Grubitzsch, H.; Modersohn, D.; Leuthold, T. & Konertz, W. (2008). Analysis of atrial fibrillatory activity from high-resolution surface electrocardiograms: Evaluation and application of a new system, *Experimental & Clinical Cardiology*, Vol. 13, No. 1, 29-35, ISSN 1205-6626

Hyvarinen, A. (1999). Fast and robust fixed point algorithms for independent component analysis. *IEEE Transactions on Neural Networks*, Vol. 10, No. 3, 626–634, ISSN 1045-9227

Hyvarinen, A.; Karhunen, J. & Oja, E. (2001). Independent Component Analysis, *Wiley*, ISBN 0-471-22131-7

Igual, J.; Llinares, R.; Guillem, M. & Millet, J. (2006). Optimal Localization of Leads in Atrial Fibrillation Episodes. *Proceedings of IEEE International Conference on Acoustics, Speech and Signal Processing, Vol. 2,* pp. 1192-1195, ISBN 1-4244-0469-X

Illanes Manriquez, A. & Zhang, Q. (2007). An algorithm for QRS onset and offset detection in single lead electrocardiogram records. *Proceedings of Annual International Conference of the IEEE Engineering in Medicine and Biology Society,* pp. 541-544, ISBN 0-14244-0788-5

Langley, P.; Bourke, J. & Murray, A. (2000). Frequency analysis of atrial fibrillation. *Proceedings of Computers in Cardiology,* pp. 65-68, ISBN 0-7803-6557-7, Cambridge, MA, USA

Langley, P.; Rieta, J.; Stridh, M.; Millet, J.; Sornmo, L. & Murray, A. (2006). Comparison of atrial signal extraction algorithms in 12-lead ECGs with atrial fibrillation. *IEEE Transactions on Biomedical Engineering,* Vol. 53, No. 2, 343–346, ISSN 0018-9294

Lemay, M.; Vesin, J.; van Oosterom, A.; Jacquemet, V. & Kappenberger, L. (2007). Cancellation of Ventricular Activity in the ECG: Evaluation of Novel and Existing Methods. *IEEE Transactions on Biomedical Engineering,* Vol. 54, No. 3, 542–546, ISSN 0018-9294

Li, X. & Zhang, X. (2007). Sequential Blind Extraction Adopting Second-Order Statistics. *IEEE Signal Processing Letters,* Vol. 14, No. 1, 58–61, ISSN 1070-9908

Llinares, R. & Igual, J. (2009). Application of constrained independent component analysis algorithms in electrocardiogram arrhythmias. *Artificial Intelligence in Medicine,* Vol., No., (to appear) page numbers (to appear), ISSN 0933-3657

Llinares, R.; Igual, J.; Millet, J. & Guillem, M. (2006). Independent component analysis of body surface potential mapping recordings with atrial fibrillation. *Proceedings of International Joint Conference on Neural Networks,* pp. 2287-2294, ISBN 0-7803-9490-9

Manios, E.; Kanoupakis, E.; Chlouverakis, G.; Kaleboubas, M.; Mavrakis, H. & Vardas, P. (2000). Changes in atrial electrical properties following cardioversion of chronic atrial fibrillation: relation with recurrence. *Cardiovascular Research,* Vol. 47, No. 2, 244-253, ISSN 0008-6363

Petrutiu, S.; Ng, J.; Nijm, G.; Al-Angari, H.; Swiryn, S. & Sahakian, A. (2006). Atrial fibrillation and waveform characterization, *IEEE Engineering in Medicine and Biology Magazine,* Vol. 25, No. 6, 24–30, ISSN 0739-5175

Pai, G. & Rawles, J. (1989). The QT interval in atrial fibrillation, *British Medical Journal,* Vol. 61, 510–513, ISSN 0959-8138

Raine, D.; Langley, P.; Murray, A.; Dunuwille, A. & Bourke J.P. (2004). Surface atrial frequency analysis in patients with atrial fibrillation: a tool for evaluating the effects of intervention. *J Cardiovasc Electrophysiol,* Vol. 15, No. 9, 1021–1026, ISSN 1045-3873

Rieta, J.; Castells, F.; Sanchez, C.; Zarzoso, V. & Millet, J. (2004). Atrial activity extraction for atrial analysis using blind source separation. *IEEE Transactions on Biomedical Engineering,* Vol. 51, No. 7, 1176– 1186, ISSN 0018-9294

Rieta, J. & Hornero (2007). Comparative study of methods for ventricular activity cancellation in atrial electrograms of atrial fibrillation. *Physiological Measurement,* Vol. 28, 925–936, ISSN 0967-3334

Sassi, R.; Corino, V. & Maniardi, L. (2007). Analysis of surface atrial signals using spectral methods for time series with missing data. *Proceedings of Computers in Cardiology*, pp. 153-156, ISBN: 978-1-4244-2533-4

Slocum, J.; Sahakian, A. & Swiryn, S. (1992). Diagnosis of atrial fibrillation from surface electrocardiograms based on computer-detected atrial activity. *Journal of electrocardiology*, Vol. 25, No. 1, 1–8, ISSN 0022-0736

Shkurovich, S.; Sahakian, A. & Swiryn, S. (1998). Detection of atrial activity from high-voltage leads of implantable ventricular defibrillators using a cancellation technique, *IEEE Engineering in Medicine and Biology Magazine*, Vol. 45, No. 2, 229–234, ISSN 0739-5175

Stambler, B.; Wood, M.; Ellenbogen, K. (1997). Antiarrhythmic actions of intravenous ibutilide compared with procainamide during human atrial flutter and fibrillation electrophysiological determinants of enhanced conversion efficacy. *Circulation*, Vol. 96, No. 12, 4298–4306, ISSN 0009-7322

Stridh, M.; Bollmann, A.; Olsson, S. & Sornmo, L. (2006): Detection and feature extraction of atrial tachyarrhythmias: a three stage method of time-frequency analysis. , *IEEE Engineering in Medicine and Biology Magazine*, Vol. 25, No. 6, 31–39, ISSN 0739-5175

Automatic Mutual Nonrigid Registration of Dense Surface Models by Graphical Model based Inference

Xiao Dong and Guoyan Zheng
ARTORG Center - ISTB, University of Bern
Switzerland
Email:guoyan.zheng@ieee.org

1. Introduction

Fully automatic nonrigid registration of shapes is highly desired for computer vision and medical image processing. For a nonrigid registration between two shapes $Shape_A$ and $Shape_B$, the ultimate goal should be to find the correspondence between subparts of the two shapes instead of to achieve a *perfect* match by applying a forced deformation without constraints on the objects. Such a correspondence assignment is usually defined and achieved as an optimization problem with a cost function abstracted as $H(S_A(\mathbf{Q}_A), S_B(Q_B), \mathbf{T}_{A\rightarrow B}, \mathbf{C}_{A\rightarrow B})$ to measure the difference of the two matched shapes, where $S_A(\mathbf{Q}_A)$ and $S_B(\mathbf{Q}_B)$ are the shape descriptors of S_A and S_B with shape parameters $\mathbf{Q}_A$ and $\mathbf{Q}_B$ in their own representation spaces, $\mathbf{T}_{A\rightarrow B}$ is a nonrigid transformation between the spatial coordinate spaces of the two shapes, and $\mathbf{C}_{A\rightarrow B}$ is the correspondence assignment between the subparts of the two shapes.

There are two ways to define the cost function $H(S_A(\mathbf{Q}_A), S_B(Q_B), \mathbf{T}_{A\rightarrow B}, \mathbf{C}_{A\rightarrow B})$. In the *robust point matching* (RPM), *active shape model*(ASM), *active appearance model* (AAM) (Cootes and Taylor, 2004), and nonrigid shape matching algorithms using the level set based contour and surface representation (Xu et al., 2001), shape signature harmonic embedding (Lee et al., 2006) and Gaussian mixture based shape models (Roy et al., 2007)(Jiang et al., 2007), the cost function is defined as

$$\begin{aligned} & H(S_A(\mathbf{Q}_A), S_B(Q_B), \mathbf{T}_{A\rightarrow B}, \mathbf{C}_{A\rightarrow B}) \\ = \;& E_{diff}(\mathbf{Q}_A), S_B(Q_B), \mathbf{T}_{A\rightarrow B}, \mathbf{C}_{A\rightarrow B}) + \gamma E_{deform}(\mathbf{T}_{A\rightarrow B}) \end{aligned} \quad (1)$$

where $E_{diff}(S_A(\mathbf{Q}_A), S_B(Q_B), \mathbf{T}_{A\rightarrow B}, \mathbf{C}_{A\rightarrow B})$ is a measurement of the shape difference between the *aligned* shapes with the nonrigid transformation $\mathbf{T}_{A\rightarrow B}$ and the correspondence assignment $\mathbf{C}_{A\rightarrow B}$, $E_{deform}(\mathbf{T}_{A\rightarrow B})$ defines the *bending energy* of the nonrigid deformation $\mathbf{T}_{A\rightarrow B}$ and γ is a factor to balance the two terms. The advantage of this approach is that both the shape difference and the bending energy are explicitly expressed and we have a wide freedom to select their definitions with different underlying physical pictures. The disadvantage is that the explicit representations of $\mathbf{T}_{A\rightarrow B}$ and $\mathbf{C}_{A\rightarrow B}$ are iteratively defined on each other, i.e., a $\mathbf{T}_{A\rightarrow B}$ can only be defined on a given $\mathbf{C}_{A\rightarrow B}$ and vice versa. This usually results in that $\mathbf{T}_{A\rightarrow B}$ and $\mathbf{C}_{A\rightarrow B}$ can only be updated iteratively during the optimization. Such an optimization strategy can only converge to local optima and it usually asks for a proper initialization.

In the shape context (Belongie et al., 2002), the spectral decomposition (Jain and Zhang, 2006) and graphical model based registration algorithms (Coughlan and Ferreira, 2002)(Caetano et al., 2004)(Rangarajan et al., 2003), both the shape difference and the bending energy of the nonrigid deformation are defined implicitly, where both of them are encoded in the relative positions between correspondent landmarks of the shapes. In such an approach, the optimization procedure aims to directly find the optimal correspondence assignment $\mathbf{C}_{A\to B}$ and the nonrigid transformation $\mathbf{T}_{A\to B}$ never appears during the optimization. The advantage of this approach is that it can lead to a fully automatic registration since the optimization does no rely on an explicit transformation $\mathbf{T}_{A\to B}$ between the two shape. The disadvantage is that usually this approach is computational expensive. In (Coughlan and Ferreira, 2002)(Caetano et al., 2004)(Zhang and Seitz, 2005)(Sun et al., 2003), graphical model based Bayesian inference was used for the purpose of point set matching, image segmentation and stereo matching. In (Xiao et al., 2007), this idea was also explored for the purpose of surface matching. One limitation of the work of (Xiao et al., 2007) is that it only matches shapes with the same number of landmarks and assumed that a correspondence assignment between the landmarks of these two shapes can always be achieved. The optimization procedure to find the optimal correspondence assignment was achieved by Gibbs sampling, which may not be efficient to explore the whole configuration space (Gibbs, 2000) and therefore apt to local optima.

This paper will explore the idea of graphical model based approach for the nonrigid surface matching of two dense surfaces. The main contributions of this paper are: (a) A cost function, which is immune to rigid transformations and robust to nonrigid shape deformations, is used to measure the difference between shapes; (b) Belief propagation is used in the optimization procedure to find the optimal correspondence assignment, which can converge efficiently for our registration purpose; (c) A hierarchical matching strategy is proposed so that it can on one hand reduce the computational complexity and on the other hand, during the matching we can always assign a sparse surface to a denser surface so that the existence of correspondent landmarks can be ensured; and (d) A parallel graphical model is constructed so that the two surfaces will mutually register to each other and also exchange local assignment information during the registration, which can accelerate the convergence of the optimization procedure and overcome local optima.

2. Graphical model based nonrigid surface matching

2.1 The cost function for nonrigid surface matching

The inputs of our system are two dense triangulated surfaces $Surf_A$,$Surf_B$ with N_A and N_B ($N_A \approx N_B$) triangle faces respectively. The surfaces can be described as $\mathbf{S}_A = [\mathbf{s}_A^0, \mathbf{s}_A^1, \ldots, \mathbf{s}_A^{N_A-1}]$ and $\mathbf{S}_B = [\mathbf{s}_B^0, \mathbf{s}_B^1, \ldots, \mathbf{s}_B^{N_B-1}]$ respectively, where $\mathbf{s}_A^i = [\mathbf{x}_A^i, \mathbf{n}_A^i]$ ($\mathbf{s}_B^i = [\mathbf{x}_B^i, \mathbf{n}_B^i]$) stands for the 3d position of the center and the normal direction of the ith face of $Surf_A(Surf_B)$.

For each landmark $\mathbf{s}_A^i$ on the surface $Surf_A$, we can compute a *shape signature* $\mathbf{d}_A^i$ of the landmark at the ith face of $Surf_A$ as

$$\mathbf{d}_A^i = [\mathbf{d}_A^{i,0}, \ldots, \mathbf{d}_A^{i,j}, \ldots, \mathbf{d}_A^{i,N_A-1}]_{j\neq i}, \mathbf{d}_A^{i,j} = [D_A^{i,j}, A_A^{i,j}, AL_A^{i,j}], \tag{2}$$

where $D_A^{i,j} = \|\mathbf{x}_A^i - \mathbf{x}_A^j\|$ is the spatial distance of landmark $\mathbf{s}_A^i$ and $\mathbf{s}_A^j$, $A_A^{i,j}$ is the angle between the normal directions $\mathbf{n}_A^i, \mathbf{n}_A^j$ of the two faces and $AL_A^{i,j}$ is the angle between the normal direction $\mathbf{n}_A^i$ and the vector connecting $\mathbf{x}_A^i$ and $\mathbf{x}_A^j$ as shown in Fig. 1(a). This shape descriptor measures the distances and angles between landmarks and vectors, therefore a spatial

shape $Surf_A(Surf_B)$ can be fully determined by the collection of all these shape signatures $\{\mathbf{d}^i_A\}(\{\mathbf{d}^i_B\})$. This shape descriptor is immune to rigid transformations. In the case of a nonrigid deformation, the landmarks and normal vectors can be regarded as connected by elastic strings and the deviation of these values can then be understood as the bending energy of the deformation. Therefore this descriptor can also handle nonrigid shape deformations.
Without losing any generality, we consider the case to register S_A to S_B. Given the shape descriptors $\{\mathbf{d}^i_A\}$ and $\{\mathbf{d}^i_B\}$, the difference between two surfaces with a given correspondence assignment between the landmarks of the surfaces $C_{A\to B}(i) = j, i = 0,1,\ldots,N_A, j = 0,1,\ldots,N_B$ can then be written as

$$H(S_A,S_B,C_{A\to B}) = \sum_i (\mathbf{d}^i_A - \widetilde{\mathbf{d}}^i_B)\Lambda(\mathbf{d}^i_A - \widetilde{\mathbf{d}}^i_B)^T \tag{3}$$

where $\widetilde{\mathbf{d}}^i_B = [\mathbf{d}_B^{C_{A\to B}(i),C_{A\to B}(0)},\ldots,\mathbf{d}_B^{C_{A\to B}(i),C_{A\to B}(j)},\ldots,\mathbf{d}_B^{C_{A\to B}(i),C_{A\to B}(N_B-1)}]$,
$\Lambda = Diag(\sigma_D^2,\sigma_A^2,\sigma_{AL}^2,\ldots,\sigma_D^2,\sigma_A^2,\sigma_{AL}^2)^{-1}$ is the covariance matrix to balance the strengths of the elastic strings that connect the landmarks. The cost function measures the difference between the shape descriptor of S_A and the shape descriptor of S_B at the correspondent landmarks.

2.2 Graphical model based correspondence assignment optimization

For the purpose of defining a 3-dimensional surface, the cost function in (3) is over-determined since its underlying graph G is a complete graph. In (Caetano et al., 2004), the authors indicated that to determine a rigid shape in $\mathbb{R}^d$, the minimal underlying graph G is *k-tree* in $\mathbb{R}^d$. A denser graph topology will improve the robustness of the representation to keep the shape with the expense of a higher computational cost. Define a graph $G = \{V,E\}$ with N_A vertices, $V = \{v_i\}$ with each vertex correspondent to one landmark in S_A and $E = \{e_{ij}\}$ with $e_{ij} = 1$ if there is an edge connecting v_i and v_j. Then a generalized representation of (3) can be given as

$$\begin{aligned} H_G(S_A,S_B,C_{A\to B}) &= \textstyle\sum_{i,j,e_{ij}=1} E_A^{i,j}(C_{A\to B}) \\ &= \textstyle\sum_{i,j,e_{ij}=1} (\mathbf{d}^{i,j}_A - \widetilde{\mathbf{d}}^{i,j}_B)\Lambda'(\mathbf{d}^{i,j}_A - \widetilde{\mathbf{d}}^{i,j}_B)^T \end{aligned} \tag{4}$$

where $\widetilde{\mathbf{d}}^{i,j}_B = \mathbf{d}_B^{C_{A\to B}(i),C_{A\to B}(j)}$, $\Lambda' = Diag(\sigma_D^2,\sigma_A^2,\sigma_{AL}^2)^{-1}$.
Accordingly a distribution $p(H_G) = \prod_{i,j,e_{ij}=1} \exp(-E_A^{i,j}(C_{A\to B}))$ can be defined and represented by a graphical model as shown in Fig. 1(b). Each vertex v^i_A represents a landmark $\mathbf{s}^i_A$ of S_A and its state is a vector $sv^i_A = [p_A^{i,0},\ldots,p_A^{i,N_B-1}]$ representing the probabilities that $\mathbf{s}^i_A$ is assigned as the correspondent landmark of the landmarks of S_B. Vertices $\{v^j_B\}$ stands for the the landmarks in S_B and its state is a vector $sv^j_B = [p_B^{j,0},\ldots,p_B^{j,N_A-1}]$ representing that $\mathbf{s}^j_B$ should be the correspondence of each landmark in S_A. The vertices $\{v^i_A\}$ are connected according to the topology of G. The potentials between $\{v^i_A\}$ encode probabilities as $\psi_A(i,j) = \exp(-\beta E_A^{i,j}(C_{A\to B}))$, where $\beta = 1/\tau$ is the inverse of the annealing temperature τ. The optimization to find the optimal correspondence assignment can then be formalized as a ML estimation to find the peak of $p(H_G)$, which can be achieved by graphical model based Bayesian inference (Coughlan and Ferreira, 2002)(Caetano et al., 2004)(Zhang and Seitz, 2005)(Sun et al., 2003). In our method, the Bayesian inference is achieved by running the belief propagation (Coughlan and Ferreira, 2002) on the graphical model as given in Fig. 1(b). When

the belief propagation converges, the state sv_A^i is then the marginal distribution of the assignment of vertex v_A^i. If the annealing template τ is low enough, then $\{sv_A^i\}$ will give a unique peak which indicates the global optimum correspondence assignment for the matching.

3. Graphical model based hierarchical mutual surface registration

It can be observed that the above described graphical model based nonrigid surface matching faces three difficulties

- The existence of correspondence assignment: In our algorithm description, we assume that the correspondent landmarks for each landmark of $Surf_A$ can always be (*uniquely*) found on $Surf_B$. For a general case where $N_A \approx N_B$, this can not always be satisfied.
- The computational complexity: To matching two surfaces with N_A and N_B faces, the computational complexity of each belief propagation iteration is $\mathcal{O}(\kappa N_A N_B^2)$, where κ is a factor related with the topology of the graphical model. The proposed algorithm is quite computational expensive for practical cases.
- The unbalanced information processing structure: In the graphical model based surface matching, the two surfaces play different roles. The graphical model is built on $Surf_A$ and the shape descriptors of the two surfaces are explored in different ways. Such an unbalanced information processing structure may lead to local optima as in the classic ICP based registration, where the correspondence is achieved by finding closest points from one data set to another. In an ideal surface matching solution, the two surfaces should be dealt with equivalently.

To overcome the above mentioned difficulties, we proposed a hierarchical mutual registration strategy, in which

- A hierarchical shape descriptor is used to describe each surface. In such a hierarchical structure, we can always match a sparse surface to a dense surface so that the existence of correspondence can be ensured.
- The computational cost on the hierarchical shape descriptor can be greatly reduced due to the fact that the matching results at coarse levels can be used as initializations for the finer levels so that the possible configurations of each landmark at finer levels can be greatly reduced.

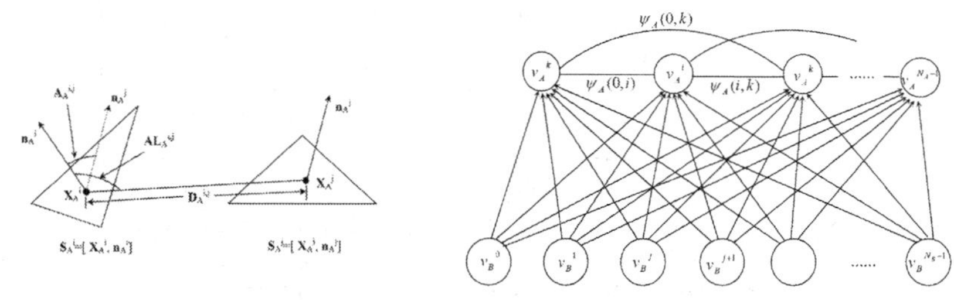

(a) The definition of the shape signature at each face of the surface

(b) The graphical models for belief propagation based nonrigid surface matching

Fig. 1. The graphical models for the registration of two surfaces taking $Surf_A$ as the template

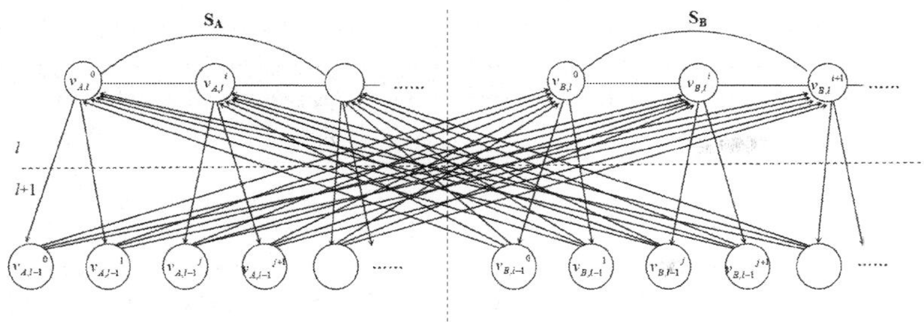

Fig. 2. The graphical model for parallel mutual registration of two hierarchically represented surfaces

- A parallel graphical model is used to achieve mutual matching of the two surfaces. During the matching procedure, the local matching result of each surface can be exchanged between surfaces so that it's more robust to local optima.

3.1 Hierarchical shape descriptors of triangulated surface meshes

To reduce the computational cost, a hierarchical coarse-to-fine strategy is used to represent each surface in L levels as $\{\mathbf{S}_{A,L-1},\ldots,\mathbf{S}_{A,1},\mathbf{S}_{A,0}\}$ and $\{\mathbf{S}_{B,L-1},\ldots,\mathbf{S}_{B,1},\mathbf{S}_{B,0}\}$. In our system a simple k-mean clustering method is used to accomplish this task. $Surf_A$ and $Surf_B$ are first segmented into $N_{A,L-1}$ and $N_{B,L-1}$ ($N_{A,L-1} \approx N_{B,L-1}$) clusters. Each cluster of $S_{A,L-1}$ ($S_{B,L-1}$) is represented as $\mathbf{s}^i_{A,L-1} = [\mathbf{x}^i_{A,L-1}, \mathbf{n}^i_{A,L-1}]$ ($\mathbf{s}^i_{B,L-1} = [\mathbf{x}^i_{B,L-1}, \mathbf{n}^i_{B,L-1}]$), where $\mathbf{x}^i_{A,L-1}$ ($\mathbf{x}^i_{B,L-1}$) is the center of the central triangle of this cluster and $\mathbf{n}^i_{A,L-1}$ ($\mathbf{n}^i_{B,L-1}$) is the mean normal direction of the faces in this cluster. Lower level representations are then obtained by further subdivide each cluster in higher level representations by k-mean clustering and each subdivided cluster can still be described by its center and normal direction. The finest level descriptors $S_{A,0}$ ($S_{B,0}$) are then S_A (S_B). To facilitate the correspondence assignment on each landmark $\mathbf{s}^i_{A,0}$ ($\mathbf{s}^i_{B,0}$)at the finest level, we build an extra representation level $S_{A,-1} = \{\mathbf{s}^i_{A,-1}\}, i = 0,1,\ldots,KN_{A,0}-1$ ($S_{B,-1} = \{\mathbf{s}^i_{B,-1}\}, i = 0,1,\ldots,KN_{B,0}-1$) by uniformly sampling K samples from each face in $S_{A,0}$ ($S_{B,0}$).

With such a hierarchical structure of each surface, we can construct hierarchical shape descriptors at each representation level as described in the previous part. The graphical model based surface matching can then be carried out to match a surface at a coarse level l to another surface at a finer level $l-1$. Due to the fact that $N_A \approx N_B$ and $N_{A,l} << N_{B,l-1}$ ($N_{B,l} << N_{A,l-1}$), the existence of correspondence can then be ensured.

3.2 Graphical model based parallel mutual registration

In the graphical model based strategy to match S_A with S_B, only the shape information of S_A encoded in $\{\psi_A(i,j)\}$ is explicitly explored. This may lead to a slow convergence and it is apt to local optima.

The idea of parallel mutual registration is stimulated from the Turbo code in communication field, which indicates that an error-correction code which satisfies two sets of constraints simultaneously can greatly improve the its performance (McEliece et al., 1998). For our purpose of nonrigid shape matching, simultaneously exploring the different shape information of the

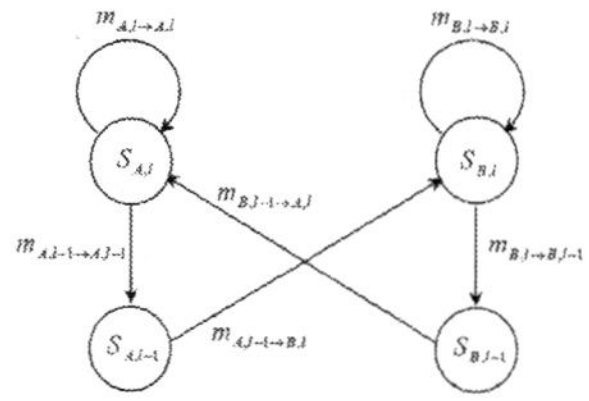

Fig. 3. Information transfer flow in the graphical model for the parallel mutual registration

two surfaces, although they are not independent since they are similar, may also improve the robustness and accelerate the convergence of our algorithm.

The graphical model for parallel mutual registration of $Surf_A$ and $Surf_B$ between representation level $l-1$ and l is a duplication of the graphical model of Fig. 1(b) as shown in Fig. 2 with extra directional edges to connect vertices representing landmarks of the same surface but at different representation levels. These edges only exist if a patch at a finer level is a subset of a patch at a coarser level.

The equivalent cost function of the parallel mutual registration scheme can be written as $H_G(S_{A,l}, S_{B,l-1}, C_{A,l\to l-1}) + H_G(S_{B,l}, S_{A,l-1}, C_{B,l\to l-1})$ with a consistency requirement on $C_{A,l\to l-1}$ and $C_{B,l\to l-1}$ encoded in the message exchange between the two subparts of Fig. 2. In the graphical model for the mutual registration, the correspondence assignment information is transferred in the graphical model as shown in Fig. 3.

3.3 Hierarchical mutual registration

The parallel registration can be carried out at each successive level of the hierarchical representation of the surfaces, where the result of belief propagation at coarse levels can be used as the initialization at finer levels. The graphical model based hierarchical mutual surface matching is summarized as in Algorithm 1.

- 1. $l = L-1$, initialize all the messages as equal distributions at all configurations.
- 2. Run the parallel mutual matching between level l and level $l-1$ with $\beta = \beta_l$ till it converges.
- 3. Using the correspondence assignment result between level l and $l-1$, initialize the correspondence assignment between level $l-1$ and $l-2$. Increase β_l to β_{l-1}, go to 2 till $l = 0$.

Algorithm 1. Graphical model based hierarchical automatic surface matching

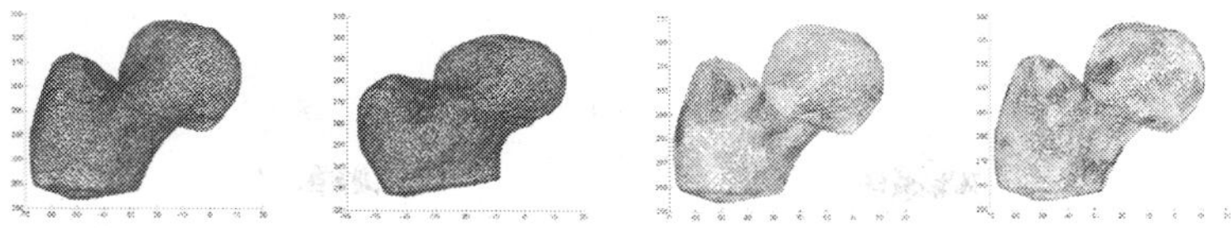

(a) Surface A (b) Surface B (c) Surface A, L=3 (d) Surface A, L=2

Fig. 4. Randomly generated surfaces from a PCA based statistical model of proximal femurs and their hierarchical representations

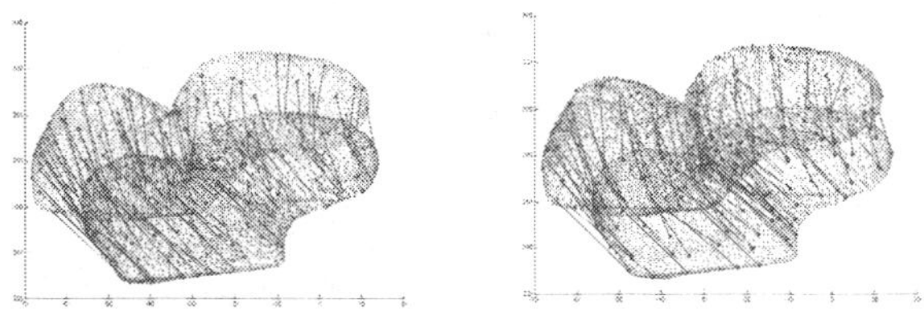

(a) Correspondence assignment between $S_{A,3}$ and $S_{B,2}$ (b) Correspondence assignment between $S_{B,3}$ and $S_{A,2}$

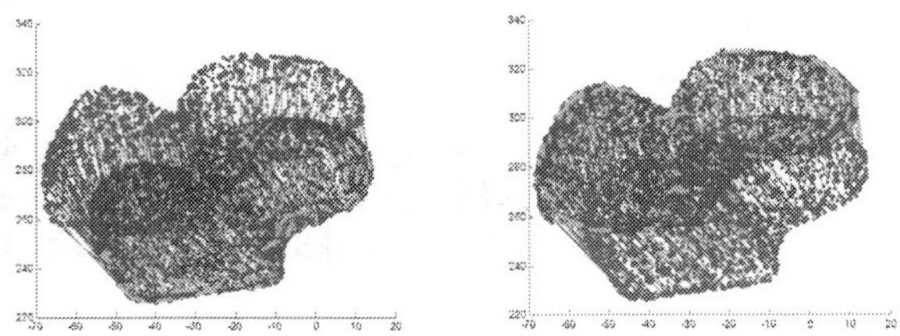

(c) Correspondence assignment between $S_{A,2}$ and $S_{B,1}$ (d) Correspondence assignment between $S_{B,2}$ and $S_{A,1}$

Fig. 5. The results of mutual registration at $l = 3$ and $l = 2$, the red lines show the correspondent landmarks on the two surfaces and the green lines show the distance between the assignment results of our algorithm and the correspondence assignment encoded in the PCA model

4. Experiments

We verified the principle of the proposed matching algorithm on a PCA based statistical model of proximal femurs including 4098 vertices and 8192 faces. Two randomly generated instances are obtained from the statistical model and one of them is further scaled by a uniform scaling of 0.9 as shown in Fig. 4(a) and 4(b). Since our matching algorithm is immune to rigid transformation, applying any rigid transformation to these surfaces will not influence the matching result. Hierarchical representations of the surfaces are constructed with $L = 3$, the first two levels ($L = 3$ and $L = 2$) of clustering results of $Surf_A$ are shown in Fig. 4(c) and 4(d).

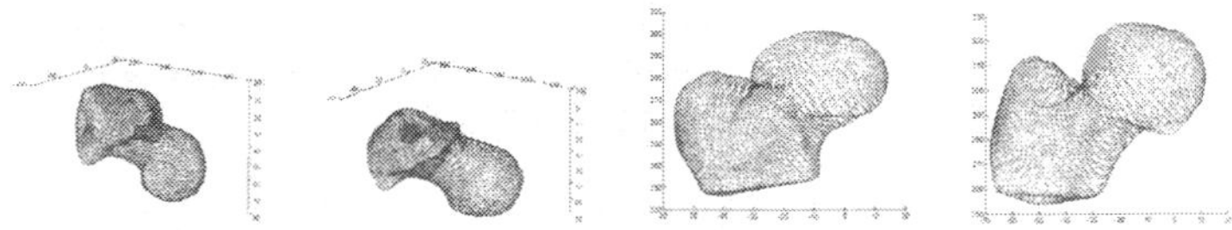

(a) The center of one patch in $S_{A,2}$ (b) Initialization of its correspondence assignment in $S_{B,1}$ (c) The center of one patch in $S_{B,2}$ (d) Initialization of its correspondence assignment in $S_{A,1}$

Fig. 6. The initialization for the mutual registration between level 2 and 1 using the assignment results at level 3

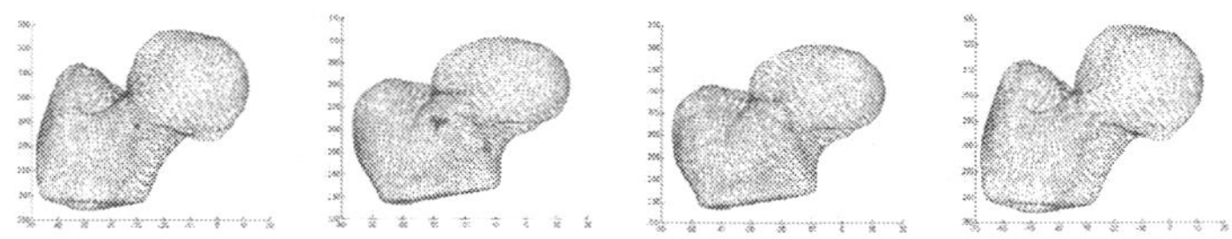

(a) (b) (c) (d)

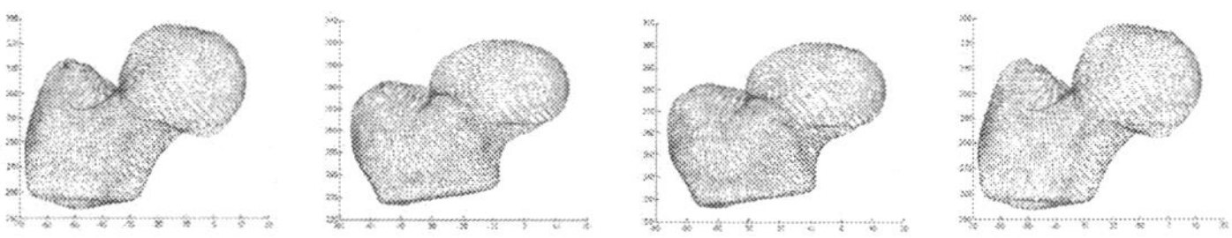

(e) (f) (g) (h)

Fig. 7. The result of mutual registration between level 2 and 1, (a)(e): centers of two patches in $S_{A,2}$; (b)(f): centers of their correspondent patches in $S_{B,1}$; (c)(g): centers of two patches in $S_{B,2}$ where most probable correspondence assignment in $S_{B,1}$ of (a)(e) are their subpatches; (d)(h): centers of the correspondent patches of (c)(g) in $S_{A,2}$; the size of the dots in (b)(d)(f)(h) represents the probability of the correspondence assignment

The correspondence assignment using the graphical model based mutual registration is then carried out on them. The underlying graph topology G is selected as a random graph, in which the degree of each node is at least 5 (connected with 5 nearest neighbours) and the average degree of one node is 10. $\Lambda' = Diag(\sigma_D^2, \sigma_A^2, \sigma_{AL}^2)^{-1}$ in (4) is selected as $\sigma_D = \mathbf{d}_{A,l}^{i,j}/4$, $\sigma_A = \sigma_{AL} = 20°$.

- The results of the mutual registration at the coarsest level $l = 3$ and $l = 2$ are shown in Fig. 5. Obviously the two surfaces are already roughly aligned at the coarsest level and this shows that the proposed algorithm does not ask for any initialization.
- The registration result at coarser level is then used to initialize the correspondence assignment at finer level as shown in Fig. 6. It can be observed that the number of candidates of each landmark at a finer level is greatly reduced due to the initialization.
- The advantage of the parallel mutual registration between the two surfaces can be observed from Fig. 7. The mutual registration can explore the shape information of two surfaces and exchange correspondence assignment information between them. This

strong constraint forces the correspondent landmarks on two surfaces to mutually assign to each other quickly. It's observed during the experiment the belief propagation at each level can converge in less than 10 iterations.

- As mentioned before, the goal of a nonrigid registration is to find optimal correspondence assignment between shapes. Since both surfaces are generated from the same PCA model, each landmark on a surface carries a point index in the PCA model. We take the landmarks with the same point index on the two surfaces as the ground truth of the correspondence assignment and then compute the registration error as the distance between the correspondent landmark obtained by our registration algorithm and the ground truth position from prior knowledge of the PCA model. The registration error is evaluated on both shapes as $2.7 \pm 2.3mm$. Of course the prior correspondence knowledge may not be the ground truth but it can be regarded as a proper reference.

5. Conclusions

In this paper we proposed a fully automatic scheme for nonrigid surface matching. The nonrigid surface matching is formalized as a graphical model based Bayesian inference and the belief propagation is used to achieve the optimization to find the optimal correspondence assignment between shapes. To further reduce the computational cost and enhance the robustness to noise and local optima, a hierarchical mutual registration strategy is implemented so that the shape information of the two surfaces can be simultaneously explored. Experiments on randomly generated surfaces from a PCA based statistical model showed the capability of the proposed algorithm to achieve an automatic nonrigid surface registration.
The proposed scheme can also be extended to incorporate other shape descriptors such as the Gaussian curvature as used in (Xiao et al., 2007) and the shape context (Belongie et al., 2002) since they can be easily modeled as local believes of each vertex in our graphical model based scheme.
One limitation of the proposed algorithm lies in the way that it handles the nonrigid deformation. Different from the commonly used TPS based *deformation energy* to set constraints on the shape deformation, our algorithm encodes a nonrigid deformation by the deformation of the subparts of a shape such as the distances and angles between landmarks. It's difficult to design a metric, which can accurately evaluate the *deformation energy*. Future work will be carried out to design better cost functions, which can measure the deformation energy more accurately by combining more shape information including local information such as curvature and deformation energies at different representation levels.

6. References

Cootes, T., Taylor, C.: Statistical models of appearance for computer vision. Technical report, University of Manchester, U.K. (2004)

Xu, C., Yezzi, A., Prince, J.: A summary of geometric level-set analogues for a general class of parametric active contour and surface models (2001)

Lee, S.M., Abbott, A.L., Clark, N.A., Araman, P.A.: A shape representation for planar curves by shape signature harmonic embedding. In: CVPR06. (2006) 1940 – 1947

Roy, A.S., Gopinath, A., Rangarajan, A.: Deformable density matching for 3d non-rigid registration of shapes. In: MICCAI 2007. (2007) 942–949

Jiang, Y.F., Xie, J., Sun, D.Q., Tsui, H.: Shape registration by simultaneously optimizing representation and transformation. In: MICCAI 2007. (2007) 809–817

Belongie, S., Malik, J., Puzicha, J.: Shape matching and object recognition using shape contexts. IEEE Transactions on Pattern Analyis and Machine Intelligence **24** (2002) 509–522

Jain, V., Zhang, H.: Robust 3d shape correspondence in the spectral domain. In: International Conference on Shape Modeling and Applications(SMI). (2006)

Coughlan, J., Ferreira, S.: Finding deformable shapes using loopy belief propagation. In: ECCV'02. (2002) 453–468

Caetano, T.S., Caeli, T., Barone, D.A.C.: An optimal probabilistic graphical model for point set matching. Technical Report Technical Report TR 04-03, University of Alberta, Edmonton, Alberta Canada (2004)

Rangarajan, A., Coughlan, J., Yuille, A.L.: A bayesian network framework for relational shape matching. In: ICCV'03. (2003) 671–678

Zhang, L., Seitz, S.M.: Parameter estimation for mrf stereo. In: CVPR'05. (2005) 288–295

Sun, J., Zheng, N.N., Shum, H.Y.: Stereo matching using belief propagation. IEEE Transactions on Pattern Analysis and Machine Interlligence **25** (2003) 1–14

Xiao, P.D., Barnes, N., Caetano, T., Lieby, P.: An MRF and Gaussian curvature based shape representation for shape matching. In: CVPR07. (2007) 17–22

Gibbs, A.L.: Bounding the convergence time of the gibbs sampler in bayesian image restroation. Biometrika **87(4)** (2000) 749–766

McEliece, R.J., MacKay, D.J.C., Cheng, J.F.: Turbo decoding as an instance of pearl's "beliefpropagation" algorithm. IEEE Journal on Selected Areas in Communications **16** (1998) 140–152

33

Intelligent and Personalised Hydrocephalus Treatment and Management

Lina Momani, Abdel Rahman Alkharabsheh and Waleed Al-Nuaimy
University of Liverpool
United Kingdom

1. Introduction

Personalised healthcare is primarily concerned with the devolution of patient monitoring and treatment from the hospital to the home. Solutions, such as body-worn sensors for clinical and healthcare monitoring, improve the quality of life by offering patients greater independence. Such solutions can go beyond monitoring to active intervention and treatment based on sensory measurement and patient feedback, effectively taking healthcare out of the hospital environment. Such personalised healthcare solutions play an increasingly important role in delivering high quality and cost-effective healthcare.

The realisation of truly autonomous systems for the personalised treatment of physiological disorders such as hydrocephalus is closer than ever. This chapter is concerned with the spreading of awareness, particularly among the biomedical engineering community e.g. organisations, companies, physicians and patients, about the possibilities that current technology offers in the area of intelligent and personalised hydrocephalus implants that seek to autonomously manage the symptoms and treat the causes in a manner specifically tuned to the individual patient. This chapter provides an insight into the workings of such a system, its pros and cons and how it can dramatically reduce patient suffering and long hospitalisation periods while increasing the quality of care that is provided.

1.1 Hydrocephalus

The human brain is surrounded by a fluid called the cerebrospinal fluid (CSF), that protects it from physical injury, keeps its tissue moist and transports the products of metabolism. This fluid is constantly produced in the parenchyma at rate of approximately 20ml.h^{-1} and drained through granulations near the sagittal sinus. If the rate of CSF absorption or drainage is consistently less than the rate of production (for a variety of reasons), the ventricles expand causing the brain to become compressed, leading to the disorder known as hydrocephalus (ASBAH, 2009), as shown in Fig. 1.

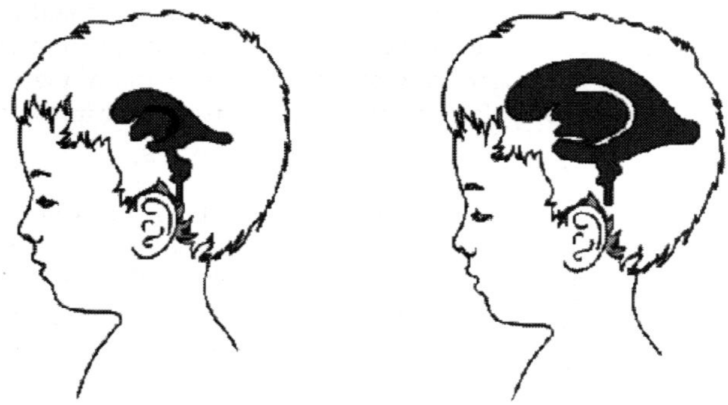

(a) (b)

Fig. 1. Schematic drawing for brain in (a) normal and (b) hydrocephalus cases, showing enlarged ventricles.

This leads to an elevation of the pressure exerted by the cranium on the brain tissue, cerebrospinal fluid, and the brain's circulating blood volume, referred to as intracranial pressure (ICP), and manifest itself in symptoms such as headache, vomiting, nausea or coma. ICP is a dynamic phenomenon constantly fluctuating in response to activities such as exercise, coughing, straining, arterial pulsation, and respiratory cycle. ICP is measured in millimeters of mercury (mmHg) and, at rest, is normally 7-15 mmHg for a supine adult, and becomes negative (averaging -10 mmHg) in the vertical position (Steiner & Andrews, 2006). Hydrocephalic patients may experience pressures of up to 120 mmHg. If left untreated, elevated ICP may lead to serious problems in the brain.

1.2 Current Treatment

Since the 1960s the usual treatment for hydrocephalus is to insert a shunting device in the patient's CSF system. This is simply a device which diverts the accumulated CSF around the obstructed pathways and returns it to the bloodstream, thus reducing ICP, and alleviating the symptoms of hydrocephalus. It consists of a flexible tube with a valve to control the rate of drainage and prevent back-flow.

These valves are passive mechanical devices that open and close depending on either the differential pressure or flow. Although there are various valve technologies and approaches, they all essentially do the same thing, which is to attempt to passively control the symptoms of hydrocephalus by assisting the body's natural drainage system. The valve is usually chosen by the surgeon on the grounds of experience, cost and personal preference.

Despite shunting developments, shunting can have complications, with different types of shunts seemingly associated with different types of complications. Shunt complications can be very serious and become life threatening if not discovered and treated early. However, due to their passive mode of operation, shunt malfunctions are generally not detected before they manifest clinically. These can be divided into issues of under-drainage, over-drainage and infection. Over-drainage and under-drainage are typical drawbacks of such shunts, where CSF is either drained in excess or less than needed, which could cause dramatic effects on the patient such as brain damage. The common cause for these two drawbacks might be an inappropriate opening/closing of the valve in respect of the duration or the timing. In other words, valve open for too short/too long periods or it opens/closes at the right timing.

Under-drainage is usually due to blockage of the upper or lower tubes of the shunt by in-growing tissue, though it can also be caused by the shunt breaking or its parts becoming disconnected from each other. The rate of blockage can be as high as 20% in the first year after insertion, decreasing to approximately 5% per year (Casey, et al., 1997), therefore, the clinical presentation of shunt blockage is usually dominated by signs of raised pressure as the brain fluid (CSF) builds up. As ICP is not readily measurable, interferences must be drawn from the symptoms presented. Sometimes the symptoms come on quickly over hour or days, but occasionally they may develop over many weeks with intermittent headache, and tiredness, change in behaviour or deterioration in schoolwork. Diagnosing shunt blockage is not always straightforward. In fact, parents can be as successful at diagnosing shunt blockage as GPs and paediatricians. Whilst additional investigations such as CT scans, X-rays and a shunt taps may help, a definitive diagnosis is sometimes only possible through surgery (ASBAH, 2009).

In the case of over-drainage, the shunt allows CSF to drain from the ventricles more quickly than it is produced. If this happens suddenly, then the ventricles in the brain collapse, tearing delicate blood vessels on the outside of the brain and causing a haemorrhage. This can be trivial or it can cause symptoms similar to those of a stroke. If the over-drainage is more gradual, the ventricles collapse gradually to become slit-like. This often interferes with shunt function causing the opposite problem, high CSF pressure, to reappear. The symptoms of over-drainage can be very similar to those of under-drainage though there are important differences.

Difficulty in diagnosing over-/under-drainage can make treatment of this complication particularly frustrating for patients and their families. It may be necessary to monitor ICP, often over 24 hours. This can be done using an external pressure monitor in the scalp connected to a recorder. Early ICP monitoring is recommended when the clinician is unable to assess the neurological examination accurately. The main concerns are the risks of infection, bleeding, device accuracy and drift of measurement over time. Thus to avoid these risks, a research work is undergoing to develop implanted pressure sensors for short and long term monitoring interrogated by telemetry (Hodgins et al., 2008).

Studies have shown that the use of an 'antisyphon device', a small button inserted into the shunt tubing, will often solve the over-drainage problem, but this does not always work. A 'programmable' or adjustable shunt is intended to allow adjustment of the working pressure of the valve without operation. The valve contains magnets, which allow the setting to be changed by laying a second magnetic device on the scalp. This is undoubtedly useful where the need for a valve of a different pressure arises, but the adjustable valve is no less prone to over-drainage than any other and it cannot be used to treat this condition (Casey et al., 1997).

One of the obvious reasons for such drawbacks is the inability of such shunts to autonomously respond to the dynamic environment. Inaccuracies and long term drift are also considered among the drawbacks of such shunts. This is mainly due to the fact that these shunts are (typically, but not always) regulated according to the differential pressure across the valves, which differs from intracranial pressure in the brain.

1.3 Motivations

Beside their documented drawbacks (Aschoff, 2001; Schley, 2004), shunts do not suit many hydrocephalus patients. This can be realised from the considerable high shunt revision and failure rates (between 30% and 40% of all shunts placed in paediatric patients fail within 1 year (Albright et al., 1988; Villavicencio et al., 2003; Piatt et al.,1993; Piatt,1995) and it is not uncommon for patients to have multiple shunt revisions within their lifetime).

Shunt insertion explicitly changes the CSF dynamics in patients with hydrocephalus, causing many to improve clinically. However, the relationship between a changed hydrodynamic state and improved clinical performance is not fully known. Therefore, further research in this area is an important challenge for the hydrocephalus research community, where development of better methods for assessment of CSF dynamic parameters as well as studies to test hypotheses on relationships between CSF dynamics and outcome after shunting is targeted. The aims are for a better understanding of hydrocephalus pathophysiology and to find new predictive tests.

Furthermore, the shunt designers had changed the shunt goal to have the option of re-establishing shunt independence step by step. This means that the statement of Hemmer "once a shunt, always a shunt" is no longer true.

Nevertheless, most patients seem to be only partially shunt-dependent, i.e. their natural drainage system still functions to some extent. The degree of shunt-dependence may range from 1% to 100%, thus draining 30-50% of CSF production may be sufficient to keep the ICP within physiological ranges, and only a few need full drainage (Aschoff, 2001). Thus the current generation of shunts do not help patients overcome the underlying problems, but on the contrary, they tend to encourage the patients to become fully shunt dependent. Research has shown however, that in some cases, shunt dependence could be reduced to less than 1% (Aschoff, 2001) which could even allow the eventual removal of the shunt (Takahashi, 2001). It is envisaged that the next generation of shunts should be able to achieve a controlled shunt arrest in the long run.

The future will bring other options related to the control of CSF production and absorption. Perhaps different valve designs will be more effective in long-term treatment and eventually the development of "smart" shunts. These will be able to react to intracranial physiology and will drain CSF in response to these changes in intracranial dynamics, rather than drain on a continuous basis (Jones & Klinge, 2008).

To address the lack of personalised treatment, the difficulty in diagnosing shunt faults, the high rate of shunt revisions, the high shunt dependency, and the lack of full understanding of shunt effect on the intracranial hydrodynamics, a personalised hydrocephalus shunting system needs to be developed. This would be tasked with the following:

- Frequent non-invasive monitoring of intracranial hydrodynamics to improve treatment outcome.
- Responding to patient symptoms and ICP readings by adjusting treatment.
- Controlling the flow of CSF through a valve of the shunting system.
- Attempting to wean patient off the treatment (shunting system).
- Wirelessly reprogramming the implanted shunting system.
- Instant diagnosis of the shunting system and detection of any fault in the early stages.

By having such system, the hospitalisation periods and patient suffering and inconvenience are reduced, the quality of treatment is improved and better understanding of intracranial hydrodynamics is established thanks to the valuable resource of ICP data.

1.4 Recent Advances

In order to achieve such a system, a mechatronic valve is needed which is electrically controlled via software. In this shunting system, the patient could play a vital role in feeding back his/her dissatisfaction, i.e. due to symptoms, regarding the treatment.

In 2005, Miethke claimed patent to a hydrocephalus valve with an electric actuating system comprising a time control system to open and close it (Miethke, 2005). The claim was that such valve would allow improved adaptation to the situation existing in a patient in the case of a hydrocephalus valve.

The intervention of a mechatronic valve provides the opportunity for different shunting systems to be developed. This type of valve can be controlled by software that can vary in its complexity and intelligence. The controlling methods could vary from a simple program that lacks any intelligence to very sophisticated and intelligent program.

Despite ICP monitoring currently being an invasive procedure, patients with hydrocephalus may need repeated episodes of monitoring months or years apart. This is a result of problems arising in which ICP readings are needed for diagnosis. The invasive nature of ICP monitoring has motivated researchers to develop a telemetric implantable pressure sensor for short- and long-term monitoring of ICP with high accuracy (Hodgins et al., 2008). Such sensor was mainly used for monitoring ICP wirelessly by the physician who could manually adjust the valve settings accordingly.

The remainder of the chapter is structured as follows: Section 2 describes the intelligent and personalised shunting system, illustrates its novelty, and lists its functions. In Section 3, the advantages and limitations of the shunting system are identified. Section 4 summaries a quick walkthrough of the shunting system, while Sections 5 and 6 present the future directions and conclusions, respectively.

2. Intelligent and Personalised Shunting System

The new generation of shunting systems are expected to overcome the drawbacks and limitations of the current shunting systems. A novel intelligent telemetric system is developed for the improved management and treatment of hydrocephalus. The intelligent system would autonomously manage the CSF flow, personalise the management of CSF flow through involving real-time intracranial pressure readings and patient's feedback, and responding to them. It also would autonomously manage and personalise the treatment of hydrocephalus, thus providing treatment that is personalised, goal-driven and reactive as well as pro-active, which gradually reduce shunt dependence and eventually establish a controlled arrest of the shunt. In addition, it would be able to monitor performance of its components, thus minimising the shunt revisions, and establish distant treatment database (e.g. computer-based patient record) and exchange treatment information, by regularly reporting the patient's record to the physician.

All these qualities can only be attained by a multi-agent approach (Momani, et al., 2008). This would also involve replacing a passive valve (commonly used in hydrocephalus shunts) with a mechatronic valve controlled by an intelligent microcontroller that wirelessly communicates with a separate smart hand-held device. The system is illustrated in Fig. 2.

This shunting system would consist of two subsystems; implantable and external (patient device). The implanted subsystem would mainly consist of ultra low power commercial microcontroller, mechatronic valve, pressure sensor and low power transceiver. This implantable shunting system would wirelessly communicate with a hand-held smartphone operated by the patient, or on the patient's behalf by a clinician or guardian. This device would have a graphical user interface and an RF interface to communicate with the user and the implantable wireless shunt respectively.

This system would also enable a physician to monitor and modify the treatment parameters wirelessly, thus reducing, if not eliminating, the need for shunt revision operations. Once implanted, such a system could lead not only to better treatment of the users of such shunts, but also allow the dynamics of this disease and the effect of shunting to be understood in greater depth.

An intelligent system, e.g. (Momani et al., 2008) , can be used to autonomously regulate the mechatronic valve according to a time-based schedule and update it based on the intracranial pressure that is measured when needed. In such system, ICP readings and other sensory inputs such as patient feedback would help in tuning the treatment and enabling the intervention of the medical practitioner to update and manually adapt the schedule. This would result in a personalised and intelligent CSF management, which leads to every patient having different management schedule according to his/her personal conditions.

2.1 Novelty

The idea of using a pressure sensor integrated into a shunt system for monitoring ICP and interrogated by telemetry is not in itself a novel idea (Ginggen, 2007; Jeong et al., 2004; Miesel & Stylos, 2001), where ICP readings used by the physician to monitor the

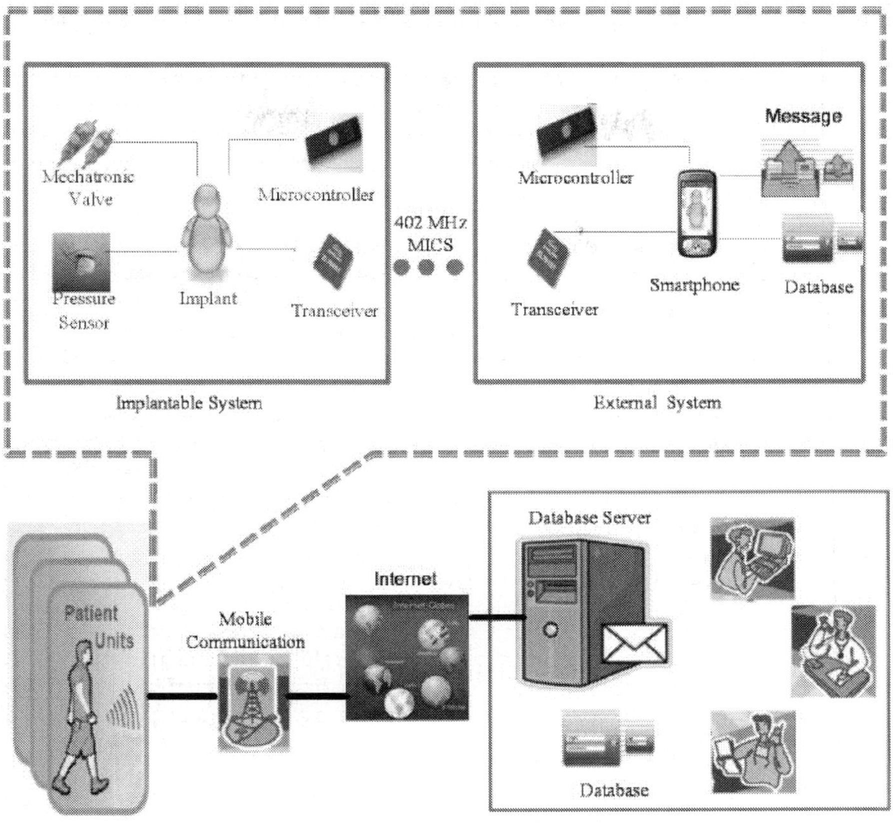

Fig. 2. Schematic diagram of the intelligent and personalised shunting system.

performance of the implanted shunt. However, the novelty in this work is in having an implantable shunting system that utilise these readings in addition to patient input as a direct feedback to instantaneously and even autonomously manage the shunt, i.e. analyse the feedback, diagnose any shunt faults and accordingly regulate the opening of a mechatronic valve. Thus an element of intelligence and personalisation would be added to the mechatronic shunting system by enabling real-time reconfiguration of the shunt parameters based on the patient's response and the ICP readings.

2.2 Strategy and Approach

The mechatronic valve is controlled by a time based schedule. The schedule would be simply the distribution of the valve state (open/close) over time. Such schedule would incur many disadvantages e.g. over-/under-drainage, if its selection is arbitrary. In order to optimise the usefulness of such a valve, its schedule should be selected in way that delivers a personalised treatment for each specific patient. Achieving such a goal is not an easy task due to the dynamic behaviour of intracranial pressure that not only varies among patients but also within individual patient with time. There are two extremes for schedule alternatives. One is a dynamic schedule that responds to the instantaneous intracranial pressure which requires an implanted pressure sensor, i.e. closed loop shunting system. The other extreme is a fixed schedule that has a fixed open frequency over 24 hours. This alternative lacks flexibility and ignores the intracranial dynamic behaviour while the first is impractical.

A schedule structure is proposed that offers a compromise between the two schedule extremes. Thus to facilitate the process of schedule selection and to add some degree of flexibility, a 24-hours schedule, shown in Fig. 3, is divided into 24 one hour sub-schedules. Each sub-schedule is identified by three parameters; the targeted hour (hr), open duration (d_{ON}) and closed duration (d_{OFF}) for that specific hour.

Treatment in the proposed shunting system is presented by a time-based valve schedule, thus dynamically modifying the schedule, would mean changing the applied treatment. Treatment would be modified in order to adapt to the individual patient and actual conditions. This modification is accomplished based on real-time inputs (e.g. symptoms delivered via patient feedback and internally measured ICP) and derived parameters such as rate of ICP change, effective opening time and figure of merits. To update the schedule, the modification is only applied on the targeted sub-schedule (hour).

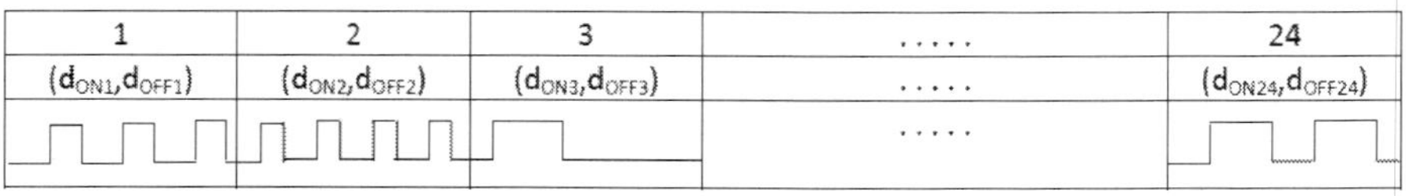

Fig. 3. A 24-hour schedule for the implanted valve.

The system acquires knowledge directly and wirelessly from the patient's satisfaction input (feedback), to make decision regarding modifying the schedule or it just records and saves patient's satisfaction for future interpretation.

Once the shunting system is implanted, the system is initially programmed by taking into consideration the empirical data patient's history, e.g. ICP data, personal information, medical history, family history.

In long run, the system should become stable and reach a state in which it adapts to the patient and deals smartly and dynamically with any changes with no need for help. As a result, these personalised schedules can be categorised according to hydrocephalus patient types so as to develop an optimum schedule for each patient's category that can be used, in future, as the initial schedule when implanting such shunts.

2.3 Functions

The intelligent shunting system will perform two main roles; management and treatment.

2.3.1 Management

This involves managing both the physiological condition and the shunting system itself. The former consists of monitoring and optimising the success of treatment, adapting the treatment to the individual and actual conditions, responding to symptoms reported via patient feedback and capturing real shunt dependency. On the other hand the latter covers the self monitoring, diagnosis and fault detection. Both of those aspects are detailed below.

A. Managing Hydrocephalus

Similar to any other shunt, the proposed shunt will aim to control ICP within the normal physiological limits. To achieve this, the following tasks are performed,

1. **Monitoring the success of treatment and its optimisation:** The shunt will routinely collect ICP readings measured by the implanted sensor, analyse them internally to check whether the current schedule succeeded in maintaining pressure within normal range. In addition, a figure of merit is calculated to help in evaluating the performance of treatment and in selecting a schedule that best suit the situation. The novelty of such function would be in it is ability to collect ICP data while the valve is closed, thus providing a valuable record of ICP for un-shunted case (without treatment) with no need to perform any additional invasive operation. Such traces are considered valuable in understanding specific-patient cases and the effect of applying different schedules, since currently physician do not perform ICP monitoring before shunting unless all other methods did not work out in diagnosing hydrocephalus due to the risks of such procedure.

2. **Adapting the treatment to the individual and actual conditions:** to successfully manage hydrocephalus, it should adapt the treatment to the needs of the specific-patient and arising circumstances. If a problem arises in the measured ICP (e.g. ICP is high), the system would respond dynamically and instantaneously by updating the valve schedule according to rules saved in the knowledge base. Initially these rules are general but with time it is revised by the shunting system to suit this particular patient.

3. **Responding to symptoms delivered via patient feedback:** Nowadays, reoccurrence of symptoms in shunted patient is usually dealt by externally monitor the ICP. Such procedure is invasive and accompanied by many risks and complications. That is why intracranial monitoring usually is the last option for un-shunted patient unless it is vital to diagnose hydrocephalus in some cases. In this system, patient feedback would be logged into the patient device to represent the type of symptom and its severity. As a result of receiving such feedback, the shunting system will investigate the cause of the symptom by checking the normality of ICP and perform self-checking for any faults in the system. And later draw a conclusion whether the cause was due to abnormality in ICP or not. In the case of any abnormality, it will respond by either modifying the valve schedule to accommodate the symptom or alerting the physician in case of faults possibilities.

The availability of such option in the proposed shunting system, spares patient from unnecessary pain, suffering and risks accompanied with the current diagnosis method. And on the contrary to current methods, this option will provide an instant diagnosing while the patient is living his/her normal life, thus no need to wait for an appointment or being hospitalised

4. **Capturing real shunt dependency:** Knowing that patients seem to be only partially shunt-dependent, the current shunts do not help in revealing the degree of dependency, but on the contrary, they tend to encourage the patients to become fully shunt dependent. Proposed shunting system can help in revealing the actual shunt dependency, thus allowing the natural drainage to keep working at its maximum power and the shunt will only give a hand when the natural drainage is overloaded.

B. Managing the Shunting System

It is important that the system functions properly so that a reasonable intracranial pressure is maintained. Currently, shunt faults are the leading cause of shunt revisions. The main shunt faults are blockage and disconnection. In an effort to detect these faults in early stages, thus avoiding any further patient inconveniences that could arise if left undetected, the proposed shunting system will perform the following preventive procedure.

1. **Self monitoring:** routinely check up if the ICP data changes in responsive manner to the valve states.
2. **Self diagnosis:** use novel fault detection measures, which are based on ICP data and valve status, to find any possibility of occurrence of any fault, determine its type (e.g. shunt blockage/disconnection/breakage or sensor dislocation/drift), and its degree.
3. **Power management:** use a real-time self wake-up method to manage the power consumption in the implanted shunt.
4. **Memory management:** use a novel method to reduce the size of stored data in the implanted shunt, thus solving a problem associated with implanted memory limitations.

2.3.2 Treatment

The goal of shunting has changed over time since it was first used. The shunt nowadays is expected to provide an option of establishing gradual shunt arrest. It is also the dream of any hydrocephalus shunted patient to regain his/her independence of the shunt and mainly rely on his/her reconditioned natural drainage system.

The capability of the proposed system to be wirelessly reprogrammed without the need for surgery and its ability to monitor the change in the intracranial hydrodynamics are essential in facilitating the shunt arrest process.

At the stage when the shunting system is fully in control of the intracranial hydrodynamics and the patient's real shunt dependency is captured, the shunting system will start achieving new objective that is reducing shunt dependency and might eventually arrest the use of the shunt (weaning).

The weaning process will involve manipulating two parameters; the length of open duration and the limits of acceptable pressure (above which ICP is considered abnormal), in away that make the patient either adapt gradually to higher level of ICP or reactivate the natural drainage to take part of the drainage process. Weaning will be implemented over stages. The length of each stage will vary based on patient response and capability to accommodate such change. For each weaning stage, the effect of modifying weaning parameters will be evaluated by routinely collecting ICP readings and patient feedback. The amount of reduction in the open duration or increase in the acceptable pressure limits will depend on parameters derived from patient's ICP data at different valve states.

3. Advantages and Limitations

The shunting system is explored and its advantages are identified. Furthermore, limitations facing implementing such system are investigated.

3.1 Advantages

Compared to the current shunts, this shunting system offers the following advantages:

- Personalising: responsive to patient needs and situation.
- Autonomous: functions without supervision or intervention.
- Reducing patient suffering, e.g. hospitalisation.
- Managing and responding to symptoms obtained from patient feedback.
- Autonomous monitoring and diagnosis of intracranial hydrodynamics.
- Potential to achieve arrest of shunt dependence.
- Wireless reprogramming; access, modify and replace current parameters.
- Ability to obtain ICP traces for patient both with and without shunt.
- Shunt self diagnosis and fault detection.
- Better understanding of hydrocephalus, intracranial hydrodynamics and the effect of shunting on them.

3.2 Limitations

The following limitations are encountered when implementing such system:

- ICP sensor inaccuracy or breakage
- Mechatronic valve intermittent problems
- Physician and patient mentality
- Technical issues
- Power limitation
- Implantable memory size limitation
- Product size limitation
- Potential faults

4. Walkthrough

A quick walk through the shunting system is summarised. It illustrates the shunt functions through an example of one day in the life of shunted hydrocephalus patient.

Bob is a hydrocephalus patient. Today, he was shunted with an intelligent shunting system. This system has been configured by the physician to suit Bob based on his medical history (including an ICP trace) and hydrocephalus type.

Once implanted, the system will attempt to initialise itself by first collecting ICP data for 24 hours and then instantiate an initial personalised 24 sub-schedules based on hourly derived parameters (e.g. average ICP and rate of change in ICP) from the collected data. Starting from the first day, the implanted shunt will perform its routine tasks; ICP monitoring, valve regulating according to the schedule, self diagnosis, and daily backup of the results.

One day Bob woke up and he was feeling drowsy. He checked if there were any alerts on his patient device (PD) but found nothing. He started to worry that there might be a problem with his shunt, thus he logged his feedback on his PD.

In the following few minutes, the intelligent agent on PD started to investigate the cause by firstly sending a request for ICP data to the implanted shunt. While waiting for a reply, it checked its database if any similar feedback that might have occurred previously at the time of the day or if such symptom is recently reoccurring.

Meanwhile, the implanted shunting system received the request and immediately initiated the ICP sensor to collect data over a period of time at different valve states. As soon as sufficient data is collected, it is sent wirelessly to the PD.

By receiving the ICP, the external shunting system (PD) starts performing analysis and calculating some derived parameters to check if the cause for such symptoms is due ICP abnormality or shunt fault. If the results of the analysis indicated that the cause of the symptom is not due to ICP abnormality or shunt fault, then a message will show up on the PD display to reassure Bob that the symptom is not ICP-related. The feedback, its time along with the ICP data and the decision made are saved to be uploaded at a later time to Bob's personal record in the central database at the hospital. On the other hand, if the results showed that the cause is due to ICP abnormality, then the intelligent system will work on modifying the schedule at that hour and track its effect for the next couple of days. A message will also show up telling Bob that the problem has been handled. Bob in either case was reassured that his shunting system was functioning properly and there was nothing to worry about.

While Bob is doing his job, the implanted shunt is regulating the valve according to a time-based schedule and at the same time perform a check up on the ICP and the shunt itself. To do this, it collects ICP data while the valve is open and closed. It checks if these data is within the acceptable limits and if not, it will alert the PD to perform modification on the schedule. The implanted shunt will also calculate some derived parameter to detect any possibility of fault occurrence in the shunt. In case any fault is detected, the implanted shunt will inform the physician through the PD, in order to take some procedures in early stage to spare Bob from unnecessary pain and suffering.

After one year of shunt experience, Bob confidence in his shunt has grown and he stopped worrying about his ICP since he knows that wherever he is, he has a personal physician that accompanies him 24 hours a day and whom will worry on his behave. Bob also pleased that he no longer has to wait for an appointment or stay in the hospital every time he had a symptom. He can now check up his ICP and shunt in minutes while having his normal life anywhere and anytime.

Two years passed on the shunting surgery. Bob is happy with his shunt, he has not experienced any symptom for long time. Thus, his shunt has recognised this progress and decided after consulting the physician to start reducing shunt dependency (shunt weaning process). First step was to reduce open duration for a selected hour based on Bob's ICP history. Bob is asked to play a vital role at this stage, by giving his feedback whenever he has symptoms, to tune and personalise the weaning process. After checking that the first step did not have harmful consequences, the shunt proceeded to its second step which is attacking a new open duration and try to reduce it. Unfortunately this time Bob could not handle the severity of the symptoms thus the shunt had to reconfigure this step to avoid any inconvenience for Bob.

After prolong period of time, Bob's shunt dependency has been reduced to minimum but unfortunately Bob's brain adaptability could not go through a complete shunt arrest. Nevertheless, Bob was really satisfied with what his shunt has done and what he is still doing and hopes that shunt arresting can be achieved in later time.

5. Future Directions

Future enhancements would include incorporating more parameters in developing and modifying the valve schedule. For example, patient daily activities (sleeping and working times, type of work (sitting, standing)) and other parameters derived from ICP traces would enhance the performance of the valve schedule if taken into consideration when deriving or modifying a schedule.

The significance of such intelligent personalised shunting system can be extended by incorporating it into a distributed network of intelligent shunts, where data mining and knowledge acquisition techniques are deployed to analyse and interpret hydrocephalus patients' data for case enquiring, treatment plan advising, and ICP classification and patient clustering. In addition it would let patients exchange and share the treatment and management process.

6. Conclusion

The realisation of truly autonomous shunting systems for personalised hydrocephalus treatment is closer than ever. This requires the use of an implanted mechatronic valve and pressure sensor, a smart hand held device, improved algorithms to analyse the inputs (e.g. ICP readings and patient feedback) and extract relevant information from raw data, and rule-based decisions controlled by local intelligence. The Management of intracranial hydrodynamics, shunt self-diagnosis, and treatment of hydrocephalus can be continuously and autonomously monitored and parameters changed as necessary by the intelligent software in the handheld device via wireless communication and data will be sent on demand to the clinician for further evaluation. Such shunting system would give hydrocephalus patients the freedom to go anywhere they like while receiving medical services and health care in a timely fashion. Visits of patients to hospitals or the doctor will be reduced to a necessary minimum, while increasing the quality of care that is provided.

7. References

Association for Spina Bifida Hydrocephalus (2009). Hydrocephalus, available online: http://www.asbah.org/.

Albright, A.L.; Haines, S.J. & Taylor, F.H. (1988). Function of parietal and frontal shunts in childhood hydrocephalus, *J Neurosurg*, vol. 69, pp. 883-886.

Aschoff, A. (2001). The evolution of shunt technology in the last decade: A critical review, presented at 3rd *International Hydrocephalus Workshop*, Kos, Greece, May 17-20th, 2001.

Casey, A. T.; Kimmings, E. J.; Kleinlugtebeld, A. D.; Taylor. W. A.; Harkness, W. F. & Hayward, R. D. (1997). The long-term outlook for hydrocephalus in childhood. (A ten-year cohort study of 155 patients), *Pediatr Neurosurg, vol.* 27, no. 2, pp. 63-70.

Ginggen, A. (2007). Optimization of the Treatment of Hydrocephalus by the Non-Invasive Measurement of the Intra-Cranial Pressure, PhD thesis, *infoscienc*, EPFL, Czech. URL : http://library.epfl.ch/theses/?nr=3757.

Hodgins, D.; Bertsch, A.; Post, N.; Frischholz, M.; Volckaerts, B.; Spensley, J.; Wasikiewicz, J. M.; Higgins, H.; Stetten, F. & Kenney, L. (2008). *IEEE Pervasive Computing*. vol. 7, no. 1, pp. 14-21, January–March 2008.

Jones, H. C. & Klinge, P. T. (2008). Hydrocephalus, In Hannover Conference 17–20th September 2008, *Cerebrospinal Fluid Res.*, 2008; vol. 5, pp. 19.

Jeong, J. S. ; Yang, S. S.; Yoon, H. J. & Jung, J. M. (2004). Micro Devices for a Cerebrospinal Fluid (CSF) Shunt System. *Sensors and Actuators A*, Vol. 110, pp. 68-76.

Kramer, L. C.; Azarow, K.; Schlifka, B. A. & Sgouros, S. (2006). *eMedicine Pediatrics*, available online: http://emedicine.medscape.com/article/937979-overview.

Miesel, K. A. & Stylos, L. (2001). Intracranial monitoring and therapy delivery control device, system and method, *United States Patent*, No. 6248080.

Miethke, C. (2005). Hydrocephalus valve, U.S. Patent 6926691, August 9, 2005.

Momani, L., Alkharabsheh, A. & Al-Nuaimy, W. (2008). Design of an intelligent and personalised shunting system for hydrocephalus, in Conf Proc 2008 IEEE Eng Med Biol Soc., Vancouver, Canada, pp. 779-782.

Piatt Jr, J.H. & Carlson, C.V. (1993). A search for determinants of cerebrospinal fluid shunt survival: retrospective analysis of a 14-year institutional experience. *Pediatr Neurosurg*, vol. 19, pp. 233-241.

Piatt Jr, J.H. (1995). Cerebrospinal fluid shunt failure: late is different from early. *Pediatr Neurosurg*, vol. 23, pp. 133-139.

Schley, D.; Billingham, J. & Marchbanks, R. J. (2004). A Model of in-vivo hydrocephalus shunt dynamics for blockage and performance diagnostics, *Mathematical Medicine and Biology*, vol. 21, no. 4, pp. 347-368, Dec. 2004.

Steiner, L. A. & Andrews, P. J. (2006). Monitoring the injured brain: ICP and CBF, *British Journal of Anaesthesia*, vol. 97, no. 1 (July 2006), pp. 26-38.

Takahashi, Y. (2001). Withdrawal of shunt systems clinical use of the programmable shunt system and its effect on hydrocephalus in children, *Childs Nerv Syst*, vol. 17, pp. 472-477, Aug. 2001.

Villavicencio, A. T.; Leveque, J.; McGirt, M. J.; Hopkins, J. S.; Fuchs, H. E. & George, T. M. (2003). Comparison of Revision Rates Following Endoscopically Versus Nonendoscopically Placed Ventricular Shunt Catheters, Surgical *Neurology*, vol. 59, no. 5, pp. 375-379.

A Simulation Study on Balance Maintenance Strategies during Walking

Yu Ikemoto, Wenwei Yu and Jun Inoue
Chiba University
Japan

1. Introduction

Recently, walking assist systems, such as robotic systems (Kawamoto et al., 2003) and functional electrical stimulation (FES) for hemiplegic walking (Yu et al., 2002; Bajd et al., 1997; Tong et al., 1998), have been widely studied for the purpose of improving activities of daily living (ADL) for paralyzed individuals. However, most systems were unable to address the perturbations resulting from uneven terrain, slips, slopes and obstacles, which frequently occur in daily-life walking; as they have not taken these perturbations into consideration, they are not yet suitable for practical use in real-life situations.

However, it is evident that humans can cope with such perturbations, especially when they cannot be predicted or perceived in advance, by means of reflexes (Zehr and Stein, 1999), which cause relatively fixed, unconscious muscular response patterns to perturbations within a short period of time ranging from several tens of ms to 200 ms.

Our ultimate goal is to realize artificial reflexes in real-world walking support systems for paralyzed individuals, whose afferent and efferent neural pathways are usually weakened, so that the reflexive system is also impaired to a certain degree. This goal requires both a qualitative and quantitative understanding of human reflexive mechanisms during walking. Reflexes of different functional organs and limbs (e.g., upper limbs (Cathers et al., 2004), hearts (Nakamura et al., 1992), and lower limbs (Zehr and Stein, 1999)), in different contexts (e.g., during flexion/extension (Cathers et al., 2004), during free fall (Bisdorff et al., 1999), and during walking (Zehr and Stein, 1999)) have been studied in the fields of kinesiology and neuroscience. It has also been shown that the flexor reflexes play an important role in locomotion, and these reflexes were implemented in several commercially available FES systems (Quintern, 2000).

Although the reflexive responses to perturbation during walking have been an object of study for quite some time (Zehr and Stein, 1999; Berger et al. 1984; Dietz et al. 1987), most studies were concerned with muscle activity recording and data analysis, through which several working hypotheses were generated. For example, electroneurograms (ENG) of high-spinal curarized cats were recorded and analyzed to show that the stimulation of flexor reflex afferents could induce a clear resetting of the locomotion rhythm (Schomburg et al, 1998). However, it is almost impossible to test this hypothesis using the same methods in humans.

Thus, the spatio-temporal relation among neuro-control mechanisms, muscle activities and physical motions remains unknown. Moreover, there is no widely accepted theory on the underlying neural mechanisms of the reflexes during walking, nor are there clear experimental results that could be directly referenced in the disciplines of physiology and motor control. However, neuro-control-level understanding and verification are necessary to artificially realize the reflexes to perturbation during walking.

Our basic hypothesis is that if the muscle activity profile of the reflexive responses to perturbation during walking can be acquired via non-invasive measurement, and if a neuromusculoskeletal walking simulation model able to present conformable behavior to human normal walking could be developed, albeit without the reflexive mechanism pre-wired (as they are still unknown), parts of the candidates for the underlying neural mechanisms can be clarified by investigating which candidate can match the measured muscle activity profile.

In our previous study (Yu et al, 2007), we investigated reflexive responses during walking through the following methods:

1) Acquiring muscle activity profiles during normal walking and slip-perturbed walking by recording and processing electromyographic (EMG) signals of several walking-related muscles in a human gait experiment.

2) Developing a central pattern generator (CPG)-based neuromusculoskeletal simulation model. Computer simulation has been employed as an approach to study the role of afferent information during human (Taga, 1994) and animal walking (Prochazka et al., 2001). In an animal study, virtual reflexes were realized by a set of if-then rules, and the gait of cat walking with and without the virtual reflexes were compared. The results showed that walking with virtual reflexes was more stable and perturbation-resistive. However, there are few studies employing a hybrid approach coupling human walking simulation with human gait experiment data.

3) Comparing joint trajectories of the simulation model with those of a human subject during normal walking to verify the simulation model's conformity with human walking.

4) Using muscle activity profiles of reflexive responses (defined as muscular-reflexive-patterns in the present study) extracted from EMG data recorded for slip-perturbed walking in the human gait experiment to construct a rapid responding pathway.

The results indicated that the simulation model could display behavior resembling that of normal human walking, and, on the occurrence of a slip-perturbation, together with the CPG-phase-modulation, the rapid muscular response could improve perturbation-resistance and maintain balance for the simulated walker.

Although these results were quite encouraging, the roles of different reflexive mechanisms have not yet been quantitatively clarified. However, understanding the roles of these functional mechanisms is not only important from the viewpoint of assistive engineering, but also for possible scientific insights into the field of motor control.

In the present study, we focused on the different roles of the reflexive muscle responses and the CPG-phase-modulation mechanism. By using the human walking simulator developed in our previous study, a series of simulation experiments were performed to investigate the roles in perturbation-resistance played by two functional mechanisms, i.e., muscular-reflexive-patterns and CPG-phase-modulation strategies, as well as the afferent feedback pre-wired in human walking models. Qualitative evaluation was performed to compare the different functional mechanisms.

For the quantitative evaluation, we used two stability criteria. One is the *Energy Stability Margin* (MESSURI et al. 1985), which is used to evaluate static postures. However, human walking and balance recovery are apparently dynamic processes, and a static stability criterion may not correctly reflect the essence of these functions. Thus, we proposed "*Energy Difference*", calculated from the rotational energy of lower limbs, to evaluate the dynamic aspect of stability.

Besides, in order to study another strategy, we tried spastic hemiplegic gait's simulation, that is one of hemiplegic gait. It suggests that spastic hemiplegic gait's simulation can consist of pes equinus and a compensated walk, and our simulated reflexive mechanisms could also improve the perturbation resistance for the spastic walking model.

2. Materials and Methods

2.1. Muscular Reflexive responses

The muscle activity profiles of reflexive responses can be extracted from EMG data recorded from slip-perturbed walking in previous human gait experiments (Cathers et al., 2004; Yu et al., 2007).

The difference between muscular activities during normal walking and perturbed walking was compared to a threshold to determine the onset of reflex responses. The threshold was defined using the mean and standard deviation of the first 2.5 s of data from the subtracted activity profile, i.e., the point at which the amplitude goes beyond mean±3 SD was considered the onset time. Additionally, for EMG recordings, the data after 2.54 s would be scanned for the onset determination. The 0.04-s gap was set according to the shortest muscle latency possible for reflex responses (Nakamura et al., 1992).

The latency data was further processed to extract muscular reflexive responses. It is noted that effective latency could not be detected for all muscles and all subjects. Thus, only the muscles for which an effective latency could be detected for more than 5 of 10 trials and more than 7 of 10 subjects were selected as the ones that should be activated during reflexive responses (Table 1). The selected muscles and their averaged latencies were designated the muscular-reflexive-patterns.

Muscles / Side	Gluteus Medius	Vastus Lateralis	Semi Tendinosus	Anterior Tibial	Gastroc Nemius
slip side	149(ms)	175 (ms)	178 (ms)	/	/
another side	143(ms)	/	88 (ms)	116 (ms)	176 (ms)

"/" indicates the side on which the muscles do not satisfy the conditions.

Table. 1. Latencies of the selected muscles.

In similar studies (Berger et al., 1984; Dietz et al., 1987), the split-belt treadmill was employed to study the corrective reactions to unpredictable one-sided deceleration and acceleration perturbations during walking. The EMG signals of two muscles, the tibialis anterior (TA) and gastrocnemius (GN), were recorded and analyzed, and our results showed the same temporal activation sequence on the contralateral side for both. That is, TA was activated first, followed by GN. TA was activated at a latency of 65 ms; however, our TA latency was 116 ms. This may have been due to differences in deceleration time; i.e., the treadmill could realize deceleration within 60 ms, whereas the deceleration time of the split-belt walking machine was 100 ms.

2.2. Simulation models

Four simulation models were developed. One was named the *Normal Walker,* which receives a command from the central nervous system and consists of a CPG model, a musculoskeletal model, and a sensory feedback module. The second one was designated the *Normal Walker with Reflex,* having the same basic elements of the *Normal Walker,* but with an additional reflex mechanism modulating the torque output from the CPG model. The third one was designated the *Spastic Walker,* having the same basic elements of the *Normal Walker,* but having pes equinus by biasing its plantarflexor neuron and compensatory actions for balance maintenance. The last one was designated the *Spastic Walker with Reflex,* having the same basic elements of the *Spastic Walker,* but with a same additional reflex mechanism as above.
The followings are the details of the four simulation models.

Normal Walker: Fig.1 shows the composition of this simulation model. The CPG was constructed as a set of coupled neural oscillators, each of which is expressed by a set of simultaneous differential equations (Matsuoka, 1985). The simultaneous differential equations are shown in eq.1. Neurons innervating lower limb muscles were mutually coupled so that their oscillations could be entrained to each other; consequently, the skeletal system controlled by the nervous system could display coordinated motion. Fig.2 shows the coupling relations between neurons.

$$\begin{aligned} \tau_n \dot{u}_n &= -u_n + \sum_s w_{ns} f_{\max}(u_s)_n - \beta v_n + z_n + feed, \\ \tau'_n \dot{v}_n &= -v_n + f_{\max}(u_n), \\ f_{\max}(\xi) &= \max(\xi, 0), \end{aligned} \tag{1}$$

where u_n is the inner state of the nth neuron, f_{max} is the output of the nth neuron, v_n is a variable representing the degree of the adaptation or self-inhibition effect of the nth neuron, z_n is an external input with a constant rate, w is the connecting weight between coupled neurons, and τ and τ' are time constants of the inner state and the adaptation effect, respectively. Neuron output $f_{\max}(u_n)$ is treated as the torque generated by the modulated muscle. Torques acting on joints were calculated as the differences of antagonistic muscle pairs.
This neural expression has also been widely used in other walking simulations (Taga, 1994; Ogihara et al., 2001). The *feed* in eq.1 can be calculated in eq.2 (Matsuoka, 1985) as

$$\begin{aligned} feed = {} & A(-X) + B_R hFg_R(-X) + B_L hFg_L(-X) \\ & + C_R hFg_R + C_L hFg_L + D(-X_d), \end{aligned} \tag{2}$$

where *feed* is a vector consisting of 14 elements corresponding to the feedback to 14 neurons (please refer to Fig. 2 for the neuron settings) and X is a vector variable expressing the state of the simulated links. (X_1, X_2), (X_3, X_4), (X_6, X_7), (X_9, X_{10}), (X_{12}, X_{13}), (X_{15}, X_{16}) and (X_{18}, X_{19}) express the positions of the center of gravity of the hip joint, left thigh, right thigh, left lower leg, right lower leg, torso and head, respectively. X_5, X_8, X_{11}, X_{14} and X_{17} express the angle of the left thigh, right thigh, left lower leg, right lower leg and torso, respectively. Correspondingly, X_{d5}, X_{d8}, X_{d11}, X_{d14} and X_{d17} stand for the angular velocity of the left thigh, right thigh, left lower leg, right lower leg and torso, respectively. hFg_R and hFg_L are two-value functions, taking a value of 1 during the stance phase and 0 during the swing phase for the right and left sides, respectively. A, B_R, B_L, C_R, C_L and D are the coefficient matrices.

Since *feed* contains pose and angle change information of the simulated links, as well as the reaction forces from the ground to the skeletal system, the interaction between the neuromusculoskeletal system and the external world could be realized. Our simulation model also employed this expression.

The weight and size of the body segments were set as follows. The head was set as a point, with a weight of 4 kgf. The torso, thigh, lower leg and foot were set as rectangles, whose width×height pairs are 0.7×0.05, 0.5×0.05, 0.6×0.05 and 0.25×0.3 m, respectively. Their weights were set as 32, 7, 4 and 1 kgf, respectively. The relative mass ratios of body segments are approximately in agreement with those of actual humans (Nakamura et al., 1992).

The model was developed using MATLAB version 7.0 software (The MathWorks, USA) and Working Model 2D version 7.0 software (MSC Software, USA). They were coupled by DDE (dynamic data exchange) protocol.

The utility of the simulation model is verified by comparing its joint trajectories during walking with those of a human subject.

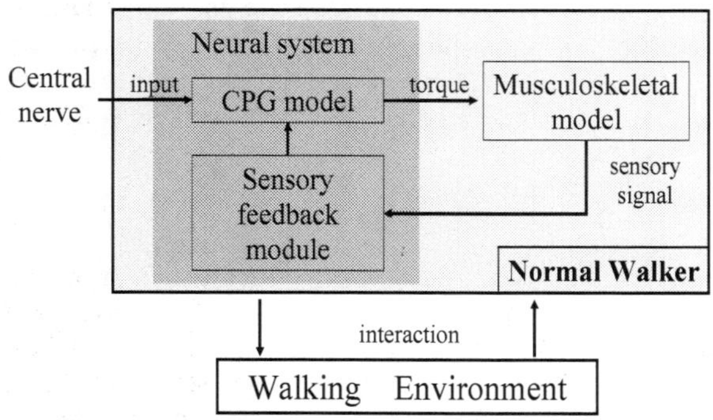

Fig. 1. the composition of *Normal Walker*

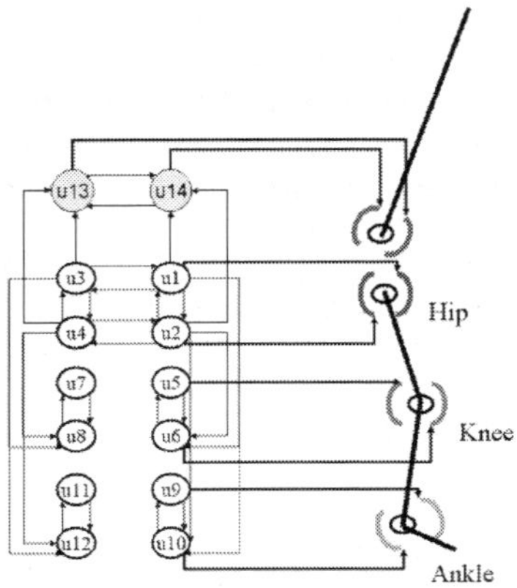

Fig. 2. The neuron-neuron and neuron-link connections

Normal Walker with Reflex: Fig.3 shows the composition of this simulation model. In order to realize the reflexive responses in the simulator, the following three points, that is, three aspects of the reflex function, should be determined:

1) Spatial aspect: the muscles that should be activated. In this study, this was decided by the muscular-reflexive-patterns described in subsection 2.1.

2) Temporal aspect: the onset timing, order of muscle activation, and interval of muscle activation. The triggering problem is addressed in a previous study on perturbation occurrence detection (Hagane et al., 2006) and will not be discussed in this paper. The order of muscle activation was again decided by the results of the measurement experiment. The interval of muscle activation was difficult to estimate from our human gait experiments, so the value is derived by an optimal search of computer simulation experiments. In this study, we used three different intervals (0.02 s, 0.05 s, and 0.09 s) because the human subject could modulate the strength of muscular reflexes suitably according to the strength of perturbation.

3) Relation to CPG output: the human walking rhythm is known to show phase-shift or "resetting" in response to external perturbation, and it is believed that such responses correct the perturbed motion and prevent the walker from falling (Yamasaki et al., 2003). Thus, in this study, after muscular reflexive activation, the CPG phase was set to be the same as that before the reflexive activation (CPG-phase-modulation). Fig.4 shows the outline of CPG-phase-modulation. The effective timing of CPG-phase-modulation (reset-time) was derived from a previous computer simulation experiment.

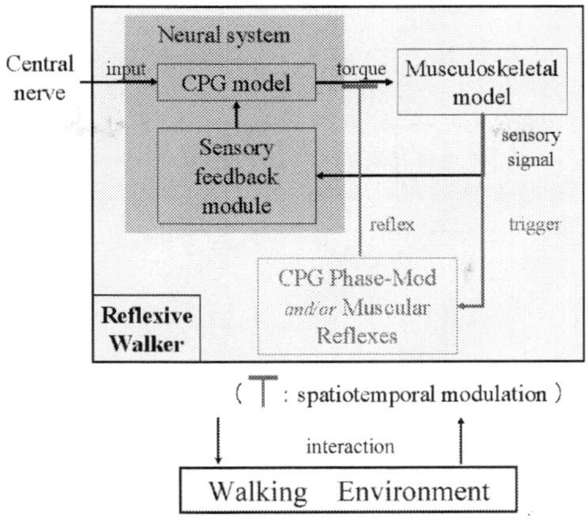

Fig. 3. The composition of *Normal Walker with Reflex*

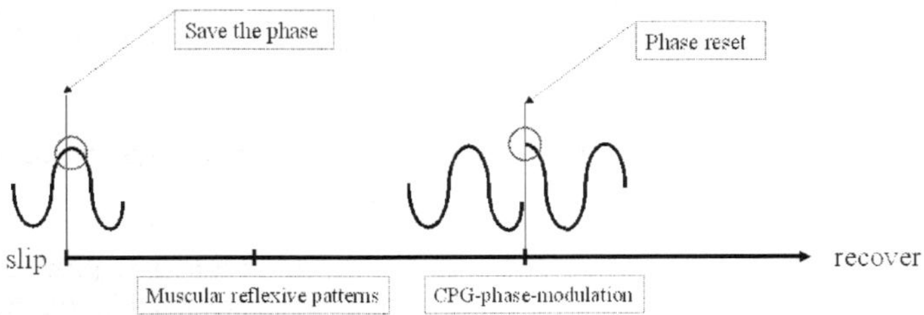

Fig. 4. CPG-phase-modulation

The slip perturbations to the simulated walkers were implemented by setting the friction coefficient to 0 for a period of time from the moment of heel strike. Different slip intervals would be used as parameters to adjust the levels of the perturbations.

If a walker was able to keep walking for 3 steps after perturbation, then its balance recovery was judged to be "successful". Otherwise, balance recovery was judged as "failed".

Phase portraits, whose horizontal axis give the angle and vertical axis gives angular velocity, were used to reveal qualitative data regarding the dynamics of the simulated walkers.

Spastic Walker: Biasing the output of the plantarflexor neuron (u10 or u12 in Fig. 2) causes pes equinus, and the model stumbles and falls. However it would keep stumbling away with compensatory actions by knee flexor and so on. So we modulated the output of the hip and knee flexors of the swing leg, so that the model could keep its balance. Appropriate parameters were decided by a trial-and-error process.

Spastic Walker with Reflex: This model has the same basic elements of the *Spastic Walker,* but also has the reflexive mechanisms explained in *Normal Walker with Reflex* section. Appropriate reflexive parameters were empirically determined. It is not so intuitive to apply the muscle activation profiles of healthy subjects to *Spastic Walker*. However, since the profiles should reflect the fundamental elements of human balance-recovery, also in order to make comparison under the similar condition, the same muscle activation profiles was applied.

2.3. Evaluation

Only the recovered/fell evaluation was unable to reflect the difference between the same "fell" or "recovered" cases. With regard to quantitative evaluation, we used two stability criteria.

Energy Stability Margin: used to evaluate static postures of a walking machine (MESSURI et al., 1985), and defined as "the potential energy gain by the change of the center of mass on the occurrence of perturbation" (Eq. 3).

$$S = M(h_{\max} - h_0) \tag{3}$$

Where M is the mass of a walking object, $h_{\max}$ is the height that a COG is changed to on the occurrence of fall, and h_0 is the current height of the COG.

Energy Difference: proposed for the dynamic evaluation of stability during walking, and defined as "the difference of the lower limb's rotational energy in swing phase between perturbed and normal walking" (Eq. 4).

$$ED = \frac{1}{2} I\omega_{perturbed}{}^{2} - \frac{1}{2} I\omega_{normal}{}^{2} \tag{4}$$

where I is a moment of inertia and ω is angular velocity of each lower limb at the time of normal and perturbed walking.

This evaluation method is unfit for *Spastic Walker* and *Spastic Walker with Reflex*, therefore is used only for *Normal Walker* and *Normal Walker with Reflex*.

3. Results and Discussion

3.1 Muscular reflexive patterns with phase modulation

Table 2 shows the balance recovery by CPG phase modulation and muscular reflexive patterns. Here, the "reset time" is a parameter of CPG phase modulation, that is, the timing at which CPG restarts from a phase memorized at the occurrence of a slip perturbation, counting from the time of the perturbation occurrence. A cross-mark (x) stands for a complete loss of its balance at the corresponding reset time and slip duration. A circle-mark (o) means that the walker ultimately recovered successfully from the corresponding perturbation, with each muscular reflexive pattern activation periods (a. 0.02 s, b. 0.05 s and c. 0.09 s).

As shown in Table 2, effective reset time that conduce balance recovery differs by slip duration, and becomes longer as slip duration increases. It is also observed that a longer muscular reflex (activation period 0.09 s) is effective for larger perturbations, and a shorter muscular reflex (activation period 0.02 s) is effective for smaller perturbations.

The first half of Fig.5 shows stable gait; however, on the occurrence of a slip perturbation at the moment of heel strike, the *Normal Walker* fell down, as shown in the latter half of the stick graph in Fig.5a.

Besides, Fig.5b shows one of the results of *Normal Walker with Reflex* successfully coping with a perturbation, in which the walker initially supported the weight with its rear leg to prevent the body from falling backwards, while simultaneously delaying the timing to move the rear leg forward for the next step, which is also observed in human gait experiments.

(a) Muscular reflexive activation period 0.02s

reset time(s)

slip duration(s)	0.1	0.12	0.14	0.16	0.18	0.2	0.22	0.24	0.26	0.28	0.3	0.32	0.34	0.36	0.38	0.4	0.42	0.44	0.46	0.48	0.5	0.52	0.54	0.56	0.58
0.1	○	○	○	○	○	○	○	○	×	×	×	×	×	×	×	×	×	×	×	×	×	○	○	×	○
0.125	○	○	○	○	○	○	○	○	○	○	×	×	×	×	×	×	×	×	×	×	○	×	×	○	×
0.15	×	×	×	×	×	○	○	○	○	○	○	○	○	○	×	○	×	×	×	×	×	○	×	×	×
0.175	×	×	×	×	×	×	×	×	×	×	×	×	×	×	×	×	×	×	×	×	×	×	×	×	×
0.2	○	○	×	×	×	×	×	×	×	×	×	×	×	×	×	×	×	×	×	×	×	×	×	×	×
0.225	×	○	○	○	○	○	×	×	×	×	×	×	×	×	×	×	×	×	×	×	×	×	○	○	×
0.25	×	×	×	×	×	×	×	×	×	×	×	×	×	×	×	×	×	×	×	×	×	×	×	×	×
0.275	×	×	×	×	×	×	×	×	×	×	×	×	×	×	×	×	×	×	×	×	×	×	×	×	×
0.3	×	×	×	×	×	×	×	×	×	×	×	×	×	×	×	×	×	×	×	×	×	×	×	×	×
0.325	×	×	×	×	×	×	×	×	×	×	×	×	×	×	×	×	×	×	×	×	×	×	×	×	×

(b) Muscular reflexive activation period 0.05s

reset time(s)

slip duration(s)	0.1	0.12	0.14	0.16	0.18	0.2	0.22	0.24	0.26	0.28	0.3	0.32	0.34	0.36	0.38	0.4	0.42	0.44	0.46	0.48	0.5	0.52	0.54	0.56	0.58
0.1	×	×	×	×	×	×	×	×	×	×	×	×	×	×	×	×	×	×	×	×	×	×	×	×	×
0.125	×	×	×	×	×	×	×	×	×	×	×	○	○	○	○	○	○	○	×	×	×	×	×	×	×
0.15	×	×	×	×	×	×	×	×	×	×	○	○	○	○	○	○	○	×	×	×	×	×	×	×	×
0.175	×	×	×	×	×	×	×	×	×	×	○	○	○	○	○	○	○	○	○	×	×	×	×	○	×
0.2	×	×	○	×	×	×	×	×	×	×	×	×	×	×	×	×	○	○	○	○	○	○	×	×	×
0.225	×	×	×	×	×	×	×	×	×	×	×	×	×	×	×	×	×	×	○	○	○	○	○	○	○
0.25	○	○	○	×	○	○	○	○	×	×	○	○	○	×	○	×	×	×	×	×	×	×	×	×	×
0.275	×	×	×	×	×	×	×	×	×	×	×	○	×	×	○	○	×	×	×	×	×	○	×	×	×
0.3	×	○	○	×	×	×	×	×	×	×	×	×	×	×	×	×	×	×	×	×	×	×	×	×	×
0.325	×	×	×	×	×	×	×	×	×	×	×	×	×	×	×	×	×	×	×	×	×	×	×	×	×

(c) Muscular reflexive activation period 0.09s

reset time(s)

slip duration(s)	0.1	0.12	0.14	0.16	0.18	0.2	0.22	0.24	0.26	0.28	0.3	0.32	0.34	0.36	0.38	0.4	0.42	0.44	0.46	0.48	0.5	0.52	0.54	0.56	0.58
0.1	×	×	×	×	×	×	×	×	×	×	×	×	×	×	×	×	×	×	×	×	×	×	×	×	×
0.125	×	×	×	×	×	×	×	×	×	×	×	×	×	×	×	×	×	×	×	×	×	×	×	×	×
0.15	×	×	×	×	×	×	×	×	×	×	×	×	×	×	×	×	×	×	×	×	×	×	×	×	×
0.175	×	×	×	×	×	×	×	×	×	×	×	×	×	×	×	×	×	×	×	×	×	×	×	×	×
0.2	×	×	×	×	×	×	×	×	×	×	×	×	×	×	×	×	×	×	×	×	×	×	×	×	×
0.225	×	×	×	×	×	×	×	×	×	×	×	×	×	×	○	○	○	○	○	○	○	○	○	○	○
0.25	○	○	○	×	×	×	×	×	×	×	×	×	×	×	×	×	○	○	○	○	○	○	○	○	○
0.275	○	○	○	○	○	○	○	○	○	○	×	○	○	○	○	○	○	×	×	○	○	×	×	×	×
0.3	○	×	×	○	○	×	×	○	○	○	○	○	×	×	×	×	×	×	×	×	×	×	×	○	○
0.325	×	×	×	○	○	○	×	○	×	○	×	○	×	×	×	×	×	×	×	×	×	×	×	×	×

Table 2. Balance recovery by CPG phase modulation and muscular reflexive patterns when slip perturbation duration changes

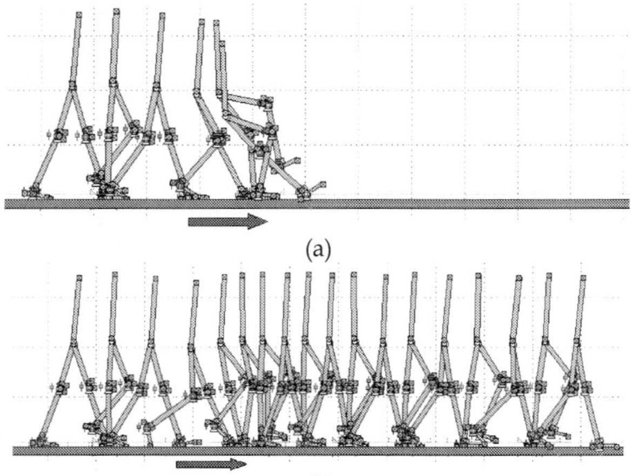

(a)

(b)

Fig. 5. Stick graphs of the *Normal Walker* and the *Normal Walker with Reflex* (arrows denote the slip period): (a) the *Normal Walker* fell down when a slip perturbation occurs; and (b) the *Normal Walker with Reflex* recovered from slip perturbation.

3.2. The roles of different regulation mechanisms

In order to examine the role of reflexive mechanisms, muscular-reflexive-patterns and CPG-phase-modulation, we evaluated the perturbed walk of each walker (*Normal Walker*, *Normal Walker* with Phase-modulation, *Normal Walker* with muscular reflex, and *Normal Walker* with both reflexes that is *Normal Walker with Reflex*) by the *Energy Stability Margin* and *Energy Difference* (see section 2.4). Five seconds of the *Energy Stability Margin* of each walker in the slip-perturbed condition (0.2-s slip) are plotted in Fig. 6. Here, slip perturbation occurs at 1 s in Fig. 6. In order to make a clear comparison, we selected an experimental condition (slip duration=0.25 s) that could lead to successful balance recovery for all 4 walkers. Note that, for the *Normal Walker*, this is the rare successful balance recovery case. Additionally, Fig. 7 shows the integration of the *Energy Stability Margin* of each walker after perturbation occurrence. Furthermore, five seconds of *Energy Difference* of each walker in the same slip perturbed condition is plotted in Fig. 8. Fig. 9 shows the integration of the *Energy Difference* of each walker after perturbation occurrence. Arrows in the figures denote points for further discussion. As shown in Figs. 6 and 8, the *Normal Walker with Reflex* has better balance recovery ability than the *Normal Walker*. It is also observed that both CPG-phase-modulation and muscular-reflexive-patterns could achieve more effective balance recovery than the *Normal Walker* (excepting the *Energy Stability Margin* value of the Phase-modulation-alone case, which will be discussed later), and the *Normal Walker with Reflex* (utilizing both mechanisms) could achieve most effective balance recovery (Figs. 7 and 9). This suggests that CPG-phase-modulation and muscular-reflexive-patterns display a cumulative effect for balance recovery.

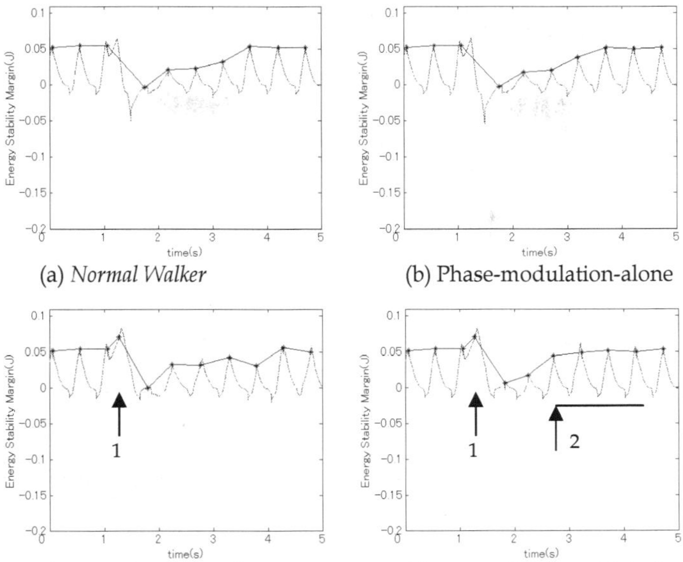

(a) *Normal Walker* (b) Phase-modulation-alone

(c) Muscular-reflex-alone (d) *Normal Walker with Reflex*

Fig. 6. *Energy Stability Margin*

Arrow 1 stands for the immediate improvement of balance after perturbation. Arrow 2 shows the beginning of recovered gait.

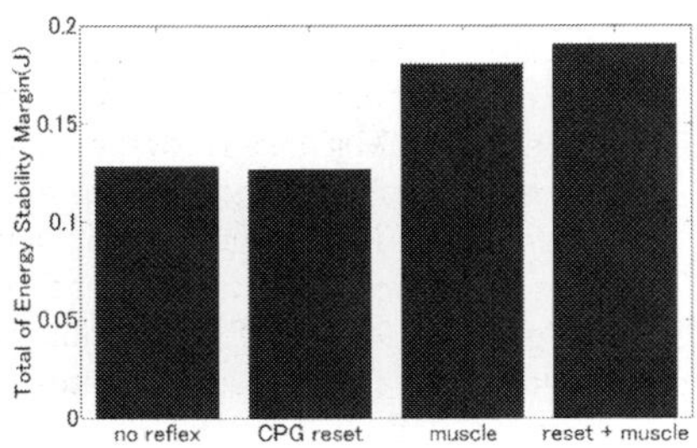

Fig. 7. Integration of *Energy Stability Margin* (from left, *Normal Walker*, *Normal Walker* with phase modulation, *Normal Walker* with muscular reflex, *Normal Walker with Reflex*)

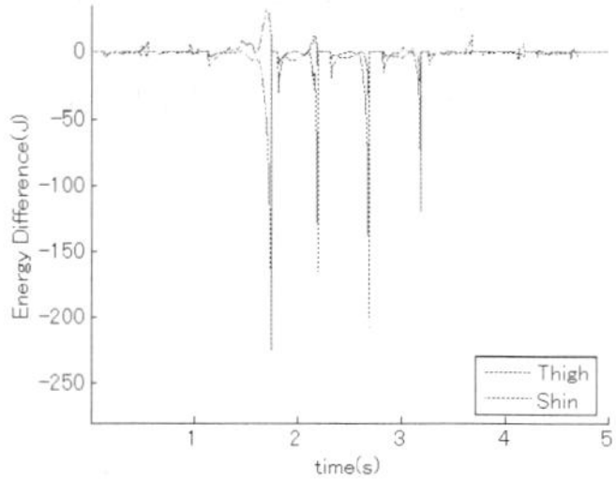

(a) *Normal Walker*

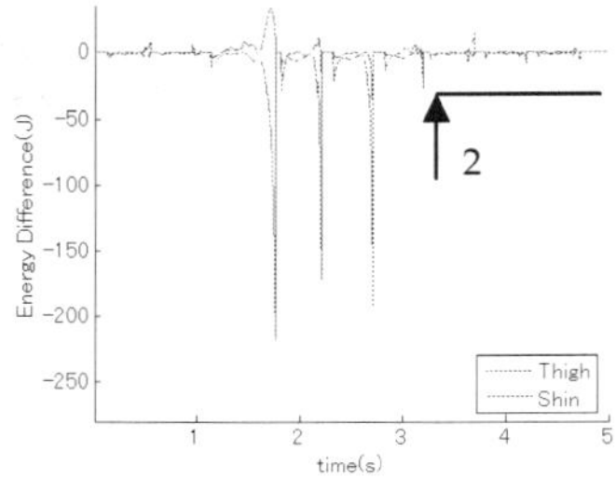

(b) Phase-modulation-alone

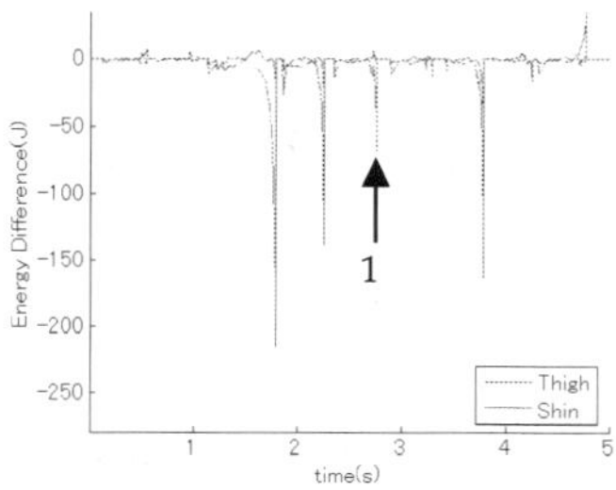

(c) Muscular-reflex-alone

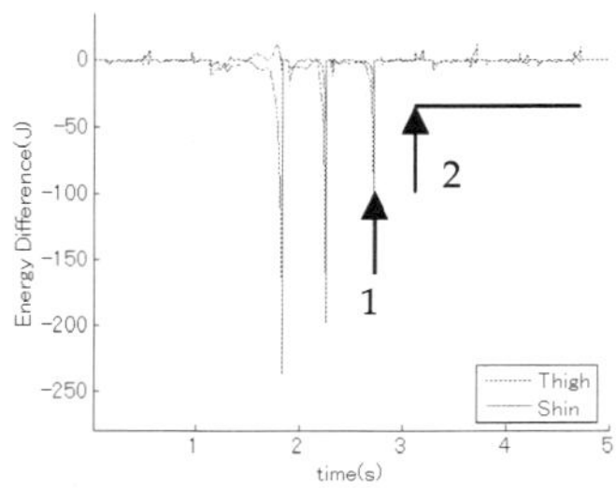

(d) *Normal Walker with Reflex*

Fig. 8. *Energy Difference*

Arrow 1 indicates the immediate improvement of balance after perturbation, by a much smaller energy difference, compared with the 4th drop in the Normal Walker case. Arrow 2 denotes the beginning of the recovered gait, where the walker possesses the same rotational energy as that of normal walking.

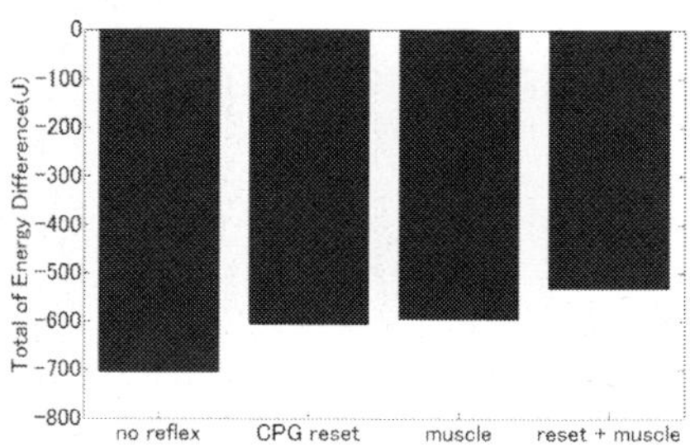

Fig. 9. Integration of *Energy Difference* (from left, *Normal Walker*, *Normal Walker* with Phase-modulation, *Normal Walker* with muscular reflex, *Normal Walker with Reflex*)

Fig. 10 (a) and (b) show the hip joint angle phase portraits of the muscular reflex alone case and the muscular reflex with phase modulation case, respectively. Note that the slip condition and activation term are same for both tests, and only the hip angle values of the perturbed side are plotted. The blue line and red lines represent the normal and perturbed walks, respectively. It was observed that the muscular reflex with phase modulation case could return back to the normal walking attractor within 1.9 s, while muscular reflex alone could lead the walker back to the normal walking attractor within 2.9 s. This result suggests that CPG-phase-modulation is effective for modulating the relationship between internal CPG and the body mechanisms enabling a fast recovery to a stable walking cycle.

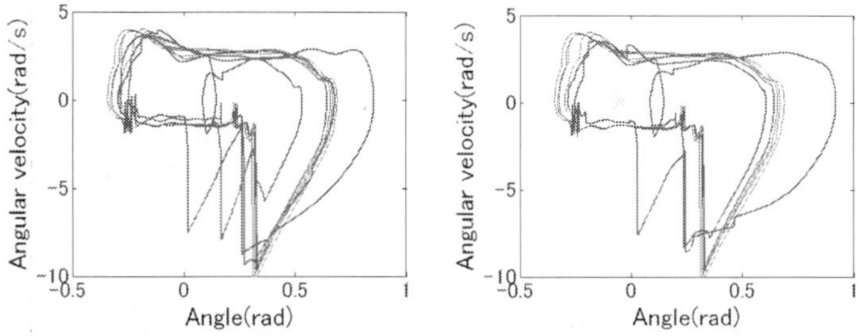

(a) Muscular reflex alone (b) With phase modulation

Fig. 10. Phase portraits of the hip joint angle (*Normal Walker*)

3.3. Spastic Gait

As the result of the experiments, *Spastic Walker* acquired a stable gait pattern. Fig.11 shows the gait of *Spastic Walker*, and Fig.12 (a) and (b) show the hip joint angle phase portraits and five seconds of Energy Stability Margin of this walker, respectively. As shown in Fig.11, *Spastic Walker* lifts its swing leg higher than *Normal Walker*, and avoids a stumbling. This result is very similar to the result of paralyzed people's gait experiment (Yu et al., 2002). Moreover, it is observed the walker has a peculiar stable limit cycle, which is different from that of *Normal Walker* (Fig.12 a). Also it is clear that the walker keeps its balance continually throughout five seconds. (Fig.12 b)

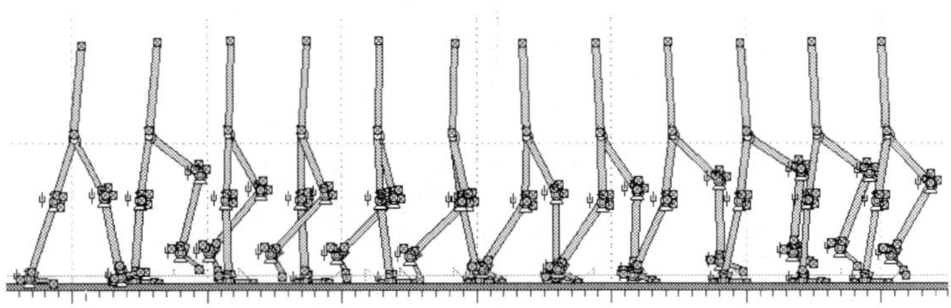

Fig. 11. Stick graph of the *Spastic Walker*

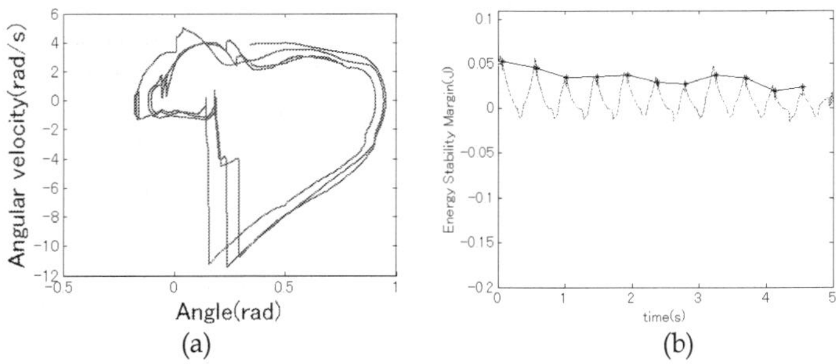

Fig. 12. (a) Phase portrait of the hip joint angle: and (b) Five seconds of the *Energy Stability Margin* of *Spastic Walker*

3.4. Recovery from slip perturbation during Spastic Gait

As anticipated, the *Spastic Walker* lost its balance and fell down on the occurrence of short-time slip perturbation (e.g. slip duration: 0.2s). However the *Spastic Walker with Reflex* was able to keep its balance for a certain period of time after the perturbation, even though not able to recover to its stable walking (Fig.13). Fig.14 shows the comparison between these two walkers. Note that the *Spastic Walker with Reflex* keeps standing position for a longer time than no-reflex case (Fig.14a; a period of 1.2s-2.0s), and has high balance stability compared with no-reflex case (Fig.14b; a period of 1.2s-1.6s).

Thus the acquired muscle activation profiles could reflect the fundamental elements of human balance-recovery, but it's not enough for a complete recovery in the case of the spastic walk. This denotes that, some additional mechanisms, other than the current reflexive mechanisms, should be explored for the balance recovery. This will be another issue for further investigation.

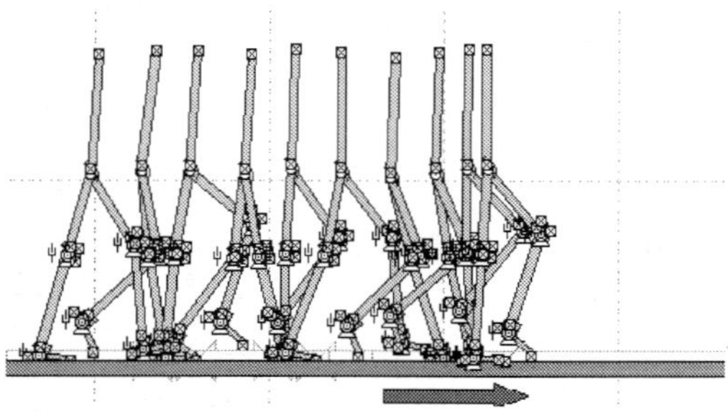

Fig. 13. Stick graph of the *Spastic Walker with Reflex* (the arrow denote the slip period): the *Spastic Walker with Reflex* kept its balance after slip perturbation.

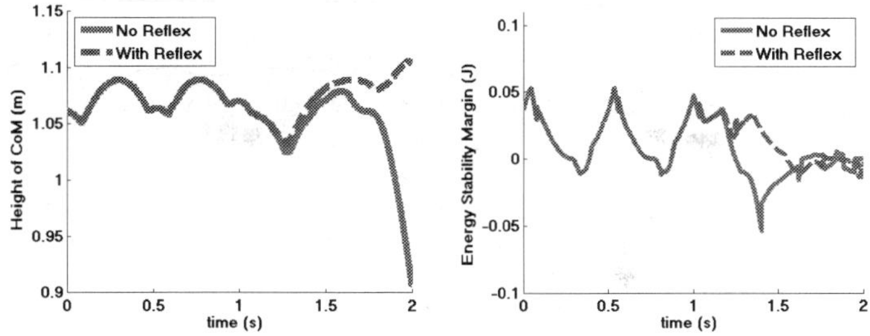

(a) (b)

Fig. 14. The comparison between the *Spastic Walker* (red line) and the *Spastic Walker with Reflex* (blue dotted line). Note that a slip perturbation occurs from 1s to 1.2s: (a) Transition of the height of CoM; and (b) Transition of *Energy Stability Margin*

4. Conclusion

In the present study, we developed four simulation models, and, through computer simulation, revealed that: 1) on the occurrence of a slip-perturbation, the rapid responding pathway could improve perturbation-resistance and maintain balance for walking; 2) using the simulation models, the roles of the muscular reflexive patterns, CPG phase modulation and afferent feedback were clarified; 3) a spastic gait can be modeled by pes equinus and appropriate compensatory muscle supports; and 4) reflexive strategies extracted from healthy subjects may contain fundamental elements of human balance recovery, thus it is available to work to some extent for spastic walkers' perturbation-resistance.

That is, feedback pathway, phase modulation, reflexive muscular patterns, and compensated gait play different but significant roles in balance recovery. Therefore, is reasonably to conclude that our model has a redundancy mechanism for walking as the human. These results demonstrated the practical possibility of realizing artificial reflexes for paralyzed individuals.

5. References

Bajd T, Stefancic M, Zmatjacic Z, Kraij A, Savrin R, Benko H, Karcnik T, Obereza P (1997) Improvement in step clearance via calf muscle stimulation. Medical & biological Engineering & Computing, Vo. 35, 113-116

Berger W, Dietz V, Quintern J (1984) Corrective Reactions to Stumbling in Man: Neuronal Co-ordination of Bilateral Leg Muscle Activity During Gait. J. Physiol 357:109-125

Bisdorff R, Bronstein AM, Wolsley C, Gresty MA, Davies A, Young A (1999) EMG responses to free fall in elderly subjects and akinetic rigid patients. J Neurol Neurosurg Psychiatry, 66: 447-455

Cathers I, O'Dwyer N, Neilson P (2004) Variation of magnitude and timing of wrist flexor stretch reflex across the full range of voluntary activation. Exp. Brain Res., 157; 324-335

Dietz V, Quintern J, Sillem M (1987) Stumbling Reactions in Man; Significance of Proprioceptive and Pre-programmed Mechanisms. J. Physiol 386:149-163

Hagane Y, Yu W, Katane T, Sekine M, Tamura T, Saitou O (2006) Detecting Perturbation Occurrence during Walking. 11th ICPE, International Conference on Precision Engineering

Kawamoto H., Kanbe S, Sankai Y (2003) Power AssistMethod for HAL-3 Estimating Operator's Intension Based on MotionInformation. Proc. of 12th IEEE Workshop on Robot and HumanI nteractive Communication (ROMAN 2003)

Mathie MJ, Celler BG, Lovell NH, Coster ACF (2004) Classification of basic daily movements using a triaxial accelerometer. Medical & biological Engineering & Computing, Vo. 42, 679-687

Mathie MJ, Coster ACF, Lovell NH, Celler BG (2003) Detection of daily physical activities using a triaxial accelerometer. Medical & biological Engineering & Computing, Vo. 41, 296-301

Matsuoka K (1985) Susteined Oscillation Generated by Mutually Inhibiting Neurons with Adaptation. Biol. Cybern. 52, 367-376

Messuri DA, Klein CA (1985) Automatic Body Regulation for Maintaing Stability of a Legged Vehicle During Rough-Terrian Locomotion. IEEE JOURNAL OF ROBOTICS AND AUTOMATION, Vol. RA-1, No. 3, September

Nakamura R, Saito H (1992) Basic Kinesiology. 4th edn. ISHIYAKU, Tokyo

Ogihara N, Yamazaki N (2001) Generation of human bipedal locomotion by a bio-mimetic neuromuscloskeletal model. Biol. Cybern. 84, 1-11

Prochazka A, Yakovenko S (2001) Locomotor control: from spring-like reactions of muscles to neural prediction. In: The Somatosensory System: Deciphering The Brain's Own Body Image. ed. Nelson, R.J. Boca Raton, CRC Press, 141-181

Quintern J (2000) Stimulation of flexor reflex afferents: a pathway to the spinal pattern generator for human locomotion? 6th Internet World Congress for Biomedical Sciences, Presentation #60

Schomburg ED, Petersen N, Barajon I, Hultborn H (1998) Flexor reflex afferents reset the step cycle during fictive locomotion in the cat. Exp. Brain Res., 122: 339-350

Taga G (1994) Emergence of bipedal locomotion through entrainment among the neuromusculoskeletal system and the environment. Physica D 75, 190-208

Tong YT, Granat MH (1998) Reliability of neural-network functional electrical stimulation gait-control system. Medical & biological Engineering & Computing, Vol. 37, 633-638

Yamasaki T, Nomura T, Sato S (2003) Possible function roles of phase resetting during walking. Biological Cybernetics, 88, 468-496

Yu W, Ikemoto Y (2007) An artificial reflex improves the perturbation-resistance of a human walking simulator. Medical and Biological Engineering and Computing, Special Issue of World Congress on Medical Physics and Biomedical Engineering 2006, springer. DOI, 10.1007/s11517-007-0255-1, 45, pp. 1095-1104

Yu W, Yamaguchi H, Yokoi H, Maruishi M, Mano Y, Kakazu Y (2002) EMG automatic switch for FES control for hemiplegics using artificial neural network. Robotics and Autonomous Systems, Vol. 40, pp. 213-224

Zehr EP, Stein RB (1999) What functions do reflexes serve during human locomotion? Elsevier Science Ltd: Progress in Neurobiology, Vol. 58, pp. 185-205

Human Facial Expression Recognition Using Fisher Independent Component Analysis and Hidden Markov Model

Tae-Seong Kim and Jee Jun Lee
Kyung Hee University, Dept. of Biomedical Engineering
Republic of Korea

1. Introduction

Facial expression recognition (FER), a special part of gesture recognition, is one of the fundamental technologies for Human Computer Interface (HCI), which allows computers or other devices to interact with humans in a similar way to human to human interactions (Mitra & Acharya, 2007). A FER system can contribute to a HCI system by responding to the expressive states of a user upon recognizing his or her emotional state from the facial images. Various approaches have been attempted to solve the FER problem so far. In one major category of approaches known as the Facial Action Units (FAU)-based FER, FAUs are identified and classified to understand facial muscle movements according to facial expressions such as joy, anger, disgust, fear, sadness, and surprise. In another category of approaches known as the emotion-specified FER, facial expressions are represented by holistic or local features and the combination of these features are used to recognize each specific expression. In general, FER involves various feature extraction and recognition or classification techniques.

Among the various feature extraction techniques, the most commonly utilized technique so far in the FER research community is Principle Component Analysis (PCA). PCA is a second-order statistical method that produces orthogonal basis of given data. In general, PC images provide global features of facial expressions. In the FAU-based FER, Padgett & Cottrell (1997) applied PCA on facial expression images to identify FAUs and to recognize facial expressions in which their best analysis was performed on the separated face regions such as eyes and mouth. Donato et al. (1999) also employed PCA for FER with their Facial Action Coding System (FACS). In the later approaches of FER, PCA is commonly augmented with Fisher Linear Discriminant (FLD) which is based on the class information which projects the data onto a subspace with the criterion that the between-class scatter of the projected data is maximized and the within-class scatter is minimized. This PCA-FLD augmentation much improved the accuracy of the classification and the performance of FER. For example, Calder et al. (2001) employed PCA and FLD using the pixel intensities of holistic face images and Dubuisson et al. (2002) performed the PCA-FLD based feature extraction on facial images to classify the expressions. However, the nature of PCA, which only relies on the second-order statics and decorrelation of data, limits the performance of

FER. To overcome this deficiency, some higher order statistical methods have been suggested lately.

As one of the higher order feature extraction techniques, lately independent component analysis (ICA) has been utilized extensively for FER tasks due to its ability to extract local features (Donato et al., 1999; Bartllet et al., 2002; Chen & Kotani, 2008; Buciu & Kotropoulos, 2003). ICA is a generalization of PCA which learns the higher order statistics of data, producing the facial features that are statistically independent to each other. It actually performs blind source separation with the assumption that the given data is a linear mixture of sources which produces statistically independent basis and coefficients (Karklin & Lewicki, 2003). For the FAU-based FER, Bartlett et al. (2002) extracted the features using ICA to classify twelve facial actions for facial expressions coding referred to as FACS. Also, Chuang & Shih (2006) utilized ICA to extract the independent features of facial expression images and recognized the upper and lower parts of FAUs and the whole face parts of FAUs. However, these works mostly focused on the successful extraction of FAUs not on the recognition of facial expressions. Also, their works encountered the limitation of AUs due to the fact that the separate facial actions do not directly draw the comparisons with human data (Calder et al., 2000). For the emotion-specified FER, Buciu et al. (2003) reported their highest recognition accuracy of 86.39% when applying ICA on the Japanese female facial expression data (Lyons et al., 1998). However, they only used the peak expressional state of each expression images to recognize the expressions while the temporal information of facial expression changes is ignored. Bartlett et al. (2002) later utilized the enhanced ICA (EICA) with the two different architectures where the first architecture finds spatially local basis images for the faces and the second produces the factorial face codes. In their proposed settings, they found that the local features of face images are sensitive to FER meanwhile the factorial code is preferred for face recognition. Later, Kwak and Pedrycz introduced the fisher version of independent component analysis (FICA) in the two different architectures similar to the way of Bartlett's, and they reported that FICA outperforms the generic ICA and EICA methods in face recognition (Kwak & Pedrycz, 2007). So far, EICA and FICA are successfully utilized for face recognition, but rarely utilized for FER.

As for the recognition techniques in FER, various distance measures such as Euclidian, Mahalonobis, and Cosine distances have been used to assign the facial data to a relevant expression class (Lyons et al., 1998). Neural network systems have been employed to extract FAUs with the Gabor wavelet based features (Tian et al., 2002). Then, a bank of Support Vector Machine (SVM) classifiers was used on the regions of facial expression images in FER (Chuang & Shih, 2006; Kotsia & Pitas, 2007). For instance, Chuang & Shih (2006) used independent components as facial expression features, and SVM was performed to extract FAUs. Recently, Hidden Markov Model (HMM), a method for dynamic and sequential event recognition, has been popularly applied for FER (Otsuka & Ohya, 1997; Aleksic & Katsaqqelos, 2006). Zhu et al. (2002) used HMM to recognize the emotions with moment invariants as their feature. In their work, they report the overall average accuracy of 96.77% where only four expressions were recognized. Cohen et al. (2003) also adopted HMMs for temporal and static modeling of FER. They used the dynamic HMM models with the facial expression features extracted using the Naïve-Bayes classifiers and they reached their best accuracy rate of 73.22% on the Cohn-Kanade database. More recently, Aleksic & Katsaqqelos (2006) introduced a FER system using multi-stream HMMs and demonstrated the best performance of 93.66%. In their system, however, only separated facial animation

parameters such as eyebrow and outer-lip were used as decision cues for FER and they trained the HMM models using FAUs as input parameters. In other words, only the spatial information was utilized for training while the temporally changing patterns are not utilized. In summary, most of these works have used static facial expression images for FER, not utilizing the information of temporal and sequential changes of facial expression features.
In this chapter, we present a novel spatiotemporal modeling approach of FER, fully dealing with sequential facial expression images analyzed with FICA and recognized with HMM (Lee et al., 2008a; Lee et al., 2008b). The fundamental differences between our method and the previous approaches are i) we focus on the sequential holistic facial images to derive local spatiotemporal features so that we can model temporally evolving spatial patterns of the facial expression feature changes and ii) we exploit the natural feature behaviors rather than finding FAUs, and lastly, iii) we come up with the spatiotemporal model of each facial expression via HMM. In our method, spatially local independent features are extracted using FICA from sequential facial expression images. These FICA features are coded of temporally changes of the spatial feature via codebook generation which provides the symbolized spatiotemporal signatures. Then, discrete HMMs are constructed and trained for dynamic FER, encoding the spatiotemporal signatures of various facial expressions. To analyze the performance of our presented approach, some conventional feature extractors including PCA, ICA, EICA, and FLD over PCA (i.e., PCA-LDA) in combination with HMM are tested. Our results show that our presented method significantly outperforms the conventional approaches.

2. Methods

2.1 System Overview

Our FER system consists of i) spatiotemporal FE feature extraction including preprocessing of sequential FE images, ii) codebook generation for temporal signature coding, iii) modeling and training of HMMs, and iv) recognition via HMMs. Fig. 1 shows the overall architecture of our FER system where, L denotes the likelihood, O the observation, and H HMM (Lee et al., 2008a).

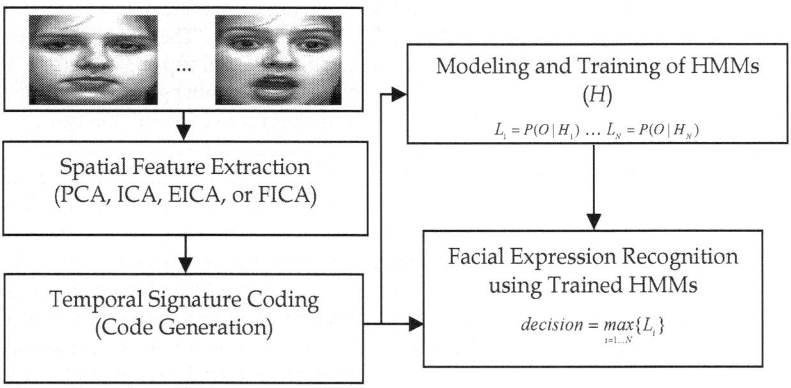

Fig. 1. Overview of our FER system.

2.2 Facial Expression Feature Extraction

The major objective of feature extraction is to find efficient FE spatial features in a lower dimensional subspace and reveal the patterns of temporal behaviors of the FE spatial features corresponding to the changes of facial expression from a neutral to a peak state of each facial expression. In preprocessing, face re-alignment, histogram equalization, and delta image generation have been performed to obtain the input images to our FER system. Then, temporally evolving spatial features are obtained in the feature extraction step.

2.2.1 Preprocessing

In preprocessing of sequential images of facial expressions, image alignment is performed first to realign the common regions of the face. In this study, we have utilized a face alignment approach described in (Zhang & Cottrell, 2004) by manually matching the eyes and mouth of the face in the designated coordinates. The facial images are scaled and translated so that the sum of square distance between the target coordinates and those of the transferred features was minimized: the triangular shape from two eyes and one mouth is scaled and translated to fit the reference location. The typical realigned image consisted of 60 by 80 pixels. Histogram equalization is then performed on the realigned images for lighting correction. Afterwards, the first frame of each input sequence is subtracted from the following frames to obtain the delta image (Donato et al., 1999), reflecting the facial expression change differences over time. Fig. 2 shows an exemplar set of a facial expression sequence of anger and the corresponding delta images.

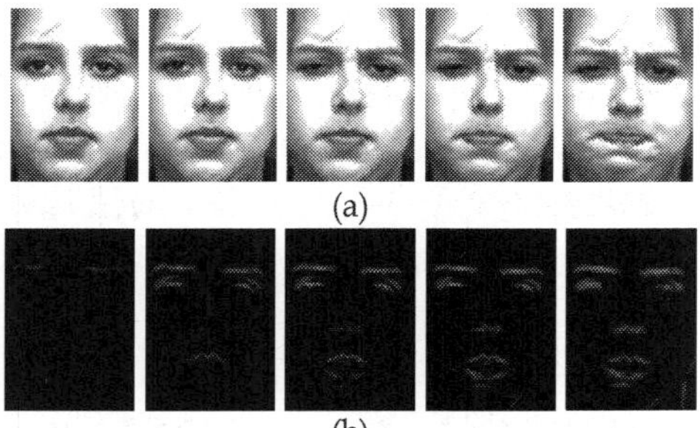

Fig. 2. Sequential facial expression images of anger: (a) a set of the aligned images and (b) the corresponding delta images.

2.2.2 Feature Extraction Using FICA

The key idea of FICA is the combination of ICA and FLD with the purpose to extract the local features such that the facial expression images are represented with them in a low dimensional space: the extracted features must be well separated in space in conjunction with temporally evolving spatial patterns. Extracting theses features via FICA consists of three fundamental stages: i) PCA is first performed for dimension reduction, ii) ICA is applied on the data in the reduced PCA subspace to find statistically independent basis features (i.e., images) for the corresponding facial expression images, and iii) FLD is finally employed to compress the features such that the similar features put close as possible and the different features put as far as possible.

For the first stage of FICA, we initially apply PCA to the data to reduce the dimension of data: PCA is a popular subspace projection method that transforms the high dimensional space to a reduced space by capturing the maximum variability which still contains the associated high order relationships. Basically, PCA basis vectors are obtained by the eigenvectors of the covariance data matrix such that

$$P^T(YY^T)P=\Lambda \tag{1}$$

where Y is the data matrix, Λ the diagonal matrix of eigenvalues, and P the orthogonal eigenvector matrix. The eigenvector associated with the largest eigenvalue indicates the axis of maximum variance and the following eigenvector with the second largest eigenvalue indicates the axis of the second largest variance. Thus, a certain number of eigenvectors associated with the higher eigenvalues defines the reduced subspace.

If we denote the image dataset as $X=(x_1,x_2,...,x_n)^T$ and its corresponding feature vectors in the reduced dimension by $V=(v_1,v_2,...,v_n)^T$. Then, the PCA algorithm finds the following feature vectors such that

$$V=XP_m \tag{2}$$

where P_m is the few selected m eigenvectors. Fig. 3 shows the PCs of the facial expression images.

As the second stage of FICA, ICA is applied to the PCA-reduced facial features to obtain statistically independent features. Basically ICA finds a linear transformation matrix to extract linear combinations of statistically independent sources from a set of random data. If we denote the observed data matrix again by $X=(x_1,x_2,...,x_n)^T$ and the sources of ICs by $S=(s_1,s_2,...,s_m)^T$. The linear ICA assumes that the data X is a linear combination of ICs such that

$$X=MS \tag{3}$$

where M is the matrix of size of $n\times m$ containing the mixing coefficients. The ICA algorithm performed on the data matrix finds an unmixing matrix W and independent source S. That is to say, the source images estimated in the rows of S are used as basis images to represent the dataset and are described as

$$U=WX \tag{4}$$

where U is an estimated independent sources and W represents the linear unmixing matrix.

Generally, ICA performance can be improved with a proper dimension reduction procedure such as PCA as a preprocessing step. ICA performed on the PCA space is also known as

EICA (Liu, 2004). Here, we apply the ICA algorithm on P_m^T which is in the reduced subspace containing the first m eigenvectors. To find the statistically independent basis images, each PCA basis image is the row of the input variables and the pixel values are observations for the variables. Thus,

$$U = W_{ICA} P_m^T \tag{5}$$

where U is the obtained basis images comprised with the coefficient W_{ICA} and the eigenvectors P_m^T. Some of the basis images are shown in Fig. 4. The reconstructed image set $\widetilde{X}$ is then described as

$$\widetilde{X} = V P_m^T = V W_{ICA}^{-1} U. \tag{6}$$

Therefore, the IC representation U can be computed by the rows of the feature vector R followed as

$$R = V W_{ICA}^{-1}. \tag{7}$$

For the final step of FICA, FLD is performed on the IC feature vectors of R. FLD is based on the class specific information which maximizes the ratio of the between-class scatter matrix and the within-class scatter matrix. The formulas for the within, S_W and between, S_B scatter matrix are defined as follows:

$$S_W = \sum_{i=1}^{c} \sum_{r_k \in C_i} (r_k - \widetilde{r}_i)(r_k - \widetilde{r}_i)^T, \tag{8}$$

$$S_B = \sum_{i=1}^{c} N_i (\widetilde{r}_i - r_m)(\widetilde{r}_i - r_m)^T \tag{9}$$

where c is the total number of classes, N_i the number of facial expression images, r_k the feature vector from all feature vector R, $\widetilde{r}_i$ the mean of class C_i, and r_m the mean of all feature vectors R.

The optimal projection W_d is chosen from the maximization of ratio of the determinant of the between class scatter matrix of the projection data to the determinant of the within class scatter matrix of the projected samples as

$$J(W_d) = |W_d^T S_B W_d| / |W_d^T S_w W_d| \tag{10}$$

where W_d is the set of discriminant vectors of S_B and S_W corresponding to the $c-1$ largest generalized eigenvalues. The discriminant ratio is derived by solving the generalized eigenvalue problem such that

$$S_B W_d = \Lambda S_W W_d \tag{11}$$

where Λ is the diagonal eigenvalue matrix. This discriminant vector W_d forms the basis of the $(c-1)$ dimensional subspace for a c-class problem.

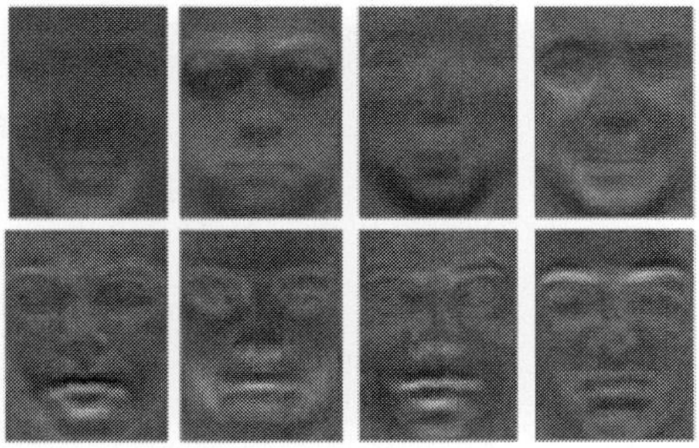

Fig. 3. Facial expression representation onto the reduced feature space using PCA. These are also known as eigenfaces.

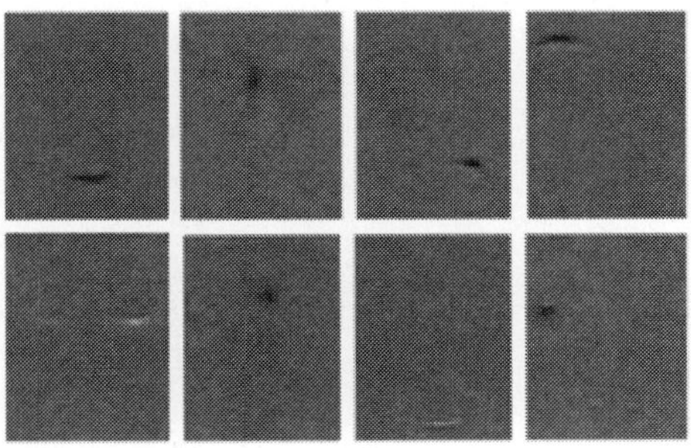

Fig. 4. Sample IC basis images.

Finally, the final feature vector G and the feature vector G_{test} for testing images can be obtained by the criterion

$$G = RW_d^T, \tag{12}$$

$$G_{test} = R_{test} W_d^T = X_{test} P_m W_{ICA}^{-1} W_d^T. \tag{13}$$

As the result of FICA, the vectors of each separated classes can be obtained. As can be seen in Fig. 5, the feature vectors associated with a specific expression are concentrated in a separated region in the feature space showing its gradual changes of each expression. The features of the neutral faces are located in the centre of the whole feature space as the origin of the facial expression, and the feature vectors of the target expressions are located in each expression region: within each expression feature region contains the temporal variations of the facial features. As shown in Fig. 6, a test sequence of sad expression is projected onto the sad feature region. The projections are evolving according to the time from $P(t_1)$ to $P(t_8)$, describing facial feature changes from the neural to the peak of sad expression.

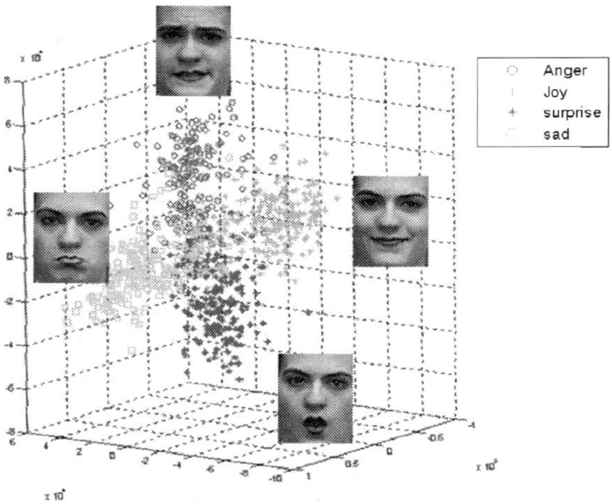

Fig. 5. Exemplar feature plot for four facial expressions.

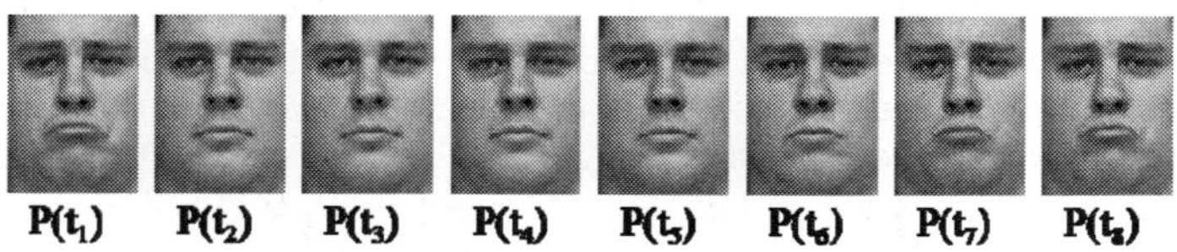

(a)

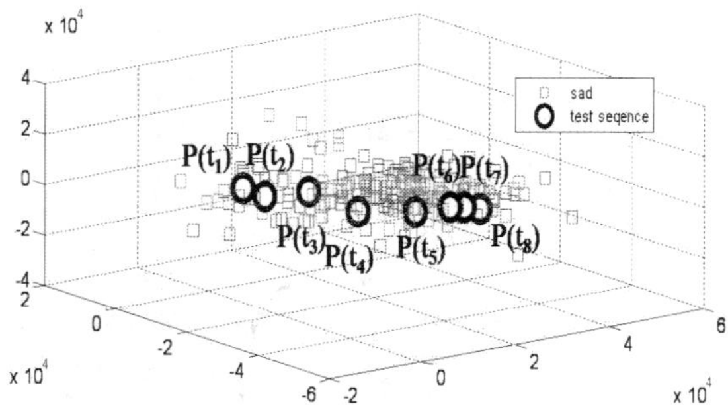

(b)

Fig. 6. (a) Test sequences of sad expression and (b) their corresponding projections onto the feature space.

2.3 Spatiotemporal Modelling and Recognition via HMM

Hidden Markov Model (HMM) is a statistical method of modeling and recognizing sequential information. It has been utilized in many applications such as pattern recognition, speech recognition, and bio-signal analysis (Rabiner, 1989). Due to its advantage of modeling and recognizing consecutive events, we also adopted HMM as a modeler and recognizer for facial expression recognition where expressions are concatenated from a neutral state to a peak of each particular expression. To train each HMM, we first perform vector quantization of training dataset of facial expression sequences to model sequential spatiotemporal signatures. Those obtained sequential spatiotemporal signatures are then used to train each HMM, learning each facial expression. More details are given in the following sections.

2.3.1 Code Generation

As HMM is normally trained with the symbols of sequential data, the feature vectors obtained from FICA must be symbolized. The symbolized feature vectors then become a codebook which is a set of symbolized spatiotemporal signature of sequential dataset, and the codebook is then regarded as a reference for recognizing the expression. To obtain the codebook, vector quantization is performed on the feature vectors from the training datasets. In our work, we utilize the Linde, Buzo and Gray (LBG)'s clustering algorithm for vector quantization (Linde et al, 1980). The LBG approach selects the first initial centroids and splits the centroids of the whole dataset. Then, it continues to split the dataset according to the codeword size.

After vector quantization is done, the index numbers are regarded as the symbols of the feature vectors to be modeled with HMMs. Fig. 7 shows the symbols of the codebook with the size of 32 as an example. The index of codeword located in the center of the whole feature space indicates the neutral faces and the other index numbers in each class feature space represents a particular expression reflecting gradual changes of an expression in time.

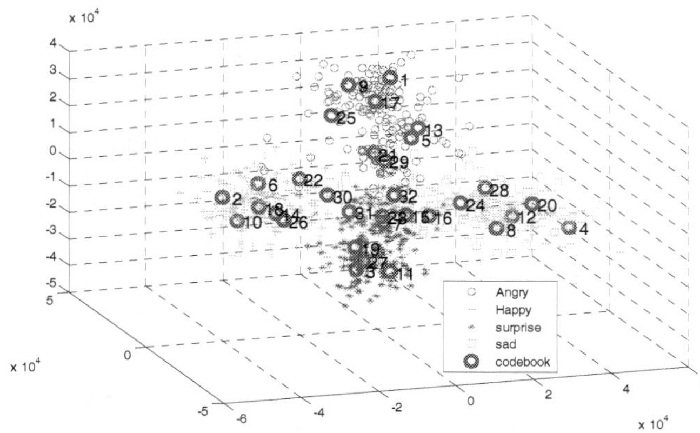

Fig. 7. Exemplary symbols of the codebook in the feature space. Only four out of six expressions are shown for clarity of presentation.

2.3.2 HMM and Training

HMM used in this work is a left-to-right model useful to model a sequential event in a system (Rabiner, 1989). Generally, the purpose of HMM is to determine the model parameter λ with the highest probability of the likelihood $\Pr(O|\lambda)$ when observing the sequential data $O=\{O_1, O_2, \cdots, O_T\}$. A HMM model is denoted as $\lambda = \{A, B, \pi\}$ and each element can be defined as follows (Zhu et al., 2002). Let us denote the states in the model by $S=\{s_1, s_2, \cdots, s_N\}$ and each state at a given time t by $Q=\{q_1, q_2, \cdots, q_t\}$. Then, the state transition probability A, the observation symbol probability B, and the initial state probability π are defined as

$$A=\{a_{ij}\},\ a_{ij}=\Pr(q_{t+1}=S_j \mid q_t=S_i),\ 1\le i, j\le N, \tag{14}$$

$$B=\{b_j(O_t)\},\ b_j=\Pr(O_t \mid q_t=S_j),\ 1\le j\le N, \tag{15}$$

$$\pi=\{\pi_j\},\ \ \pi_j=\Pr(q_1=S_j). \tag{16}$$

In the learning step, we set the variable, $\xi_t(i,j)$, the probability of being in the state q_i at time t and the state q_j at time $t+1$, to re-estimate the model parameters, and we also define the variable, $\gamma_t(i)$, the probability of being in the state q_i at time t as follows

$$\xi_t(i,j)=\frac{\alpha_t(i)a_{ij}b_j(O_{t+1})\beta_{t+1}(j)}{\Pr(O \mid \lambda)}, \tag{17}$$

$$\gamma_t(i)=\sum_{j=1}^{N}\xi(i,j) \tag{18}$$

where $\alpha_t(i)$ is the forward variable and $\beta_t(i)$ is the backward variable such that

$$\alpha_1(i)=\pi_i b_i(O_1),\ \ (1\le i\le q) \tag{19}$$

$$\alpha_{t+1}(j)=[\sum_{i=1}^{N}\alpha_t(i)a_{ij}]b_j(O_{t+1}),\ \ (t=1,2,\ldots,T-1) \tag{20}$$

$$\beta_T(i)=1,\ \ (1\le i\le q) \tag{21}$$

$$\beta_t(i)=\sum_{j=1}^{N}a_{ij}b_j(O_{t+1})\beta_{t+1}(i).\ \ (t=T-1, T-2, \ldots, 1) \tag{22}$$

Using the variables above, we can estimate the updated parameters A and B of the model of λ via estimating probabilities as follows

$$\bar{a}_{ij} = \frac{\sum_{t=1}^{T-1} \xi_t(i,j)}{\sum_{t=1}^{T-1} \gamma_t(i)}, \tag{23}$$

$$\bar{b}_j(k) = \frac{\sum_{\substack{t=1 \\ O_t=k}}^{T-1} \gamma_t(i)}{\sum_{t=1}^{T-1} \gamma_t(i)} \tag{24}$$

where $\bar{a}_{ij}$ is the estimated transition probability from the state i to the state j and $\bar{b}_j(k)$ the estimated observation probability of symbol k from the state j.

When training each HMM, a training sequence is projected on the FICA feature space and symbolized using the LBG algorithm. The obtained symbols of training sequence are compared with the codebook to form a proper symbol set to train the HMM. Table 1 describes the examples of symbol set for some expression sequences. Symbols in the first two frames are revealing the neutral states whose symbols are on the center of the whole feature subspace and the symbols are assigned into each frame as each expression gradually changes to its target state.

After training the model, the observation sequences $O=\{O_1, O_2, \cdots, O_T\}$ from a video dataset are evaluated and determined by the proper model with the likelihood $\Pr(O|\lambda)$. The likelihood of the observation O given the trained model λ can be determined via the forward variable in the form

$$\Pr(O|\lambda) = \sum_{i=1}^{N} \alpha_T(i) \; . \tag{25}$$

The criterion for recognition is the highest likelihood value of each model. Figs. 8 and 9 show the structure and transition probabilities for the anger case before and after training with the codebook size of 32 as an example.

Expression	Frame 1	Frame 2	Frame 3	Frame 4	Frame 5	Frame 6	Frame 7	Frame 8
Joy	24	32	30	30	14	14	10	10
Sad	32	32	24	16	13	12	4	12
Angry	21	21	13	9	7	8	22	25
Surprise	23	34	34	26	19	19	27	27

Table 1. Example of codebook symbols of the training expression data.

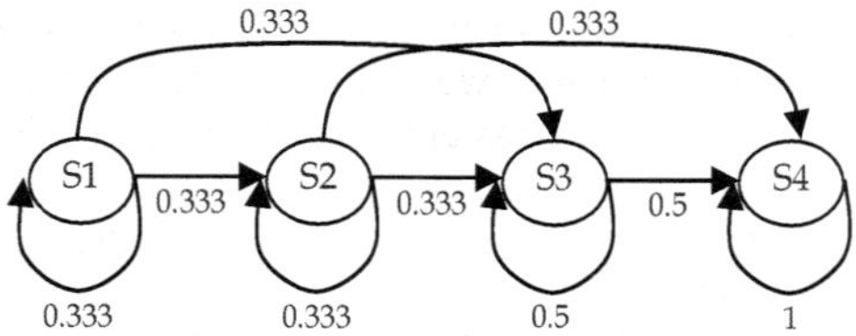

Fig. 8. HMM structure and transition probabilities for anger before training.

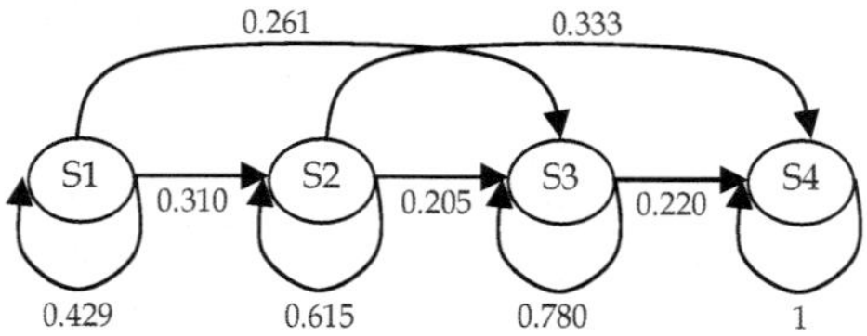

Fig. 9. HMM structure and transition probabilities for anger after training.

3. Experimental Setups

To assess the performance of our FER system, a set of comparison experiments were performed with each feature extraction method including PCA, generic ICA, PCA-LDA, EICA, and FICA in combination with the same HMMs. We recognized six different, yet commonly tested expressions: namely, anger, joy, sadness, surprise, fear, and disgust. The following subsections provide more details.

3.1 Facial Expression Database

The facial expression database used in our experiment is the Cohn-Kanade AU-coded facial expression database consisting of facial expression sequences with a neutral expression as an origin to a target facial expression (Cohn et al., 1999). The image data in the Cohn-Kanade AU-coded facial expression database displays only the frontal view of the face and each subset is comprised of several sequential frames of the specific expression. There are six universal expressions to be classified and recognized. Facial expressions include 97 subjects with the subsets of some expressions. For data preparation, 267 subsets of 97 subjects which contain 8 sequences per expression are selected. A total of 25 sequences of anger, 35 of joy, 30 of sadness, 35 of surprise, 30 of fear, and 25 of disgust sequences are used in training and for the testing purpose, 11 of anger, 19 of joy, 13 of sadness, 20 of surprise, 12 of fear, 12 of disgust subsets are used.

3.2 Recognition Setups for RGB Images

From the database mentioned above, we selected 8 consecutive frames from each video sequences. The selected frames are then realigned with the size of 60 by 80 pixels. Afterwards, histogram equalization and delta image generation were performed for the feature extraction. A total of 180 sequences from all expressions were used to build the feature space.

As we tried to assess our FER system, we applied a total of 180 and 87 image sequences for training and testing respectively. Next, we performed the experiments to empirically determine the optimal number of features and the size of the codebook. To do this, we tested a range of feature numbers selected in the PCA step. Once the optimal number of features was determined, the experiment for the size of the codebook was conducted. We test the performance with the different sizes (2^n, n=4, 5, 6) of the codebook for vector quantization along with HMM in order to determine the optimal settings.
Finally, we compared the different feature extraction methods under the same HMM structure. Previously, PCA and ICA have been extensively explored due to its strong ability of building a feature space, and PCA-LDA has been one of the good feature extractor because of the LDA classifier that finds out the best linear discrimination from the PCA subspace. In this regard, our FICA results have been compared with the conventional feature extraction methods namely PCA, generic ICA, EICA, and PCA-LDA based on the results for the optimal number of features with the same codebook size, and HMM procedure.

3.3 Recognition Setups for Depth Images

Some drawbacks associated with RGB images are known that they are highly affected by lighting conditions and colors causing the distortion of the facial shapes. As one way of overcoming these limitations is the use of depth images. These depth images generally reflect 3-D information of facial expression changes. In our study, we performed preliminary studies of testing depth images and examined their performance for FER. Fig. 10 shows a set of facial expression of surprise from a depth camera called Zcam (www.3dvsystems.com). We tested only four basic expressions in this study: namely, anger, joy, sadness, and surprise using the method presented in the previous section (Lee et al., 2008b).

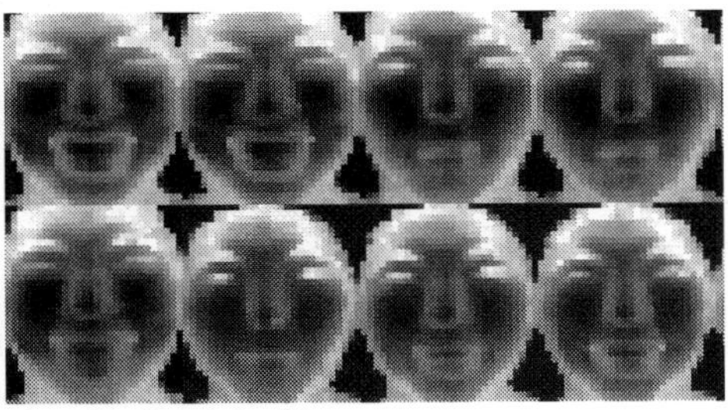

Fig. 10. Depth facial expression images of joy.

4. Experimental Results

Before testing the presented FER system, the system requires setting of two parameters: namely the number of features and the size of codebook. In our experiments, we have tested the eigenvectors in the range from 50 to 190 with the training data and have decided empirically 120 as the optimal number of eigenvectors since it provided the best overall recognition rate. As for the size of the codebook, we have tested the codebook size of 16, 32, and 64, and then decided 32 as the optimal codebook size since it provided the best overall recognition rate for the test data (Lee et al., 2008a).

4.1 Recognition via RGB Images

For recognition comparison between FICA and four other types of conventional feature extraction methods including PCA, ICA, EICA, and PCA-LDA, all extraction methods mentioned above were implemented with the same HMMs for recognition of facial expressions. The results from each experiment in this work represent the best recognition rate with the empirical settings of the selected number of features and the codebook size. For the PCA case, we computed eigenvectors of all the dataset and selected 120 eigenvectors to train the HMMs. As shown in Table 2, the recognition rate using the PCA method was 54.76%, the lowest recognition rate. Then, we employed ICA to extract the ICs from the dataset. Since the ICA produces the same number of ICs as the number of original dimensions of dataset, we empirically selected 120 ICs with the selection criterion of kurtosis values for each IC for training the model. The result of ICA method in Table 3 shows the improved recognition rate than the result of PCA. We also compared the EICA method. We first chose the proper dimension in the PCA step, and processed ICA from the selected eigenvalues to extract the ECIA basis. The results are presented in Table 4, and the total mean of recognition rate from EICA representation of facial expression images was 65.47% which is higher than the generic ICA and PCA recognition rates. Moreover, the best conventional approach PCA-LDA was performed for the last comparison study and it achieved the recognition rate of 82.72% as shown in Table 5. Using the settings above, we conducted the experiment of FICA method implemented with HMMs, and it achieved the total mean of recognition rate, 92.85% and expression labeled as surprise, happy, and sad were recognized with the high accuracy from 93.75% to 100% as shown in Table 6.

Label	Anger	Joy	Sadness	Surprise	Fear	Disgust
Anger	30	0	20	0	10	40
Joy	4	48	8	8	28	4
Sad	0	6.06	81.82	12.12	0	0
Surprise	0	0	0	68.75	12.50	18.75
Fear	0	8.33	50	8.33	33.33	0
Disgust	0	8.33	25	0	0	66.67
Average	54.76					

Table 2. Person independent confusion matrix using PCA (unit : %).

Label	Anger	Joy	Sadness	Surprise	Fear	Disgust
Anger	30	0	10	30	10	20
Joy	4	60	0	0	36	0
Sad	0	6.06	87.88	6.06	0	0
Surprise	0	0	12.50	81.25	0	6.25
Fear	0	25	25	8.33	33.33	8.33
Disgust	0	8.33	25	0	0	66.67
Average	59.86					

Table 3. Person independent confusion matrix using ICA.

Label	Anger	Joy	Sadness	Surprise	Fear	Disgust
Anger	60	0	0	0	20	20
Joy	4	72	8	4	12	0
Sad	0	6.06	87.88	6.06	0	0
Surprise	0	0	12.50	81.25	0	6.25
Fear	0	16.67	16.67	8.33	50	8.33
Disgust	25	8.33	25	0	0	41.67
Average	65.47					

Table 4. Person independent confusion matrix using EICA.

Label	Anger	Joy	Sadness	Surprise	Fear	Disgust
Anger	60	0	10	0	0	30
Joy	0	88	0	0	8	4
Sad	0	6.06	87.88	6.06	0	0
Surprise	0	0	0	93.75	6.25	0
Fear	0	8.33	8.33	8.33	75	0
Disgust	0	0	0	0	8.33	91.67
Average	82.72					

Table 5. Person independent confusion matrix using PCA-LDA.

Label	Anger	Joy	Sadness	Surprise	Fear	Disgust
Anger	80	0	0	0	0	20
Joy	0	96	0	0	4	0
Sad	0	0	93.75	0	6.25	0
Surprise	0	0	0	100	0	0
Fear	0	8.33	0	0	91.67	0
Disgust	0	0	0	0	8.33	91.67
Average	92.85					

Table 6. Person independent confusion matrix using FICA.

As mentioned above, the conventional feature extraction based FER system produced lower recognition rate than the recognition rate of our method, 92.85%. Fig. 11 shows the summary of recognition rate of the conventional compared against our FICA-based method.

4.2 Recognition via Depth Images

A total of 99 sequences were used with 8 images in each sequence, displaying the frontal view of the faces. A total of 15 sequences for each expression were used in training, and for the testing purpose, 10 of anger, 10 of joy, 8 of surprise, and 11 of sadness subsets were used. We empirically selected 60 eigenvectors for dimension reduction, and test the performance with the codebook size of 32. On the data set of RGB and depth facial expressions of the same face, we applied our presented system to compare the FER performance. Table 7 and 8 show the recognition results for each case. More details are given in Lee at al. (2008b).

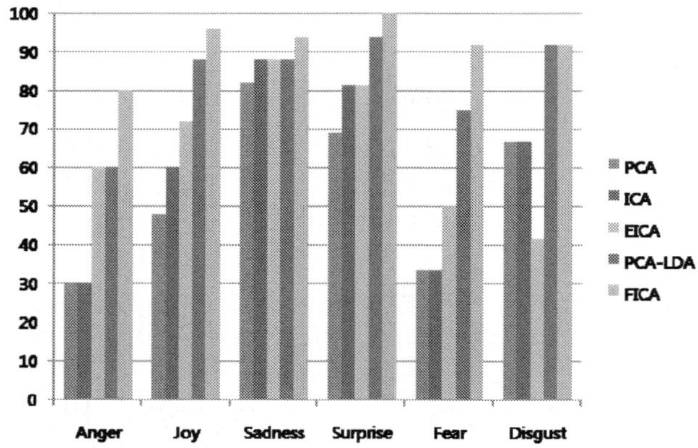

Fig. 11. Recognition rate of facial expressions using the conventional feature extraction methods and the presented FICA feature extraction method.

Label	Anger	Joy	Sadness	Surprise
Anger	100	0	20	0
Joy	10	90	0	0
Sadness	9.09	9.09	81.82	0
Surprise	12.5	12.5	0	75
Average	86.5			

Table 7. Person independent confusion matrix using the sequential RGB images (unit :%).

Label	Anger	Joy	Sadness	Surprise
Anger	100	0	0	0
Joy	0	100	0	0
Sadness	0	0	100	0
Surprise	0	0	0	100
Average	100			

Table 8. Person independent confusion matrix using the sequential depth images.

5. Conclusion

In this work, we have presented a novel FER system utilizing FICA for facial expression feature extraction and HMM for recognition. Especially in the framework of FICA and HMM, the sequential spatiotemporal feature information from holistic facial expressions is modeled and used for FER. The performance of our presented method has been investigated on sequential datasets of six facial expressions. The result shows that FICA can extract optimal features which are well utilized in HMM, outperforming all other conventional feature extraction methods. We have also applied the presented system to 3-D depth facial expression images and showed its improved performance. We believe that our presented

FER system should be useful toward real-time recognition of facial expressions which could be also useful in many other applications of HCI.

6. Acknowledgement

This research was supported by the MKE (Ministry of Knowledge Economy), Korea, under the ITRC (Information Technology Research Center) support program supervised by the IITA (Institute of Information Technology Advancement) (IITA-2009-(C1090-0902-0002)).

7. Reference

Aleksic, P. S. & Katsaggelos, A. K. (2006). Automatic facial expression recognition using facial animation parameters and multistream HMMs, *IEEE trans. Information and Security*, Vol. 1, Nol. 1, pp. 3-11, ISSN. 1556-6013

Bartlett, M. S.; Donato, G. ; Movellan, J. R.; Hager, J. C.; Ekman, P. & Sejnowski, T. J. (1999). Face Image Analysis for Expression Measurement and Detection of Deceit, *Proceedings of the 6th Joint Symposium on Neural Computation*, pp. 8-15

Bartlett, M. S.; Movellan, J. R. & Sejnowski, T. J. (2002). Face Recognition by Independent Component Analysis, *IEEE trans. Neural Networks*, Vol. 13, No. 6, pp. 1450-1464, ISSN. 1045-9227

Buciu, I.; Kotropoulos, C. & Pitas, I. (2003). ICA and Gabor Representation for Facial Expression Recognition, *Proceedings of the IEEE*, pp. 855-858

Calder, A. J.; Young, A. J.; Keane, J. & Dean, M. (2000). Configural information in facial expression perception, *Journal of Experimental psychology, Human Perception and Performance. Human perception and performance*, Vol. 26, No. 2, pp. 527-551

Calder, A. J.; Burton, A. M.; Miller, P.; Young, A. W. & Akamatsu, S. (2001). A principal component analysis of facial expressions, *Vision Research*, Vol.41, pp. 1179-1208

Chen, F. & Kotani, K. (2008). Facial Expression Recognition by Supervised Independent Component Analysis Using MAP Estimation, *IEICE trans. INF. & SYST.*, Vol. E91-D, No. 2, pp. 341-350, ISSN. 0916-8532

Chuang, C.-F. & Shih, F. Y. (2006). Recognizing Facial Action Units Using Independent Component Analysis and Support Vector Machine, *Pattern Recognition*, Vol. 39, No. 9, pp. 1795-1798, ISSN. 0031-3203

Cohen, I.; Sebe, N.; Garg, A; Chen, L. S. & Huang, T. S. (2003). Facial expression recognition from video sequences: temporal and static modeling, *Computer Vision and Image Understanding*, Vol. 91, ISSN. 1077-3142

Cohn, J. F.; Zlochower, A.; Lien, J. & Kanade, T. (1999). Automated face analysis by feature point tracking has high concurrent validity with manual FACS coding, pp. 35-43, *Psychophysiology*, Cambridge University Press

Danato, G.; Bartlett, M. S.; Hagar, J. C.; Ekman, P. & Sejnowski, T. J. (1999). Classifying Facial Actions, IEEE Trans. Pattern Analysis and Machine Intelligence, vol. 21(10), pp. 974-989

Dubuisson, S.; Davoine, F. & Masson, M. (2002). A solution for facial expression representation and recognition, *Signal Processing: Image Communication*, Vol. 17, pp. 657-673

Lee, J. J.; Uddin, M. D. & Kim, T.-S. (2008a). Spatiotemporal human facial expression recognition using fisher independent component analysis and Hidden Markov Model, *Proceedings of the IEEE Int. Conf. Engineering in Medicine and Biology Society, pp. 2546-2549*

Lee, J. J.; Uddin, M. D.; Truc P. T. H. & Kim, T.-S. (2008b). Spatiotemporal Depth Information-based Human Facial Expression Recognition Using FICA and HMM, *Int. Conf. Ubiquitous Healthcare, IEEE, Busan, Korea*

Lyons, M.; Akamatsu, S.; Kamachi, M. & Gyoba, J. (1998). Coding facial expressions with Gabor wavelets, *Proceedings of the Third IEEE Int. Conf. Automatic Face and Gesture Recognition*, pp. 200-205

Rabiner, L. R. (1989). A Tutorial on Hidden Markov Models and Selected Applications in Speech Recognition, *Proceedings of the IEEE*, Vol. 77, No. 2, pp. 257-286

Linde, Y.; Buzo, A. & Gray, R. (1980). An Algorithm for Vector Quantizer Design, *IEEE Transaction on Communications*, Vol. 28, No. 1, pp. 84–94, ISSN. 0090-6778

Liu, C. (2004). Enhanced independent component analysis and its application to content based face image retrieval, *IEEE trans. Systems, Man, and Cybernetics*, Vol. 34, No. 2, pp. 1117-1127

Karklin, Y. & Lewicki, M. S. (2003). Learning higher-order structures in natural images, *Netw. Comput. Neural Syst.*, Vol. 14, pp. 483-499

Kwak, K. C. & Pedrycz, W. (2007). Face recognition using an enhanced independent component analysis approach, *IEEE Trans. Neural Network*, Vol. 18, pp. 530-541, ISSN. 1045-9227

Kotsia, I. & Pitas, I. (2007). Facial expression recognition in image sequences using geometric deformation features and support vector machine, *IEEE trans. Image Processing*, Vol. 16, pp. 172-187, ISSN. 1057-7149

Mitra, S. & Acharya, T. (2007). Gesture Recognition: A survey, *IEEE Trans. Systems, Man, and Cybernetics*, Vol. 37, No. 3, pp. 331-324, ISSN. 1094-6977

Otsuka, T. & Ohya, J. (1997). Recognizing multiple person's facial expressions using HMM based on automatic extraction of significant frames from image sequences. *Proceedings of the IEEE Int. Conf. Image Processing*, pp. 546-549

Padgett, C. & Cottrell, G. (1997). Representation face images for emotion classification, *Advances in Neural Information Processing Systems*, vol. 9, Cambridge, MA, MIT Press

Tian, Y,-L.; Kanade, T. & Cohn, J. F. (2002). Evaluation of Gabor wavelet based facial action unit recognition in image sequences of increasing complexity, *Proceedings of the 5th IEEE Int. Conf. Automatic Face and Gesture Recognition*, pp. 229-234

Zhang, L. & Cottrell, G. W. (2004). When Holistic Processing is Not Enough: Local Features Save the Day, *Proceedings of the Twenty-sixth Annual Cognitive Science Society Conference*

Zhu, Y.; De Silva, L. C. & Ko, C. C. (2002). Using moment invariants and HMM in facial expression recognition, *Pattern Recognition Letters*, Vol. 23, pp. 83-91, ISSN. 0167-8655

Requirements and solutions for advanced Telemedicine applications

George J. Mandellos, George V. Koutelakis, Theodor C. Panagiotakopoulos, Michael N. Koukias and Dimitrios K. Lymberopoulos
Wire Communication Laboratory, Electrical & Computer Engineering Department, University of Patras, GR 265 04 Panepistimioupoli - Rion Greece

1. Introduction

Telemedicine, as the term means, is the provision of medicine and the exchange of heath-care information at a distance. Moreover, it is the use of advanced telecommunication and information technologies to transmit and exchange health information and provide health care services across geographic, time, social and cultural barriers [Vikas Singh, 2006]. It includes both, the clinical (diagnosis, treatment, medical records and prevention of disease) and academic medicine (research, continuous education, knowledge exchange, evaluation and training). In general, telemedicine is not a new technology, but term encompassing diverse information and communication technologies aiming to offer health-related activities wherever and whenever these are needed or requested.

Telemedicine is the only solution to several situations of healthcare provision. Two of the major cases, where there is no alternative to telemedicine, are emergencies and lack of expertised and/or experienced medical staff either in rural areas of developing countries or across the majority of the health care network of underdeveloped countries.

Many published studies [C. Weston et al., 1994] have shown that an early and specialized pre-hospital management of emergency cases contributes to the patient's survival. Especially in cases of serious injuries, spinal cord or internal organs trauma, the way that injured persons are treated and transported as well as the time period of their transportation is crucial. This is where telemedicine can contribute to an initial diagnosis, initial treatment during the patient's transportation and proper preparation at the hospital's premises for the patient's in-hospital treatment. Furthermore, in rural areas and in some occasions at health centres where primary care is provided, there is a lack either in medical staff or in specific expertise of the existing medical staff. In such cases, telemedicine is of great importance, as it eliminates the need for transportation, where in some cases such as islands cannot be easy. In addition it offers cost savings and immediate treatment administered by the expertised physician lying at a central hospital.

Despite the fact that telemedicine seems to be a necessity in several cases and has a huge impact both in personal and social level, there are many obstacles that need to be overcome so that an effective, efficient and cost effective telemedicine application is realized.

Generally, the problems telemedicine providers and consumers have to deal with are summarized in three major categories, juridical, financial and technological. On the other hand, telemedicine is not always easy to be implemented or supported, because a long list of factors affects its evolution.
This chapter will mainly focus on the technological problems, aiming to provide efficient and effective solutions. Taking into account the fact that telemedicine is realized by the fusion of communication and information technologies, the provided solutions will involve two directions. First, towards the communication part, which forms the platform for any kind of e-health application and, second the information structuring structure offering adaption to the medical treatment demands, each health related incident sets.
Before the comprehensive analysis of the problems and requirements of telemedicine, as well as the technological solutions adopted by several telemedicine applications, we consider that the presentation of some information, regarding general attributes of telemedicine, is quite necessary. For this reason, the next section will report on the types of telemedicine, the reasons why telemedicine is not only being implemented, but seems to be the only solution in several occasions, the telemedicine applications and the players having either a major or less important role in several levels, spanning from the design to the market analysis of telemedicine systems and applications.

2. General attributes of telemedicine

2.1. Types of telemedicine

Telemedicine sessions can be distinguished according to the interaction taking place between the clients and the expert and the type of the exchanged information.
The two types of interaction are the Real-time (synchronous) and the Store and Forward (asynchronous).
In Real-time telemedicine, a synchronous interaction between providers/patients/ healthcare professionals at distant locations is established, using some kind of communication technology providing audio/visual/data exchange and wireless or microwave signals. This type of telemedicine often renders increased accuracy and offers better assessment of the overall patient's health condition resulting, among other things, in more satisfied patients. Keep in mind that patients' satisfaction is a key factor so that telemedicine will be integrated in our everyday life, as stated in many researches existing in the literature. The main disadvantage is that the parties involved must be scheduled, because in the real-time telemedicine usually two healthcare providers are involved, so they both need to be available at the same time. In Real-time telemedicine, apart from video-conferencing, peripheral sensing devices (biosignal measurement devices) can also be attached to the patient or to the equipment, in order to offer the ability of remote interactive examination. This type of telemedicine is used most often in accidents, psychiatry, internal medicine, rehabilitation, cardiology, paediatrics, obstetrics and gynaecology as well as neurology.
The Store and Forward or prerecorded (asynchronous) technology involves the acquisition of medical data (images, bio-signals) and its transmission by the referrer to a medical expert for consultation, evaluation or other purposes, at a convenient time. This type of telemedicine does not require simultaneous communication between the referrer and the healthcare professional in real time. E-mail is a common example. The diagnostic accuracy is

lower related to the real-time telemedicine, because the expert evaluates the data with a delay and he doesn't interact with the patient while care is provided, but it has advantages considering hardware and software complexity, cost and convenience. This type of telemedicine is often used in radiology, pathology and dermatology.
The type of information exchanged between the parties during a telemedicine session can be comprised of data, audio, video or a combination of them. Data includes patient's demographic information, biosignal measurements acquired through sensors connected to the patient and peripheral devices, etc. Audio includes the conversation (voice signals) between the two parties. Video includes still images and/or video pictures concerning the medical incident.

2.2. Necessity of telemedicine

A significant percentage of emergency cases are due to car crash accidents and coronary artery diseases. Statistics for car accidents in USA and Europe prove that many thousands of people loose their lives and many more drivers or passengers are severely injured. Studies performed in Greece, a country with a very high death rate due to car crashes, proved that most of the fatal injuries in accidents happened far away from any competent healthcare institution, thus resulting in long response times [Mandellos et al., 2004]. The long response time (ambulance arrival, transportation time, evaluation time and treatment initiation) [Mandellos et al., 2004] leads a significant percentage of victims caused by accidents in rural roads to die on the scene, or during the transportation [A. G. Heriot et al., 1993]. Some of the above cases had a 50% chance of survival, if adequate pre-hospital care existed.
Heart disease is another common example of high death rates in emergency cases, since two thirds of all patients die before reaching the central hospital [T. Evans, 1998]. The delay in administering the appropriate therapy [T. Kereiakes et al., 1990] comes either from the patient's failure to recognize the seriousness of his symptoms and seek emergency care, or the needed pre-hospital evaluation and transport time, or the time required for diagnosis and initiation of treatment in the hospital.
The above show the great necessity of telemedicine in emergencies. The emergency cases comprise a major case, among many others, where telemedicine can play an extremely vital role. Airplanes, ships, rural areas and disaster areas constitute some other important cases where telemedicine appears to be either the only or the most efficient and effective solution.
Moreover, the use of telemedicine offers several benefits in the traditional healthcare network as it:

- Increases the accessibility of and to professional caregivers
- Increases the quality, efficiency and continuity of healthcare to patients
- Increases the focus on preventive medicine through early intervention
- Reduces the overall cost of healthcare both for care providers and consumers
- Reduces the unnecessary transfer of patients to regional hospitals
- Enables the education and training for both medical stuff and citizens, and improves the medical knowledge
- Provides services to remote areas in case of natural calamities, disasters and military and space operations.
- Enables the patient's remote monitoring
- Reduces the time needed for diagnosis extraction and patient treatment.
- Leads to a rapid response time in pre-hospital actions.

2.3. Telemedicine applications

Because of the above benefits telemedicine has, telemedicine is utilized for providing various services that spawns numerous specialties and can be broadly categorized as home-based care, telepsychiatry, teleradiology, general telemedicine, telecardiology, teleconsultation, telemedicine in disaster areas teledermatology, ambulatory and emergency care, telepathology, self-care teledentistry and telesurgery.

In order to be applied to the above fields, telemedicine applications use the same basic components, e.g. capturing infrastructure, communication media, processing equipment to display, process and manage the information and deliver feedback.

The used infrastructure to capture the necessary information includes a Biosignal Acquisition Module, for biosignal acquisition through sensors connected to the patient and peripheral devices, and in some cases a Digital Camera, for patient's digital image or video capturing. The processing module such as a Personal Computer or Personal Digital Assistant from the patient's side integrates the acquired data (biosignals, demographics, videos, geolocation, etc.) in order to be transmitted. On the expert's side it displays the received data and gives the necessary tools to doctor in order to evaluate them. The communication medium connecting the telemedicine parties makes use of various communication technologies such as POTS networks (PSTN or ISDN), GSM cellular phone networks, 2g, 2.5g and 3g networks, Bluetooth and RF technologies, Satellite Systems, LAN, WLAN, WiMAX, Home/Personal/Body Area Networks, Mobile ad-hoc networks or MANET's.

Also, optional equipment (GPS receiver, microscope, etc) can be used so that various incidents can be managed through telemedicine.

2.4. The players involved

Telemedicine is a very complicated scheme. The implementation of a telemedicine application requires the cooperation, among different type of players. There are directly and indirectly involved players who can be categorized in the following categories:

- Healthcare consumers (especially patients)
- Health professionals (experts, family doctors, nurses, paramedic, obstetrician, etc.)
- Other professionals involved in the wider area of healthcare (directors, researchers, epidemics, technicians, IT engineers, statistician, etc.)
- Hospitals and health centers
- Communication companies
- Complementary (non-medical) services suppliers
- Infrastructure manufacturers and suppliers
- Hardware and network manufacturers
- Universities and research institutes
- Insurance companies
- Pharmaceutical companies
- Health ministry
- Health management organizations
- Organizations for standardizing and licensing.

The above list shows one of the major intrinsic difficulties in establishing a telemedicine application, as it needs a huge effort put on management, administration and cooperation among different types of participants.

3. Potential problems and requirements

Telemedicine is not always easy to be implemented or supported. Our long experience as a telemedicine R&D group of University of Patras, during design, development and implementation of several projects since 1992, and the cooperation with the players involved demonstrated a long list of factors affecting the evolution of the telemedicine. Generally, we can divide them in three main categories, juridical, financial and technological. Although these categories do not have clear border against each other, they can be broadly classified into the following groups:

3.1. Juridical problems

Medical malpractice liability. Medical Malpractice Liability is a big case for healthcare providers with iniquitous costs because of penalties. The nature of telemedicine, the communication network interruptions, and the errors caused by hardware failures during the transportation makes it vulnerable to malpractice lawsuits. In many countries, there is a significant uncertainty regarding whether malpractice insurance policies cover services provided by telemedicine. Telemedicine networks that cross border lines for example in countries line US, create additional uncertainties regarding the state where a malpractice lawsuit may be litigated and the law that will be used. Is the law to be considered in the state of the provider, the patient, or in another state which covers the network?

Absence of legislative regulations on attribution of responsibilities. In some countries like Greece there aren't legislative regulations to define the telemedicine service operation. A major barrier in this case is who is the responsible on the telemedicine incident evaluation, the local paramedic or the remote expert? Another barrier is the financial of the people involved in a telemedicine session.

Absence of Licensing and Credentialing. It is a consequence of the above absence of a suitable law for telemedicine services.

Absence of rights. Usually, the ambulance staffs have not the required advanced theoretical knowledge and experience to handle emergency situations. Moreover, it is not certified to provide medical care without a medical expert's advice. On the other hand, expert physicians such as cardiologists, neurosurgeons, orthopaedics cannot participate in ambulance staff for financial aspects or practical reasons.

3.2. Financial problems

Cost and Reimbursement for Telemedicine Services. Often telemedicine services are established during research projects. Most of the telemedicine projects around the world are still funded by state or federal grants. Although the communication costs and the cost of the basic equipment generally are falling, many public and private payers are reluctant to set standard for payment or reimbursement because of the uncertainty inherent in telemedicine because of its evolving nature and lack of conclusive evidence of its effectiveness and range of applications.

Telecommunication regulations - limitations. The limited competition for telecommunication services in some areas caused by country regulations leads to a significantly decreased number of available network types. So the absence of competition keeps the communication cost high.
Equipment costs. The majority of the already existing hardware and software components designed for telemedicine purposes have a relatively high cost which most of the people cannot afford.

3.3. Technological problems

Closed Systems. There is a significant number of telemedicine services used by healthcare providers. Many of them are provided by closed systems without offering interoperability with other medical systems (such as Electronic Health Record Systems).
Wide range of telemedicine. Telemedicine lies across a wide range of medical activities resulting in redundancies, lack of interoperability, cost sharing and incompatibilities between systems.
Communication Networks. The limited competition for telecommunication services in rural areas and islands leads to a significantly decreased number of available network types (such as GSM, 3G, etc.) in the above areas. Also, the available signal strength in those areas is rather limited and the frequent interruptions or even the signal absence in some areas (caused by the geomorphology) during a telemedicine session render telemedicine unavailable.
User refusal against new technologies. People do not want to involve any new technologies in their life, especially when they are constrained by thirds (e.g. profession guidelines). So they are negative in the introduction of new equipment and claim legislative and financial reasons in order to abstain.
Telemedicine resources. In order a telemedicine system to be able to serve a wide area of medical cases, it needs various interconnected medical devices. The barrier here is whether this equipment is sufficient to meet clinical standards and whether its usage inhibits healthcare professionals from using it. Some times the quality and resolution of radiographic images transmitted doesn't meet the standards. Another factor is the lack of know how in order to make a proper use of the equipment's features. Telemedicine, in most occasions, requires expensive infrastructure and highly complex setup which is a limiting factor for small providers and physician clinics or health centres established in small islands.
Information structuring. With respect to the information structuring we highlight the following:
Variability of incidents served by telemedicine. A telemedicine system can be addressed to serve various incident types (patients suffering from heart diseases, pneumonics, several injuries etc.). Every single incident requires a different collection of diverse vital signs or relative information in order to determine the condition of the transported patient.
The absence of a protocol able to handle all the selected data in order to allow the interoperability between Medical Information Systems. There are many protocols handling an information subtotal.
The capability of scalable user access depending on his type/specialty. Telemedicine systems as they are applied in a wide area of activities have to introduce control processes, in order to keep the information confidentiality.

4. Methods for structuring, processing, archiving and transmitting the medical information

The successful design, implementation and utilization of a telemedicine system needs the resolution of several problems listed in the previous section. Resolving the aforementioned problems is often a very difficult task demanding the cooperation of various social groups. Being engineers we will focus on providing solutions to the technological problems not addressing the other two groups (i.e. juridical and financial)

In order to overcome some of the technological limitations, we adopt solutions that will be presented in the following paragraphs. These solutions have been succesfully implemented in a telemedicine system [Mandellos et al., 2008 (a)] resulted by a project tuned by the Greek Information Society and the Greek Ministry of Defense. This telemedicine system (fig. 1) supports diverse types of endpoints including moving transports (MT) (such as ambulances, ships, planes, etc.), handheld devices and fixed units, using diverse communication networks. The above telemedicine system targets to the improved pre-hospital patient treatment. Although vital sign transmission has the priority against other services provided by the telemedicine system (videoconference, remote management, voice calls etc.), a predefined algorithm controls provision, switching and QoS of the other potential services. A distributed database system controlled by a central server, aims to manage patient attributes, exams and incidents handled by several Telemedicine Coordination Centers (TCC). Doctors and other mecical personnel are able to participate for observation purposes, during the incident evaluation through workstations in TCCs or through Regional Teleconference Rooms (RTRs).

4.1 Bandwidth limitations lead to the adoption of an adaptive protocol

In many medical incidents, the correct diagnosis depends on the amount and type of data relative to patient's health state [Mandellos et al., 2008 (a)]. In some cases the referring doctor needs to know more data for the patient's state from those provided by the acquired measurements. Such data are patient's demographic data, mnemonic and medical history, patient's allergy state, patient's ancestry, etc. These data affect the correct treatment (e.g. pharmaceutical allergy precludes some drugs) or the patient's handling (e.g. blood transfusion is prohibited by some religions; patient must be treated separately from other patients if he suffers from infectious diseases or has sensitive immunizer system). The doctor, takes different measurements on patient's Vital Signs (for cardiac diseases he takes an ElectroCardioGram - ECG, for pulmonary diseases he takes measurements of blood oxygen saturation - SPO_2 while on other cases he takes body's temperature (TEMP), non invasive blood pressure (NiBP), etc) depending on patient's symptoms. Consequently, the total amount of data collected during an incident could have diverse length type compared to another incident.

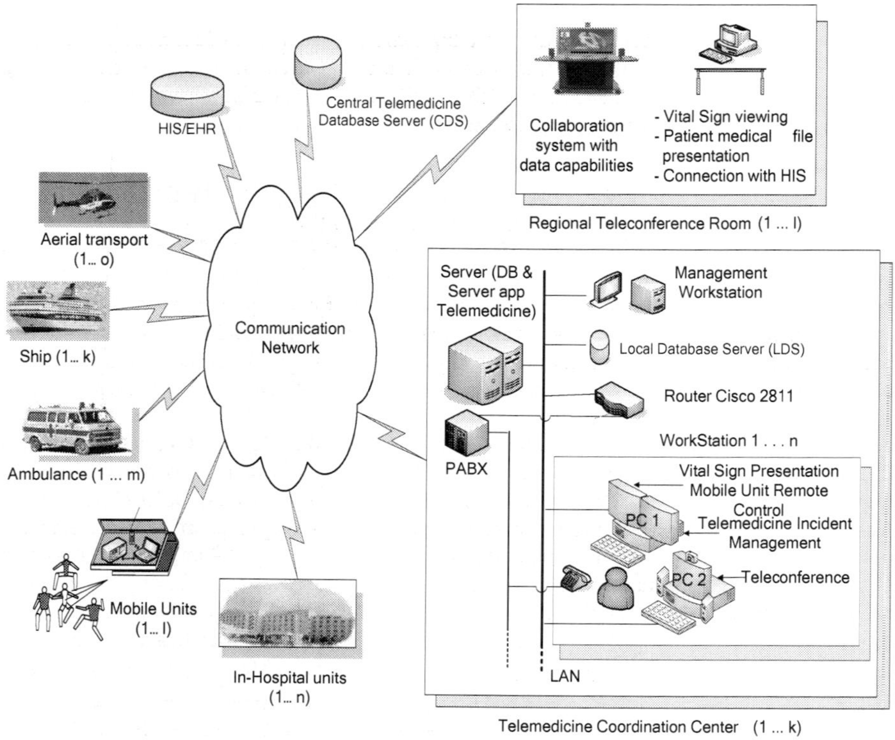

Fig. 1. General structure of a Telemedicine System.

This diversity of data led to the necessity of an adaptive protocol in order to minimize the required transmission time, the recovery time and finally the storage space. Authors have proposed some extensions in order the new protocol to be able to handle more data based on the file format of SCP-ECG protocol [Health Informatics, 2002] which handles a basic set of demographics data and also ECG measurements. The new protocol is referred as e-SCP-ECG+ protocol [Mandellos et al., 2008 (b)]. The finally used protocol has significant changes and constitutes a newer version of the aforementioned protocol. This version made extensions in order all types of data collected during an incident to be handled. The protocol consists of a sections collection, each of them handling different types of data. A main section is defined to control critical data on other sections (e.g. existence, offset, length, etc.). Thus, the protocol's structure permits the handling only of the existing data.

The data handled by the latest protocol version covers patient demographic data, ancestry data, profession data, mnemonic and medical history, a quick description of the incident, a first diagnosis, allergy state and measurements on ECG, SPO_2, NiBP, TEMP, Heart Rate and CO_2.

The user has the ability to manage the acquired data such as user inputs and Medical Monitor (MM) measurements and define the data set describing each incident via a PC

connected between MM and communication media. Afterwards, the formatted data can be transmitted to the TCC.
The new expanded protocol can be used in a big variety of medical incidents. The possibility to manage only the data that characterize each medical incident has the advantage of minimal possible volume of data, which results in a high flexibility regarding their management and in a very fast transmission.

4.2. Communication network instability or absence in many areas leads to the adoption of an alternative communication media structure

The reassurance of a stable communication between Mobile Units (MU) and TCCs, with the best possible quality regarding the available networks at the various access points is very important. It is more than obvious that the transmission of vital signs to the TCC is required by all means, so that the paramedical staff of the MT can offer crucial treatment the soonest possible. For this purpose, communication capabilities using multiple networks of diverse physical media are developed to guarantee the successful vital signs transmission under all circumstances (Fig. 1).
The development focused on mobile communications due to the fact that a patient transportation is taking place. GPRS offers wider geographical area coverage but low transmission rates. Mobile Asymmetric Digital Subscriber Line (M-ADSL) clearly offers higher transmission rates with lower cost but it lacks in geographical area coverage. In the occasions where the system was installed at ships transporting patients from islands to central hospitals of the mainland (University hospitals or other central hospital), satellite modems are used. The choice of the wireless network is mainly based on the offered Quality of Service (QoS) and not only on its availability. Moreover, priorities are embedded regarding the choice of the wireless network. The designation of the network to be used for call transfers and transactions is made depending on these priorities and the available networks. Thus, the result is a single network connection based on a priority algorithm (as mentioned above) that will host (in contrast with the previous pilot operation of the project) all the communications used to handle a single incident.
In any communication between MUs and TCCs two different and independent calls (C1 and C2) are made from the MU to the TCC. C1 call enables vital signs transfer and C2 call enables either telephone communication via an ordinary telephone set (wired or wireless) or communication via teleconference, where, depending on the available bandwidth, text, voice and video transmission will be possible in a respective hierarchical way. In all cases one or more connections are used within the same transmission media, to circulate all the information (data, voice and video) regarding a single incident.
Moreover, priorities are designated regarding the kind of data that must be transferred each time, when the available bandwidth is inefficient. Examples of validations (demarcation of situations/behaviour) carried out by this transmission sub-system according to these priorities are the following:

- In a GPRS network in case of low bandwidth only vital signs transmission is accomplished. If bandwidth is sufficient, text is also transmitted.
- In a wireless LAN (IEEE 802.11 a/b/g) or satellite modem in case bandwidth reaches low rates high priority is given to vital signs transmission in regard of teleconference.

It is obvious by the examples given above that in every case the bandwidth is not efficient, transmission of crucial medical information i.e. vital signs, has priority against the delivery of any other service offered by the telemedicine system.
Using the adaptive protocol described above, the vital signs transmission is performed by means of transferring packets of a fixed time period (e.g. 10 sec) from the MU to the TCC. These vital signs packets include all the acquired vital signs from the patient for the respective period of time. The application developed provides the potential to define the period of time in which transmitted vital signs are partitioned. Thus, it is possible to adjust the size of each transmitted packet. Detection of low bandwidth results in a larger packet size in order to limit the transactions with the database and prevent a possible flood in the network connection. This adjustment will result in a higher delay imported at the beginning of the real time transmission due to the initial control-process of the first large sized packet. Detection of high bandwidth results in a smaller packet size accompanied with lower delay imported to the transmission due to a fast initial control-process of the first small sized packet. The size of the vital signs packet can be dynamically adjusted depending on a periodically measurement of the available bandwidth.

4.3. A call management application controls the productive telemedicine system's operation

Each TCC hosts one Management Workstation (MW), three Treatment Workstations (TWs), as well as one Local Database Server (LDS) for storing the whole of incident data. The MW in its turn hosts a call management application, which is responsible the control and management of incoming calls from the MTs to the TCCs and the already established connections between them. When a call arrives at the TCC, optical and sound alerts are enabled to the MW to inform of the data arrival. MW selects a TW in order to handle the incident. The call management application enables TCC's administrator to route an incoming call to the TCC to a workstation, redirect an already established session from one workstation to another, to connect or disconnect any endpoint in an active session, to invite participants, etc.
Apart from these functionalities, the call management application provides control and management of the wider established telemedicine network outside the physical area of the TCC. It offers endpoint management (i.e. insertion, deletion, modification etc.), teleconference administration and management of users (i.e. insertion, deletion, access level designation and access data modification of users authorized to access TWs, MWs, RTRs and MUs).
The latest part, of which the call management application is responsible, is the maintenance of the telemedicine system. Through this application, the administrator is able to start/stop/restart the proxy servers which consist the intermediates of the communication between MUs and TWs. Furthermore, it provides the functionality to flag several types of incidents that either were not properly handled (e.g. due to connection loss between TCC's and MUs) or lack information and need further identification. These incidents are then handled in an offline mode by any willing TW, where the diagnostic reports are filled and the overall incident information is sent to the LDS.

4.4. Multiple TCCs

In order to ensure that a call initiated by a MU, will be served by a workstation in a TCC, in all cases, we established 3 networked TCCs. There were many occasions where all the TWs of a specific TCC were engaged while calls where arriving in this TCC. Furthermore, there were cases where the LDS of a TCC crashed or communications were broken due to various reasons. This led as to establish multiple TCC's in different central hospitals, not only to offer the ability of simultaneous handling of a relatively high number of telemedicine incidents, but also to be able to cope with such problems. So, in case all workstations in the referral TCC aren't able to treat a telemedicine call due to the reasons mentioned above, a predefined algorithm reroutes the call to another TCC which has available workstations.

4.5. Distributed database system

The information management in the telemedicine applications mainly follows an hierarchical structure represented by three basic information entities: Patient - Incident - Exams (Vital signs, still images and short time patient video). The archiving systems implemented by different TCCs result in a distributed system regarding the storage of information at the each TCC that any telemedicine-related information is being collected. A central database connects with peripheral databases located at the TCCs and this central database is responsible for the integration and coordination of the telemedicine databases.

Each Exam can be considered as a complete part of an Incident. Consequently, Exams are related only to one TCC and the attributes of one Incident are stored in its LDS. The different Incidents that comprise one Patient are often related to different TCCs. Thus, the Central Database Server (CDS) of the Telemedicine System is designed to keep records of the attributes of Patients and Incidents. However, the whole content of the Exams that is related to an Incident is stored in the LDS of the TCC that handled it. Inside the CDS, a reference connects user to the proper LDS of a TCC, which keeps the Exams data.

Thus, Exams remain locally stored, yet they appear as a reference link in the CDS of the Telemedicine. Each access of a LDS comes through the CDS and consequently any query related to Exams data is assigned to the proper LDS located at the respective TCC. The choice of the proper LDS is made regarding the attributes of the TCC that is related to the requested Incident.

Central telemedicine database should communicate with either the central Hospital Information System (HIS) or an Electronic Health Record (EHR) system in order to update the patient data corresponding to a telemedicine incident (Fig. 1). Central database also updates the HIS/EHR for possible changes to data regarding already registered patients or even registers new patients to the HIS/EHR whenever this is required during a patient identification process. Communication between central telemedicine database and HIS/EHR is accomplished exchanging the appropriate Health Level 7 (HL7) messages on occasion.

The distributed database can be implemented with robust grid database server software installed on a cluster of database servers. At the central telemedicine server, suitable proxy server software should be installed. This proxy server has the responsibility to perform the communication between the telemedicine system and the HIS/EHR. The proxy server undertakes to send and receive the (HL7) messages for the communication between the CDS and the HIS/EHR.

4.6. The necessity of participation more than one expert or educational reasons leads to the establishment of multiple RTRs

The designed Telemedicine System also defines a number or RTRs. A RTR is consisted of a collaborating system with data capabilities and a PC for vital sign viewing, patient medical file presentation and connection with the HIS. The RTR offers the capability of participation both in on-line incident evaluation and off-line incident's data observation. A RTR is able to connect or disconnect at any point in time during an active session.

This application can serve either for multi-expertise discussion on a specific incident or for educational purposes. For instance, practitioners in central hospitals, medical staff in secondary and primary care provision facilities could observe an incident while it is actually treated and receive feedback regarding the treatment methodology or specific medical information.

5. Factors confining the intensity of telemedicine systems' usage

During the previous decade the implementation of many Telemedicine systems begun aiming at connection remote regions with the nearest big hospitals or creation a Telemedicine network that is expanded in a wider geographic area. Telemedicine systems are also implemented aiming at the development of a national telemedicine network, which will be able to use the telecommunication infrastructure of a country in order to provide the capability of smooth enterprise operation regardless of the consequences.

Many telemedicine systems are implemented only as pilot applications. The results of the pilot operation of such systems range from moderately until to satisfactory enough. Nevertheless, most of these systems are abandoned after the end of the pilot use period or maybe the end of an extra short period of use. The factors, that such systems either are often not used in the desirable level or even in certain times are abandoned, can be summarised in the followings:

- Lack of specialised personnel for the enterprise operation of telemedicine systems.
- Complexity of the use case scenarios especially in that cases that two scenarios of telemedicine operation (real time - store and forward) are combined in the same information system.
- Lack of financing for sufficient service level agreements that would support and guarantee the sufficient operation of telemedicine systems
- Insufficient planning of the designed telemedicine solution viability, e.g. short-sighted risk analysis or not ensured essential economic support for the further enterprise operation of such a project.
- Design of autonomous telemedicine systems. No efficient collaboration with other hospital information systems, which participate in the management of the medical incident, is forecasted. Furthermore no collaboration of the designed telemedicine system with other existing telemedicine systems is taken into account. That means weakness of the implemented system to be interoperable.
- Many doctors and some patients are critical regarding the change of the traditional way of medical incidents' management, especially when an urgent incident takes place. This disposal of doctors (mainly) is often related with the lack of sufficient support in the problems appeared in the enterprise operation.

- Absence of a central institution for the management and exploitation of the telemedicine units. Lack of a central exploitation scenario for telemedicine. The extension of the fragmented telemedicine information systems in an integrated national telemedicine system, with the central responsibility and coordination of the corresponding Health Ministry is demanded. Only such an integrated system, which connects all the regional units of telemedicine with the central hospitals and allocates proper infrastructure and personnel for these hospitals in order to serve telemedicine incidents, can meet the requirements efficiently.

6. Conclusion

It is clear that telemedicine, when used correctly, enables health care provision where traditional health networks could hardly or were unable to do so and also improves the quality of the already existing healthcare services. There are several occasions, where telemedicine seems to be better than traditional methods such as the exchange of health-related information allowing a more accurate, faster and easier access to information. On the other hand many issues remain to be solved in order to telemedicine to be developed as a significant means of providing healthcare and be considered as an integral part of the mainstream healthcare. Coordinated and strategic planning, evaluation of the cost-effectiveness of telemedicine projects, funding and reimbursement are only some of the wide ranged needs of a process through which telemedicine services are commercially acceptable and harmonic integrated in the existing healthcare delivery in a significant degree.

Telemedicine, like all medicine, is constantly evolving. The growth and integration of new and emerging information and communication technologies into healthcare delivery surely holds great potential for all players. While the population of the elderly grows and chronic diseases are diffusing the requirements and expectations of citizens from the tomorrow health systems are evolving from the proper treatment and service provided in health centres to the provision of a more protective (proactive self-care), reachable (i.e. at home, at work, while travelling abroad) and high-quality health advice and assistance. Modern healthcare services are expected to be available around the clock, seven days a week, so that systems with pervasive access and near-absolute fault tolerance are indispensable. With introduction of new technologies in healthcare, the clinical practices are changing too, requiring healthcare professionals to collaborate across disciplines and organisational boundaries. Thus providers are looking for ways to deliver health services to the patient as promptly and as locally as possible, while supporting contact and collaboration between healthcare professionals and patients throughout the care episode.

With respect to these requirements from the tomorrow worldwide health systems, designed and developed frameworks should support a two-fold paradigm shift in health delivery:

- from symptom-based to preventive healthcare, and
- from hospital-centred to person-centred health systems.

Homecare and individualized monitoring systems are considered the segment with the greatest potential for financial and clinical impact in the forthcoming years, being considered a serious solution for life quality improvement by healthcare purchasers. Currently, the information level, penetration and usage rate is very much dependent on country development level. By assessing, evaluating and validating such systems in a clinically approved setup in more than one country around the world will improve acceptability of such systems at worldwide level, followed by market and business opportunities for innovative companies, and could help lower the costs of care.

7. References

Health Informatics - Standard Communication Protocol - Computer assisted electrocardiography, CEN/TC251, prEN 1064:2002.

T. Evans, (1998). "Cardiac arrests outside hospital", *British Medical Journal,* vol. 316, Apr. 1998, pp. 1031-1032, ISSN: 0007-1447

A. Heriot, (1993). "Delay in presentation after myocardial infraction", *J. R. Soc. Med,* vol. 86, Nov. 1993, pp. 62-64, ISSN 0141-0768.

D. Kereiakes, D. Weaver, J. Anderson et al. (1990). "Time delays in the diagnosis and treatment of acute myocardial infraction: a tale of eight cities", *American Heart Journal,* vol. 120, Oct. 1990, pp. 773-780, ISSN: 0002-8703.

G. Mandellos, D. Lymperopoulos, M. Koukias, A. Tzes, N. Lazarou, and C. Vagianos, (2004). "A Novel Mobile Telemedicine System for Ambulance Transport. Design and Evaluation", *26th Annual International Conference of the IEEE Engineering in Medicine and Biology Society,* pp. 3080-3083, ISBN: 0-7803-8439-3, San Fransisco, California, Sept. 2004, IEEE, New Jersey.

G. Mandellos, G. Koutelakis, Th. Panagiotakopoulos, A. Koukias, M Koukias, D. Lymperopoulos, (2008) (a). "Dynamic Biosignal Management and Transmission during Telemedicine Incidents Handled by Mobile Units over Diverse Network Types", *30th Annual International Conference of the IEEE Engineering in Medicine and Biology Society,* pp. 2852-2856, ISBN: 978-1-4244-1814-5, Vancouver, British Columbia, Canada, Aug. 2008, IEEE, New Jersey.

G. Mandellos, M Koukias, D. Lymperopoulos, (2008) (b). "Dynamic Structuring the e-SCP-ECG+ protocol for multi vital-sign handling", *8th International Conference on Bioinformatics and BioEngineering,* Oct. 2008, Athens, Greece.

C. Weston, W. Penny, and D. Julian, (1994). "Guidelines for the early management of patients with myocardial infraction", *British Medical Journal,* vol. 308, Mar. 1994, pp. 767-771, ISSN: 0007-1447

Vikas Singh, (2009). "Telemedicine & Mobile Telemedicien System: An Overview", *Health Information Systems,* 2006. Available from: http://works.bepress.com/cgi/viewcontent.cgi?article=1001&context=vikas_singh retrieved on May 11, 2009.